CEN
Review Manual

THIRD EDITION

Emergency Nurses Association

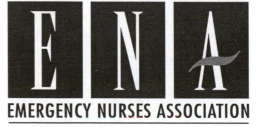

EMERGENCY NURSES ASSOCIATION

KENDALL/HUNT PUBLISHING COMPANY
4050 Westmark Drive   Dubuque, Iowa 52004

TABLE OF CONTENTS

ACKNOWLEDGEMENTS

Lead Editor

Susan A. Barnason, PhD, RN, CEN, CCRN, CS
Associate Professor
College of Nursing
University of Nebraska Medical Center
Lincoln, NE

Section Editors

Kathleen Carlson, RN, MSN, CEN
Patient Care Manager
New York United Hospital Medical Center
Port Chester, NY

Vicky A. Garcia, RN, MSN
Clinical Educator
Methodist Specialty and Transplant Hospital
San Antonio, TX

Catherine T. Kelly, PhD, RN, ANP, CEN, CCRN
Professor - Nursing
SUNY @ Ulster
Stone Ridge, NY

Benjamin Marett, RN, MSN, CEN, COHN-S, CNA
Clinical Nurse Specialist
Emergency Care Consultants of the Carolinas, Inc.
Rock Hill, SC

Susan W. Somerson, RN, MSN, CRNP, CEN
Nurse Practitioner
Frankford Health Care System
Philadelphia, PA

Contributing Authors

Sherri-Lynne A. Almeida, RN, MSN, MEd, DrPH, CEN
Vice President, Client Services
Team Health Southwest
Houston, TX

Rita T. Anderson, RN, CEN
Staff Nurse, Emergency Department
Westchester Medical Center
Valhalla, NY

Mary M. Bailey, RN, BSN, CEN
Trauma Education Coordinator
Albert Einstein Medical Center
Philadelphia, PA

Joie Harris Bertram, RN, MSN, CEN, CNRN
Clinical Nurse Specialist - ED
Porter Memorial Health System
Valparaiso, IN

Michelle C. Bridge, RN, MSN, CEN, NREMTB, CFNP
Family Nurse Practitioner
Instructor, EMS
Newark, DE

Beth A. Broering, RN, MSN, CEN, CCRN
Trauma Clinical Nurse Specialist
Inova Fairfax Hospital
Falls Church, VA

Elizabeth A. Coyne, RN, MSN, CRNP, CEN
Nurse Practitioner
Methodist Hospital
Division of Thomas Jefferson Hospital
Philadelphia, PA

Laura M. Criddle, MS, RN, CEN, CCRN, CFRN
Emergency Trauma and Neuro Clinical Nurse
   Specialist
Oregon Health and Sciences University
Portland, OR

Thomas Culwell, RN, BSN, CEN, CCRN, CFRN, LP
Faculty, University of Texas Health Science Center
   at San Antonio
Civilian Training Officer, San Antonio EMS
San Antonio, TX

Jan Daubener, RN, MSN
Professional Search Consultant
Exec Quest Inc.
Statesville, NC

Rita A. Dello Stritto, RN, PhDc, CNS, ENP, CEN
Emergency Nurse Practitioner
Brazos Emergency Physician Associates
Houston, TX

Darcy R. Egging, RN, MS, CS-ANP, CEN
Nurse Practitioner
Valley Emergency Care Delnor Hospital
Geneva, IL

Diane L. Gurney, RN, MS, CEN
Trauma Coordinator / Educator
Cape Cod Hospital Emergency Center
Hyannis, MA

Patti M. Heckman, BSN, RN, CEN, CFRN, CMTE
Transport Coordinator
Methodist Children's Hospital of South Texas
San Antonio, TX

T. Randall Huey, RN, MS, CEN
Clinical Educator, Emergency Services
Wellstar Health System
Marietta, GA

Stacey R. Ingram, RN, BSN, CEN
RN Unit Supervisor, Emergency Department
Saint Mary's Regional Medical Center
Reno, NV

Kathleen S. Jordan, RN, MS, FNP-C
Nurse Practitioner
Mid-Atlantic Emergency Medicine Associate
Charlotte, NC

Susan E. Kaplan, RN, CEN, SANE
Staff Nurse, Emergency Department
University Massachusetts Memorial Health Care
Worcester, MA

Helen Keating, RN, BSN, CEN
Staff Nurse Emergency Department
St. Luke's / Roosevelt Hospital Center
New York, NY

Debora E. Klingman, RN, CEN
Charge Nurse, Emergency Department
Horton Medical Center
Middletown, NY

Cathy Norton Lind, RN, MSN, CEN, FNP
Director of Emergency Services
The Brookdale University Hospital and Medical Center
Brooklyn, NY

Anne P. Manton, Ph.D., RN
Associate Professor
Fairfield University School of Nursing
Fairfield, CT

Susan J. McAllen, RN, BSN, CEN
Staff Nurse, Emergency Department
Montefiore Hospital and Medical Center
Bronx, NY

Estelle R. MacPhail, RN, MS, CEN
Director Emergency Services
Southern N.H. Medical Center
Nashua, NH

Catherine L. McJannet, RN, MN, CEN
Associate Professor of Nursing
Southwestern College
Chula Vista, CA

Jessie M. Moore, RN, MSN, CEN
Clinical Nurse Specialist
Midstate Medical Center
Meriden, CT

Claudia M. Niersbach, JD, RN, EMT-P
Assistant Corporation Counsel
Department of Law, Torts Division
City of Chicago
Chicago, IL

Sharon M. Pierce-Peabody, RN, MS, FNP
Westmount, Quebec, Canada

Sally Boyle Quinn, RN, MSN, CEN
Clinical Nurse
Temple University Hospital
Philadelphia, PA

Denise R. Ramponi, RN, MSN, CRNP, CEN
NP / PA Emergency Department Supervisor
Heritage Valley Health System
Beaver, PA

Doris A. Rasmussen, MSN, RN, CCRN, CEN, CS,
  CCNS
Clinical Nurse Specialist
Lincoln, NE

Joan Rembacz, RN, MS, CCRN, TNS, CCNS
TNS / Trauma Coordinator
Provena St. Joseph Hospital
Elgin, IL

Pierre Joseph Richard, RN, BSN, CCRN, EMT/P
Clinical Resource Coordinator
Saint Francis Hospital
Poughkeepsie, NY

Mary T. Schmidt Roth, BSN, MS, MPH, CCRN, FNPC
Nurse Practitioner
Jamaica Hospital
Jamaica, NY

Carole L. Rush, RN, MEd, CEN
Injury Prevention Specialist and Emergency Staff Nurse
Calgary Health Region
Calgary, Alberta, Canada

Debra A. Seguin, RN, MN, CCRN, CEN
Clinical Nurse - Emergency Services
William Beaumont Hospital
Royal Oak, MI

Susan B. Sheehy, RN, MSN, MS, CEN, FAAN
Editor-in-Chief, PEPID-RN
Boston, MA

Magen M. Silcox, RN, MS, CEN
Clinical Educator
Lexington Medical Center
West Columbia, SC

Michelle A. Silliker, FNP-C, CEN
Family Nurse Practitioner
Olean General Hospital and Olean Medical Group
Olean, NY

Michelle A. Tracy, RN, CPN, MA
Registered Nurse Level III
University of Rochester Medical Center
Rochester, NY

Ann Marie Tyrell, RN, MS, CEN
Network Director of Emergency Services
New Hanover Regional Medical Center
Wilmington, NC

Jean B. Will, EdD, RN, MSN, CEN, EMT-P
Associate Professor
MCP Hahnemann University
Philadelphia, PA

E. Marie Wilson, RN, MPA
Consultant
Riverside Solutions
Westbrook, CT

Mary Ellen Wilson, RN, MS, CEN, FNP
Clinical Educator, Emergency Services
New Hanover Health Network
Wilmington, NC

Diane M. Salentiny Wrobleski, MS, RN, CEN
Clinical Nursing Education Specialist
Mayo Medical Center
Rochester, MN

Copy Editor

Marcia Ringel
Ridgewood, NJ

A special thanks to the following work group members who made the first and second editions of the CEN Review Manual possible.

First Edition

Patricia Epifanio, RN, MS, CEN
Anne Manton, RN, MS, CEN
Kathleen Kelly Carlson, RN, MSN, CEN
Benjamin Marett, RN, MSN, CEN, CNA

Second Edition

Lorene Newberry, RN, MS, CEN
Sue Barnason, RN, PhD, CEN, CCRN
Kathleen Kelly Carlson, RN, MSN, CEN
Zeb Koran, RN, MSN, CEN, CCRN
Benny Marett, RN, MSN, CEN, CNA, COHN

CHAPTER 1

Introduction

What is the CEN?

The Certification Examination for Emergency Nurses is developed and administered by the Board of Certification for Emergency Nurses (BCEN). Upon successfully completing the certification examination, the emergency nurse earns the Certified Emergency Nurse (CEN) credential. The Emergency Nurses Association recognizes the CEN as representing a knowledge level required to deliver competent emergency nursing care.

Why Should I Be Certified as a CEN?

Emergency nursing certification promotes professionalism and assures the public that the Certified Emergency Nurse possesses essential knowledge to function competently. The CEN promotes high-quality emergency nursing care by:

- Establishing knowledge, requirements, and achievements necessary for certification in nursing;
- Measuring the attainment of a defined body of emergency nursing knowledge;
- Encouraging participation in continuing education for emergency nursing;
- Promoting professional development and career advancement; and
- Recognizing nurses who have met the requirements of the CEN examination (BCEN, 2001).

What is the Purpose of the CEN Review Manual?

Like previous editions of the *Certified Emergency Nurse (CEN) Review Manual*, this third edition is intended to serve as a preparatory aid for nurses who plan to take the CEN examination. The manual is intended for use by both first-time certifying nurses and by nurses who are preparing for recertification.

The main focus of the manual is to provide a means of self-assessment in the topic areas found in the CEN examination itself. Another purpose is to provide a review and overview of emergency nursing knowledge by presenting an explanation (rationale) for each of the four multiple-choice answers to every question—the three incorrect ones as well as the single correct one.

How is the CEN Review Manual constructed?

The *CEN Review Manual* contains 1,100 new questions, unique to this edition, written by emergency nursing experts throughout the country. The content of the questions represents and reinforces current standards and practices in the Emergency Department setting.

The format of the *CEN Review Manual* has changed somewhat. Each of the five chapters in the text that contains a simulated test consists of 150 questions. In addition, two tests of 175 questions each are provided on the enclosed CD-ROM. A new feature introduced with this edition is that every sample test has been carefully constructed to contain the same proportion of items in each content category as the CEN examination itself. (In the past, each chapter contained questions in discrete subject areas, or content categories.) As a result, your score, which you will post in the charts provided, should clearly indicate any subject areas in which you would benefit from further study. The answer key reveals the content category of each question.

How Can Using the CEN Review Manual Help Me?

Using the manual will help you to:

- identify the subject areas in which you are strong or weak so that you can study for the certification exam most efficiently;
- work toward a high or improved score on the certification exam;
- assist you in passing the exam; and
- enhance your knowledge of how to manage many specific situations that may arise in clinical practice.

What Are Some Other Advantages of Using the CEN Review Manual?

You can derive many benefits from reading the three chapters that follow this introduction and precede the practice examinations themselves, which begin in Chapter 6.

- **Test blueprint.** Chapter 2 explains the BCEN test blueprint on which the CEN examination is based.
- **Test preparation.** Use Chapter 3 as a general review of strategies in preparing for the certification examination.
- **Nursing process and diagnosis.** Chapter 4 provides an overview of the nursing process, including the use of nursing diagnoses in emergency nursing practice. This section delineates ways in which nursing process is integrated into CEN testing questions.

This edition of the *CEN Review Manual* not only includes five traditional paper-and-pencil sample tests but also offers a new feature: computerized versions of simulated tests. Each of the two computerized simulation examinations contains 175 items—25 more than each practice examination in the text, and the same number as is found on the exam itself. Taking these sample tests on a computer will simulate the experience of actually taking the CEN examination online.

Timers built into the computerized tests establish the same time constraints as the actual examination: 3 hours. If you choose to send your computerized responses to ENA, you will receive a score sheet containing the correct answers and rationales to the computerized tests. In addition, you will gain the important bonus of continuing education verification, earning 3.6 CECH per completed examination. Chapter 11 provides more information on the continuing education opportunity offered by the computerized simulated tests.

This manual can be used in several different ways. Choose whichever best suit your needs as you prepare for the CEN examination. This book provides an overview of the CEN blueprint, practice exams representative of content areas on the CEN examination, methods for self-assessment of your areas of CEN content knowledge, and an opportunity to take computer-based simulation tests. Make this manual work for you as a fine resource in preparing for the CEN examination.

REFERENCES

Board of Certification for Emergency Nursing. (2001). *International certification examination for emergency nursing (Candidate Handbook)*. Des Plaines, IL: Author.

Emergency Nurses Association (ENA). (2000). *CEN review manual* (2nd ed.). Park Ridge, IL: Author.

CHAPTER 2

Test Blueprint

Emergency nursing certification provides a method to measure attainment of a defined body of knowledge that an emergency nurse requires to function at the "competent" level (BCEN, 1997). Measurement of this knowledge through a certification examination stimulates the application of knowledge to clinical practice.

The basis for any certifying examination is a test blueprint, which reflects specific content areas covered in the examination. The use of a test blueprint assures the consistent application of emergency nursing knowledge and minimizes variability in the measurement of that knowledge.

The Board of Certification for Emergency Nursing determines the components of the test blueprint for the CEN exam. The test blueprint is revised periodically to assure that the test remains an accurate reflection of emergency nursing knowledge. The test blueprint used as the basis for the CEN examination is protected by copyright held by the Board of Certification for Emergency Nursing.

Clinical and professional practice are the cornerstones of the CEN test blueprint. Clinical knowledge is the dominant content area covered within the CEN exam. The test blueprint does not address age-specific knowledge. Knowledge required for various age groups is tested within each content area or dimension of the examination. Therefore, age-specific content is distributed throughout the exam. Similarly, nursing process is integrated into all aspects of the test blueprint and tested within each content area or dimension of the test.

Content Area/ Dimension of CEN Examination	Content-Specific Topics
Clinical Pathophysiology by System	• Cardiovascular Emergencies • Gastrointestinal Emergencies • Obstetric, Genitourinary, and Gynecological Emergencies • Maxillofacial and Ocular Emergencies • Neurological Emergencies • Orthopedic Emergencies and Wound Management • Psychosocial Emergencies • Respiratory Emergencies
Patient Care Management	• Education • Disaster • Patient Care Delivery • Stabilization and Transfer
Environmental & Toxicology	• Environmental Emergencies (e.g., heat/cold injuries, submersion injuries) • Acute poisonings and intake of substances of abuse
Shock & Multisystem Trauma	• Shock States • Critically Injured Patients
Medical	• Communicable and Infectious Disease Emergencies • Endocrine Emergencies • Specific Medical Emergencies (e.g., Reye's syndrome, gout, coma, fluid and electrolyte emergencies)
Professional Issues	• Standards of Practice • Research • Legal Issues • Professional Performance

REFERENCES

Board of Certification for Emergency Nursing. (2001). *International certification examination for emergency nursing (Candidate Handbook)*. Des Plaines, IL: Author.

Emergency Nurses Association (ENA). (2000). *CEN review manual* (2nd ed.). Park Ridge, IL: Author.

CHAPTER 3

Test-Taking Strategies

When you decide to take the CEN certification examination, it is important that you begin to prepare both your mind and your emotions for success. Maintaining strong study habits and positive attitudes will help to strengthen your efforts.

Test Anxiety

Most people have experienced anxiety associated with taking a test. Anxiety is a response to an event perceived as a threat. Anxiety is an involuntary response based on fear. Feeling mild anxiety before taking a test can actually be helpful by providing the adrenaline needed to remain alert and perform well. What should be avoided is a level of anxiety so high that it interferes with the ability to recall the information that is needed to make decisions in determining the answers to the test questions.

One way to minimize testing-related anxiety is to identify the reasons you are feeling anxious and then to analyze them, confront them, and change them. In addition, the better you are prepared for the testing situation, the more confident you will be with the process.

Preparing for the CEN Test

Since 2000, the CEN exam has been offered in a computer-based testing (CBT) format as well as the traditional paper one. Usually the CBT version of the CEN is administered in a small testing center in which each candidate sits in a private cubicle.

Absolutely no prior computer experience is necessary for taking a CBT examination. Before the CEN examination begins, each candidate reviews a tutorial program that explains how to take the test online. Once the candidate feels comfortable with the computer, he or she can begin to take the exam.

The CBT version of the CEN examination must be completed within 3 hours. (Completing the tutorial program before the test begins is not included in this time period.) The CEN examination comprises 175 multiple-choice questions; of which 150 items are scored and 25 items are pretest questions that are later used to determine whether certain questions should be used on future examinations. Upon completing the examination, the examinee receives a report that not only identifies the total score as passing or failing but also provides a subscore in each major subject area.

TEST BLUEPRINT

Preparation for a test like the CEN exam begins with determining what material you will be required to know. The BCEN provides a blueprint for the test items on the CEN examination. Review the blueprint in Chapter 2 of this manual to become aware of the broad content areas of the CEN.

ORGANIZING AND USING RESOURCES

Once you know the broad content areas to be covered on the CEN examination, gather emergency nursing resources that will be useful as you prepare. Examples include textbooks on emergency nursing, the Core Curriculum for Emergency Nursing, and journal articles on content related to the topics in the CEN test blueprint. A quick way to review your emergency nursing resources is to read their headings and subheadings.

Take notes on central ideas. The act of writing will help you organize your thoughts and to remember the material. Describe key concepts and explain how information ties together. Jot down important names, relationships, and formulas and examples that will jog your memory as you review them. Flash cards can be helpful memory joggers.

Then rewrite your notes and organize them into major categories that make sense to you. Organizing your notes based on the CEN test blueprint may also be useful.

PACING YOURSELF

Cramming as the examination date nears usually increases anxiety. Developing a study plan in advance and using it over time is far more effective and less stressful. Determine how much material you must cover before your CEN examination is scheduled. Plot a time line on a calendar. By doing this, you will gain a realistic perspective for reviewing your materials and resources. Be sure to allow extra time in your plan for the more difficult content areas and for areas with which you are less familiar than others.

Overstudy! When you believe you have retained 100% of the material, study for another 25%. Scrupulously following your study and review schedule will prevent procrastination and let you relax on occasion without guilt.

Part of your strategy for review may include joining a CEN study group or taking a formal CEN review course. All members of the study group should have an equal grasp of the material. Coming into the study group with baseline knowledge will guard against inadvertently learning incorrect information. Study groups can provide a forum in which to think out loud, clear up misunderstandings, and put together relationships between facts. Group discussion will reinforce your long-term memory, too.

STRATEGIES FOR TAKING MULTIPLE-CHOICE EXAMINATIONS

Read the stem of each question first. Then answer each item on the exam in your head, searching for the closest answer among the choices given. Some general test-taking tips:

- Eliminate any answers that are obviously wrong. This tactic is especially helpful when you are unsure of the correct answer.
- Do not eliminate an answer unless you know what every word means.
- Implausible answers may be partly right.
- Most responses are correct in themselves but are not related to the stem of the question.
- Don't read between the lines. Well-written certification questions are intended to be straightforward.
- Read each question carefully.

- Try to reason out the answers to tough questions.
- Look for clues in an answer. Analyze the wording in a question's stem. The correct answer is often the one that uses words similar to those in the question.
- Choose the closest answer—the one that is definitely better than the rest.
- Often questions that ask about a hypothetical psychosocial situation are related to how the nurse should deal with a patient's emotional response. The correct answer is often the one related to accepting the patient's feelings.
- It is usually best to follow your first impulse in determining your response to a question.
- Make an educated guess. Doing this increases your odds of answering correctly from 0% to 25% when you aren't sure of the answer.
- Don't look for any pattern to correct items on the exam. Letters (A, B, C, or D) that precede the correct answers on the certification examination are chosen at random.

THE NIGHT BEFORE AND THE DAY OF THE EXAM

The night before your exam, get a good night's rest. On the day of your scheduled CEN examination, take essential materials (e.g., photo identification, admission ticket). Psych yourself into a mood to succeed. Imagine yourself doing well on the CEN exam. You will have spent plenty of time preparing for the event. Believe that you will remain calm and perform well.

USING PRACTICE EXAMINATIONS FOR TESTING ASSESSMENT

Another major strategy for success on the CEN certification examination is to take practice examinations that simulate the experience. Besides helping you to identify areas of emergency nursing content that you will want to review before taking the examination, taking practice examinations can motivate you and enhance your confidence.

In certification examinations like the CEN, all test items are of the multiple-choice variety. They contain a stem followed by several options. The stem presents a problem or asks a question. Options are potential answers to the questions. Options include both the correct answer and the distractors (incorrect answers). While all the options often seem plausible, the correct answer represents the best response to the question.

By taking practice examinations, you will identify strengths and weaknesses in your emergency nursing knowledge while gleaning insight into your own test response patterns. After you have completed a practice CEN examination, reread the items that you answered incorrectly and ask yourself the questions on the following grid. Consider using some of the strategies identified to enhance future performance when taking an examination or test.

Contributing Factors: Why do you think you answered item incorrectly?	Possible Strategies
Did I really know the right answer, but marked it incorrectly on the scoring sheet?	• Take time to review your answers after you have marked your scoring sheet to ensure that you have marked the item you intended.
Did I not have the knowledge to answer the question?	• Review the rationale for the correct response, which usually contains succinct information to help you fill gaps in your ED knowledge base. • Read the reference list at the end of the manual. You can use these references to update or refresh your knowledge of particular content areas.
Did I misunderstand the question?	• After reading the rationale, reread the stem of the question and all distractors. Does the correct answer now make sense to you or do you have a knowledge gap?
Did I miss a key word or concept in the stem (body of the question)?	• After reading the rationale, reread the stem of the question and all distractors. Does the correct answer now make sense to you or do you have a knowledge gap?
Did I change my answer?	• If you find that you often change your answers on a test or exam, determine whether or not the changed answer tends to be correct. • If you tend to change incorrect answers to correct ones, it may be to your advantage to continue this practice. • If you tend to change correct answers to incorrect ones, reevaluate the usefulness of this practice.

REFERENCES

Condon, V. M., & Drew, D. E. (1995). Improving examination performance using exam analysis. *Journal of Nursing Education, 34*(6), 254–261.

Emergency Nurses Association (ENA). (2000). *CEN review manual* (2nd ed.). Park Ridge, IL: Author.

Nugent, P. M., & Vitale, B. A. (1993). *Test success: Test-taking techniques for beginning nursing students*. Philadelphia: F. A. Davis.

CHAPTER 4

Nursing Process

· ·

This manual provides you with questions and answers, rationales for the correct and incorrect answers, and references to help you prepare for the CEN examination. As you study, remember that the entire nursing process, including nursing diagnosis, is an integral part of emergency nursing and therefore of the examination.

Nursing Process

The steps of the nursing process provide the framework for the essential components of emergency nursing practice. These steps are assessment or data gathering, analysis and/or nursing diagnosis, planning, intervention, and evaluation. It has been suggested that reassessment is another critical step in the nursing process.

Assessment

Assessment is defined as the "systematic collection of data about the patient's actual or risk for health care problems and needs" (Jordan, p. 12). Two types of information are included in assessment: subjective data and objective data.

Subjective data represent information offered by the patient or others. This information may include descriptions of the current health concern or concerns, the patient's report of past medical history, and events and perceptions surrounding the precipitating event that brought the patient to seek treatment. Caregivers, friends, and bystanders may provide subjective data, especially when patients cannot provide such information themselves.

Objective data include vital signs, other physical findings, and nursing observations. Emergency nursing assessment differs from usual nursing assessment in that it begins with a primary assessment. Included in the primary assessment is the determination of the patient's airway, breathing, and circulatory status (ABCs). If the primary assessment identifies any area of concern, attention is given to correcting life-threatening conditions before the assessment is continued.

Once the primary assessment has been completed and emergent problems, if any, have been identified and addressed, a secondary assessment is performed. Secondary assessment is a systematic head-to-toe examination of the patient in search of signs of illness or injury. Particular attention is paid to areas of concern that the patient has expressed.

Both subjective and objective assessment is an ongoing process in emergency nursing. Assessment is an ongoing process throughout the patient's stay in the emergency setting.

Analysis and Nursing Diagnosis

When initial data collection has been completed, the next phase of the nursing process calls for the nurse to analyze all assessment data in order to identify and prioritize the patient's actual or potential health problems. To conclude the analysis, the nurse creates a "label" (diagnosis) that describes the problem or problems that the nurse has identified. The North American Nursing Diagnosis Association (NANDA) defines nursing diagnosis as "a clinical judgment about individual, family or community responses to actual or potential health problems or life processes. A nursing diagnosis provides the basis for selection of nursing interventions to achieve outcomes for which the nurse is accountable" (NANDA, p. 245).

"Making a nursing diagnosis," NANDA states, "requires analysis, synthesis, and accuracy in interpreting and making sense of complex clinical data. This critical thinking process allows the nurse to make decisions about desired outcomes and interventions needed to help achieve those outcomes" (NANDA, p. vii).

In essence, nursing diagnoses are those descriptions or definitions of a patient's problem or problems for which the nurse is held responsible. While the satisfactory resolution of many health problems requires a collaborative effort—and indeed, nurses are actively involved in the treatment of the patient's medical diagnosis—medical and nursing diagnoses differ. A nursing diagnosis is based on the priorities of care delivery by the nurse. Multiple nursing diagnoses may be applicable to the patient, but the nurse and patient must prioritize the diagnoses in order to plan care that will be most effective.

Planning

Once the analysis has been completed and the diagnoses prioritized, the nurse must develop a plan of care. In busy emergency settings, it is not unusual for this plan or components of it to be unwritten. It is clear, however, that the nurse must formulate a plan in order to proceed with the appropriate interventions for a particular patient. The plan includes the patient's priorities as well as the nurse's.

Implementation

Implementation of the plan follows the priorities already established. The interventions should be patient oriented, goal directed, and based on established psychological and/or physiological principles. The nurse selects interventions based on the likelihood of success in achieving desired outcomes.

Interventions can be independent or collaborative. Independent interventions are those activities that s/he is licensed to implement and responsible for implementing, based on the nurse's education and experience. In many instances these are the interventions selected to resolve or moderate identified nursing diagnoses. Collaborative interventions are those activities performed by the nurse in conjunction with members of other health care disciplines. For example, if the patient's nursing diagnosis is pain, independent nursing interventions might include positioning and anxiety reduction, while collaborative interventions might include administration of pain medications. Administration of pain medication is a collaborative intervention because the nurse may not administer the medication until a physician has written an order for it.

Evaluation

As the plan is being developed and implemented, the nurse must be aware of the outcome that is desired as a result of the intervention(s) to be made. The evaluation component of the nursing process is the time when the nurse assesses the attainment of the desired outcome as a result of the intervention(s). The criteria by which the efficacy of the intervention will be measured should be predetermined as part of the plan of care. Criteria should be outcome focused and based on patient response.

If the interventions suggested above for relief of pain are implemented, certain outcomes are expected to result; for example, "Patient will experience pain relief within 30 minutes." Evaluation in this case would consist of the nurse's assessment of the patient for present pain status 30 to 40 minutes after the intervention had been made and comparing that to the level of pain experienced before the interventions took place. If satisfactory pain relief has been accomplished, the steps of the nursing process should be repeated. In this way, additional assessment data, analysis/nursing diagnosis, or interventions as result of ongoing assessment may lead to a more satisfactory outcome.

Reassessment

Emergency patients should be reassessed regularly while they are in the emergency setting. The analysis and/or nursing diagnosis should be reviewed, and additional independent and collaborative interventions would be implemented if planned outcomes had been achieved or if changes were noted in reassessment. Following these steps, the patient's response to the interventions would be once again evaluated. The steps of the nursing process should be repeated as frequently as needed to meet the goals established by the patient and nurse.

Documentation

All nursing assessments, nursing diagnoses, interventions, and evaluation must be documented. "Unless the nurse can document his or her thinking in a manner other nurses and healthcare providers can interpret, that thinking process is invisible. Accurately naming and reporting the results of the nurse's critical thinking helps other caregivers know a patient's needs and how the plan of care will meet those needs. Using standardized nursing language to document the nurse's thinking in an efficient way to achieve interdisciplinary understanding" (NANDA, p. vii).

It is important to consider all steps of the nursing process in preparing documentation, both for legal reasons and to ensure clear communication to other caregivers.

REFERENCES

Jordan, K. S. (Ed.). (2000). *Emergency nursing core curriculum* (5th ed.). Philadelphia: W. B. Saunders.

North American Nursing Diagnosis Association. (2001). *Nursing diagnosis: Definitions & classifications.* Philadelphia: Author.

CHAPTER 5

Using the CEN Review Manual

This manual is organized into 11 chapters. The first five provide information on ways you can prepare to take the CEN examination. You are encouraged to read these five brief chapters before you start to take the practice tests that start in Chapter 6.

Chapter 1 answers questions that nurses ask about the CEN examination and how to prepare for it. Chapter 2 describes the test blueprint concept and the content areas contained in the CEN exam, which are based on the BCEN test blueprint. Chapter 3 contains information and strategies to maximize test-taking skills for the CEN exam. Nursing process and nursing diagnosis are the dual focus of Chapter 4, with an emphasis on how these concepts are integrated into the CEN exam. The current chapter will help you benefit optimally from using the practice examinations as a method of CEN test preparation.

Getting the Most Out of the Practice CEN Examinations

Five chapters in this manual consist of practice CEN tests that contain 150 questions each and are of equal difficulty. General subjects (content categories) in these practice exams are proportional to those in the CEN test blueprint.

Blank answer sheets for the practice examinations are provided at the end of Chapter 11. Follow the steps below to develop strategies that can assist you in assessing your emergency nursing knowledge. What you learn in these self-assessments will serve as the basis for implementing additional test-taking strategies.

1. Upon completing a written practice examination, turn to the section of the practice examination that contains the correct answers and explanations (rationales) for every multiple-choice answer, the wrong ones as well as the right ones.
2. Indicate on your answer sheet whether each of your answers was correct or incorrect.
3. Count the total number of items that you answered correctly. Plot your score on the graph. Observe your total score against the Self-Diagnostic Profile section at the end of the chapter containing each practice test. Then refer to Figure 1 in that section.

    Your goal is to achieve a score of 70% or more, for which you must answer more than 105 items correctly. Each 20% segment of the grid represents 30 questions. Once you have calculated the percentage of your correct responses, plot your score.

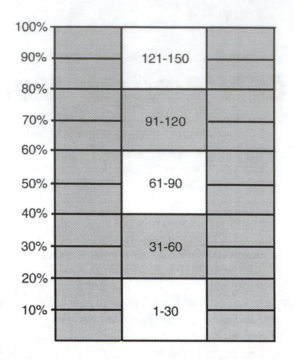

Figure 1: Total Score Grid

4. For each question that you answered **incorrectly**, indicate on your answer sheet the major category of the test blueprint that is being evaluated by the test item:
    *   Cardiovascular
    *   Gastrointestinal
    *   GU/GYN/OB
    *   Maxillofacial & Ocular
    *   Neurological
    *   Orthopedics & Wound Care
    *   Psychosocial
    *   Respiratory
    *   Patient Care Management
    *   Substance Abuse/Toxicology/ Environmental
    *   Shock & Multi-System Trauma
    *   General Medical
    *   Professional Issues
5. Count the total number of **incorrectly answered** items in each category. Plot this number on the graph, with placement based on the appropriate content area within the Self-Diagnostic Profile section of the chapter. A bar graph represents the number of items for each content area. Each section on a bar represents one item.

For example, if you missed three items on cardiovascular content, you would fill in three squares on the cardiovascular bar. This would mean that you answered approximately 23% of the items incorrectly.

Refer to Figure 2. If you have answered more than 30% of the questions in any content area incorrectly, you should see this discovery as a cue that you should focus your studying efforts on this content area more intensively.

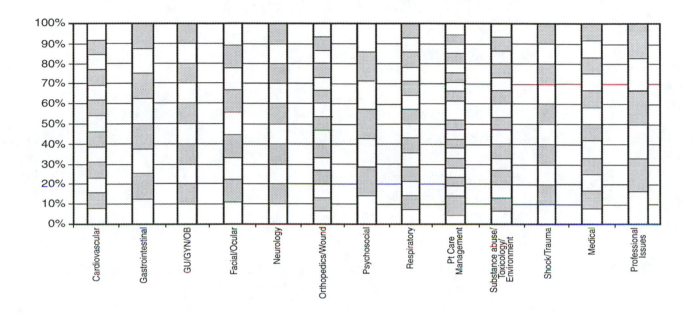

Figure 2: Content-Specific Score Grid

Using the Rationale Section of the CEN Review Manual

Another very useful aspect of this manual is the rationale section that follows each practice exam. To enhance your preparation for the CEN, read the rationales for each correct answer and each incorrect answer (distractor). By reviewing these materials, you are using a highly effective study technique to reinforce your emergency nursing knowledge.

Another strategy using the rationale section to identify content knowledge with which you may be insufficiently familiar is to home in on items that you have answered incorrectly. Determine whether the content is really unfamiliar to you or if there was some other reason that you answered the item incorrectly. Studying the rationales carefully may provide you with enough review of content. If not, you may decide to use other resources to review the areas in which your emergency nursing knowledge is least strong.

Summary

This manual can serve as an invaluable study aid as you prepare to take the CEN examination. You may discover additional strategies for using the manual constructively besides those described in this and previous chapters.

Review the manual and reflect on your own learning preferences. Then use the manual to prepare for the CEN exam. Good luck!

Practice Examination 1

1. Acute coronary syndrome includes which of the following conditions?
   A. Atrial fibrillation
   B. Left bundle branch block
   C. Chest pain
   D. Unstable angina

2. Which of the following is the expected outcome for a patient treated for acute coronary syndrome?
   A. Reduced fatigue
   B. Relief of chest pain or angina
   C. Muffled heart sounds
   D. Increased jugular venous pressure

3. How is tenecteplase (TNKase) administered for acute myocardial infarction?
   A. Bolus plus infusion intravenously
   B. Infused over 60 minutes intravenously
   C. Single bolus given over 5 seconds intravenously
   D. Two intravenous boluses given 30 minutes apart

4. A 55-year-old female presents to the ED with intermittent chest pain of 4 hours' duration. She is pain free at the time of admission. She is on hormone replacement therapy and stopped smoking 2 weeks ago after a 30-pack-year history. The most appropriate triage and management for this patient would be:
   A. emergent; cardiac workup.
   B. nonemergent; admission to chest pain unit.
   C. urgent; clinic referral.
   D. nonemergent; sent home.

5. A 78-year-old male presents with a chief complaint of dizziness for the past 3 to 4 days. Patient reports that he had a myocardial infarction 8 years ago, at which time a permanent pacemaker was implanted. He denies chest pain. Initial vital signs are BP 168/88 mmHg, pulse 78/min apically, and respirations 18/min. What is your interpretation of the following ECG rhythm strip?

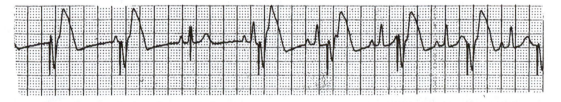

   A. 1:1 ventricular pacing
   B. Dual-chambered pacemaker (DDD) with appropriate sensing
   C. Ventricular pacing with loss of capture
   D. Atrial pacing with loss of sensing

6.   A 54-year-old male presents to the ED with a chief complaint of chest pain. His previous hospital record reveals that 4 weeks ago he had a coronary stent inserted and underwent angioplasty of the left anterior descending (LAD) coronary artery. His chest pain presentation suggests the possibility of coronary restenosis. Which leads on a 12-lead electrocardiogram would you examine for ST segment changes associated with restenosis?
A. I, AVL
B. II, III, AVF
C. V_2, V_3
D. V_5, V_6

7.   Which of the following conditions would be represented by an elevated ST segment in all leads except AVR and V_1?
A. Acute anterior myocardial infarction
B. Pericarditis
C. Myocardial ischemia
D. Cardiac tamponade

8.   Which of the following assessment findings is associated with pericardial tamponade?
A. Tracheal deviation
B. Muffled heart sounds
C. Increased venous return
D. Paradoxical pulse ≤5 mm Hg

9.   In the presence of myocardial damage, which of the following cardiac biomarkers remains elevated for the longest time?
A. CK/MB
B. C-reactive protein
C. Myoglobin
D. Troponin

10.   In the early setting of an acute myocardial infarction, beta blockers have been found to be useful because they:
A. decrease myocardial oxygen consumption.
B. improve venous return
C. increase contractility
D. limit the infarct to subendocardial damage

11.   The patient for whom you are caring presents with the following rhythm and suddenly becomes *unresponsive*. Your first action after establishing "pulselessness" is to:

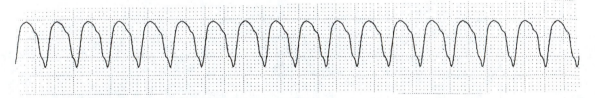

A. defibrillate at 200 joules.
B. charge the paddles for synchronized cardioversion.
C. give bretylium tosylate (Bretylol).
D. give lidocaine hydrochloride (Xylocaine) by bolus and start a drip.

12. A 35-year-old male in severe cardiopulmonary distress was admitted to the ED by ambulance. On presentation, he was pale and tachycardic and had bilateral crackles, a low-grade temperature, and a loud systolic murmur. History revealed that he is a smoker, takes medication for hypertension, and recently underwent cardiac catheterization, which was negative for significant coronary disease. A presumptive diagnosis of infective endocarditis was made. Which of the following was the most likely predisposing factor contributing to infective endocarditis?
   A. Acute myocardial infarction
   B. Heart catheterization procedure
   C. Hypertension
   D. Smoking history

13. If a patient who is being managed for chest pain in the ED is allergic to aspirin, what alternative antithrombotic agent can be used?
   A. Acetylsalicylic acid ("baby aspirin") 80 mg chewed
   B. Ticlopidine hydrochloride (Ticlid) 250 mg orally
   C. Enoxaparin (Lovenox) 1 mg/kg subcutaneously
   D. Eptifibatide (Integrelin) infusion intravenously

14. A patient who is experiencing panic-level anxiety:
   A. is able to process information.
   B. may exhibit psychotic behavior.
   C. has a wide perceptual field.
   D. can effectively communicate his or her needs.

15. A 35-year-old woman has just been brought into the ED by the police after having been sexually assaulted. The patient is alert. Initial assessment reveals bruises and abrasions on her face, breasts, arms, and hands. She makes minimal eye contact with the nurse and speaks only when asked a question. What is the most appropriate action for the emergency nurse to take?
   A. Escort the patient to the bathroom for a shower and contact a social worker.
   B. Notify the emergency physician that a vaginal examination must be done immediately.
   C. Accompany the patient to a private treatment area and explain the sexual assault examination process.
   D. Once the patient is in the treatment area, let her alone to compose her thoughts about the incident so that an accurate police report can be filed.

16. A 24-year-old first-year male law student is brought to the ED by police after being found running naked on the highway. Triage assessment reveals an extremely active young man who rhymes his sentences while speaking. There is no correlation between assessment questions posed by the triage nurse and verbal responses from the patient. Vital signs are within normal limits. No obvious injuries are present. The ED nurse is aware that the following illness may mimic a psychiatric disorder:
   A. Infection
   B. Cardiovascular insult
   C. Splenic injury
   D. Anaphylaxis

17. A 13-year-old male is brought to the ED by EMS, police. and school officials after having drawn a picture of himself holding a gun to his class. He is withdrawn and does not interact freely with the triage nurse. School officials report that this is not the first time this student has received attention for his behavior and that his grandmother refuses to acknowledge that he is having emotional problems. The most appropriate action for the triage nurse to take at this time is to:
    A. place the patient in a quiet, secure environment.
    B. search the patient for a gun.
    C. notify the patient's grandmother immediately.
    D. assess the patient for signs of agitation and aggression.

18. When a psychotic patient is experiencing visual hallucinations of bugs on the bed in the ED, the ED nurse should:
    A. brush the "bugs" from the bed sheets.
    B. put the patient in a regular patient room, close to the nurses' station.
    C. assure the patient that the "bugs" will not hurt him or her.
    D. reorient the patient to reality.

19. The priority nursing interventions for a suicidal patient in the ED include:
    A. placing the patient in a private area.
    B. talking to the patient about any suicide plans.
    C. implementing a "no-suicide" safety contract.
    D. praising the patient's positive attributes.

20. Which of the following is the priority nursing diagnosis for a patient who has come or been brought to the ED after attempted suicide?
    A. Impaired verbal communication
    B. Anxiety
    C. Risk for injury
    D. Altered thought processes

21. An unrestrained female driver is brought into the ED by EMS. Paramedics report that she was driving an old car without airbags and that the steering wheel was bent. The patient is awake and alert, with a Glasgow Coma Scale (GCS) of 15. She is pale and anxious, with labored respirations. She states that another driver cut her off at an intersection. You note paradoxical chest wall movement and suspect a flail chest. Which of the following would be your primary concern for this patient?
    A. Pulmonary contusion
    B. Deep-vein thrombosis
    C. Facial lacerations
    D. Concurrent thoracic vertebral fracture

22. The priority intervention for a patient with suspected tension pneumothorax is:
    A. endotracheal intubation.
    B. needle thoracentesis.
    C. two large-bore IVs.
    D. covering the wound with an occlusive dressing.

23. A patient is evaluated after receiving severe chest injuries in a motor vehicle crash (MVC) and presents with severe dyspnea, increasing subcutaneous emphysema of the neck, and decreased breath sounds on auscultation. What nursing diagnosis is a priority for this patient?
    A. Fluid volume deficit
    B. Impaired gas exchange
    C. Ineffective airway clearance
    D. Body image disturbance

24.   You are caring for a patient who has been diagnosed with hyperventilation. What is another common symptom related to this condition?
A. Seizures
B. Chest pain
C. Carpopedal spasms
D. Fever

25.   Patient teaching for a patient with emphysema should include:
A. the importance of being vaccinated each year against pneumococcal disease.
B. the need for prophylactic antibiotic therapy when a family member becomes ill.
C. the need for adequate hydration to reduce mucus tenacity.
D. the importance of smoking cessation to reverse structural changes caused by the disease.

26.   A patient with chronic obstructive pulmonary disease is treated with a sustained-release oral theophylline preparation. Which of the following conditions would predispose the patient most to theophylline toxicity?
A. Diabetes mellitus
B. Congestive heart failure
C. Asthma
D. Renal disease

27.   A 40-year-old male involved in a house fire presents, conscious, to the ED with dyspnea, sooty sputum, and a brassy cough. He is receiving 100% oxygen via nonrebreather reservoir mask. The ED nurse should FIRST:
A. check for burn percentage.
B. prepare for intubation.
C. assess airway and breathing.
D. start fluid resuscitation.

28.   Which of these children is at highest risk for foreign body aspiration?
A. A 7-year-old with gastroenteritis
B. A 4-year-old with rhinitis
C. A 2-year-old with a history of chickenpox (varicella) exposure
D. A 6-year-old with a history of cerebral palsy

29.   An obese 36-year-old female presents to your ED with sudden onset of left-sided chest pain and shortness of breath. She is diaphoretic, pale, and in acute respiratory distress. She denies any trauma, fever, nausea, or vomiting. Past medical history is unremarkable except that she was placed on birth control pills 6 months ago. Initial vital signs are BP 100/60 mmHg, pulse 118/min, and respirations 36/min. The priority nursing diagnosis for this patient is:
A. fluid volume deficit.
B. anxiety.
C. pain, alteration in comfort.
D. impaired gas exchange.

30.   What diagnostic test or tests does a patient with noncardiogenic pulmonary edema require?
A. Ventilation/perfusion scan
B. Fiberoptic endoscopy and pulse oximetry
C. ECG and chest radiograph
D. Chest radiograph and ABG

31. The triad involved with heroin-induced pulmonary edema is hypoxia, stupor, and:
    A. hypertension.
    B. mydriasis.
    C. miosis.
    D. arrhythmias.

32. Which of the following patients is at high risk for possible aspiration?
    A. A 25-year-old male with mycoplasma pneumonia
    B. A 42-year-old female with gastroesophageal reflux disease
    C. A 16-year-old male with alcohol intoxication
    D. An 84-year-old female with decreased mental status

33. Which of the following patients would most likely present with pleural effusion?
    A. A 19-year-old thin male with sudden onset of sharp chest pain and reporting shortness of breath that began today
    B. A 26-year-old male with a stab wound to the chest and a chest tube in place
    C. A 6-year-old female with fever and cough
    D. A 62-year-old female 7 days after undergoing coronary bypass surgery

34. The ED nurse should expect a child with bronchiolitis to be admitted when the patient has:
    A. an oxygen saturation of 90, respiratory rate of 70, retractions, and fatigue.
    B. an oxygen saturation of 95, mild wheezing, and patchy infiltrate on x-ray and is drinking well.
    C. an oxygen saturation of 96, respiratory rate of 34, mild wheezing, and a positive nasal aspirate for respiratory syncytial virus.
    D. an oxygen saturation of 92, respiratory rate of 36, mild retractions, and mild wheezing.

35. A 12-year-old presents with fever, ear pain, and diarrhea. The child is diagnosed with otitis media. Which of the following is an ominous complication of acute otitis media?
    A. Intracranial complications
    B. Lateral sinus thrombosis
    C. Cholesteatoma
    D. Perforated tympanic membrane

36. Which of the following statements about Bell's palsy is true?
    A. It is caused by paralysis of the tenth cranial nerve.
    B. It is idiopathic unilateral facial paralysis.
    C. It is progressive in nature and eventually affects the entire body.
    D. Onset is usually seen in the second decade of life.

37. A patient presents with decreased vision in the left eye that began with flashes of light. The patient describes the process of vision loss as "a curtain lowering over the eye." There is no evidence of trauma to the eye and the patient denies any pain. The patient's signs and symptoms suggest:
    A. Corneal abrasion
    B. Acute angle-closure glaucoma
    C. Retinal detachment
    D. Central retinal artery occlusion

38. A tripod fracture is another name for what type of fracture?
    A. Le Fort I fracture
    B. Le Fort II fracture
    C. Orbit fracture
    D. Zygomatic fracture

39.   Discharge instructions for the parent of a child with conjunctivitis should emphasize:
      A. how to apply an eye patch properly.
      B. possible side effects of steroid drops.
      C. exercises to strengthen the extraocular muscles.
      D. ways to prevent the spread of disease.

40.   Before performing ear irrigation, the nurse must:
      A. evaluate the patient's hearing.
      B. visualize the integrity of the tympanic membrane.
      C. instill anesthetic otic drops.
      D. administer medication to prevent vertigo.

41.   If a cerebral spinal fluid leak is suspected, the nurse should test nasal drainage for the presence of:
      A. nitrites.
      B. glucose.
      C. ketones.
      D. potassium.

42.   Treatment of a patient with a corneal abrasion includes antibiotic drops *and*:
      A. narcotic analgesia and soft contact lenses.
      B. cycloplegic drops and nonsteroidal anti-inflammatory eye drops.
      C. repeated application of topical anesthesia with narcotic analgesia.
      D. soft contact lenses with eye patch.

43.   Treatment of a child with croup should include:
      A. humidified oxygen, antipyretics, and antibiotics.
      B. humidified oxygen, antibiotics, and epinephrine.
      C. hydration, steroids, and racemic epinephrine.
      D. hydration, epinephrine, and sedation.

44.   A 71-year-old man is brought to the ED by his family. Family members state that he must have had a stroke because he woke up this morning paralyzed on the left side and unable to speak clearly. The emergency physician will not be able to see this patient for 10 minutes. Initial nursing intervention should include which of the following actions?
      A. Arterial blood gases
      B. Bedside blood glucose test
      C. Physical exam for signs of abuse
      D. Preparation for thrombolytics

45.   Intravenous propranolol (Inderal) has been ordered for your patient with thyroid storm. This drug is used to:
      A. keep the heart rate under 100.
      B. control hypertension.
      C. decrease tremulousness.
      D. stimulate thyroxine production.

46.   The patient with thyroid storm is at increased risk of death from:
      A. hyperthermia.
      B. hypotension.
      C. infection.
      D. heart failure.

47. Patients with myxedema coma need to be monitored carefully for:
    A. hypertension.
    B. supraventricular tachycardia.
    C. hyperventilation.
    D. hypothermia.

48. A 6-year-old boy is brought to the triage desk by his aunt. He has had fever and cough for 3 days and now has a red rash. The aunt does not know other details of the child's health history. Your first action as triage nurse should be to:
    A. contact the child's parents for permission to treat.
    B. institute isolation precautions with the child immediately.
    C. obtain vital signs and examine the rash.
    D. ask the aunt to wait her turn, since several other patients are waiting.

49. The incubation period for chickenpox is:
    A. 1 to 3 days.
    B. 2 to 4 days.
    C. 7 to 10 days.
    D. 10 to 20 days.

50. While working a shift in the ED, a nurse receives a call from the mother of a pediatric patient seen 4 days ago for scabies. The mother states that she used the medication as prescribed and washed all clothing and bedding in hot water. The child is still complaining of itching and is scratching himself during the night, but the rash seems to be gone. The nurse should advise the mother to:
    A. bring the child back to the ED for a checkup.
    B. pick up a refill of the medication and treat the child again.
    C. relaunder clothes and bedding, using very hot water and a hot dryer.
    D. be aware that itching is common for about 7 days even if the infection has been cured.

51. During treatment of diabetic ketoacidosis, including fluid replacement and insulin, the patient must be closely monitored for:
    A. hypokalemia.
    B. hyperphosphatemia.
    C. hypernatremia.
    D. hyperkalemia.

52. A male patient is brought to the ED by ambulance from a homeless shelter, where staff had been unable to awaken him. He is lying supine on the stretcher, receiving high-flow oxygen by nonrebreather mask. He is unresponsive to pain, with a regular respiratory rate of 18 and warm, dry, pale skin. His radial pulse is 90 and full. No other history is available. The priority nursing diagnosis for this patient is:
    A. ineffective airway clearance.
    B. impaired gas exchange.
    C. fluid volume deficit.
    D. impaired tissue perfusion.

53. A 65-year-old man is brought to the ED by his friends, who say that he has had vomiting and diarrhea for 2 days and is now unable to walk. The only other history they know is that he "gives himself a shot every morning." The patient looks ill, with flushed face and rapid, deep respirations. He moans and moves when touched, but is unable to answer any questions. Initial vital signs are BP 98/70 mmHg, pulse 100/min, and respirations 28/min. Skin is cool and dry. The pulse oximeter does not

register. While troubleshooting, you note that the patient's hands are very cold. What is your priority for this patient?
A. Obtain orthostatic (postural) vital signs.
B. Take a rectal temperature.
C. Attach the pulse oximeter to his toe.
D. Cover his hands with warm packs.

54. Which nursing diagnosis best describes the most immediate life-threatening problem for a patient with hyperglycemic, hyperosmolar, nonketotic coma (HHNC)?
A. Fluid volume deficit
B. Fluid volume excess
C. Impaired gas exchange
D. Altered cerebral tissue perfusion

55. The ED nurse has verbal orders to give ceftriaxone (Rocephin) 250 mg IM to a young man with gonorrhea. He has no allergies. His only significant medical history is hemophilia. The nurse should:
A. give the medicine as ordered, using lidocaine to mix the powder.
B. give the medicine as ordered and have the patient wait 1 hour so that he can be monitored for bleeding.
C. ask the physician to write the order on the chart, to avoid a medication error.
D. question the drug route, reminding the physician that the patient has hemophilia.

56. Upper motor neuron disease can be detected by:
A. dilated pupils.
B. a brisk patellar reflex.
C. a positive Babinski (plantar) reflex.
D. slow, irregular breathing.

57. Kernig's sign is:
A. low back or posterior thigh pain on hip flexion with gradual knee extension.
B. neck flexion that results in hip and knee flexion.
C. dilated pupils and rapid, shallow respirations.
D. brisk reflexes followed by decerebrate posturing.

58. A 36-year-old male patient presents to the ED with complaints of severe headache and blurred vision. On physical examination, his head and upper chest are flushed and diaphoretic. His lower extremities are pale and cool to the touch. Initial vital signs are BP 190/110 mmHg, pulse 40/min, and respirations 24/min. He had a spinal cord injury 2 years ago and is paralyzed below the nipple line. Your priority intervention would be to:
A. initiate IV access and provide pain relief as ordered.
B. administer antihypertensive medications as ordered.
C. place the patient in a darkened, quiet room.
D. insert a urinary catheter.

59. A young teenager is seen in the ED after being involved in a bicycle crash. He is unresponsive and has severe facial lacerations with moderate edema. He is found to have a subdural hematoma. Before intubation, lidocaine (Xylocaine) 25 mg is administered. The ED nurse should evaluate the effect of this medication by:
A. noting a transient decrease in intracranial pressure.
B. observing for decreased ventricular ectopy.
C. monitoring for pupil changes.
D. noting an increase in heart rate.

60.   A patient with a closed head injury is given 100 g of mannitol (Osmitrol). The expected outcome from this infusion is:
A. increased sensitivity of the cranial nerves.
B. increased urinary output.
C. decreased gastric motility.
D. decreased osmolarity of glomerular filtrate.

61.   A basilar artery migraine headache is manifested by:
A. nausea and vomiting, auditory issues, and frontal pain.
B. ataxia, confusion, and slurred speech.
C. seizure activity, hypertension, and tachycardia.
D. bilateral visual disturbances, paresthesias, and confusion.

62.   A 29-year-old male presents to the ED with ipsilateral nasal congestion, rhinorrhea, lacrimation, papillary changes, a droopy eyelid, and conjunctival injection, coupled with pain behind one eye. He will probably be treated for:
A. tension headache.
B. cluster headache.
C. temporal arteritis.
D. subarachnoid hemorrhage.

63.   A 59-year-old male patient presents to the ED with complaints of severe headache, blurred vision, and restlessness. He is alert and oriented. Pupils are equal and reactive to light. Initial vital signs are BP 168/100 mmHg, pulse 90/min, and respirations 18/min. He complains of neck pain on physical examination. Based on your assessment, you anticipate a diagnosis of:
A. meningitis.
B. migraine headache.
C. subarachnoid hemorrhage.
D. stroke in evolution.

64.   A patient is transferred to the ED from an outlying hospital. The patient has been diagnosed with an epidural hematoma by CT scan at the primary hospital. Upon admission, the patient is unconscious. Initial vital signs are BP 160/80 mmHg, pulse 46/min, and respirations 18/min. Breathing is being controlled with a bag valve mask. As the ED nurse, you should prepare for:
A. a lumbar puncture to determine the amount of blood loss.
B. insertion of an intracranial pressure (ICP) monitor and admission to the ICU.
C. transfer to the OR.
D. potential organ donation.

65.   A 45-year-old male presents to the ED with complaints of severe pain and burning around the left eye, pain in the left side of the head, increased tearing, and nausea. You note ptosis of the left eye, which is red. The patient states that these symptoms started approximately 30 minutes before arrival. This patient's symptoms are most commonly associated with:
A. cluster headache.
B. tension headache.
C. intracerebral neoplasm.
D. optic neuritis.

66. A patient presents to the ED complaining of left wrist swelling and tenderness after a fall. The wrist is swollen and ecchymotic. X-rays confirm a navicular fracture. Treatment of this type of fracture includes:
    A. open reduction and internal fixation.
    B. daily, gentle range-of-motion exercises to preserve function.
    C. immobilization with a splint for 2 weeks.
    D. immobilization with a cast for 12 weeks.

67. A radial head subluxation has been successfully reduced in a 2-year-old boy. Which of the following statements by the mother indicates a proper understanding of discharge instructions?
    A. "He will grow out of this."
    B. "I will ask his pediatrician to apply a splint tomorrow."
    C. "This may happen again; it can't be avoided."
    D. "I will ask my pediatrician to order a magnetic resonance imaging (MRI) scan."

68. When a thumb spica splint is being applied, the hand should be positioned as if holding:
    A. a paper clip.
    B. a soda can.
    C. a pencil.
    D. up a wall.

69. A mother brings her 5-year-old child to the ED after the child was bitten by a mouse in the kitchen of their home. Which of the following statements about rabies post exposure prophylaxis (RPEP) is true?
    A. It is not indicated in this situation.
    B. It may be able to be withheld if the mouse can be captured and observed for 10 days.
    C. It should be started immediately.
    D. The child should have a rabies antibody titer drawn 10 days later. If the values are elevated, RPEP should be started.

Questions 70–73

A 14-year-old boy is brought to the ED by his parents after he was taken down in a hard tackle during a football scrimmage. He complains of left shoulder pain. A deformity of the left clavicle is visible.

70. The priority nursing assessment is to evaluate:
    A. the peripheral nerves.
    B. breath sounds.
    C. brachial pulse.
    D. pain.

71. X-rays confirm a clavicular fracture. The nurse should be most alert for serious underlying injuries if the fracture is:
    A. located in the medial aspect of the clavicle.
    B. displaced.
    C. located in the middle third of the clavicle.
    D. angulated.

72. Orders for this patient include the application of a figure 8 support. After this device has been applied, the nurse should evaluate:
     A. sensation over the clavicle.
     B. ulnar pulse.
     C. shoulder range of motion.
     D. thumb abduction.

73. Which of the following statements indicates the patient's appropriate understanding of home care for a fracture of the clavicle?
     A. "I will take the support off when I go to sleep."
     B. "I will apply ice to the area."
     C. "I can remove the support to shower."
     D. "I can take the support off after 7 days."

Questions 74–76

A 24-year-old sanitation worker presents to the ED holding 3 amputated fingers in a soiled cloth. The patient is awake, alert, and oriented, but appears to be anxious and upset. Upon examination of the affected hand, you note that the first, second, and third fingers are missing. The hand is swollen, ecchymotic, and bleeding profusely from the stumps.

74. The nurse should FIRST:
     A. apply direct pressure to the stumps to control bleeding.
     B. administer an oral antibiotic.
     C. reapproximate the amputated digits and hold them in place with a pressure dressing.
     D. place the amputated digits in sterile water.

75. Bleeding of the stumps has been controlled. The next priority should be given to treatment of the amputated fingers. The nurse should:
     A. scrub the digits with iodine solution and place them in a plastic bag.
     B. flush the digits with mild soap solution, then soak them in sterile saline.
     C. wrap the digits in dry gauze and place them directly on dry ice.
     D. wrap the digits in moist gauze, insert them in a plastic bag, and place the bag on ice.

76. Diagnostic x-ray films should be taken of:
     A. the affected hand with stumps.
     B. the affected hand with stumps and the amputated fingers.
     C. the affected hand with stumps, the amputated fingers, and the forearm.
     D. the affected hand and the opposite hand for comparison.

77. A patient presents with pain in the sole of her foot after stepping on a nail. Initial assessment includes:
     A. an x-ray.
     B. a computed tomography (CT) scan.
     C. a magnetic resonance imaging (MRI) scan.
     D. an ultrasound scan.

78. A middle-aged woman walks slowly into triage. She reports that someone pulled out a chair as she was preparing to sit down, causing her to fall on a concrete floor. Pain is present but tolerable when she stands or lies down, but intense when she sits. The nurse should suspect a fracture of the:
     A. symphysis pubis.
     B. ischial ramus.
     C. iliac crest.
     D. acetabulum.

79.　A 25-year-old male complains of pain, swelling, and cuts on his hand after being involved in a fight. During your triage assessment, the most important question to ask is:
　　A. "When was your last tetanus shot?"
　　B. "How did you get the cuts on your hand?"
　　C. "When did this happen?"
　　D. "Do you have any other medical problems?"

80.　Posterior shoulder dislocation is most likely the result of which mechanism?
　　A. Seizure
　　B. Motor vehicle collision
　　C. Fall
　　D. Assault

81.　A 48-year-old male presents at the ED complaining of an acute onset of epigastric abdominal pain radiating to the back. A quick assessment reveals a history of hyperlipidemia and hypertension treated by medications that include thiazide diuretics. The patient has hypotension and cool, clammy skin and is tachycardic. The priority intervention for this patient is to:
　　A. order laboratory tests, including amylase and lipase.
　　B. prepare to administer morphine for relief of pain.
　　C. administer intravenous fluids and electrolytes.
　　D. prepare for ultrasonography as a diagnostic evaluation tool.

82.　Which of the following signs/symptoms is commonly associated with viral gastroenteritis?
　　A. Persistent vomiting
　　B. Increased urinary output
　　C. Hypoactive bowel sounds
　　D. Bloody stools

83.　A 32-year-old female arrives in the ED complaining of abdominal pain. She states that she has a history of Crohn's disease. What description of recent bowel activity should lead the nurse to suspect that the patient is experiencing another episode of Crohn's disease?
　　A. Clay-colored stools
　　B. Melena
　　C. Bright-red blood
　　D. Diarrhea

84.　The patient is being discharged with a diagnosis of hiatal hernia and has discharge instructions to take an antacid. The ED nurse will instruct the patient that some antacids produce diarrhea and some produce constipation. Antacids that have a laxative effect contain:
　　A. aluminum.
　　B. calcium
　　C. magnesium.
　　D. sodium.

85.　Diagnostic peritoneal lavage (DPL) that has been performed on your patient is positive for blood and fecal matter. The trauma surgeon is concerned that this patient may have incurred an injury to the:
　　A. liver.
　　B. stomach.
　　C. pancreas.
　　D. colon.

86. A 12-year-old boy complaining of left shoulder pain and malaise presents to the ED with his mother. As you are escorting the boy alone to x-ray, he confides that he was "beaten up" by 3 other boys 2 days ago and hit in the "belly," when his left shoulder started to "hurt." Your next action should be to:
   A. advise him he should tell his mother.
   B. continue to take him for his shoulder films.
   C. take him back to the treatment area immediately.
   D. take him directly to the computed tomography (CT) scanner.

87. A woman brings her 4-week-old male infant to the ED, stating that he has had increased projectile vomiting over the last week. In addition, the infant's stools have decreased in frequency and amount. On physical exam, peristaltic waves are noted in the upper right quadrant along with an olive-size mass. The ED nurse recognizes that the priority nursing intervention is to:
   A. administer intravenous fluids and electrolytes.
   B. administer rectal promethazine HCl (Phenergan) 12.5 mg.
   C. prepare for the administration of a barium enema.
   D. prepare for nasogastric intubation.

88. Heartburn is a common manifestation of esophageal disease. Which of the following statements about heartburn is true?
   A. Heartburn is often experienced with postural changes.
   B. The symptoms of heartburn can be relieved by lying down.
   C. The symptoms of heartburn can be relieved by drinking ample fluids.
   D. Heartburn is not affected by cigarette smoking.

89. A 55-year-old male presents to the ED complaining of right flank pain (rated at 8/10) for 3 hours. He is diaphoretic and restless. Initial vital signs are BP 164/92 mmHg, pulse 96/min, respirations 20/min, oxygen saturation 96%, and temperature 98.4° F (36.9° C). The patient has no past history of similar pain. Your planning and determination of urgency of care for this patient are based on ruling out which of the following medical conditions FIRST?
   A. Renal colic
   B. Abdominal aortic aneurysm
   C. Costochondritis
   D. Acute diverticulitis

90. A 64-year-old patient has unstable atrial fibrillation at a rate of 134 with associated chest pain and some shortness of breath. The physician orders ibutilide (Corvert) to be given to the patient intravenously. Initial vital signs are BP 124/70 mmHg, pulse 134/min, respirations 22/min, oxygen saturation 95%, and temperature 97.4° F (36.9° C). Knowing the side effects of ibutilide, the ED nurse places at the bedside and is prepared to give which of the following medications?
   A. Epinephrine (Adrenalin)
   B. Potassium
   C. Naloxone (Narcan)
   D. Magnesium

91. A 25-year-old college student took 25 tablets of Dimetapp as a suicidal gesture approximately 3 hours ago. The patient presents to the ED alert and oriented x 4 (slightly drowsy). Initial vital signs are BP 110/70 mmHg, pulse 76/min, respirations 18/min, oxygen saturation 95%, and temperature 97.9° F (36.6° C). The most effective way to manage this patient's toxic emergency is to:
   A. give syrup of ipecac.
   B. perform gastric lavage.

    C. give activated charcoal.

    D. give polyethylene glycol–electrolyte solution (GoLytely).

92. A 4-year-old male has a foreign body in his throat that is partially obstructing the airway. His color is pink. He has no altered level of consciousness and does not appear to be in acute distress. While you await the transport team that is coming to transport this child to a children's hospital, in what position should he be placed?

    A. Prone with face to side

    B. Supine

    C. Any position in which he feels comfortable

    D. Secured upright

93. Your 2-year-old patient has been diagnosed with croup and has not responded to saline mist respiratory treatment. After racemic epinephrine treatment, as ordered by the physician, the child's respiratory condition improves dramatically. How long should this child be monitored in the ED before discharge?

    A. One hour

    B. Two hours

    C. Four hours

    D. Six hours

94. An 84-year-old male presents to the ED reporting diffuse abdominal pain (now rated at 10/10) for the past 2 days. The pain had a slow onset and is described as aching and constant. The patient has a history of atrial fibrillation (now well controlled) and appears to be slightly dehydrated. Initial vital signs are BP 166/88 mmHg, pulse 94/min, respirations 24/min, oxygen saturation 95%, and temperature 98.2° F (36.8° C). Examination of the abdomen reveals an abdomen that is soft and nontender, with bowel sounds present. The patient has had a computed tomography (CT) scan of the abdomen, which was negative. All lab test results are within normal limits. The rectal exam is heme negative. What condition do you suspect?

    A. Appendicitis

    B. Mesenteric ischemia

    C. Cholecystitis

    D. Diverticulitis

95. The priority treatment of choice for a methanol overdose is:

    A. Ethanol IV

    B. Activated charcoal PO

    C. Polyethylene glycol–electrolyte solution (GoLytely) PO

    D. Flumazenil (Romazicon) IV

96. Consent rates for organ donation are highest when the request is made by the:

    A. ED nurse.

    B. hospital chaplain.

    C. Organ Procurement Organization (OPO) coordinator in conjunction with the hospital staff.

    D. primary intensive care unit nurse and the attending physician.

97. The full emergency operations preparation cycle includes:

    A. planning, education, drills, and evaluation.

    B. scene management, hospital management, and city management.

    C. meetings, assembling reference notebooks, and construction of facilities.

    D. training exercises and critiquing.

98. Parents bring their 5-day-old infant to the ED for what they call "poor feeding." Mom reports that the baby was breastfeeding well until the previous evening. Your triage exam reveals a term female infant who is pale, slightly mottled, and listless, with poor muscle tone. Initial vital signs are HR 160, respirations 44/min with mild retractions, and rectal temperature 100.8° F (37.9° C). Capillary refill is 3 seconds centrally and 4 seconds peripherally. After the infant has been placed in a treatment room, oxygen is provided blow-by. The next intervention should be to:
    A. give acetaminophen and place a urine bag on the infant.
    B. do an Accu-Chek and give the infant a bottle of 5% dextrose in water.
    C. establish IV access and collect blood for a CBC, blood culture, electrolytes, and a bedside Accu-Chek.
    D. prepare for intubation and establish IV access.

99. Which of the following statements about children's pain is true?
    A. Behavioral manifestations reflect pain intensity.
    B. Children may not admit to having pain.
    C. Narcotics are more likely to cause respiratory depression in children than in adults.
    D. It is not possible to evaluate pain in nonverbal children.

100. Discharge instructions to the parents of a child who has had a febrile seizure should include:
    A. instructions to prevent future seizures by treating fever with cool baths.
    B. reassurance that febrile seizures do not cause brain damage.
    C. a discussion of the side effects of phenytoin (Dilantin).
    D. reassurance that febrile seizures do not last beyond adolescence.

101. A 4-year-old male fell from a moving all-terrain vehicle (ATV) and has multiple injuries. He has been stabilized in your ED and will be transported to a regional pediatric hospital for ongoing evaluation and treatment. A pediatric transport team is flying in to pick up and transport the patient. Which of the following interventions is NOT appropriate in preparing the patient's family for his transport?
    A. Explain why the patient needs to be transferred.
    B. Provide the family with maps and directions to the receiving facility.
    C. Send the family to the receiving facility as soon as possible so they can be there when the patient arrives.
    D. Caution the family to observe all traffic laws in traveling to the accepting facility.

102. Equipment in the transport environment should have which of the following characteristics?
    A. Electrically powered, with the ability to function on battery power for 10-minute intervals.
    B. Portable, combining several functions in a single piece of equipment.
    C. Able to be placed on a small shelf or the floor while in transit for better visibility and accessible to the transport crew.
    D. Weigh no more than 15 lb.

Questions 103 and 104

A patient with an acute myocardial infarction and severe cardiac failure has been stabilized in a small metropolitan ED. The patient is on 3 vasoactive drips and 1 antiarrhythmic drip, has an intra-aortic balloon pump inserted, and is intubated with ventilatory support. The patient is to be transferred to the ED of a cardiac specialty center on the opposite side of the same city as the sending facility, 30 miles away. Copies of the patient's records and x-rays are to be sent with the patient. The sending facility has secured an accepting physician and administrative acceptance of the patient by the receiving facility. An advanced life-support (ALS) ambulance with 2 paramedic caregivers and a basic emergency medical technician driver is performing the transport.

103.   This case constitutes an Emergency Medical Treatment and Active Labor Act (EMTALA) violation because:
   A. A transfer from one ED to another violates EMTALA.
   B. The transport crew is not properly trained for a patient who is this acutely ill.
   C. The accepting physician is not qualified to care for a patient who is this acutely ill.
   D. The benefits of the transfer do not outweigh the risks.

104.   The most appropriate mode of transport is:
   A. ground ambulance; routine transfer.
   B. ground ambulance; emergency transfer.
   C. rotor-wing air ambulance transfer.
   D. fixed-wing air ambulance transfer.

105.   A patient is transported to a hospital by helicopter. The aircraft has side doors for patient access. The nose of the helicopter is at 12 o'clock. The crew states that a "hot offload" is indicated. The best approach to the aircraft as its rotors are still turning is:
   A. standing upright from the 1 o'clock position.
   B. crouching from the 5 o'clock position.
   C. standing upright from the 7 o'clock position.
   D. crouching from the 11 o'clock position.

106.   A patient arrives in the ED 10 minutes after having been pulled from a frozen pond. The patient is pulseless, apneic, and unresponsive and has a temperature of 77° F (25° C). The cardiac monitor indicates ventricular fibrillation. Which of the following combinations of modes of care is most appropriate?
   A. Defibrillate at 200, 300, and 360 joules and begin cardiopulmonary resuscitation (CPR).
   B. Begin CPR and warming.
   C. Begin CPR, start an IV, and give epinephrine, followed by defibrillation at 360 joules.
   D. Begin CPR and insert a nasogastric tube.

107.   A passenger train has derailed. First responders indicate that at least 56 people have been injured. A nurse has gone in an ambulance to assist with care at the scene. Which of the following patients is the highest priority for treatment and transport ("red" category)?
   A. A 75-year-old with femur, tibia, and fibula fractures; pale, moist skin; and pelvic tenderness and mobility on palpation.
   B. A 45-year-old with a metal rod impaled in the right forearm. The arm is neurovascularly intact. The patient is ambulatory.
   C. A 63-year-old with second-degree and third-degree burns over 95% of body surface areas. The patient is unconscious and has a thready pulse.
   D. A 25-year-old with pain in the left lateral lower chest and a 5-inch laceration in the left forearm. The wound squirts blood when uncovered. The patient is controlling the bleeding by applying pressure with a bandanna. Skin is pink and dry.

108.   A 55-year-old woman in congestive heart failure states that she had a heart transplant 3 years ago. The patient denies chest pain. Which of the following statements best describes why she is not having chest pain?
   A. Her sensitivity to pain is diminished because she is taking multiple antirejection medications.
   B. Atherosclerosis, which contributes to coronary artery clot, spasm, and chest pain, will not develop from the transplant.
   C. She may never experience chest pain. Heart transplant recipients have a denervated organ.
   D. Her perception of pain is affected by her perception of her heart as belonging to someone else.

109. A 155-lb (70.5-kg) patient with a massive anteroseptal myocardial infarction develops cardiogenic shock. The physician orders dopamine at (Intropin) 8 mcg/kg/min. Two 200-mg ampules of dopamine (Intropin) are added to 250 ml of D5W. The drip factor is 60 gtt/ml. The appropriate flow rate in gtt/min is:
    A. 12
    B. 16
    C. 21
    D. 30

110. A medication recommended for delirium tremens is:
    A. Atenolol (Tenormin) 50–100 mg PO
    B. Chlordiazepoxide (Librium) 25–100 mg PO
    C. Lorazepam (Ativan) 1–5 mg PO, IV, IM
    D. Clonidine (Catapres) 0.1–0.4 mg PO

111. Rocky Mountain spotted fever can be very difficult to diagnose in its early stages. Patients infected with rickettsiae generally visit a physician in the first week of their illness, following an incubation period of about 5 to 10 days after a tick bite. The early clinical presentation of Rocky Mountain spotted fever is nonspecific and may resemble a variety of other infectious and noninfectious diseases. Which of the following is the classic triad of findings for this disease?
    A. Fever, nausea, muscle pain
    B. Rash, muscle pain, severe headache
    C. History of tick bite, abdominal pain, diarrhea
    D. Fever, rash, history of tick bite

112. Which of the following is the major clinical forms of human anthrax?
    A. Cutaneous and inhalation
    B. Inhalation and gastrointestinal
    C. Cutaneous and gastrointestinal
    D. Cutaneous, inhalation, and gastrointestinal

113. Symptoms of a systemic reaction to a snake bite include:
    A. hypertension.
    B. GI disturbances.
    C. petechiae.
    D. decreased salivation.

114. A 7-year-old boy arrives in the ED stating that he was bitten on the foot while playing outside. He is screaming with pain at the bite mark, nauseated, and weak. He describes severe abdominal pain and spasms in his leg. You suspect that he has been bitten by a:
    A. tick.
    B. black widow spider.
    C. wasp.
    D. brown recluse spider.

115. Which of the following statements is true about human bites?
    A. Human bites have a decreased risk for cellulitis.
    B. Human bites have the highest rate of infection of all bite injuries.
    C. A person who has been bitten by another person should receive antibiotics if signs of infection are present.
    D. Human bites rarely cause deep tissue injury.

116. Early symptoms of anthrax pneumonia include:
    A. abrupt onset, elevated temperature, productive cough.
    B. insidious onset, mild fever, nonproductive cough.
    C. abrupt onset, high fever, productive cough.
    D. fever, chills, cough, hemoptysis.

117. An appropriate nursing diagnosis for a patient who has been bitten by a brown recluse spider bite is:
    A. impaired verbal communication.
    B. impaired gas exchange.
    C. pain related to muscle spasm.
    D. impaired skin integrity.

118. A 56-year-old man with a known history of depression arrives in your ED complaining of nausea, vomiting, and severe headache. He has severe hypertension. Which type of medication can cause a hypertensive crisis?
    A. Tricyclics
    B. Barbiturates
    C. Sedative-hypnotics
    D. Monoamine oxidase (MAO) inhibitors

119. Female patients older than 50 years who are taking antipsychotic medications are at risk for which side effect?
    A. Endocrine changes
    B. Tardive dyskinesia
    C. Photosensitivity
    D. Orthostatic hypotension

120. A medication used for controlling the ventricular response rate of a patient with supraventricular tachycardia is:
    A. atropine.
    B. isoproterenol (Isuprel).
    C. labetalol (Normaline).
    D. verapamil (Calan).

121. Which of the following would be a CONTRAINDICATION for the administration of activated charcoal?
    A. Hyperactive bowel sounds
    B. Elevated blood pressure
    C. Acetaminophen (Tylenol) toxicity
    D. Vitamin toxicity

122. A patient presents to the ED complaining of fever, chills, headache, and extreme exhaustion. He states that he has been feeling ill since his return from Africa 2 days ago. On examination, you note that the patient has a very swollen, tender lymph gland accompanied by pain. You suspect that the patient has:
    A. African sleeping sickness.
    B. ehrlichiosis.
    C. plague.
    D. Chagas' disease.

123.   Which of the following is the leading cause of vector-borne infectious illness in the United States?
    A. Lyme disease
    B. Yellow fever
    C. Dengue fever
    D. West Nile virus

124.   A 6-year-old child is brought to the ED by his mother 15 minutes after having been stung in the forearm by a bee. On examination, a 2-cm circular lesion that is red, swollen, and tender is observed. The ED nurse knows that this is:
    A. probably an infection.
    B. an anaphylactic reaction.
    C. a normal reaction.
    D. an indication of serum sickness.

125.   The Emergency Medical Treatment and Active Labor Act (EMTALA) includes which of the following situations?
    A. A visitor in the hospital lobby
    B. A hospital employee reporting for work
    C. A woman in labor arriving at the hospital by taxicab
    D. An injured lawn care worker whose condition the physician determines to be stable

126.   According to EMTALA, when a patient is transferred to another facility, the sending facility must provide:
    A. copies of a complete listing of charges from the sending facility.
    B. insurance information and worker's compensation information if the patient was injured on the job.
    C. a certificate signed by the physician confirming that benefits of the transfer outweigh the risk of transfer.
    D. a complete listing of the patient's valuables and personal belongings.

127.   In a negligence suit, the plaintiff must prove four key elements in a court of law: duty to the patient, breach of duty by the health care professional, injury resulting from the breach, and:
    A. inadequate education and training of the health care professional.
    B. breach of duty is the proximate cause of injury.
    C. documentation inadequate to fully describe the situation that resulted in injury.
    D. incident report incomplete when retrieved by the plaintiff's attorney.

128.   Hospitals that violate EMTALA provisions are subject to:
    A. fines by the federal government.
    B. a waiver of the CLIA (Clinical Laboratory Improvement Act) permit.
    C. a complete audit by OSHA.
    D. immediate closure until an investigation is completed.

129.   When reviewing a medical record, you note the following documentation: "Patient condition deteriorated and physician notified at 1800." Which of the following statements about this documentation is correct?
    A. The notation is too short.
    B. Abbreviations should be used whenever possible.
    C. Military time is not acceptable in a patient chart.
    D. Specifics are missing from the description.

130. Which of the following situations is considered an exception to required parental consent for treatment of a 14-year-old patient?
A. Unemancipated minors
B. Elevated alcohol level
C. Gonorrhea
D. Commission of a crime

Questions 131–134

A 17-year-old female presents to the ED with a chief complaint of left-sided pelvic pain. The patient states that the pain started suddenly 3 hours ago and has become constant, sharp, and very severe. Her last menstrual period was approximately 6 weeks ago, but she has been spotting for several days. The patient states that she is sexually active. Initial vital signs are BP 120/70 mmHg, pulse 128/min, respirations 22/min, and temperature 100° F (37.8° C). You suspect ectopic pregnancy.

131. Additional information that you should obtain includes the presence of any risk factors. Risk factors for the development of an ectopic pregnancy include:
A. a history of pelvic inflammatory disease (PID).
B. fertility drug use.
C. previous tubal ligation.
D. all of the above.

132. What is the appropriate triage category for this patient?
A. Urgent
B. Emergent
C. Nonurgent
D. Referral to fast track

133. The most accurate diagnostic test for an ectopic pregnancy includes:
A. quantitative urinary BhCG.
B. transvaginal ultrasound.
C. a complete blood count (CBC).
D. serum electrolyte levels.

134. The most appropriate nursing diagnosis for this patient is:
A. fear.
B. pain.
C. risk for fluid volume deficit.
D. risk for injury.

Questions 135–137

A 39-year-old female presents to the ED with the chief complaints of vaginal bleeding, cramping pelvic pain, and low back pain for several hours. The patient states that she is 8 weeks pregnant by dates. Her pregnancy has been confirmed by a quantitative BhCG in her physician's office. This is her fourth pregnancy and she has 3 children. Her second pregnancy resulted in the birth of twins. She had a spontaneous abortion 1 year ago. She states that she has been using 1 pad per hour for the past several hours but has not passed any blood or tissue.

135. When documenting the patient's pregnancy history, the ED nurse should write:
A. gravida 4, para 3, abortion 1, living 3.
B. gravida 5, para 3, abortion 1, living 3.
C. gravida 5, para 2, abortion 1, living 3.
D. gravida 4, para 2, abortion 1, living 3.

136.   The physical examination reveals a moderate amount of uterine bleeding without clots or tissue. The cervix is closed. Transvaginal ultrasound reveals an intrauterine pregnancy with a gestational age of approximately 7 weeks and with positive fetal cardiac motion. The patient's condition is classified as a(n):
    A. complete abortion.
    B. threatened abortion.
    C. incomplete abortion.
    D. missed abortion.

137.   You are preparing the patient to be discharged to home, accompanied by her husband. Discharge teaching should include all of the following EXCEPT:
    A. Maintain bed rest for the remainder of the pregnancy.
    B. Avoid the use of tampons. Use sanitary pads only.
    C. Pelvic rest until bleeding and cramping subside.
    D. Return to the ED or obstetrician if bleeding or pain increases.

138.   Which of the following nursing interventions would be a priority for the ED patient with hyperemesis gravidarum?
    A. Infusion of D5W at a rate of 150 ml/hour.
    B. Evaluating baseline laboratory studies of serum electrolytes.
    C. Monitoring urinary output and dipstick urine for ketones.
    D. Administering antiemetics as ordered.

139.   Risk factors for the development of hypertension during pregnancy include:
    A. maternal age greater than 40 years.
    B. African-American heritage.
    C. multiple gestation.
    D. all of the above.

140.   A 34-year-old female presents to the ED after having been involved in a motor vehicle collision. She is 34 weeks pregnant and has sustained blunt trauma to the chest and abdomen. All of the following interventions are appropriate EXCEPT:
    A. Initiate high-flow oxygen.
    B. Elevate the backboard 15 degrees in the left lateral position.
    C. Initiate 2 large-bore IVs with normal saline or Ringer's lactate solution.
    D. Perform a pelvic exam to assess for possible uterine bleeding.

141.   The goals in treating all forms of shock include:
    A. restoration of anaerobic metabolism.
    B. restoration of oxygenation and tissue perfusion.
    C. administration of dopamine (Intropin) to reverse acidosis.
    D. administration of D5W for fluid volume resuscitation.

142.   Which stage of shock results in widespread cellular destruction and does not respond to any form of aggressive treatment?
    A. Compensated (nonprogressive) shock
    B. Uncompensated (progressive) shock
    C. Irrefractory shock
    D. Irreversible (refractory) shock

143. Assessment of the patient in shock should include which of the following in the primary survey?
    A. Abdominal sounds
    B. Level of consciousness
    C. Areas of deformity
    D. Complete neurologic exam

144. Typical vital sign changes that occur in uncompensated (progressive) shock include:
    A. a widening pulse pressure.
    B. bradycardia.
    C. decreased capillary refill time.
    D. narrowed pulse pressure.

145. A 78-year-old patient who was involved in a major car crash was brought to your ED. The paramedics' report states that she was trapped in the vehicle and sustained a left femur fracture as well as closed fractures of the left forearm and pelvis. You expect this patient to be in hypovolemic shock because:
    A. older adults are normally anemic and the fractures have contributed to blood loss.
    B. closed forearm fractures can cause significant blood loss in any trauma patient.
    C. impaired response to physiologic changes causes older adults to tolerate blood loss less well.
    D. the systemic body failure common in older adults makes them poor candidates for resuscitation.

146. A 42-year-old male patient presents via ambulance with a chief complaint of vomiting blood. Vital signs are BP 70/palpation, HR 128/min, and respirations 38/min. The patient's level of consciousness is confused. You conclude that your patient has which category of volume loss/hemorrhage?
    A. Class I
    B. Class II
    C. Class III
    D. Class IV

147. Your 36-year-old trauma patient has been diagnosed with a severe liver laceration. Initial vital signs are BP 82/palpation, pulse 126/min, and respirations 34/min. His level of consciousness is "confused." As the ED nurse, you anticipate that volume replacement will include:
    A. 0.3% normal saline.
    B. 0.9% normal saline.
    C. lactated Ringer's solution and blood products.
    D. 3% normal saline.

148. Blood products that are about to be administered to a patient with hemorrhagic shock should be warmed to prevent:
    A. a transfusion reaction.
    B. metabolic alkalosis.
    C. hypokalemia.
    D. hypothermia.

149. How much crystalloid should be given per bolus for the pediatric patient presenting in shock?
    A. 10 ml/kg
    B. 20 ml/kg
    C. 25 ml/kg
    D. 40 ml/kg

150.   Your trauma patient remains in shock despite aggressive fluid resuscitation. You note a distended abdomen and dropping blood pressure. Your patient is too unstable to be sent for a computed tomography (CT) scan. You anticipate that the physician will perform or order:

A.   a flat plate x-ray of the abdomen.

B.   diagnostic peritoneal lavage (DPL).

C.   a peritoneal tap.

D.   a pleural needle decompression.

Practice Examination 1

1. Acute coronary syndrome includes which of the following conditions?
    A. Atrial fibrillation
    B. Left bundle branch block
    C. Chest pain
    D. UNSTABLE ANGINA

Rationale:

    D. Acute coronary syndrome includes acute myocardial infarction (AMI), both Q-wave and non-Q wave AMI, and unstable angina.
    A. Atrial fibrillation is not a category in acute coronary syndrome.
    B. While left bundle branch block may be associated with an acute myocardial infarction, it is not a category in acute coronary syndrome.
    C. Chest pain is not considered a category for acute coronary syndrome.

Content Category: Cardiovascular

Reference: Roettig & Tanabe, 2000; p. 8.

2. Which of the following is the expected outcome for a patient treated for acute coronary syndrome?
    A. Reduced fatigue
    B. RELIEF OF CHEST PAIN OR ANGINA
    C. Muffled heart sounds
    D. Increased jugular venous pressure

Rationale:

    B. Relief of chest pain is the primary focus of interventions to abort or minimize effects of acute coronary syndrome.
    A. You do not have sufficient assessment information to indicate fatigue as a factor. Reflect on the primary presenting symptom of acute coronary syndrome.
    C. Muffled heart sounds would not be an expected finding with acute coronary syndrome.
    D. If the patient has heart failure subsequent to acute myocardial infarction, jugular venous pressure may be increased. However, the expected outcome would be decreased or normalized jugular venous pressure.

Content Category: Cardiovascular

Reference: Roettig & Tanabe, 2000; p. 8; Barnason, 1998; pp .459–514.

3. How is tenecteplase (TNKase) administered for acute myocardial infarction?
    A. Bolus plus infusion intravenously
    B. Infused over 60 minutes intravenously
    C. SINGLE BOLUS GIVEN OVER 5 SECONDS INTRAVENOUSLY
    D. Two intravenous boluses given 30 minutes apart

Rationale:

C. Single bolus dosing. No additional infusion is needed after the bolus dose.
A. A bolus plus infusion intravenously is needed to administer alteplase (Activase).
B. An infusion over 60 minutes intravenously is required with streptokinase (Streptase).
D. Two IV boluses 30 minutes apart is the method for administering reteplase (Retavase) as a fibrin-olytic agent.

Content Category: Cardiovascular

Reference: Roettig & Tanabe, 2000; p. 24.

4. A 55-year-old female presents to the ED with intermittent chest pain of 4 hours' duration. She is pain free at the time of admission. She is on hormone replacement therapy and stopped smoking 2 weeks ago after a 30-pack-year history. The most appropriate triage and management for this patient would be:
    A. EMERGENT; CARDIAC WORKUP.
    B. nonemergent; admission to chest pain unit.
    C. urgent; clinic referral.
    D. nonemergent; sent home.

Rationale:

A. Patient's atypical chest pain, prodromal symptoms, and risk factors place her at high risk for acute coronary syndrome. Hormone replacement therapy does not provide absolute protection against coronary artery disease in women.
B. Inappropriate, considering history and risk factors.
C. Inappropriate, considering history and risk factors.
D. Inappropriate, considering history and risk factors.

Content Category: Cardiovascular

Reference: Jairath, 2001; pp. 17–28; Bahr, 1998.

5. A 78-year-old male presents with a chief complaint of dizziness for the past 3 to 4 days. Patient reports that he had a myocardial infarction 8 years ago, at which time a permanent pacemaker was implanted. He denies chest pain. Initial vital signs are BP 168/88 mmHg, pulse 78/min apically, and respirations 18/min. What is your interpretation of the following ECG rhythm strip?

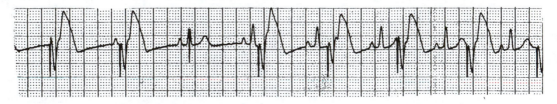

    A. 1:1 ventricular pacing
    B. Dual-chambered pacemaker (DDD) with appropriate sensing
    C. VENTRICULAR PACING WITH LOSS OF CAPTURE
    D. Atrial pacing with loss of sensing

Rationale:

C. Note the loss of a captured ventricular beat following the pacer spike on the ECG rhythm strip.

A. A pacer spike is not consistently followed by ventricular depolarization on the ECG.

B. There is no consistent evidence of atrial and/or ventricular pacing followed respectively by atrial and/or ventricular depolarization on the ECG.

D. Incorrect.

Content Category: Cardiovascular

Reference: Reynolds & Apple, 2001; p. 121.

6. A 54-year-old male presents to the ED with a chief complaint of chest pain. His previous hospital record reveals that 4 weeks ago he had a coronary stent inserted and underwent angioplasty of the left anterior descending (LAD) coronary artery. His chest pain presentation suggests the possibility of coronary restenosis. Which leads on a 12-lead electrocardiogram would you examine for ST segment changes associated with restenosis?

A. I, AVL
B. II, III, AVF
C. V_2, V_3
D. V_5, V_6

Rationale:

C. The leads V_2, V_3 reflect the left anterior descending artery, associated with ECG changes of an anterior myocardial infarction.

A. The leads I, AVL reflect circumflex artery and lateral wall changes.

B. The leads II, III, AVF reflect right coronary changes.

D. The leads V_5, V_6 reflect the left circumflex and right coronary arteries.

Content Category: Cardiovascular

References: Casey et al., 1998; p. 330; Staudenmayer et al., 1999; p. 623.

7. Which of the following conditions would be represented by an elevated ST segment in all leads except AVR and V_1?

A. Acute anterior myocardial infarction
B. PERICARDITIS
C. Myocardial ischemia
D. Cardiac tamponade

Rationale:

B. The ECG findings associated with pericarditis are elevation of ST segments except for aVR and V_1.

A. Acute changes would appear in the ECG segments corresponding with the affected portion of the myocardium (e.g., anterior, lateral).

C. Ischemic changes would appear as ST segment depressions in ECG segments corresponding with areas of myocardial ischemia.

D. Cardiac tamponade is not demonstrated by ST segment elevation on an ECG.

Content Category: Cardiovascular

Reference: Barnason, 1998; pp. 459–514.

8.   Which of the following assessment findings is associated with pericardial tamponade?
      A. Tracheal deviation
      B. MUFFLED HEART SOUNDS
      C. Increased venous return
      D. Paradoxical pulse = 5 mm Hg

Rationale:

      B. On auscultation of the chest, muffled and distant heart sounds are noted in patients with peri-
          cardial tamponade.
      A. Tracheal deviation is not a finding associated with tamponade. It is more classically associated
          with tension pneumothorax.
      C. Tamponade usually causes restricted contractility of the heart, which causes decreased cardiac
          output and therefore decreased, not increased, venous return.
      D. In order for paradoxical pulse to be significant, it must be = 10 mm Hg. A significant paradoxical
          pulse can be associated with pericardial tamponade. Paradoxical pulse refers to a decrease of sys-
          tolic blood pressure from expiration to inspiration.

Content Category: Cardiovascular

Reference: Barnason, 1998; pp. 459–514.

9.   In the presence of myocardial damage, which of the following cardiac biomarkers remains elevated
      for the longest time?
      A. CK/MB
      B. C-reactive protein
      C. Myoglobin
      D. TROPONIN

Rationale:

      D. Troponin levels remain elevated for up to 7 days.
      A. CK/MB levels usually normalize after 48 to 72 hours.
      B. C-reactive protein in not a biomarker for myocardial "injury."
      C. Myoglobin usually normalizes 8 hours after an injury.

Content Category: Cardiovascular

Reference: Staudenmayer et al., 1999; p. 627.

10.   In the early setting of an acute myocardial infarction, beta blockers have been found to be useful
       because they:
       A. DECREASE MYOCARDIAL OXYGEN CONSUMPTION.
       B. improve venous return
       C. increase contractility
       D. limit the infarct to subendocardial damage

Rationale:

       A. The effects of cardioselective beta blockers to reduce myocardial workload cause myocardial
           oxygen consumption to be decreased as well.
       B. Beta blockers do not act to increase venous return.
       C. Cardioselective beta blockers reduce contractility, thereby reducing myocardial workload.
       D. While the cardioselective action of beta blockade reduces infarct "size," this effect does not nec-
           essarily limit the amount of damage to subendocardial versus complete transmural infarction.

Content Category: Cardiovascular

Reference: Staudenmayer et al., 1999; p. 628.

11.   The patient for whom you are caring presents with the following rhythm and suddenly becomes *unresponsive*. Your first action after establishing "pulselessness" is to:

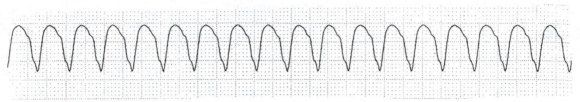

A. DEFIBRILLATE AT 200 JOULES.
B. charge the paddles for synchronized cardioversion.
C. give bretylium tosylate (Bretylol).
D. give lidocaine hydrochloride (Xylocaine) by bolus and start a drip.

Rationale:

A. Treat this rhythm as unconscious ventricular tachycardia.
B. This action would be appropriate only if the patient remained conscious and was markedly hypotensive and refractory to medications.
C. Incorrect.
D. Incorrect.

Content Category: Cardiovascular

Reference: American Heart Association, 2000; pp. I-1–I-384.

12.   A 35-year-old male in severe cardiopulmonary distress was admitted to the ED by ambulance. On presentation, he was pale and tachycardic and had bilateral crackles, a low-grade temperature, and a loud systolic murmur. History revealed that he is a smoker, takes medication for hypertension, and recently underwent cardiac catheterization, which was negative for significant coronary disease. A presumptive diagnosis of infective endocarditis was made. Which of the following was the most likely predisposing factor contributing to infective endocarditis?
A. Acute myocardial infarction
B. HEART CATHETERIZATION PROCEDURE
C. Hypertension
D. Smoking history

Rationale:

B. Invasive diagnostic procedures can precipitate the development of infective endocarditis.
A. The patient did not present with a new AMI and the recent heart catheterization was normal.
C. Hypertension is not considered a contributing cause for infective endocarditis.
D. Smoking history is not considered to predispose infective endocarditis.

Content Category: Cardiovascular

Reference: Barnason, 1998; pp. 459–514.

13.   If a patient who is being managed for chest pain in the ED is allergic to aspirin, what alternative antithrombotic agent can be used?
    A.   Acetylsalicylic acid ("baby aspirin") 80 mg chewed
    B.   TICLOPIDINE HYDROCHLORIDE (TICLID) 250 MG ORALLY
    C.   Enoxaparin (Lovenox) 1 mg/kg subcutaneously
    D.   Eptifibatide (Integrelin) infusion intravenously

Rationale:

B.   Ticlid can be administered in place of aspirin as an alternative antithrombotic agent in a patient who has a known aspirin allergy.

A.   Regardless of dose, patient will still have an allergy to aspirin, which is therefore contra-indicated.

C.   Enoxaparin is a low-molecular-weight heparin. It is an anticoagulant, not an antithrombotic agent.

D.   Integrelin is a IIb/IIIa glycoprotein inhibitor. It is not a substitute for an antithrombotic agent.

Content Category: Cardiovascular

Reference: Roettig & Tanabe, 2000; p. 20.

14.   A patient who is experiencing panic-level anxiety:
    A.   is able to process information.
    B.   MAY EXHIBIT PSYCHOTIC BEHAVIOR.
    C.   has a wide perceptual field.
    D.   can effectively communicate his or her needs.

Rationale:

B.   In a person who is experiencing panic-level anxiety, disorganization of the personality is taking place. In this state, the patient has difficulty relating to others, has distorted perceptions and loss of rational thought, and may experience hallucinations or delusions.

A.   A person experiencing panic is unable to focus on any details or to complete even simple tasks with direction. Misperceptions are common. At panic levels, the focus is on self and the patient is unable to process external stimuli.

C.   A person experiencing mild anxiety is attentive and has a wide perceptual field. The perceptual field narrows as the anxiety level increases.

D.   A person experiencing panic is unable to communicate verbally in a clear manner and often has difficulty functioning.

Content Category: Psychosocial

References: Townsend, 1999; pp. 423–428; Videbeck, 2001; p. 264; ENA, Core Curriculum, 2000; pp. 347–351.

15. A 35-year-old woman has just been brought into the ED by the police after having been sexually assaulted. The patient is alert. Initial assessment reveals bruises and abrasions on her face, breasts, arms, and hands. She makes minimal eye contact with the nurse and speaks only when asked a question. What is the most appropriate action for the emergency nurse to take?
   A. Escort the patient to the bathroom for a shower and contact a social worker.
   B. Notify the emergency physician that a vaginal examination must be done immediately.
   C. ACCOMPANY THE PATIENT TO A PRIVATE TREATMENT AREA AND EXPLAIN THE SEXUAL ASSAULT EXAMINATION PROCESS.
   D. Once the patient is in the treatment area, let her be alone to compose her thoughts about the incident so that an accurate police report can be filed.

Rationale:

   C. Remaining with the patient throughout the sexual assault examination process permits a trust relationship to develop between nurse and patient. Minimizing the number of interactions with various staff members will reduce the patient's anxiety about the process.
   A. The patient should not shower or change her clothes until the sexual assault examination is completed. A shower could destroy potential valuable evidence.
   B. Timeliness of the examination is unimportant. This is not the first action to be taken by the emergency nurse. Evidence collection may occur up to 72 hours after the assault.
   D. The patient should be afforded a comforting, compassionate environment of care that is provided by the emergency nurse. The patient should not be left alone except by her own request.

Content Category: Psychosocial

Reference: ENA, Core Curriculum, 2000; pp. 463–464.

16. A 24-year-old first-year male law student is brought to the ED by police after being found running naked on the highway. Triage assessment reveals an extremely active young man who rhymes his sentences while speaking. There is no correlation between assessment questions posed by the triage nurse and verbal responses from the patient. Vital signs are within normal limits. No obvious injuries are present. The ED nurse is aware that the following illness may mimic a psychiatric disorder:
   A. INFECTION
   B. Cardiovascular insult
   C. Splenic injury
   D. Anaphylaxis

Rationale:

   A. Infection of the central nervous system may produce behavioral changes.
   B. Cardiovascular insult may produce some changes in mental status if hypoxia is extreme.
   C. Splenic injury with significant hypovolemia resulting in severe hypoxia may produce behavioral changes. However, this patient shows no signs of physical injury.
   D. As with significant trauma or cardiovascular insult, a shock state will produce hypoxia-driven behavioral changes. This patient demonstrates no evidence of anaphylaxis.

Content Category: Psychosocial

References: ENA, Core Curriculum, 2000; pp. 360–363; Kitt et al., 1995; pp. 457–462.

17.   A 13-year-old male is brought to the ED by EMS, police. and school officials after having drawn a picture of himself holding a gun to his class. He is withdrawn and does not interact freely with the triage nurse. School officials report that this is not the first time this student has received attention for his behavior and that his grandmother refuses to acknowledge that he is having emotional problems. The most appropriate action for the triage nurse to take at this time is to:
   A. place the patient in a quiet, secure environment.
   B. search the patient for a gun.
   C. notify the patient's grandmother immediately.
   D. ASSESS THE PATIENT FOR SIGNS OF AGITATION AND AGGRESSION.

Rationale:

   D. Assessment for signs of impending agitation and aggression will assist the nurse in placing the patient in an appropriate treatment area and in maintaining a safe environment of care.
   A. While safety and security are paramount, assessing for signs of violent behavior will help the nurse to develop an appropriate therapeutic milieu.
   B. Weapons search is conducted by law enforcement personnel if the patient is in custody.
   C. Notifying the family is the responsibility of school officials. If the family has not been contacted, this can be done after the assessment for impending agitation and aggression has been done.

Content Category: Psychosocial

References: Kitt et al., 1995; pp. 460–462; Varcarolis, 1998; pp. 304–312.

18.   When a psychotic patient is experiencing visual hallucinations of bugs on the bed in the ED, the ED nurse should:
   A. brush the "bugs" from the bed sheets.
   B. put the patient in a regular patient room, close to the nurses' station.
   C. assure the patient that the "bugs" will not hurt him or her.
   D. REORIENT THE PATIENT TO REALITY.

Rationale:

   D. Reorientation to the reality of being sick and in the ED is necessary and reassures the patient that the staff is available to help.
   A. Participating in the hallucination is nontherapeutic and reinforces the hallucination as reality. Instead, the nurse must address the underlying stressor.
   B. A patient who is experiencing hallucinations should be placed in a safe, secure room that contains a minimal amount of extra equipment or furniture.
   C. While it is important to reinforce that the nurses will keep the patient safe, communicating that the bugs are real would only reinforce the patient's hallucinations.

Content Category: Psychosocial

Reference: Stuart & Laraia, 1998; p. 474.

19.   The priority nursing interventions for a suicidal patient in the ED include:
   A. placing the patient in a private area
   B. TALKING TO THE PATIENT ABOUT ANY SUICIDE PLANS
   C. implementing a "no-suicide" safety contract.
   D. praising the patient's positive attributes.

Rationale:

   B. Talking about a patient's suicide plans—including the means, location, and time—is a necessary part of a lethality assessment. Such a discussion does not introduce the idea to commit suicide.

A. A form of supervision, either one to one or by uninterrupted observation, is necessary for a suicidal patient in the ED until a physician's order has removed the need for such supervision.

C. A no-suicide or safety contract is an appropriate intervention for psychiatric inpatients or outpatients. In the ED, however, a more appropriate action would be to determine the patient's suicide plans and to place the patient on one-to-one or constant visual supervision.

D. Artificial praise is usually recognized as such by the patient and often lowers the patient's already low self-esteem.

Content Category: Psychosocial

References: Stuart & Laraia, 1998; p. 395; Videbeck, 2001; pp. 367–371.

20. Which of the following is the priority nursing diagnosis for a patient who has come or been brought to the ED after attempted suicide?
    A. Impaired verbal communication
    B. Anxiety
    C. RISK FOR INJURY
    D. Altered thought processes

Rationale:

C. Safety is the priority for the patient in the emergent situation following an attempted suicide.

A. Impaired verbal communication usually characterizes the patient with an underlying physiological condition such as a cerebrovascular accident.

B. Although a patient may experience anxiety after a suicide attempt, this is not the priority diagnosis.

D. While altered thought processes may be present, this is not the priority diagnosis.

Content Category: Psychosocial

Reference: ENA, Core Curriculum, 2000; pp. 360–363.

21. An unrestrained female driver is brought into the ED by EMS. Paramedics report that she was driving an old car without airbags and that the steering wheel was bent. The patient is awake and alert, with a Glasgow Coma Scale (GCS) of 15. She is pale and anxious, with labored respirations. She states that another driver cut her off at an intersection. You note paradoxical chest wall movement and suspect a flail chest. Which of the following would be your primary concern for this patient?
    A. PULMONARY CONTUSION
    B. Deep-vein thrombosis
    C. Facial lacerations
    D. Concurrent thoracic vertebral fracture

Rationale:

A. Approximately 75% of patients with blunt chest trauma experience some degree of underlying pulmonary contusion because of the amount of mechanical energy that has been transferred to the chest.

B. The development of a deep-vein thrombosis can be a late complication after trauma and is not the primary concern for this patient.

C. Facial lacerations are not a priority for this patient. Because she is talking to you and has a GCS of 15, she has a patent airway.

D. A concurrent thoracic vertebral fracture may be present. However, the primary concern is to maintain effective breathing.

Content Category: Respiratory

References: ENA, Core Curriculum, 2000; pp. 4–5, 123–125, 348, 585–586; Newberry, 1998; pp. 296–297.

22.   The priority intervention for a patient with suspected tension pneumothorax is:
    A. endotracheal intubation.
    B. NEEDLE THORACENTESIS.
    C. two large-bore IVs.
    D. covering the wound with an occlusive dressing.

Rationale:

    B. Decompression by needle thoracotomy with a 12-gauge to 16-gauge needle in the second inter-
        costal space in the midclavicular line on the affected side is the treatment of choice for tension
        pneumothorax.
    A. Although endotracheal intubation may be needed in the patient who has tension pneumotho-
        rax, the buildup of pressure on the affected side must be resolved first.
    C. Insertion of 2 large-bore IV's is an important intervention to support circulation of the trauma
        victim, but life-threatening inadequate ventilation must be addressed first.
    D. Tension pneumothorax is not associated with an open sucking chest wound. Therefore, an
        occlusive dressing is not indicated.

Content Category: Respiratory

References: Kidd et al., 2000; pp. 668–669; ENA, Core Curriculum, 2000; pp. 8–11, 385.

23.   A patient is evaluated after receiving severe chest injuries in a motor vehicle crash (MVC) and pre-
    sents with severe dyspnea, increasing subcutaneous emphysema of the neck, and decreased breath
    sounds on auscultation. What nursing diagnosis is a priority for this patient?
    A. Fluid volume deficit
    B. Impaired gas exchange
    C. INEFFECTIVE AIRWAY CLEARANCE
    D. Body image disturbance

Rationale:

    C. You suspect a tracheobronchial injury, which is a tear in a large airway structure; therefore, air-
        way obstruction can occur. Airway is the first priority in caring for this patient.
    A. There is no evidence of severe bleeding or a fluid volume deficit.
    B. Gas exchange may be a potential threat, but a patent airway is the priority.
    D. There is a potential for a body image disturbance. This problem can be addressed after airway,
        breathing, and circulation have been assessed and maintained.

Content Category: Respiratory

References: ENA, Trauma Manual, 2000; p. 122; Newberry, 1998; pp. 297–298; Blansfield et al., 1999;
            pp. 265–266; Tintinalli, 2000; p. 1685.

24.   You are caring for a patient who has been diagnosed with hyperventilation. What is another com-
    mon symptom related to this condition?
    A. Seizures
    B. Chest pain
    C. CARPOPEDAL SPASMS
    D. Fever

Rationale:

C. Carpopedal spasms occur as a result of a decrease in carbon dioxide due to hyperventilation, which causes tetanylike activity in the muscles of the hands and feet. These symptoms will resolve as the patient's carbon dioxide level returns to normal.

A. Seizures or involuntary movements relating to abnormal electrical brain activity are not associated with hyperventilation.

B. Chest pain associated with respiratory symptoms usually represents a different medical problem, such as angina or myocardial infarct, and is very rarely associated with hyperventilation.

D. Fever can be associated with some type of infectious process, but not with hyperventilation.

Content Category: Respiratory

References: ENA, Core Curriculum, 2000; pp. 569–570; Newberry, 1998; pp. 475–476.

25. Patient teaching for a patient with emphysema should include:
   A. the importance of being vaccinated each year against pneumococcal disease.
   B. the need for prophylactic antibiotic therapy when a family member becomes ill.
   C. THE NEED FOR ADEQUATE HYDRATION TO REDUCE MUCUS TENACITY.
   D. the importance of smoking cessation to reverse structural changes caused by the disease.

Rationale:

C. Adequate hydration contributes to good bronchial hygiene.

A. Pneumococcal vaccination should be obtained, but is not needed every year.

B. Prophylactic antibiotic therapy has led to bacterial resistance. Its use is controversial.

D. Smoking cessation will not reverse alveolar structural changes caused by emphysema, although it will help decrease inflammatory processes.

Content Category: Respiratory

References: Newberry, 1998; pp. 431–451; Kitt et al., 1995; pp. 188–200; ENA, Core Curriculum, 2000; pp. 559–566.

26. A patient with chronic obstructive pulmonary disease is treated with a sustained-release oral theophylline preparation. Which of the following conditions would predispose the patient most to theophylline toxicity?
   A. Diabetes mellitus
   B. CONGESTIVE HEART FAILURE
   C. Asthma
   D. Renal disease

Rationale:

B. Congestive heart failure slows the metabolism of drugs such as theophylline that are predominantly cleared by the liver and can lead to early development of toxicity.

A. Diabetes does not affect the absorption or distribution of theophylline preparation and therefore will not predispose the patient to toxicity levels.

C. While theophylline use in asthma is less common than it once was, no sequelae of the disease contribute to the development of toxic levels if the drug is used.

D. Renal disease does not affect the development of theophylline toxicity to any extent and is not a contraindication for its use.

Content Category: Respiratory

References: Newberry, 1998; pp. 431–451; Kitt et al., 1995; pp.188–200, 508; ENA, Core Curriculum, 2000; pp. 559–566.

27.   A 40-year-old male involved in a house fire presents, conscious, to the ED with dyspnea, sooty sputum, and a brassy cough. He is receiving 100% oxygen via nonrebreather reservoir mask. The ED nurse should FIRST:
A. check for burn percentage.
B. prepare for intubation.
C. ASSESS AIRWAY AND BREATHING.
D. start fluid resuscitation.

Rationale:

C. Assessing airway and breathing is the priority. Dyspnea, sooty sputum, and brassy cough are signs of an inhalation injury. The patient with an inhalation injury is at risk for edema and obstruction of the airway.
A. Checking for burn percentage is important, especially for calculating fluid resuscitation formula, but the highest priorities are airway patency and ventilatory status.
B. Intubation equipment should be readily available, but assessing airway and breathing is always the initial response.
D. Fluid resuscitation may be an important part of the patient's management, but the first response is always to assess airway and breathing.

Content Category: Respiratory

Reference: Rosen et al., 1998; p. 947.

28.   Which of these children is at highest risk for foreign body aspiration?
A. A 7-year-old with gastroenteritis
B. A 4-year-old with rhinitis
C. A 2-year-old with a history of chickenpox (varicella) exposure
D. A 6-YEAR-OLD WITH A HISTORY OF CEREBRAL PALSY

Rationale:

D. A 6-year-old with cerebral palsy is at greater than normal risk for aspiration because the medical condition causes a decrease in or loss of protective reflexes.
A. A 7-year-old male with a history of gastroenteritis is older than the age group in which aspiration of a foreign body is common.
B. Rhinitis is an inflammation of the nasal mucosa. It does not involve potential loss of protective reflexes and is not associated with foreign body aspiration.
C. Exposure to chickenpox, which causes a rash that ends with lesions that are crusted over, would cause no potential loss of protective reflexes or association with a foreign body aspiration.

Content Category: Respiratory

Reference: ENA, Core Curriculum, 2000; pp. 139, 157, 259.

29.   An obese 36-year-old female presents to your ED with sudden onset of left-sided chest pain and shortness of breath. She is diaphoretic, pale, and in acute respiratory distress. She denies any trauma, fever, nausea, or vomiting. Past medical history is unremarkable except that she was placed on birth control pills 6 months ago. Initial vital signs are BP 100/60 mmHg, pulse 118/min, and respirations 36/min. The priority nursing diagnosis for this patient is:
A. fluid volume deficit.
B. anxiety.
C. pain, alteration in comfort.
D. IMPAIRED GAS EXCHANGE.

Rationale:

D. Impaired gas exchange occurs in pulmonary embolus because ventilation exceeds perfusion. The occluded vessel is unable to provide blood flow to the pulmonary capillaries past the blockage. The patient should be closely monitored for hypoxia.

A. There is a high risk for fluid volume deficit if there is a major obstruction to the pulmonary circulation, causing hypotension. In that case, fluid resuscitation would be necessary. Impaired gas exchange would remain the priority.

B. Anxiety is a consideration because of the patient's unstable condition, questionable outcome and SOB. While it is important to provide reassurance and support, impaired gas exchange must be the first priority.

C. Pain related to a pulmonary embolus, causing an alteration in the patient's comfort, should definitely be addressed; however, impaired gas exchange remains the priority.

Content Category: Respiratory

Reference: Newberry, 1998; pp. 202–204.

30. What diagnostic test or tests does a patient with noncardiogenic pulmonary edema require?
    A. Ventilation/perfusion scan
    B. Fiberoptic endoscopy and pulse oximetry
    C. ECG and chest radiograph
    D. CHEST RADIOGRAPH AND ABG

Rationale:

D. Chest radiographic and arterial blood gas measurements should be done. The chest radiograph will identify pulmonary infiltrates and the amount of edema present. The ABG will reveal the patient's acid-base condition and oxygenation status and aid in treatment, especially in determining baseline status and being able to trend therapeutic interventions.

A. A ventilation/perfusion (V/Q) scan is used in diagnosing pulmonary embolus.

B. Fiberoptic endoscopy may be done to visualize the area directly if airway edema is suspected. Pulse oximetry is done on all patients with respiratory compromise. A chest radiograph and arterial blood gases will provide the information of highest priority.

C. An ECG should be done to make sure there are no abnormalities after the ABG has been drawn because this patient is presenting with a pulmonary problem.

Content Category: Respiratory

Reference: Rosen et al., 1998; p.1446.

31. The triad involved with heroin-induced pulmonary edema is hypoxia, stupor, and:
    A. hypertension.
    B. mydriasis.
    C. MIOSIS.
    D. arrhythmias.

Rationale:

C. Miosis, contraction of the pupil, occurs in 90% of patients presenting with acute opiate overdose, as occurs with heroin. Miosis completes the triad in heroin-induced pulmonary edema.

A. Hypotension, not hypertension, usually occurs.

B. Mydriasis (dilation of the pupil) is not seen in heroin overdose. It would be more likely to be seen in a patient with an overdose of tricyclic antidepressants.

D. Arrhythmias can occur in heroin overdose, but it is usually secondary to hypoxia.

Content Category: Respiratory

References: Rosen et al., 1998; p.1385; Sondhi et al., 2001; pp. 30–32.

32.   Which of the following patients is at high risk for possible aspiration?
A. A 25-year-old male with mycoplasma pneumonia
B. A 42-year-old female with gastroesophageal reflux disease
C. A 16-year-old male with alcohol intoxication
D. AN 84-YEAR-OLD FEMALE WITH DECREASED MENTAL STATUS

Rationale:

D. An elderly patient with decreased mental status is more likely to present with problems of maintaining an open airway. Patients are less likely to position themselves to prevent the tongue from falling back over the airway or the tongue may fall back secondary to loss of muscle control.
A. Mycoplasma pneumonia in a young person can frequently be treated with antibiotics on an outpatient basis. Aspiration would not occur in this patient.
B. Gastroesophageal reflux disease is associated with heartburn and chest discomfort rather than actual vomiting. Therefore, the airway is not placed at risk.
C. A young male with alcohol intoxication but without actual poisoning will most likely be able to maintain an airway.

Content Category: Respiratory

Reference: ENA, Core Curriculum, 2000; p. 139.

33.   Pleural effusion would most likely present in which of the following patients?
A. A 19-year-old thin male with sudden onset of sharp chest pain and reporting shortness of breath that began today
B. A 26-year-old male with a stab wound to the chest and a chest tube in place
C. A 6-year-old female with fever and cough
D. A 62-YEAR-OLD FEMALE 7 DAYS AFTER UNDERGOING CORONARY BYPASS SURGERY

Rationale:

D. A 62-year-old female 7 days after undergoing coronary bypass surgery is at risk for pneumonia, a common cause of pleural effusion.
A. A 19-year-old male with sudden onset of sharp chest pain accompanied by shortness of breath may have a pulmonary embolism or spontaneous pneumothorax. Although pulmonary embolism is associated with pleural effusion, it is too early for it to develop.
B. A 26-year-old with a stab wound and a chest tube should not have an effusion. The chest tube would prevent an effusion from developing.
C. A 6-year-old with fever and cough could have pneumonia, but that is not the most likely choice among those presented. Many children with fever and cough have viral upper respiratory infections.

Content Category: Respiratory

Reference: ENA, Core Curriculum, 2000; p 570.

34.   The ED nurse should expect a child with bronchiolitis to be admitted when the patient has:
A. AN OXYGEN SATURATION OF 90, RESPIRATORY RATE OF 70, RETRACTIONS, AND FATIGUE.
B. an oxygen saturation of 95, mild wheezing, and patchy infiltrate on x-ray and is drinking well.

C. an oxygen saturation of 96, respiratory rate of 34, mild wheezing, and a positive nasal aspirate for respiratory syncytial virus.

D. an oxygen saturation of 92, respiratory rate of 36, mild retractions, and mild wheezing.

Rationale:

A. The patient with an oxygen saturation rate of 90, respiratory rate of 70, retractions, and fatigue is exhibiting signs of continued respiratory distress and requires admission for continued monitoring and treatment.

B. The patient with an oxygen saturation of 92, mild retractions and wheezing, and a respiratory rate of 36, may benefit from continued treatment in the ED to improve saturations. This patient would most likely be discharged after stabilization.

C. The patient with an oxygen saturation of 96, respiratory rate of 36, and mild wheezing does not have respiratory compromise, which requires admission even though the RSV is positive.

D. The patient who has an oxygen saturation of 95 and mild wheezing and who is drinking well is not in great respiratory distress, even though the chest x-ray is abnormal.

Content Category: Respiratory

References: ENA, Core Curriculum, 2000; p. 563; Newberry, 1998; pp. 725–730.

35. A 12-year-old presents with fever, ear pain, and diarrhea. The child is diagnosed with otitis media. Which of the following is an ominous complication of acute otitis media?
    A. Intracranial complications
    B. LATERAL SINUS THROMBOSIS
    C. Cholesteatoma
    D. Perforated tympanic membrane

Rationale:

B. Lateral sinus thrombosis is an ominous complication of otitis media. It is caused by spread of the infection in the mastoid and lateral sinus. Clinical findings are similar to those of otitis media and mastoiditis.

A. Intracranial complications are more likely in chronic otitis media than in the disease's acute form.

C. Cholesteatoma is a serious complication associated with chronic otitis media.

D. Although perforation is a potential complication, it is not so ominous as lateral sinus thrombosis.

Content Category: Maxillofacial/Ocular

Reference: Urdaneta & Lucchesi, 2000; pp.1518–1526.

36. Which of the following statements about Bell's palsy is true?
    A. It is caused by paralysis of the tenth cranial nerve.
    B. IT IS IDIOPATHIC UNILATERAL FACIAL PARALYSIS.
    C. It is progressive in nature and eventually affects the entire body.
    D. Onset is usually seen in the second decade of life.

Rationale:

B. Bell's palsy is an idiopathic (cause unknown) unilateral facial nerve paralysis of cranial nerve VII. Symptoms include rapid onset with occasional ear and facial pain.

A. Bell's palsy is caused by paralysis of cranial nerve VII.

C. Bell's palsy affects only the facial area.

D. Bell's palsy is most common in patients over age 40.

Content Category: Maxillofacial/Ocular

References: Olson, 2000; pp. 673–688; Peacock, 2000; pp.1526–1532.

37. A patient presents with decreased vision in the left eye that began with flashes of light. The patient describes the process of vision loss as "a curtain lowering over the eye." There is no evidence of trauma to the eye and the patient denies any pain. The patient's signs and symptoms suggest:
    A. Corneal abrasion
    B. Acute angle-closure glaucoma
    C. RETINAL DETACHMENT
    D. Central retinal artery occlusion

Rationale:

    C. Retinal detachment is a painless condition in which the patient characteristically sees flashes of light followed by a curtainlike decease in vision. Often, patients complain of dark spots or floaters.
    A. Corneal abrasion is associated with a significant amount of pain. The patient has denied having pain.
    B. Patients with acute angle-closure glaucoma complain of headaches, nausea, vomiting, and halos around light.
    D. Central retinal artery occlusion produces a sudden loss of vision. Retinal detachment causes progressive vision loss.

Content Category: Maxillofacial/Ocular

References: Egging, 2000; pp. 689–706; Rhee & Pyfer, 1999; pp. 366–369.

38. A tripod fracture is another name for what type of fracture?
    A. Le Fort I fracture
    B. Le Fort II fracture
    C. Orbit fracture
    D. ZYGOMATIC FRACTURE

Rationale:

    D. A tripod fracture is an extensive fracture of the zygomatic process. It consists of a fracture through the frontozygomatic suture and the maxillary process of the zygoma. Fracture lines pass through the inferior orbital floor, the inferior orbital rim, the lateral wall of the maxillary sinus, and the zygomatic arch.
    A. Le Fort I is a horizontal fracture in the body of the maxilla.
    B. Le Fort II is called a pyramidal fracture because it incorporates the central maxilla, nasal area, and ethmoid bones.
    C. Orbit fracture is a fracture of the orbit of the eye

Content Category: Maxillofacial/Ocular

References: Gisness, 1998; pp. 373–387; Munter & McGuirk, 1997; pp. 4–23.

39. Discharge instructions for the parent of a child with conjunctivitis should emphasize:
    A. how to apply an eye patch properly.
    B. possible side effects of steroid drops.
    C. exercises to strengthen the extraocular muscles.
    D. WAYS TO PREVENT THE SPREAD OF DISEASE.

Rationale:

    D. Conjunctivitis is a highly contagious infection. Family members should be instructed in strategies to prevent the spread of infection.
    A. Eye patching is not indicated for conjunctivitis.
    B. Antibiotic drops, not steroids, are prescribed for conjunctivitis.
    C. Conjunctivitis is an infection of the conjunctiva. There is no involvement of the muscles; therefore, exercises are of no use in this patient.

Content Category: Maxillofacial/Ocular

Reference: Egging, 1998; pp. 689–706.

40. Before performing ear irrigation, the nurse must:
    A. evaluate the patient's hearing.
    B. VISUALIZE THE INTEGRITY OF THE TYMPANIC MEMBRANE.
    C. instill anesthetic otic drops.
    D. administer medication to prevent vertigo.

Rationale:

B. Before the ear is irrigated, the tympanic membrane must be ascertained to be intact.
A. Hearing assessment is best performed under optimal conditions. The need to remove a potential obstruction would present conditions that were less than optimal.
C. Instilling an anesthetic solution may be necessary for some patients, but is not mandatory.
D. Medications to prevent vertigo are not usually required for ear irrigation.

Content Category: Maxillofacial/Ocular

Reference: Olson, 1998; pp. 673–688.

41. If a cerebral spinal fluid leak is suspected, the nurse should test nasal drainage for the presence of:
    A. nitrites.
    B. GLUCOSE.
    C. ketones.
    D. potassium.

Rationale:

B. Glucose is a normal finding in cerebral spinal fluid. Cerebral spinal fluid should not be draining from any orifice.
A. Nitrites are not found in cerebral spinal fluid.
C. Ketones are not found in cerebral spinal fluid.
D. Potassium is not found in cerebral spinal fluid.

Content Category: Maxillofacial/Ocular

Reference: Begley & Newberry, 1998; pp. 525–535.

42. Treatment of a patient with a corneal abrasion includes antibiotic drops *and*:
    A. narcotic analgesia and soft contact lenses.
    B. CYCLOPLEGIC DROPS AND NONSTEROIDAL ANTI-INFLAMMATORY EYE DROPS.
    C. repeated application of topical anesthesia with narcotic analgesia.
    D. soft contact lenses with eye patch.

Rationale:

B. Cycloplegic drops may be indicated to help relieve the pain from ciliary spasm. Nonsteroidal anti-inflammatory eye drops assist with pain relief.
A. Nonnarcotic analgesia can be sufficient to control pain. Soft contact lenses are contraindicated.
C. Continuous topical anesthesia impairs healing and is contraindicated in corneal abrasions; non-narcotic analgesia is appropriate for the severity of the pain.
D. Soft contact lenses are contraindicated. Eye patches have been shown to impair healing because they decrease oxygen tension to the cornea and can increase eye pain.

Content Category: Maxillofacial/Ocular

References: Buttaravoli & Stair, 2000; Cohen et al., 1999; pp. 19–52.

43.   Treatment of a child with croup should include:
   A. humidified oxygen, antipyretics, and antibiotics.
   B. humidified oxygen, antibiotics, and epinephrine.
   C. HYDRATION, STEROIDS, AND RACEMIC EPINEPHRINE.
   D. hydration, epinephrine, and sedation.

Rationale:

   C. Hydration should be provided by the least invasive route possible to replace insensible water losses from respiratory distress and fever. The literature clearly demonstrates the clinical benefits of steroid use in moderate to severe croup. Steroids should be given within 1 hour of presentation to induce vasoconstriction of the edematous mucosa. All children who receive racemic epinephrine should also receive steroids. Racemic epinephrine is the mainstay of treatment for moderate to severe croup because it decreases airway edema, most likely by vasoconstriction of the boggy mucosal vessels.
   A. Supplemental humidified oxygen should be given to children with croup. Antipyretics should be given for fever to decrease the required minute ventilation and work of breathing. Antibiotics are NOT indicated for patients with a diagnosis of croup because almost all cases are viral.
   B. Supplemental humidified oxygen should be given to children with croup. Antibiotics are NOT indicated for patients with a diagnosis of croup because almost all cases are viral. Racemic epinephrine is the mainstay of moderate to severe croup treatment.
   D. Hydration should be provided by the least invasive route to replace insensible water losses from respiratory distress and fever. Racemic epinephrine is the mainstay of moderate to severe croup treatment. Children with croup should NOT be sedated except in the course of rapid-sequence intubation.

Content Category: Maxillofacial/Ocular

Reference: Cordle & Relich, 2000; pp. 879–890.

44.   A 71-year-old man is brought to the ED by his family. Family members state that he must have had a stroke because he woke up this morning paralyzed on the left side and unable to speak clearly. The emergency physician will not be able to see this patient for 10 minutes. Initial nursing intervention should include which of the following actions?
   A. Arterial blood gases
   B. BEDSIDE BLOOD GLUCOSE TEST
   C. Physical exam for signs of abuse
   D. Preparation for thrombolytics

Rationale:

   B. Signs and symptoms of stroke are sometimes caused by hypoglycemia. A bedside blood glucose test can rapidly determine whether low blood sugar is the problem.
   A. Blood gas analysis is usually reserved for situations in which respiratory failure or metabolic abnormality is suspected.
   C. While a physical examination might be useful if one suspected head injury caused by abuse, it is not part of the initial intervention.
   D. Thrombolytic therapy for acute stroke must be started within 3 hours of onset of symptoms. Since the patient awoke with symptoms, it is impossible to determine when those symptoms began; therefore, he is not a candidate for thrombolytic therapy.

Content Category: General Medical

References: Peabody, 2000; pp. 227–274; Ragland, 1996; pp. 939–972; Wood, 1998; pp. 593–610.

45. Intravenous propranolol (Inderal) has been ordered for your patient with thyroid storm. This drug is used to:
    A. KEEP THE HEART RATE UNDER 100.
    B. control hypertension.
    C. decrease tremulousness.
    D. stimulate thyroxine production.

Rationale:

A. Tachycardia is a major problem in thyroid storm. Propranolol is used to keep the heart rate under 100, in order to maintain cardiac output.
B. Hypertension is rarely significant; more often the patient with thyroid storm is hypotensive. Propranolol would not be the first drug of choice to control hypertension.
C. Tremulousness does not need drug treatment.
D. Too much thyroxine is the problem in thyroid storm. Propylthiouracil is the medication used to block synthesis of thyroxine and tri-iodothyronine. Propranolol may slow the conversion of T-4 to T-3, but this is not its primary use.

Content Category: General Medical

References: Peabody, 2000; pp. 227–274; Ragland, 1996; pp. 939–972; Wood, 1998; pp. 593–610.

46. The patient with thyroid storm is at increased risk of death from:
    A. hyperthermia.
    B. hypotension.
    C. infection.
    D. HEART FAILURE.

Rationale:

D. Heart failure is a common cause of death in thyroid storm. Increased amounts of thyroid hormones cause increased heart rate and blood pressure, which in turn may lead to cardiac decompensation and heart failure.
A. Hyperthermia is a problem in thyroid storm, but it can usually be controlled with acetaminophen (Tylenol) and other cooling measures.
B. Hypotension can also be controlled with fluids and medications.
C. While infection may be a precipitating cause of thyroid storm, patients with infections are not at risk for developing infection as a result of thyroid storm.

Content Category: General Medical

References: Peabody, 2000; pp. 227–274; Ragland, 1996; pp. 939–972; Wood, 1998; pp. 593–610.

47. Patients with myxedema coma need to be monitored carefully for:
    A. hypertension.
    B. supraventricular tachycardia.
    C. hyperventilation.
    D. HYPOTHERMIA.

Rationale:

D. Hypothermia is a common problem due to slowed metabolism from hypothyroidism. Temperature is usually above 95° F (35° C).
A. In myxedema coma, hypotension is common. Hypertension would be seen only in the presence of a concurrent problem.

B. Bradycardia, not tachycardia, occurs with severe hypothyroidism.

C. Patients with myxedema coma may have tongue swelling (macroglossia), which interferes with ventilation. This in addition to depressed metabolism causes hypoventilation rather than hyperventilation.

Content Category: General Medical

References: Peabody, 2000; pp. 227–274; Ragland, 1996; pp. 939–972; Wood, 1998; pp. 593–610.

48.   A 6-year-old boy is brought to the triage desk by his aunt. He has had fever and cough for 3 days and now has a red rash. The aunt does not know other details of the child's health history. Your first action as triage nurse should be to:

A. contact the child's parents for permission to treat.

B. INSTITUTE ISOLATION PRECAUTIONS WITH THE CHILD IMMEDIATELY.

C. obtain vital signs and examine the rash.

D. ask the aunt to wait her turn, since several other patients are waiting.

Rationale:

B. Measles (rubeola) must be considered when there is a history of fever and cough followed by the appearance of a red rash. There are many causes of fever and rash in children; however, given the lack of immunization history and the extremely contagious nature of rubeola, safe practice necessitates immediate isolation precautions to prevent potential spread of the disease to other patients and staff.

A. Unless the aunt is legal guardian, the parents should be contacted. However, that can wait until after the child has been isolated.

C. Vital signs and examination of the rash should be done once the child is in a room away from other people.

D. This child has a potentially contagious illness and should not wait in an area where he might infect others. If he does not appear very ill, he can probably safely await treatment in an isolated area.

Content Category: General Medical

References: Cosby, 1998; pp. 721–741; Peabody, 2000; pp. 227–274; Weinstock & Catapano, 1996; pp. 668–673.

49.   The incubation period for chickenpox is:

A. 1 to 3 days.

B. 2 to 4 days.

C. 7 to 10 days.

D. 10 TO 20 DAYS.

Rationale:

D. The incubation period is 10 to 20 days. Until the varicella vaccine is more widely administered, emergency nurses will continue to be asked about chickenpox.

A. The contagious period starts 1 to 3 days before the rash appears.

B. Two to 4 days is the incubation period for scarlet fever.

C. The shortest incubation time is 10 days.

Content Category: General Medical

References: Cosby, 1998; pp. 721–741; Peabody, 2000; pp. 227–274; Weinstock & Catapano, 1996; pp. 668–673.

50.   While working a shift in the ED, a nurse receives a call from the mother of a pediatric patient seen 4 days ago for scabies. The mother states that she used the medication as prescribed and washed all clothing and bedding in hot water. The child is still complaining of itching and is scratching himself during the night, but the rash seems to be gone. The nurse should advise the mother to:
A. bring the child back to the ED for a checkup.
B. pick up a refill of the medication and treat the child again.
C. relaunder clothes and bedding, using very hot water and a hot dryer.
D. BE AWARE THAT ITCHING IS COMMON FOR ABOUT 7 DAYS EVEN IF THE INFECTION HAS BEEN CURED.

Rationale:

D. Itching often continues for up to 7 days. Patients should not be retreated without a physician's order.
A. At this time there is no reason to bring the child back to the ED as long as the nurse believes that the mother followed instructions. The fact that the rash seems to be gone is a good indication that treatment was appropriate.
B. Retreatment is probably not necessary and should be done only on a physician's order.
C. One laundering is sufficient. If the child requires retreatment, laundry must be redone at that time.

Content Category: General Medical

References: Cosby, 1998; pp. 721–741; Peabody, 2000; pp. 227–274. Salluzzo, 1996; pp. 856–867.

51.   During treatment of diabetic ketoacidosis, including fluid replacement and insulin, the patient must be closely monitored for:
A. HYPOKALEMIA.
B. hyperphosphatemia.
C. hypernatremia.
D. hyperkalemia.

Rationale:

A. Hypokalemia develops rapidly during treatment with insulin. As glucose enters the cells in the presence of insulin, free fatty acid release and gluconeogenesis decrease. Hydrogen ions are returned to the extracellular environment in exchange for potassium, significantly depleting extracellular potassium levels. Hypokalemia may result in life-threatening dysrhythmias.
B. Phosphate levels may appear elevated at the onset of treatment because of prerenal azotemia and insulin deficiency. In reality, osmotic diuresis leads to a total body depletion. Several hours into treatment, the patient may develop hypophosphatemia.
C. The patient often has hyponatremia from fluid loss at the start of treatment. Replacement of fluids with normal saline returns sodium levels to normal but does not induce hypernatremia.
D. At the onset of treatment, most patients have relative extracellular hyperkalemia because of the buffer mechanism by which hydrogen ions are transferred into the cell in exchange for potassium. As the pH rises during treatment, potassium moves back into the cell, resulting in hypokalemia.

Content Category: General Medical

References: Peabody, 2000; pp. 227–274; Ragland, 1996; pp. 939–972; Wood, 1998; pp. 593–610.

52.   A male patient is brought to the ED by ambulance from a homeless shelter, where staff had been unable to awaken him. He is lying supine on the stretcher, receiving high-flow oxygen by nonrebreather mask. He is unresponsive to pain, with a regular respiratory rate of 18 and warm, dry, pale skin. His radial pulse is 90 and full. No other history is available. The priority nursing diagnosis for this patient is:

A. INEFFECTIVE AIRWAY CLEARANCE.
B. impaired gas exchange.
C. fluid volume deficit.
D. impaired tissue perfusion.

Rationale:

A. Regardless of the cause of this man's coma, he is at grave risk for airway obstruction and aspiration because he is positioned on his back. Comatose patients lack the ability to control tongue and jaw muscles and have ineffective swallowing. Ineffective airway clearance is the highest priority.

B. Comatose patients may have impaired gas exchange; however, this patient has normal respirations and is receiving high-flow oxygen.

C. Fluid volume deficit may be a problem, but the patient's skin is warm and dry and he has adequate peripheral circulation as evidenced by a full radial pulse.

D. The presence of a full radial pulse indicates that the patient's blood pressure is at least 80mm systolic, a level that provides minimal adequate tissue perfusion. His pulse, respiratory rate, and skin condition also support the likelihood of acceptable tissue perfusion.

Content Category: General Medical

References: Henry, 1996; pp. 225–233; Wood, 1998; pp. 593–610.

53.   A 65-year-old man is brought to the ED by his friends, who say that he has had vomiting and diarrhea for 2 days and is now unable to walk. The only other history they know is that he "gives himself a shot every morning." The patient looks ill, with flushed face and rapid, deep respirations. He moans and moves when touched, but is unable to answer any questions. Initial vital signs are BP 98/70 mmHg, pulse 100/min, and respirations 28/min. Skin is cool and dry. The pulse oximeter does not register. While troubleshooting, you note that the patient's hands are very cold. What is your priority for this patient?

A. Obtain orthostatic (postural) vital signs.
B. TAKE A RECTAL TEMPERATURE.
C. Attach the pulse oximeter to his toe.
D. Cover his hands with warm packs.

Rationale:

B. Every patient should have a temperature taken in the ED. That is especially true in this case because of the severity of the man's condition. Older people are particularly susceptible to concomitant problems; his skin is not warm, even though his face is flushed; and the pulse oximeter won't register, probably because of cold hands. He had a rectal temperature of 92° F (33° C) in addition to the primary diagnosis of diabetic ketoacidosis.

A. While obtaining orthostatic vital signs is often very useful, doing so requires the patient's cooperation. His vital signs already indicate a potentially serious problem.

C. The patient has marginal vital signs. Since circulation to the legs and feet is sacrificed early during cardiovascular compromise, it is unlikely that the toe will have adequate blood flow to register on the probe. The earlobe is perhaps the second choice until the hands are warm.

D. Warm packs are a nice idea, but this patient is seriously ill. The reason for his cold hands needs to be investigated before treatment is begun for that problem.

Content Category: General Medical

Reference: Sedlak, 1998; pp. 113–127.

54. Which nursing diagnosis best describes the most immediate life-threatening problem for a patient with hyperglycemic, hyperosmolar, nonketotic coma (HHNC)?
    A. FLUID VOLUME DEFICIT
    B. Fluid volume excess
    C. Impaired gas exchange
    D. Altered cerebral tissue perfusion

Rationale:

A. Patients with HHNC have blood glucose levels greater than 800mg/dl, causing osmotic diuresis and profound dehydration. Patients with this illness are often elderly and already have decreased cardiac and renal function. Severe dehydration further impairs those functions.

B. HHNC patients are volume depleted, not overloaded. However, they need to be closely monitored for fluid volume excess during treatment.

C. This illness is primarily a vascular volume problem. Unless the patient has underlying pulmonary disease or anemia, gas exchange will probably be adequate. Patients are at risk, however, for ineffective airway clearance.

D. Altered cerebral tissue perfusion is a problem, but not immediately life threatening unless the airway is obstructed. Once volume replacement has occurred, the patient's level of consciousness should normalize. During treatment, patients may develop cerebral edema because the blood-brain barrier does not allow rapid exchange of fluids, solutes, and medications.

Content Category: General Medical

References: Peabody, 2000; pp. 227–274; Ragland, 1996; pp. 939–972; Wood, 1998; pp. 593–610.

55. The ED nurse has verbal orders to give ceftriaxone (Rocephin) 250 mg IM to a young man with gonorrhea. He has no allergies. His only significant medical history is hemophilia. The nurse should:
    A. give the medicine as ordered, using lidocaine to mix the powder.
    B. give the medicine as ordered and have the patient wait 1 hour so that he can be monitored for bleeding.
    C. ask the physician to write the order on the chart, to avoid a medication error.
    D. QUESTION THE DRUG ROUTE, REMINDING THE PHYSICIAN THAT THE PATIENT HAS HEMOPHILIA.

Rationale:

D. A patient with hemophilia should never be given an IM injection unless factor replacement is given for several days. Many oral medications are effective in treating gonorrhea. A busy ED physician might easily forget that the patient has an underlying problem. This situation parallels one in which the physician inadvertently orders a medication to which the patient is allergic.

A. The drug, dose, route, and use of lidocaine are appropriate, but not in a patient with hemophilia.

B. If a patient with hemophilia is given an IM injection, s/he must receive factor replacement immediately and for several days thereafter.

C. It is always a good idea to have a written order for medications, but in this case the medication error would still exist.

Content Category: General Medical

References: Eberst, 1996; pp. 983–986; Newberry, 2000; pp. 275–317.

56. Upper motor neuron disease can be detected by:
     A. dilated pupils.
     B. a brisk patellar reflex.
     C. A POSITIVE BABINSKI (PLANTAR) REFLEX.
     D. slow, irregular breathing.

Rationale:

     C. A positive Babinski, also known as a plantar reflex, exhibited by dorsiflexion of the great toe and fanning of the other toes, may indicate upper motor neuron disease. It may also be elicited when a person is unconscious after a drug overdose, alcohol intoxication, or seizure.
     A. Dilated pupils are not indicative of upper motor neuron disease.
     B. A brisk patellar reflex is not indicative of upper motor neuron disease.
     D. A slow, irregular breathing pattern is not indicative of upper motor neuron disease.

Content Category: Neurology

Reference: Snyder, 2000; pp. 275–317.

57. Kernig's sign is:
     A. LOW BACK OR POSTERIOR THIGH PAIN ON HIP FLEXION WITH GRADUAL KNEE EXTENSION.
     B. neck flexion that results in hip and knee flexion.
     C. dilated pupils and rapid, shallow respirations.
     D. brisk reflexes followed by decerebrate posturing.

Rationale:

     A. Kernig's sign is a meningeal sign that may be indicative of meningitis. The cause is a stretch of the meninges as demonstrated by low back pain or posterior thigh pain on hip flexion with gradual knee extension.
     B. Neck flexion that results in hip and knee flexion is not a sign of meningitis.
     C. Dilated pupils and rapid, shallow respirations are not indicative of meningeal irritation.
     D. Brisk reflexes with posturing are also not present with meningeal irritation.

Content Category: Neurology

Reference: Sheehy & Lenehan, 1999.

58. A 36-year-old male patient presents to the ED with complaints of severe headache and blurred vision. On physical examination, his head and upper chest are flushed and diaphoretic. His lower extremities are pale and cool to the touch. Initial vital signs are BP 190/110 mmHg, pulse 40/min, and respirations 24/min. He had a spinal cord injury 2 years ago and is paralyzed below the nipple line. Your priority intervention would be to:
     A. initiate IV access and provide pain relief as ordered.
     B. administer antihypertensive medications as ordered.
     C. place the patient in a darkened, quiet room.
     D. INSERT A URINARY CATHETER.

Rationale:

     D. Autonomic dysreflexia may occur in spinal cord–injured patients with injury above the T6 level. Noxious stimuli cause massive reflex stimulation of the sympathetic nerves below the level of injury, resulting in vasoconstriction; cool, pale skin; and a rise in blood pressure. A reflex slowing of the heart and vasodilation above the level of injury occur. The most common noxious stimuli are a distended bladder and fecal impaction.

A. Relieving the noxious stimuli will reduce blood pressure and vasodilation, causing the headache to resolve.

B. Hypertension will resolve once the inciting stimuli have been relieved.

C. The noxious stimuli must be identified and corrected quickly to relieve the sympathetic discharge.

Content Category: Neurology

References: Snyder, 2000; pp. 275–317; Hickey, 1997; pp. 419–465.

59. A young teenager is seen in the ED after being involved in a bicycle crash. He is unresponsive and has severe facial lacerations with moderate edema. He is found to have a subdural hematoma. Before intubation, lidocaine (Xylocaine) 25 mg is administered. The ED nurse should evaluate the effect of this medication by:

A. NOTING A TRANSIENT DECREASE IN INTRACRANIAL PRESSURE.

B. observing for decreased ventricular ectopy.

C. monitoring for pupil changes.

D. noting an increase in heart rate.

Rationale:

A. Administration of lidocaine (Xylocaine) 25 mg before intubation of the head-injured patient causes a very transient (2–3 min.) decrease in intracranial pressure (ICP). Intubation may cause an increase in ICP, which may be prevented with the administration of lidocaine.

B. Lidocaine may be used to decrease ventricular ectopy, but at a higher dose than 25 mg for a teenager.

C. Lidocaine does not cause pupil changes.

D. Lidocaine does not cause increased heart rate.

Content Category: Neurology

Reference: Sheehy & Lenehan, 1999.

60. A patient with a closed head injury is given 100 g of mannitol (Osmitrol). The expected outcome from this infusion is:

A. increased sensitivity of the cranial nerves.

B. increased urinary output.

C. decreased gastric motility.

D. DECREASED OSMOLARITY OF GLOMERULAR FILTRATE.

Rationale:

D. Mannitol (Osmitrol) serves as a osmotic diuretic and acts by increasing osmolarity of glomerular filtrates, which raise the osmotic pressure of fluid in the renal tubules. This action increases urinary output, assisting with decreasing intracranial pressure.

A. Although mannitol does assist with the decrease in intracranial pressure, it does not have an effect on the sensitivity of the cranial nerves. Improvement may be noted in cranial nerve function as elevated intracranial pressure is decreased.

B. Mannitol increases the osmolarity of glomerular filtrate, thus increasing urinary output by decreasing the absorption of water and electrolytes.

C. Mannitol does not have a direct effect on decreasing gastric motility. Side effects of nausea, vomiting, and diarrhea have been described.

Content Category: Neurology

Reference: Skidmore-Roth, 2001; pp. 586–587.

61.   A basilar artery migraine headache is manifested by:
A.   nausea and vomiting, auditory issues, and frontal pain.
B.   ataxia, confusion, and slurred speech.
C.   seizure activity, hypertension, and tachycardia.
D.   BILATERAL VISUAL DISTURBANCES, PARESTHESIAS, AND CONFUSION.

Rationale:

D.   Migraine headaches are often thought to be caused by arterial spasms. Basilar artery migraines are located near the occipital region of the brain, affecting vision, sensation, balance, and thought processes.
A.   Nausea and vomiting may be present along with auditory issues, but frontal pain does not accompany basilar artery migraine.
B.   Ataxia, confusion, and slurred speech are generally not seen with basilar migraine.
C.   Seizures are not common with migraine headaches.

Content Category: Neurology

Reference: Snyder, 2000; pp. 275–317.

62.   A 29-year-old male presents to the ED with ipsilateral nasal congestion, rhinorrhea, lacrimation, papillary changes, a droopy eyelid, and conjunctival injection, coupled with pain behind 1 eye. He will probably be treated for:
A.   tension headache.
B.   CLUSTER HEADACHE.
C.   temporal arteritis.
D.   subarachnoid hemorrhage.

Rationale:

B.   Cluster headaches occur more often in men than in women. The patient is typically in his late 20s and complains of an excruciating sharp pain behind or near one eye. The patient may also experience diaphoresis and facial flushing. The cluster headache may be precipitated by extreme heat or cold to the face, excitement, flashing lights, alcohol use, or sleep. The leading theory is that the cause is a spasm of an intracavernous carotid artery affected by a dysfunctional hypothalamus.
A.   The patient's symptoms do not suggest tension headache.
C.   The patient's symptoms do not suggest temporal arteritis.
D.   The patient's symptoms do not suggest subarachnoid hemorrhage.

Content Category: Neurology

Reference: Snyder, 2000; pp. 275–317.

63.   A 59-year-old male patient presents to the ED with complaints of severe headache, blurred vision, and restlessness. He is alert and oriented. Pupils are equal and reactive to light. Initial vital signs are BP 168/100 mmHg, pulse 90/min, and respirations 18/min. He complains of neck pain on physical examination. Based on your assessment, you anticipate a diagnosis of:
A.   meningitis.
B.   migraine headache.
C.   SUBARACHNOID HEMORRHAGE.
D.   stroke in evolution.

Rationale:

C. Subarachnoid hemorrhage is bleeding into the subarachnoid space from a ruptured intracranial aneurysm or atrioventricular malformation (AVM) or is associated with advanced atherosclerosis. These headaches are frequently described as "the worst headache in my life." Meningeal signs and nuchal rigidity occur because blood is irritating to the arachnoid and pia mater.

A. Meningitis is an infection of the meninges that may present with throbbing headache, meningeal signs, and nuchal rigidity, but hypertension is unlikely.

B. Meningeal signs and nuchal rigidity are not associated with migraine headaches.

D. Stroke in evolution describes the progressive development of deficits over a period of time. Meningeal signs are commonly associated with stroke in evolution.

Content Category: Neurology

References: Boss, 1998; pp. 510–571; Snyder, 2000; pp. 275–317.

64. A patient is transferred to the ED from an outlying hospital. The patient has been diagnosed with an epidural hematoma by CT scan at the primary hospital. Upon admission, the patient is unconscious. Initial vital signs are BP 160/80 mmHg, pulse 46/min, and respirations 18/min. Breathing is being controlled with a bag valve mask. As the ED nurse, you should prepare for:
   A. a lumbar puncture to determine the amount of blood loss.
   B. insertion of an intracranial pressure (ICP) monitor and admission to the ICU.
   C. TRANSFER TO THE OR.
   D. potential organ donation.

Rationale:

C. An epidural hematoma is bleeding between the skull and dura mater resulting from a blow to the head. A torn middle meningeal artery with arterial bleeding leads to a rapidly forming hematoma, with associated morbidity and mortality greater than 50%. Rapid surgical intervention and efforts to decrease intracranial pressure are considered the best treatment.

A. A lumbar puncture is not indicated for a patient with a diagnosed epidural bleed, since bleeding is taking place between the skull and the dura mater.

B. Insertion of an ICP monitor would be considered for this patient, but the patient would need treatment before being admitted to the ICU.

D. Although epidural hematomas carry a high mortality and morbidity, all treatment options should be considered.

Content Category: Neurology

References: Snyder, 2000; pp. 275–317; Sheehy & Lenehan, 1998; p. 395.

65.   A 45-year-old male presents to the ED with complaints of severe pain and burning around the left eye, pain in the left side of the head, increased tearing, and nausea. You note ptosis of the left eye, which is red. The patient states that these symptoms started approximately 30 minutes before arrival. This patient's symptoms are most commonly associated with:

A. CLUSTER HEADACHE.
B. tension headache.
C. intracerebral neoplasm.
D. optic neuritis.

Rationale:

A. Cluster headaches occur primarily in men aged 20 to 50 years. The name is derived from the occurrence of several attacks during the day for a period of days followed by a long period of remission. Cluster headaches are characterized by severe unilateral tearing, burning, and periorbital or temporal pain that lasts for 30 minutes to 2 hours. Associated symptoms include lacrimation, reddening of the eye, nasal stuffiness, eyelid ptosis, and nausea. Pain may be referred to the midface and teeth.

B. Tension headaches are mild to moderate bilateral headaches with a sensation of a tight band or pressure around the head. These headaches, the most common type, occur in both men and women.

C. Clinical manifestations of intracerebral tumor result from the invasion and destruction of local tissue as well as from increased intracranial pressure. Focal deficits depend on the tumor site. Clinical manifestations of increased intracranial pressure include headache, vomiting, papilledema, unsteady gait, and diminishing cognitive function.

D. Optic neuritis is a presenting complaint in approximately 25% of persons with multiple sclerosis. The condition, which evolves rapidly, is a result of optic nerve demyelination. Subjective symptoms are blurring, foggy or hazy vision, and impaired color perception. Central visual acuity, color vision deficit, and visual field deficits occur.

Content Category: Neurology

Reference: Boss, 1998; pp. 510–571.

66.   A patient presents to the ED complaining of left wrist swelling and tenderness after a fall. The wrist is swollen and ecchymotic. X-rays confirm a navicular fracture. Treatment of this type of fracture includes:

A. open reduction and internal fixation.
B. daily, gentle range-of-motion exercises to preserve function.
C. immobilization with a splint for 2 weeks.
D. IMMOBILIZATION WITH A CAST FOR 12 WEEKS.

Rationale:

D. A navicular fracture generally occurs after a fall on an outstretched hand that leads to a direct blow to the hand. The fracture is typically immobilized for 12 weeks.

A. Open reduction and internal fixation repair are not warranted for emergency management of this fracture.

B. Navicular fractures must be immobilized in a spica position to decrease the risk of avascular necrosis.

C. Two weeks of splinting would be inadequate for navicular healing.

Content Category: Orthopedics/Wound Care

Reference: Walker, 2000; pp. 501–535.

67. A radial head subluxation has been successfully reduced in a 2-year-old boy. Which of the following statements by the mother indicates a proper understanding of discharge instructions?
    A. "HE WILL GROW OUT OF THIS."
    B. "I will ask his pediatrician to apply a splint tomorrow."
    C. "This may happen again; it can't be avoided."
    D. "I will ask my pediatrician to order a magnetic resonance imaging (MRI) scan."

Rationale:

A. Radial head subluxation usually occurs in children under 6 years of age. As the child grows older, the structures in the elbow begin to fit more tightly, offering less opportunity for subluxation.
B. There is no need to immobilize the arm after successful reduction.
C. Radial head subluxation may recur if the arm is pulled or yanked. Avoiding these maneuvers can prevent a recurrence.
D. There is no indication for MRI after radial head subluxation.

Content Category: Orthopedics/Wound Care
Reference: Greene & Luck, 1997; pp. 550–668.

68. When a thumb spica splint is being applied, the hand should be positioned as if holding:
    A. a paper clip.
    B. A SODA CAN.
    C. a pencil.
    D. up a wall.

Rationale:

B. The thumb should be held in a somewhat abducted position for a thumb spica splint. Asking the patient to hold an imaginary soda can facilitates abduction.
A. Holding a paper clip would cause the thumb to adduct.
C. Holding a pencil also causes adduction.
D. Holding up a wall would place the thumb in extension

Content Category: Orthopedics/Wound Care
Reference: Rosen et al., 1999.

69. A mother brings her 5-year-old child to the ED after the child was bitten by a mouse in the kitchen of their home. Which of the following statements about rabies post exposure prophylaxis (RPEP) is true?
    A. IT IS NOT INDICATED IN THIS SITUATION.
    B. It may be able to be withheld if the mouse can be captured and observed for 10 days.
    C. It should be started immediately.
    D. The child should have a rabies antibody titer drawn 10 days later. If the values are elevated, RPEP should be started.

Rationale:

A. Rabies is not transmitted by mice, squirrels, or other small rodents. Therefore, RPEP is generally not indicated for such an exposure.
B. Observation of the biting animal is recommended for dogs or cats if the animal's vaccination history is unknown or incomplete.
C. RPEP is not recommended after bites by small rodents.
D. Rabies antibody titer drawn 10 days later will not provide useful information. RPEP is most effective when started within 10 days of the bite.

Content Category: Orthopedics/Wound Care

Reference: Talan et al., 1999; pp. 590–596.

Questions 70–73

A 14-year-old boy is brought to the ED by his parents after he was taken down in a hard tackle during a football scrimmage. He complains of left shoulder pain. A deformity of the left clavicle is visible.

70.   The priority nursing assessment is to evaluate:
    A. the peripheral nerves.
    B. BREATH SOUNDS.
    C. brachial pulse.
    D. pain.

Rationale:

    B. Breath sounds should be assessed to rule out underlying pneumothorax or hemothorax.
    A. Peripheral nerve function should be assessed, but this is not a priority assessment.
    C. Peripheral pulses should be assessed, but assessment of breath sounds is a higher priority.
    D. Clavicle fractures can be painful and distressing to parent and child. Nevertheless, pain should be addressed only after airway, breathing, and circulation have been evaluated.

Content Category: Orthopedics/Wound Care

Reference: Rosen et al., 1999.

71.   X-rays confirm a clavicular fracture. The nurse should be most alert for serious underlying injuries if the fracture is:
    A. LOCATED IN THE MEDIAL ASPECT OF THE CLAVICLE.
    B. displaced.
    C. located in the middle third of the clavicle.
    D. angulated.

Rationale:

    A. Although rare, clavicle fractures near the sternum carry the greatest potential for damage to underlying structures.
    B. Fractures of the clavicle are frequently displaced, but this rarely has any significance or sequelae.
    C. Fractures of the clavicle are most commonly found in the middle third of the clavicle. These are infrequently associated with underlying injuries.
    D. Fractures of the clavicle are often angulated but generally do well without reduction.

Content Category: Orthopedics/Wound Care

References: Rosen et al., 1999; Johnson, 1997; pp. 71–123.

72.   Orders for this patient include the application of a figure 8 support. After this device has been applied, the nurse should evaluate:
    A. sensation over the clavicle.
    B. ulnar pulse.
    C. shoulder range of motion.
    D. THUMB ABDUCTION.

Rationale:

    D. Incorrect application of the figure 8 support can cause injury to the radial nerve. The nurse should ensure that there is no evidence of radial nerve injury.

    A. Application of the figure 8 support should not alter sensation over the clavicle.

    B. While the vascular status of the arm should be assessed, the radial or brachial pulses are the preferred sites.

    C. Movement of the shoulder in the immediate post injury period is painful and need not be performed.

Content Category: Orthopedics/Wound Care

References: Rosen et al., 1999; Johnson, 1997; pp. 71–123; Stern, 1997.

73.   Which of the following statements indicates the patient's appropriate understanding of home care for a fracture of the clavicle?

    A. "I will take the support off when I go to sleep."

    B. "I WILL APPLY ICE TO THE AREA."

    C. "I can remove the support to shower."

    D. "I can take the support off after 7 days."

Rationale:

    B. Applying ice to the area will decrease pain and swelling.

    A. The support should be worn for sleep.

    C. The support should continue to be worn and the patient encouraged to take sponge baths rather than showers.

    D. Timing for removal should be dictated by the follow-up provider.

Content Category: Orthopedics/Wound Care

Reference: James, 1998; pp. 325–357.

Questions 74–76

A 24-year-old sanitation worker presents to the ED holding 3 amputated fingers in a soiled cloth. The patient is awake, alert, and oriented, but appears to be anxious and upset. Upon examination of the affected hand, you note that the first, second, and third fingers are missing. The hand is swollen, ecchymotic, and bleeding profusely from the stumps.

74.   The nurse should FIRST:

    A. APPLY DIRECT PRESSURE TO THE STUMPS TO CONTROL BLEEDING.

    B. administer an oral antibiotic.

    C. reapproximate the amputated digits and hold them in place with a pressure dressing.

    D. place the amputated digits in sterile water.

Rationale:

    A. Direct pressure should be applied to control bleeding without causing further tissue damage. A pressure dressing may be used.

    B. Antibiotics will be included in the plan of care, but more likely intravenous antibiotics than the oral kind. This patient should receive nothing by mouth and be prepared for reimplantation surgery.

    C. Amputated body parts should be wrapped in sterile gauze, moistened with saline, and placed in a plastic bag, which should be placed in an airtight container on ice. Attempting to reapproximate the stumps could cause additional injury.

    D. The amputated digits should not be immersed directly in any solution.

Content Category: Orthopedics/Wound Care

Reference: Walker, 2000; pp. 501–535.

75. Bleeding of the stumps has been controlled. The next priority should be given to treatment of the amputated fingers. The nurse should:
    A. scrub the digits with iodine solution and place them in a plastic bag.
    B. flush the digits with mild soap solution, then soak them in sterile saline.
    C. wrap the digits in dry gauze and place them directly on dry ice.
    D. WRAP THE DIGITS IN MOIST GAUZE, INSERT THEM IN A PLASTIC BAG, AND PLACE THE BAG ON ICE.

Rationale:

   D. The amputated part should be wrapped in sterile saline–moistened gauze and placed in a plastic bag inside an airtight container, which should then be placed on ice.
   A. The amputated part should not be cleansed with iodine solution or any other abrasive cleansing agent. Doing so would cause increased cellular damage.
   B. The amputated part should never be soaked in any solution or fluid. Doing so would cause increased cellular damage and limit the likelihood of successful reimplantation.
   C. The amputated part should never be wrapped in dry gauze. Doing so would cause tissue and cellular damage.

Content Category: Orthopedics/Wound Care

Reference: Walker, 2000; pp. 501–535.

76. Diagnostic x-ray films should be taken of:
    A. the affected hand with stumps.
    B. THE AFFECTED HAND WITH STUMPS AND THE AMPUTATED FINGERS.
    C. the affected hand with stumps, the amputated fingers, and the forearm.
    D. the affected hand and the opposite hand for comparison.

Rationale:

   B. The affected hand with stumps and the amputated fingers should be x-rayed to determine the severity of damage and the probability of successful reimplantation.
   A. Not only the affected hand but also the amputated parts should be x-rayed.
   C. There is no need to x-ray the forearm unless further damage is considered or observed or the patient has a forearm complaint.
   D. There is no need to x-ray the opposite hand unless other damage is assessed.

Content Category: Orthopedics/Wound Care

Reference: Walker, 2000; pp. 501–535.

77. A patient presents with pain in the sole of her foot after stepping on a nail. Initial assessment includes:
    A. AN X-RAY.
    B. a computed tomography (CT) scan.
    C. a magnetic resonance imaging (MRI) scan.
    D. an ultrasound scan.

Rationale:

A. An x-ray is the first step to rule out the presence of a foreign body.
B. CT and MRI show the contrast between soft tissue and differentiating densities.
C. MRI cannot be used with metal objects or with substances such as gravel because doing so produces artifact.
D. Ultrasound can identify objects as small as 1 mm × 2 mm. Ultrasound can be used if plain films are negative and the index of suspicion for a foreign body is high.

Content Category: Orthopedics/Wound Care
Reference: Wahl et al., 1996; pp. 317–322.

78. A middle-aged woman walks slowly into triage. She reports that someone pulled out a chair as she was preparing to sit down, causing her to fall on a concrete floor. Pain is present but tolerable when she stands or lies down, but intense when she sits. The nurse should suspect a fracture of the:
A. symphysis pubis.
B. ISCHIAL RAMUS.
C. iliac crest.
D. acetabulum.

Rationale:

B. The ischial ramus, one of the bones used for sitting down, would logically be injured in a case like this. This type of fracture is normally stable, permitting ambulation.
A. The symphysis would more likely be injured if the patient had fallen forward onto the lower abdomen.
C. An iliac crest fracture would be expected if the patient had fallen laterally onto the hip.
D. The patient with an acetabular fracture usually cannot ambulate.

Content Category: Orthopedics/Wound Care
Reference: Rosen et al., 1999.

79. A 25-year-old male complains of pain, swelling, and cuts on his hand after being involved in a fight. During your triage assessment, the most important question to ask is:
A. "When was your last tetanus shot?"
B. "HOW DID YOU GET THE CUTS ON YOUR HAND?"
C. "When did this happen?"
D. "Do you have any other medical problems?"

Rationale:

B. The triage nurse must be concerned that any patients who have been involved in a fight with lacerations or abrasions may have incurred a human bite. Human bites, particularly those of the hand, are at high risk for infection.
A. Asking about the date of the patient's last tetanus shot should be part of routine questioning of anyone who has incurred a laceration, burn, abrasion, avulsion, or bite.
C. Asking when the event took place should be part of routine questioning of anyone who visits the ED with an injury.
D. Asking whether a patient has any other medical problems should be part of routine questioning of anyone who visits the ED.

Content Category: Orthopedics/Wound Care
References: Simon & Slobodkin, 1996; pp. 1217–1225; Strauss, 1999; pp. 487–536.

80. Posterior shoulder dislocation is most likely the result of which mechanism?
     A. SEIZURE
     B. Motor vehicle collision
     C. Fall
     D. Assault

Rationale:

   A. A seizure cause sudden internal rotation during the tonic phase.
   B. Motor vehicle collision is not a mechanism for posterior dislocation.
   C. Fall is not a mechanism for posterior dislocation.
   D. Assault is not a mechanism for posterior dislocation.

Content Category: Orthopedics/Wound Care

Reference: Bailey, 1998; pp. 415–447.

81. A 48-year-old male presents at the ED complaining of an acute onset of epigastric abdominal pain radiating to the back. A quick assessment reveals a history of hyperlipidemia and hypertension treated by medications that include thiazide diuretics. The patient has hypotension and cool, clammy skin and is tachycardic. The priority intervention for this patient is to:
     A. order laboratory tests, including amylase and lipase.
     B. prepare to administer morphine for relief of pain.
     C. ADMINISTER INTRAVENOUS FLUIDS AND ELECTROLYTES.
     D. prepare for ultrasonography as a diagnostic evaluation tool.

Rationale:

   C. The administration of IV fluids and electrolytes is the priority intervention for any patient with hypotension; cool, clammy skin; and tachycardia. In this case, the patient is suspected to have acute pancreatitis. Among patients with this condition, 5% die of the acute effects of peripheral vascular collapse. Large losses of fluid occur in the retroperitoneal spaces, peripancreatic spaces, and abdominal cavity.
   A. Laboratory tests such as those for amylase and lipase levels are important in the diagnostic evaluation of pancreatitis. However, they are not the nurse's priority when a patient presents with possible hypotension and shock.
   B. Morphine is not the drug of choice in pancreatitis. Meperidine (Demerol) would be the drug of choice for pain relief because it causes fewer spasms in the sphincter of Oddi.
   D. A CAT scan would be more useful, because more sensitive, than an ultrasound scan for detecting an enlarged pancreas. The diagnosis of pancreatitis would not override the intervention of IV fluids.

Content Category: Gastrointestinal

References: Porth, 1998; pp. 769–771; ENA, 1994; pp. 29–45.

82. Which of the following signs/symptoms is commonly associated with viral gastroenteritis?
     A. PERSISTENT VOMITING
     B. Increased urinary output
     C. Hypoactive bowel sounds
     D. Bloody stools

Rationale:

    A. Vomiting for six to eight hours is the usual course of viral gastroenteritis. Persistent vomiting for longer than twelve hours in the child or adult needs to be investigated and evaluated.

    B. Decreased urinary output is normally found with gastroenteritis related to the mild dehydration state.

    C. Hyperactive bowel sounds are normally found with gastroenteritis.

    D. Bloody stools is usually indicative of infectious diarrhea or bacterial gastroenteritis requiring treatment, or more serious disease states, such as diverticulitis.

Content Category: Gastrointestinal

References: Reilly, 1991; pp. 843–847; Soud & Rogers, 1998; pp. 333–362; Wyatt et al., 1999; pp. 516–533.

83.   A 32-year-old female arrives in the ED complaining of abdominal pain. She states that she has a history of Crohn's disease. What description of recent bowel activity should lead the nurse to suspect that the patient is experiencing another episode of Crohn's disease?

    A. Clay-colored stools

    B. Melena

    C. Bright-red blood

    D. DIARRHEA

Rationale:

    D. Crohn's disease is an inflammatory process of the bowel that causes frequent diarrhea.

    A. Clay-colored stools would be indicative of a biliary obstruction.

    B. Melena represents bleeding of the upper intestine.

    C. The presence of bright-red blood is usually related to bleeding of the lower intestine.

Content Category: Gastrointestinal

References: Kidd et al., 2000; pp. 107–108; Newberry, 1998; p. 545.

84.   The patient is being discharged with a diagnosis of hiatal hernia and has discharge instructions to take an antacid. The ED nurse will instruct the patient that some antacids produce diarrhea and some produce constipation. Antacids that have a laxative effect contain:

    A. aluminum.

    B. calcium

    C. MAGNESIUM.

    D. sodium.

Rationale:

    C. Antacids that contain magnesium have a laxative effect.

    A. Antacids that contain calcium have a constipating effect.

    B. Antacids that contain aluminum have a constipating effect.

    D. Antacids do not contain sodium.

Content Category: Gastrointestinal

Reference: Hodgson & Kizor, 2000; pp. 1077–1079.

85.   Diagnostic peritoneal lavage (DPL) that has been performed on your patient is positive for blood and fecal matter. The trauma surgeon is concerned that this patient may have incurred an injury to the:
A. liver.
B. stomach.
C. pancreas.
D. COLON.

Rationale:

D. A DPL obtained in a patient with an injury to the bowel or colon is positive for blood and fecal matter.
A. In a patient who has incurred a liver injury, a DPL is usually positive for blood but not for fecal matter.
B. A DPL performed on someone who has had a stomach injury may be positive for blood or undigested food matter, but not for fecal material. Instilled DPL fluid could be aspirated from the nasogastric tube.
C. In a patient who has had a pancreatic injury, peritoneal lavage is positive for amylase, but not for fecal material, and usually not for blood unless other structures have been damaged as well.

Content Category: Gastrointestinal

References: ENA, Core Curriculum, 2000; pp. 49–53, 149; Black & Matassarin-Jacobs, 1997; p. 2531.

86.   A 12-year-old boy complaining of left shoulder pain and malaise presents to the ED with his mother. As you are escorting the boy alone to x-ray, he confides that he was "beaten up" by 3 other boys 2 days ago and hit in the "belly," when his left shoulder started to "hurt." Your next action should be to:
A. advise him he should tell his mother.
B. continue to take him for his shoulder films.
C. TAKE HIM BACK TO THE TREATMENT AREA IMMEDIATELY.
D. take him directly to the computed tomography (CT) scanner.

Rationale:

C. Kehr's sign, a frequent sign of a splenic injury after blunt trauma, is referred pain to the left shoulder from irritation of the peritoneum because of bleeding. This patient should indeed be brought immediately back to a treatment area and a physician should be notified.
A. Advising the young man to tell his mother about his situation may be appropriate later. The priority would be to control potential hemorrhage.
B. Continuing with the shoulder films before the patient is further assessed and ABCs supported would not be a nursing priority. The shoulder pain may be Kehr's sign, not a shoulder injury.
D. Taking the patient directly to the CT scanner without further assessment and notifying an emergency physician would not be in the patient's best interest. He patient would not be prepared for the abdominal scan he needs and parental consent would not be given. Since further assessment has not been completed, the patient's status could change quickly, with potential occult bleeding.
Category Content: Gastrointestinal

References: ENA, Core Curriculum, 2000; pp. 49–53; Newberry, 1998; p. 404.

87.   A woman brings her 4-week-old male infant to the ED, stating that he has had increased projectile vomiting over the last week. In addition, the infant's stools have decreased in frequency and amount.

On physical exam, peristaltic waves are noted in the upper right quadrant along with an olive-size mass. The ED nurse recognizes that the priority nursing intervention is to:
A. ADMINISTER INTRAVENOUS FLUIDS AND ELECTROLYTES.
B. administer rectal promethazine HCl (Phenergan) 12.5 mg.
C. prepare for the administration of a barium enema.
D. prepare for nasogastric intubation.

Rationale:

A. Administration of IV fluids and electrolytes is vital in preventing dehydration and electrolyte imbalances that occur with bowel obstruction (pyloric stenosis) in infant males, as is commonly seen at age 2 to 10 weeks.
B. Administration of promethazine is not indicated, since the vomiting is related to bowel obstruction. The possible need to insert a nasogastric tube makes it unwise to administer promethazine.
C. Administration of barium enema is commonly indicated in Hirschsprung's disease, but not in pyloric stenosis. A barium swallow can usually confirm the presence of pyloric stenosis.
D. While it may be necessary to insert a nasogastric tube, the priority is to administer fluids as part of the primary survey.

Content Category: Gastrointestinal

References: Newberry, 1998; pp. 537–535; Wyatt et al., 1999; pp. 516–533.

88. Heartburn is a common manifestation of esophageal disease. Which of the following statements about heartburn is true?
A. HEARTBURN IS OFTEN EXPERIENCED WITH POSTURAL CHANGES.
B. The symptoms of heartburn can be relieved by lying down.
C. The symptoms of heartburn can be relieved by drinking ample fluids.
D. Heartburn is not affected by cigarette smoking.

Rationale:

A. Heartburn is often experienced with postural changes such as bending, stooping, or lifting.
B. Heartburn symptoms are best relieved by standing up, not by lying down.
C. Heartburn is exacerbated, not relieved, by drinking ample fluids.
D. Cigarette smoking exacerbates heartburn.

Content Category: Gastrointestinal

Reference: Black & Matassarin-Jacobs, 1997; pp. 1734, 1737–1741.

89. A 55-year-old male presents to the ED complaining of right flank pain (rated at 8/10) for 3 hours. He is diaphoretic and restless. Initial vital signs are BP 164/92 mmHg, pulse 96/min, respirations 20/min, oxygen saturation 96%, and temperature 98.4° F (36.9° C). The patient has no past history of similar pain. Your planning and determination of urgency of care for this patient are based on ruling out which of the following medical conditions *first*?
A. Renal colic
B. ABDOMINAL AORTIC ANEURYSM
C. Costochondritis
D. Acute diverticulitis

Rationale:

B. Abdominal aortic aneurysm should be the first condition ruled out in any patient over age 50 whose first-time presentation has the appearance of renal colic. The risk for weakened blood vessels increases with age.

A. Renal colic may be a potential diagnosis, but an abdominal aortic aneurysm must be ruled out first. A urine dipstick or urinalysis may demonstrate hematuria, which is strongly indicative of renal colic. Even so, the patient should be given a spiral CT of the abdomen to show the aorta as well as the kidneys, ureters, and bladder. If a spiral CT of the abdomen is not available, alternative diagnostic studies must be done to visualize the abdominal aorta.

C. Costochondritis does not usually make the patient diaphoretic or restless or induce such a high pain rating (8/10). Costochondritis is usually characterized by muscular pain of the chest that is associated with movement.

D. Acute diverticulitis is not usually associated with flank pain.

Content Category: Patient Care Management

Reference: ENA, Core Curriculum, 2000.

90. A 64-year-old patient has unstable atrial fibrillation at a rate of 134 with associated chest pain and some shortness of breath. The physician orders ibutilide (Corvert) to be given to the patient intravenously. Initial vital signs are BP 124/70 mmHg, pulse 134/min, respirations 22/min, oxygen saturation 95%, and temperature 97.4° F (36.9° C). Knowing the side effects of ibutilide, the ED nurse places at the bedside and is prepared to give which of the following medications?
A. Epinephrine (Adrenalin)
B. Potassium
C. Naloxone (Narcan)
D. MAGNESIUM

Rationale:

D. Magnesium would be used either prophylactically before the ibutilide is given or in the event of ibutilide-induced torsade de pointes, which occurs in approximately 10% of patients who receive ibutilide.

A. Epinephrine (Adrenalin) is used for acute anaphylaxis and cardiac arrest.

B. Potassium would not be used in connection with ibutilide unless it was coincidentally being used for hypokalemia.

C. Naloxone (Narcan) would not be used, since no opioids have been given.

Content Category: Patient Care Management

References: ENA, Core Curriculum, 2000; American Heart Association, 2000.

91. A 25-year-old college student took 25 tablets of Dimetapp as a suicidal gesture approximately 3 hours ago. The patient presents to the ED alert and oriented x 4 (slightly drowsy). Initial vital signs are BP 110/70 mmHg, pulse 76/min, respirations 18/min, oxygen saturation 95%, and temperature 97.9° F (36.6° C). The most effective way to manage this patient's toxic emergency is to:
A. give syrup of ipecac.
B. perform gastric lavage.
C. GIVE ACTIVATED CHARCOAL.
D. give polyethylene glycol–electrolyte solution (GoLytely).

Rationale:

C. Activated charcoal is the initial treatment of choice for an overdose in a patient who has not taken a medication containing a heavy metal (such as lithium or iron), sustained-release medications, or alcohol. The action of charcoal is to bind with the toxin and decrease absorption.

A. Syrup of ipecac is not an appropriate choice in a patient who took medication 3 hours previously. Ipecac is generally not favored by toxicologists because it removes only about 50% of the pills and forces more medication into the small intestine, where it is absorbed. Vomiting may potentiate aspiration.

    B. Gastric lavage is also generally not favored by toxicologists for patients with a 3-hour history of ingestion. The lavage action forces any medication that remains in the stomach into the duodenum, where it is rapidly absorbed.

    D. GoLytely is used for gut decontamination, which is usually reserved for patients who have not taken sustained-release medications or medications containing a heavy metal (such as lithium or iron).

Content Category: Patient Care Management

Reference: ENA, Core Curriculum, 2000.

92. A 4-year-old male has a foreign body in his throat that is partially obstructing the airway. His color is pink. He has no altered level of consciousness and does not appear to be in acute distress. While you await the transport team that is coming to transport this child to a children's hospital, in what position should he be placed?

    A. Prone with face to side

    B. Supine

    C. ANY POSITION IN WHICH HE FEELS COMFORTABLE

    D. Secured upright

Rationale:

    C. Allow the child to choose his own position. He will most likely choose the position that maximizes breathing. When the airway is compromised, a child is likely to choose a tripoding or sniffing position.

    A. Forcing the child into any position may cause him to become very upset and may therefore compromise the airway. The position that maximizes the airway is upright sniffing or tripoding position, which the child would most likely choose if permitted to do so.

    B. See A.

    D. See A.

Content Category: Patient Care Management

Reference: ENA, Core Curriculum, 2000.

93. Your 2-year-old patient has been diagnosed with croup and has not responded to saline mist respiratory treatment. After racemic epinephrine treatment, as ordered by the physician, the child's respiratory condition improves dramatically. How long should this child be monitored in the ED before discharge?

    A. One hour

    B. TWO HOURS

    C. Four hours

    D. Six hours

Rationale:

    B. The child should be monitored for at least 2 hours after racemic epinephrine treatment because of the potential for rebound respiratory distress within that window.

    A. One hour would not be long enough to monitor the child.

    C. Two hours is the recommended minimum. If the patient's condition warrants longer observation, the time may be extended.

    D. Two hours is the recommended minimum. If the patient's condition warrants longer observation, the time may be extended.

Content Category: Patient Care Management

Reference: ENA, Core Curriculum, 2000.

94.   An 84-year-old male presents to the ED reporting diffuse abdominal pain (now rated at 10/10) for the past 2 days. The pain had a slow onset and is described as aching and constant. The patient has a history of atrial fibrillation (now well controlled) and appears to be slightly dehydrated. Initial vital signs are BP 166/88 mmHg, pulse 94/min, respirations 24/min, oxygen saturation 95%, and temperature 98.2° F (36.8° C). Examination of the abdomen reveals an abdomen that is soft and nontender, with bowel sounds present. The patient has had a computed tomography (CT) scan of the abdomen, which was negative. All lab test results are within normal limits. The rectal exam is heme negative. What condition do you suspect?
A. Appendicitis
B. MESENTERIC ISCHEMIA
C. Cholecystitis
D. Diverticulitis

Rationale:

B. This patient is at risk for mesenteric ischemia based on his circulatory problems and age. The history and the negative results for all tests represent a classic presentation for mesenteric ischemia.

A. Appendicitis usually produces a fever, altered bowel elimination pattern, abnormal abdominal physical findings, and elevated WBC and might be seen on the CT of the abdomen.

C. Cholecystitis usually presents with a more localized area of pain, may be accompanied by elevated WBC and elevated amylase and lipase levels, and may be seen on CT of the abdomen.

D. Diverticulitis involves a more localized area of pain, may produce elevated WBC, and may be seen on CT of the abdomen.

Content Category: Patient Care Management

Reference: ENA, Core Curriculum, 2000.

95.   The priority treatment of choice for a methanol overdose is:
A. ETHANOL IV
B. Activated charcoal PO
C. Polyethylene glycol–electrolyte solution (GoLytely) PO
D. Flumazenil (Romazicon) IV

Rationale:

A. Ethanol IV is the treatment of choice because it competes with ethanol at the receptor sites and prevents the conversion of the ingested methanol to formaldehyde.

B. Activated charcoal PO does not bind with alcohol and therefore would be ineffective.

C. GoLytely would not be used for gut decontamination because it is typically not indicated with this type of overdose.

D. Romazicon is used as an antagonist for benzodiazepines because it reverses their action at the receptor sites.

Content Category: Patient Care Management

References: ENA, Core Curriculum, 2000; Snyder, 1993.

96.   Consent rates for organ donation are highest when the request is made by the:
A. ED nurse.
B. hospital chaplain.
C. ORGAN PROCUREMENT ORGANIZATION (OPO) COORDINATOR IN CONJUNCTION WITH THE HOSPITAL STAFF.
D. primary intensive care unit nurse and the attending physician.

Rationale:

C. Organ Procurement Organization (OPO) staff working with hospital staff are the best choice for requesting consent for donation from patients' family members for many reasons. These include the OPO staff's training and experience, the greater amount of time they can spend with families, and their belief that the process helps donor families. Because OPO staff are often perceived to be "on the outside," the consent rate improves when they work in conjunction with hospital staff. Numerous studies have shown that when procurement coordinators are involved in the approach for donation, donation increases by almost 50%.

A. A family request for donation is particularly sensitive to problems of timing and coordination. A lone clinician who is well intentioned but inexperienced and unfamiliar with the family request process can easily disrupt and irreparably damage that process. A key skill that OPO staff members provide is restraint; they move ahead only when the family is ready. The process often takes more time than nurses and physicians in a busy department can spare. Many health care professionals view the request for donation as negative for the donor's family, an attitude that may provoke emotional distress in the family. This attitude decreases the health care provider's comfort level in making the request, a condition that can lead to an insensitive, task-oriented approach or no approach at all.

B. The primary role of the hospital chaplain in this setting is to support the patient's family. The transition to donation can more easily be made by the OPO coordinator.

D. Health care professionals may be too busy with immediate concerns to spend the time needed with family that is often required as they decide whether to grant permission for organ donation.

Content Category: Patient Care Management

Reference: Ehrle et al., 1999; pp. 21–33.

97. The full emergency operations preparation cycle includes:
    A. PLANNING, EDUCATION, DRILLS, AND EVALUATION.
    B. scene management, hospital management, and city management.
    C. meetings, assembling reference notebooks, and construction of facilities.
    D. training exercises and critiquing.

Rationale:

A. Planning, education, drills, and evaluation make up the emergency operations preparation cycle, starting at any point and completing the full cycle.

B. Scene management, hospital management, and city management are components of communitywide emergency operations planning.

C. Meetings, assembling reference notebooks, and construction of facilities are some of the tasks that may be required for emergency operations planning.

D. Training exercises and critiquing are components of the education portion of the emergency operations preparation cycle.

Content Category: Patient Care Management

Reference: Newberry, 1998; p. 205.

98.   Parents bring their 5-day-old infant to the ED for what they call "poor feeding." Mom reports that the baby was breastfeeding well until the previous evening. Your triage exam reveals a term female infant who is pale, slightly mottled, and listless, with poor muscle tone. Initial vital signs are HR 160, respirations 44/min with mild retractions, and rectal temperature 100.8° F (37.9° C). Capillary refill is 3 seconds centrally and 4 seconds peripherally. After the infant has been placed in a treatment room, oxygen is provided blow-by. The next intervention should be to:
   A. give acetaminophen and place a urine bag on the infant.
   B. do an Accu-Chek and give the infant a bottle of 5% dextrose in water.
   C. ESTABLISH IV ACCESS AND COLLECT BLOOD FOR A CBC, BLOOD CULTURE, ELECTROLYTES, AND A BEDSIDE ACCU-CHEK.
   D. prepare for intubation and establish IV access.

Rationale:

   C. The next treatment priority is to secure IV access and simultaneously draw blood for lab work, especially a CBC with differential, a blood culture, and blood for a bedside Accu-Chek.
   A. Incorrect.
   B. Incorrect.
   D. Incorrect.

Content Category: Patient Care Management

Reference: ENA, 1999; p. 254.

99.   Which of the following statements about children's pain is true?
   A. Behavioral manifestations reflect pain intensity.
   B. CHILDREN MAY NOT ADMIT TO HAVING PAIN.
   C. Narcotics are more likely to cause respiratory depression in children than in adults.
   D. It is not possible to evaluate pain in nonverbal children.

Rationale:

   B. To avoid an injection or a procedure they fear, children may not admit to having pain.
   A. Children with more active, resisting behaviors may rate pain lower than children with passive, accepting behaviors. A child's developmental level, coping abilities, and temperament influence pain behavior.
   C. Narcotics are no more dangerous for children than for adults.
   D. Several scales have been developed that use changes in behavioral and physiologic parameters to measure pain in nonverbal children.

Content Category: Patient Care Management

References: ENA, 1999; Wong, 1999; p. 1151.

100.   Discharge instructions to the parents of a child who has had a febrile seizure should include:
   A. instructions to prevent future seizures by treating fever with cool baths.
   B. REASSURANCE THAT FEBRILE SEIZURES DO NOT CAUSE BRAIN DAMAGE.
   C. a discussion of the side effects of phenytoin (Dilantin).
   D. reassurance that febrile seizures do not last beyond adolescence.

Rationale:

   B. Parents are often concerned about the possibility of brain damage in a child who is having febrile seizures.
   A. Cool baths are not helpful in treating fever and may cause rebound fever.
   C. Dilantin is not used to treat febrile seizures.
   D. Febrile seizures rarely occur in school-age children.

Content Category: Patient Care Management

Reference: Wong, 1999.

101.   A 4-year-old male fell from a moving all-terrain vehicle (ATV) and has multiple injuries. He has been stabilized in your ED and will be transported to a regional pediatric hospital for ongoing evaluation and treatment. A pediatric transport team is flying in to pick up and transport the patient. Which of the following interventions is NOT appropriate in preparing the patient's family for his transport?

A. Explain why the patient needs to be transferred.

B. Provide the family with maps and directions to the receiving facility.

C. SEND THE FAMILY TO THE RECEIVING FACILITY AS SOON AS POSSIBLE SO THEY CAN BE THERE WHEN THE PATIENT ARRIVES.

D. Caution the family to observe all traffic laws in traveling to the accepting facility.

Rationale:

C. Do NOT allow the family to leave the hospital until the child leaves.

A. Explaining the reason for the transfer reduces the family's stress, confusion, and uncertainty.

B. Giving the family maps and directions is helpful.

D. Gently caution the family to observe traffic laws at this stressful time.

Content Category: Patient Care Management

Reference: ENA, 1999; p. 261.

102.   Equipment in the transport environment should have which of the following characteristics?

A. Electrically powered, with the ability to function on battery power for 10-minute intervals.

B. PORTABLE, COMBINING SEVERAL FUNCTIONS IN A SINGLE PIECE OF EQUIPMENT.

C. Able to be placed on a small shelf or the floor while in transit for better visibility and accessible to the transport crew.

D. Weigh no more than 15 lb.

Rationale:

B. Equipment in the transport setting should be lightweight and portable and should combine several functions in a single piece of equipment. For example, some cardiac monitors can also be used to perform noninvasive blood pressure monitoring, invasive pressure monitoring, pulse oximetry, and end-tidal carbon dioxide monitoring.

A. Transport equipment needs to be battery powered or electrically powered with battery backup that will last from 1 to 2 times the estimated duration of transport.

C. Transport equipment should be secured at all times. Placing it loose on the floor or small shelf is dangerous, as unsecured items can become projectiles when the vehicle rapidly starts and stops, performs quick turns, or experiences turbulence.

D. Equipment in the transport setting should be lightweight, although a specific weight is difficult to name. An isolette for neonatal transport easily weighs more than 15 lb.

Content Category: Patient Care Management

References: Jaimovich & Vidyasagar, 1996; p. 469; Holleran, 1996; p. 105.

Questions 103 and 104

A patient with an acute myocardial infarction and severe cardiac failure has been stabilized in a small metropolitan ED. The patient is on 3 vasoactive drips and 1 antiarrhythmic drip, has an intra-aortic balloon pump inserted, and is intubated with ventilatory support. The patient is to be transferred to the ED of a cardiac specialty center on the opposite side of the same city as the sending facility, 30 miles away. Copies of the patient's records and x-rays are to be sent with the patient. The sending facility has secured an accepting physician and administrative acceptance of the patient by the receiving facility. An advanced life-support (ALS) ambulance with 2 paramedic caregivers and a basic emergency medical technician driver is performing the transport.

103.   This case constitutes an Emergency Medical Treatment and Active Labor Act (EMTALA) violation because:
  A.   A transfer from one ED to another violates EMTALA.
  B.   THE TRANSPORT CREW IS NOT PROPERLY TRAINED FOR A PATIENT WHO IS THIS ACUTELY ILL.
  C.   The accepting physician is not qualified to care for a patient who is this acutely ill.
  D.   The benefits of the transfer do not outweigh the risks.

Rationale:

  B.   Transfer legislation mandates that the transfer personnel and equipment be appropriate for the degree of illness or injury of each patient. A crew consisting only of a driver and 2 paramedics does not provide adequate support for a patient who is receiving intensive-care-level care, including multiple titratable drips, assisted ventilation, and intra-aortic balloon counterpulsation. The transport crew should include at least 1 nurse or physician who is experienced in caring for intensive-care patients of this type.
  A.   The Emergency Medical Treatment and Active Labor Act (EMTALA) sets no limitations on which area of a hospital can send or receive a transfer patient.
  C.   Not true. The accepting facility has a cardiac specialty center.
  D.   The benefits do outweigh the risks. The small facility that provided initial treatment for the patient sought out a cardiac specialty center for transfer.

Content Category: Patient Care Management

References: Moy, 2000; pp. 88–90, 110; Holleran, 1994; pp. 104–105.

104.   The most appropriate mode of transport is:
  A.   ground ambulance; routine transfer.
  B.   ground ambulance; emergency transfer.
  C.   ROTOR-WING AIR AMBULANCE TRANSFER.
  D.   fixed-wing air ambulance transfer.

Rationale:

  C.   The patient is very ill. The hospitals are on opposite sides of the city. A rotor-wing air ambulance (helicopter) is most appropriate, as it will minimize out-of-hospital time considerably.
  A.   Emergency or critical care transfer is appropriate; a routine transfer is not.
  B.   Ground transfer would be inappropriate unless air transportation would be significantly delayed.
  D.   Although a fixed-wing air ambulance moves quickly, such transport involves additional delays of ground transport from the hospital to the airport on both ends of the trip. For a transfer across a city, rotor-wing transport is more appropriate. Fixed-wing transport is usually reserved for transporting patients farther than 150 miles.

Content Category: Patient Care Management

References: Jaimovich & Vidyasagar, 1996; pp. 69–73; Holleran, 1994; pp. 105–107; Holleran, 1996; pp. 95–97.

105.   A patient is transported to a hospital by helicopter. The aircraft has side doors for patient access. The nose of the helicopter is at 12 o'clock. The crew states that a "hot offload" is indicated. The best approach to the aircraft as its rotors are still turning is:
   A. standing upright from the 1 o'clock position.
   B. crouching from the 5 o'clock position.
   C. standing upright from the 7 o'clock position.
   D. CROUCHING FROM THE 11 O'CLOCK POSITION.

Rationale:

   D. Personnel should approach helicopters in a crouched position. Personnel approaching helicopters should approach the nose (12 o'clock position) directly or from no more than 45° to the right or left of the nose.
   A. Standing upright is inappropriate. The 1 o'clock position is acceptable.
   B. Personnel should approach the nose (12 o'clock position) directly or from no more than 45° to the right or left of the nose. The aircraft should not be approached from the rear.
   C. Standing upright is inappropriate.

Content Category: Patient Care Management

Reference: McCloskey & Orr, 1995; p. 652.

106.   A patient arrives in the ED 10 minutes after having been pulled from a frozen pond. The patient is pulseless, apneic, and unresponsive and has a temperature of 77° F (25° C). The cardiac monitor indicates ventricular fibrillation. Which of the following combinations of modes of care is most appropriate?
   A. Defibrillate at 200, 300, and 360 joules and begin cardiopulmonary resuscitation (CPR).
   B. BEGIN CPR AND WARMING.
   C. Begin CPR, start an IV, and give epinephrine, followed by defibrillation at 360 joules.
   D. Begin CPR and insert a nasogastric tube.

Rationale:

   B. Severely hypothermic patients warrant CPR (part of which is airway control), warming, and monitoring of temperature and cardiac rhythm.
   A. Patients with severe hypothermia should not be defibrillated until warm.
   C. Patients with severe hypothermia should not be defibrillated until warm.
   D. CPR is necessary, but the insertion of a nasal gastric tube is not appropriate initially. Warming, an extremely important aspect of initial care, was omitted from this answer.

Content Category: Patient Care Management

Reference: Holleran, 1994; pp. 190–192.

107.   A passenger train has derailed. First responders indicate that at least 56 people have been injured. A nurse has gone in an ambulance to assist with care at the scene. Which of the following patients is the highest priority for treatment and transport ("red" category)?

A. A 75-YEAR-OLD WITH FEMUR, TIBIA, AND FIBULA FRACTURES; PALE, MOIST SKIN; AND PELVIC TENDERNESS AND MOBILITY ON PALPATION.

B. A 45-year-old with a metal rod impaled in the right forearm. The arm is neurovascularly intact. The patient is ambulatory.

C. A 63-year-old with second-degree and third-degree burns over 95% of body surface areas. The patient is unconscious and has a thready pulse.

D. A 25-year-old with pain in the left lateral lower chest and a 5-inch laceration in the left forearm. The wound squirts blood when uncovered. The patient is controlling the bleeding by applying pressure with a bandanna. Skin is pink and dry.

Rationale:

A. An unstable pelvic fracture with signs of shock warrants immediate intervention to decrease the chances of death. This patient is the first priority.

B. A stable patient with an arm injury and neurovascular intactness is not first priority. This patient is currently minor ("green" category), but should be monitored for deterioration to delayed ("yellow") or critical ("red") categories.

C. An unconscious burn patient with burns to more than 80% to 90% of the body and a thready pulse is considered terminal ("black" category). This patient is the lowest priority.

D. A stable patient with a controlled arterial bleed and left lateral lower chest pain is currently delayed ("yellow" category). Part of the concern is the potential for injuries in the left lower chest and left upper abdomen.

Content Category: Patient Care Management

Reference: Holleran, 1994; p. 82.

108.   A 55-year-old woman in congestive heart failure states that she had a heart transplant 3 years ago. The patient denies chest pain. Which of the following statements best describes why she is not having chest pain?

A. Her sensitivity to pain is diminished because she is taking multiple antirejection medications.

B. Atherosclerosis, which contributes to coronary artery clot, spasm, and chest pain, will not develop from the transplant.

C. SHE MAY NEVER EXPERIENCE CHEST PAIN. HEART TRANSPLANT RECIPIENTS HAVE A DENERVATED ORGAN.

D. Her perception of pain is affected by her perception of her heart as belonging to someone else.

Rationale:

C. Heart transplant recipients receive a denervated organ. Therefore, pain receptors are not connected. These patients may never experience chest pain. It is important to know that the first sign of myocardial infarction in the transplant patient is congestive heart failure.

A. Taking multiple antirejection medications does not diminish sensitivity to pain.

B. Atherosclerosis can develop in the transplanted heart, usually starting about 5 years after the transplant.

D. Patient perception of the transplanted heart is not an issue, since the heart does not have any pain receptors.

Content Category: Patient Care Management

Reference: ENA, Core Curriculum, 2000; p. 498.

109. A 155-lb (70.5-kg) patient with a massive anteroseptal myocardial infarction develops cardiogenic shock. The physician orders dopamine (Intropin) at 8 mcg/kg/min. Two 200-mg ampules of dopamine (Intropin) are added to 250 ml of D5W. The drip factor is 60 gtt/ml. The appropriate flow rate in gtt/min is:

   A. 12
   B. 16
   C. **21**
   D. 30

   [ed: please replace the letter "x" with multiplication symbol in lines 2, 7, and 9 of the first section (C) below]

Rationale:

   C. Calculate the concentration of mcg/ml:
   200 mg amp $\times$ 2 = 400 mg = 400,000 mcg/250 ml
   400,000 mcg/250 ml = 1600 mcg/ml
   Convert pounds to kilograms:
   155 lb = 70 kg
   Calculate the dose per kilogram:
   70 kg $\times$ 8 mcg = 560 mcg
   Calculate drops per minute:
   569 $\times$ 60 = 33,600 divided by 1600 = 21 gtt/min

   A. This flow rate will deliver 4.6 mcg/kg/min.
   B. This flow rate will deliver 6.1 mcg/kg/min.
   D. This flow rate will deliver 11.4 mcg/kg/min.

Content Category: Patient Care Management

References: ENA, Core Curriculum, 2000; p. 798–799; Skidmore-Roth, 1994; p.1073.

110. A medication recommended for delirium tremens is:
   A. Atenolol (Tenormin) 50–100 mg PO
   B. Chlordiazepoxide (Librium) 25–100 mg PO
   C. LORAZEPAM (ATIVAN) 1–5 MG PO, IV, IM
   D. Clonidine (Catapres) 0.1–0.4 mg PO

Rationale:

   C. Lorazepam (Ativan) 1–5 mg PO, IV, IM is recommended for delirium tremens.
   A. Atenolol (Tenormin) provides symptomatic relief for minor alcohol withdrawal.
   B. Chlordiazepoxide (Librium) 25–100 mg PO helps to sedate a patient during minor alcohol withdrawal.
   D. Clonidine (Catapres) 0.1–0.4 mg PO is recommended for minor alcohol withdrawal and gives symptomatic relief.

Content Category: Substance Abuse/Toxicology/Environment

Reference: Newberry, 1998.

111.   Rocky Mountain spotted fever can be very difficult to diagnose in its early stages. Patients infected with rickettsiae generally visit a physician in the first week of their illness, following an incubation period of about 5 to 10 days after a tick bite. The early clinical presentation of Rocky Mountain spotted fever is nonspecific and may resemble a variety of other infectious and noninfectious diseases. Which of the following is the classic triad of findings for this disease?
   A.   Fever, nausea, muscle pain
   B.   Rash, muscle pain, severe headache
   C.   History of tick bite, abdominal pain, diarrhea
   D.   FEVER, RASH, HISTORY OF TICK BITE

Rationale:

   D.   As identified in the literature, this is the classic triad of findings for Rocky Mountain spotted fever. The rash first appears 2 to 5 days after the onset of fever. This normally occurs 5 to 10 days after a tick bite. Younger patients usually develop the rash earlier than older patients. Most often it begins as small, flat, pink, non-itchy spots on the wrists, forearms, and ankles. These spots turn pale when pressure is applied and eventually become raised on the skin. The characteristic red, spotted (petechial) rash of Rocky Mountain spotted fever is usually not seen until the sixth day or later after onset of symptoms. This type of rash occurs in 35% to 60% of patients with the disease. The rash involves the palms or soles in as many as 50% to 80% of patients; however, this distribution may not occur until late in the course of disease.

   A.   The early clinical presentation of Rocky Mountain spotted fever is nonspecific and may resemble a variety of other infectious and noninfectious diseases. These symptoms may be present initially after an incubation period of 5 to 10 days.

   B.   The characteristic rash is a later sign of Rocky Mountain spotted fever. The rash first appears 2 to 5 days after the onset of fever. This normally occurs 5 to 10 days after a tick bite. Muscle pain and severe headache present early in the course of disease

   C.   Abdominal pain and diarrhea are late symptoms of Rocky Mountain spotted fever and do not occur in all patients.

Content Category: Substance Abuse/Toxicology/Environment

References: Abramson & Givner, 1999; 539–540; Archibald & Sexton, 1995; pp.1122–1125.

112.   Which of the following is the major clinical forms of human anthrax?
   A.   Cutaneous and inhalation
   B.   Inhalation and gastrointestinal
   C.   Cutaneous and gastrointestinal
   D.   CUTANEOUS, INHALATION, AND GASTROINTESTINAL

Rationale:

   D.   *Cutaneous:* Most (about 95%) anthrax infections occur when the bacterium enters a cut or abrasion on the skin, such as when the person is handling contaminated wool, hides, leather, or hair products (especially goat hair) of infected animals. Skin infection begins as a raised itchy bump that resembles an insect bite but within 1 to 2 days develops into a vesicle and then a painless ulcer, usually 1–3 cm in diameter, with a characteristic black necrotic area in the center. Lymph glands in the adjacent area may swell. About 20% of untreated cases of cutaneous anthrax result in death. With appropriate antimicrobial therapy, however, deaths are rare.

   Inhalation: Initial symptoms may resemble those of a common cold. After several days, the symptoms may progress to severe breathing problems and shock. Inhalation anthrax is usually fatal.

Gastrointestinal: The GI disease form of anthrax may follow the consumption of contaminated meat and is characterized by an acute inflammation of the intestinal tract. Initial signs and symptoms of nausea, loss of appetite, vomiting, and fever are followed by abdominal pain, vomiting of blood, and severe diarrhea. Intestinal anthrax results in death in 25% to 60% of cases.

A. This answer omits the intestinal form of anthrax.
B. This answer omits the cutaneous form of anthrax.
C. This answer omits the inhalation form of anthrax.

Content Category: Substance Abuse/Toxicology/Environment

References: Smego et al., 1998; pp. 97–102; Suffin et al., 1998; pp. 97–102; Centers for Disease Control, 1999; p. 4.

113.   Symptoms of a systemic reaction to a snake bite include:
A. hypertension.
B. GI DISTURBANCES.
C. petechiae.
D. decreased salivation.

Rationale:

B. Systemic reactions to a snakebite include nausea, vomiting, diaphoresis, syncope, and a metallic or rubber taste. Patients may experience paralysis, difficulty speaking, and visual disturbances as well.
A. Although fear may raise the blood pressure, hypotension is most often noted as a systemic reaction to envenomation.
C. Petechiae may be noted as a local reaction to snakebite.
D. Increased salivation, muscle twitching, and epistaxis may develop as a result of snakebite.

Content Category: Substance Abuse/Toxicology/Environment

Reference: Newberry, 1998.

114.   A 7-year-old boy arrives in the ED stating that he was bitten on the foot while playing outside. He is screaming with pain at the bite mark, nauseated, and weak. He describes severe abdominal pain and spasms in his leg. You suspect that he has been bitten by a:
A. tick.
B. BLACK WIDOW SPIDER.
C. wasp.
D. brown recluse spider.

Rationale:

B. The black widow spider bite is neurotoxic. Systemic symptoms include nausea, vomiting, hypertension, increased temperature, and hyperactive reflexes. People who have been bitten by black widow spiders may also have respiratory difficulties, headache, syncope, and chest and abdominal pain or spasms.
A. A tick bite may cause mild stinging at the site, but it does not cause neurotoxic effects.
C. A wasp sting is a severe, painful sensation and may cause anaphylaxis. Muscle cramping is not common with a wasp sting.
D. The brown recluse spider emits a cytotoxic venom. Symptoms can include local edema, erythema, local ischemia, and tissue necrosis.

Content Category: Substance Abuse/Toxicology/Environment

Reference: Newberry, 1998; pp. 632–633.

115.   Which of the following statements is true about human bites?
A.   Human bites have a decreased risk for cellulitis.
B.   HUMAN BITES HAVE THE HIGHEST RATE OF INFECTION OF ALL BITE INJURIES.
C.   A person who has been bitten by another person should receive antibiotics if signs of infection are present.
D.   Human bites rarely cause deep tissue injury.

Rationale:

B.   Human bites have the highest rate of infection and tissue damage of all bite injuries. The human mouth may harbor over 40 potential pathogens.
A.   Human bites have an increased risk for cellulitis.
C.   Treatment of human bites is similar to that of other bite injuries with the exception that people with human bites should always receive prophylactic antibiotics.
D.   Human bites are frequently accompanied by tissue injuries caused by the mouth's crushing ability.

Content Category: Substance Abuse/Toxicology/Environment
Reference: Newberry, 1998; pp. 632–633.

116.   Early symptoms of anthrax pneumonia include:
A.   abrupt onset, elevated temperature, productive cough.
B.   INSIDIOUS ONSET, MILD FEVER, NONPRODUCTIVE COUGH.
C.   abrupt onset, high fever, productive cough.
D.   fever, chills, cough, hemoptysis.

Rationale:

B.   Insidious onset, mild fever, and nonproductive cough are early manifestations of anthrax pneumonia.
A.   Abrupt onset, elevated temperature, and productive cough are symptoms of pneumococcal pneumonia.
C.   Staphylococcal pneumonia manifests itself with abrupt onset, high fever, and productive cough, which is often bloody with purulent sputum.
D.   Streptococcal pneumonia often causes a fever greater than 102.2° F, chills, cough, and pharyngitis.

Content Category: Substance Abuse/Toxicology/Environment
Reference: Newberry, 1998.

117.   An appropriate nursing diagnosis for a patient who has been bitten by a brown recluse spider bite is:
A.   impaired verbal communication.
B.   impaired gas exchange.
C.   pain related to muscle spasm.
D.   IMPAIRED SKIN INTEGRITY.

Rationale:

D.   Impaired skin integrity is a nursing diagnosis for a patient who has been bitten by a brown recluse spider, whose venom is considered cytotoxic and causes edema, skin inflammation, and tissue destruction.
A.   Verbal communication would not be affected by the bite unless it involved the airway structures.

B. Gas exchange would not be affected unless airway structures were involved in the envenomation.

C. Muscle spasms are commonly seen with bites by black widow spiders but not with those by brown recluse spiders.

Content Category: Substance Abuse/Toxicology/Environment

Reference: ENA, Core Curriculum, 2000.

118.   A 56-year-old man with a known history of depression arrives in your ED complaining of nausea, vomiting, and severe headache. He has severe hypertension. Which type of medication can cause a hypertensive crisis?
  A. Tricyclics
  B. Barbiturates
  C. Sedative-hypnotics
  D. MONOAMINE OXIDASE (MAO) INHIBITORS

Rationale:

D. MAO inhibitors inhibit the breakdown of tyramine. Tyramine buildup in the blood can lead to a hypertensive crisis.

A. Tricyclics can cause hypotension, but not hypertension.

B. Barbiturates can cause hypotension, but not hypertension.

C. Sedative-hypnotics can cause hypotension, but not hypertension.

Content Category: Substance Abuse/Toxicology/Environment

References: ENA, Core Curriculum, 2000; Oman et al., 2001.

119.   Female patients older than 50 years who are taking antipsychotic medications are at risk for which side effect?
  A. Endocrine changes
  B. TARDIVE DYSKINESIA
  C. Photosensitivity
  D. Orthostatic hypotension

Rationale:

B. Women over age 50 who are taking antipsychotics can develop tardive dyskinesia, consisting of rhythmic involuntary movements of the tongue, face, and mouth with protrusion of the tongue and chewing movements. These can progress to irreversible movements.

A. Endocrine changes such as weight gain and edema can occur in any patient who is taking an antipsychotic medication.

C. All patients who are taking antipsychotics should be protected from ultraviolet light.

D. Orthostatic hypotension can occur in any patient who is taking an antipsychotic medication. Such medications should be used cautiously in elderly patients and in those who have cardiovascular disease.

Content Category: Substance Abuse/Toxicology/Environment

Reference: Newberry, 1998.

120. A medication used for controlling the ventricular response rate of a patient with supraventricular tachycardia is:
   A. atropine.
   B. isoproterenol (Isuprel).
   C. labetalol (Normaline).
   D. VERAPAMIL (CALAN).

Rationale:

   D. Verapamil (Calan) is a calcium channel blocker that is used in patients with supraventricular tachycardias as well as rapid heart rates caused by atrial fibrillation, atrial flutter, or atrial tachycardia.
   A. Atropine is used in bradycardia dysrhythmias to block stimulation of the vagus nerve.
   B. Isoproterenol (Isuprel), a beta-adrenergic agonist, may be used to increase cardiac rate.
   C. Labetalol (Normodyne) is a selective adrenergic blocker used for hypertension.

Content Category: Substance Abuse/Toxicology/Environment
Reference: Newberry, 1998.

121. Which of the following would be a CONTRAINDICATION for the administration of activated charcoal?
   A. Hyperactive bowel sounds
   B. Elevated blood pressure
   C. ACETAMINOPHEN (TYLENOL) TOXICITY
   D. Vitamin toxicity

Rationale:

   C. Patients with acetaminophen (Tylenol) toxicity may be treated with N-acetylcysteine (NAC). The charcoal binds with NAC and deactivates it.
   A. Diminished bowel sounds, not hyperactive bowel sounds, are a contraindication to using activated charcoal.
   B. Blood pressure is not affected by the administration of activated charcoal.
   D. Activated charcoal would be indicated in a patient with a vitamin toxicity to absorb any vitamin products that remain in the stomach or intestine.

Content Category: Substance Abuse/Toxicology/Environment
Reference: Newberry, 1998.

122. A patient presents to the ED complaining of fever, chills, headache, and extreme exhaustion. He states that he has been feeling ill since his return from Africa 2 days ago. On examination, you note that the patient has a very swollen, tender lymph gland accompanied by pain. You suspect that the patient has:
   A. African sleeping sickness.
   B. ehrlichiosis.
   C. PLAGUE.
   D. Chagas' disease.

Rationale:

   C. The typical sign of the most common form of human plague is a swollen and very tender lymph gland, accompanied by pain. The swollen gland is called a bubo. Bubonic plague should be suspected with the development of a swollen gland, fever, chills, headache, and extreme exhaustion and if the patient has a history of possible exposure to infected rodents, rabbits, or fleas. A person usually becomes ill with bubonic plague 2 to 6 days after being infected.

A. A bite by the tsetse fly is often painful and can develop into a red sore (chancre). Fever, severe headaches, irritability, extreme fatigue, swollen lymph nodes, and aching muscles and joints are common symptoms of sleeping sickness. Some people develop a skin rash. Progressive confusion, personality changes, slurred speech, seizures, and difficulty in walking and talking occur when infection has invaded the central nervous system.

B. The early clinical presentations of ehrlichiosis may resemble nonspecific signs and symptoms of various other infectious and noninfectious diseases. Patients with ehrlichiosis generally visit a physician in the first week of illness after an incubation period of about 5 to 10 days after the tick bite. Initial symptoms usually include fever, headache, malaise, and muscle aches. Other signs and symptoms may include nausea, vomiting, diarrhea, cough, joint pains, confusion, and occasionally rash.

D. Acute symptoms of Chagas' disease occur in only about 1% of cases. Most people who have been infected do not seek medical attention. The most recognized symptom of acute Chagas' infection is the Romaña's sign: swelling of the eye on one side of the face, usually at the bite wound or where feces were rubbed into the eye. Other symptoms are usually not specific for Chagas' disease infection. These symptoms may include fatigue, fever, enlarged liver or spleen, and swollen lymph glands. Sometimes a rash, loss of appetite, diarrhea, and vomiting occur. In general, symptoms last for 4 to 8 weeks and then disappear even without treatment.

Content Category: Substance Abuse/Toxicology/Environment

References: Campbell & Dennis, 1998; pp. 975–983; Farmer, 1995; pp. 438–448; Kirchoff, 1996; pp. 517–532.

123. Which of the following is the leading cause of vector-borne infectious illness in the United States?
   A. LYME DISEASE
   B. Yellow fever
   C. Dengue fever
   D. West Nile virus

Rationale:

A. Lyme disease is a rapidly emerging vector-borne infectious disease in the United States. More than 128,000 cases have been reported to US health authorities since 1982, when a systematic national surveillance was initiated. Lyme disease now accounts for more than 95% of all reported vector-borne illness in the US.

B. Yellow fever occurs only in Africa and South America. In South America, sporadic infections occur almost exclusively in forestry and agricultural workers from occupational exposure in or near forests.

C. The incidence of dengue fever is variable, depending on epidemic activity. Globally, an estimated 50 to 100 million cases of dengue fever and several hundred thousand cases of dengue hemorrhagic fever are diagnosed per year.

D. West Nile virus has been described in Africa, Europe, the Middle East, west and central Asia, Oceania (subtype Kunjin), and, most recently, North America.

Content Category: Substance Abuse/Toxicology/Environment

Reference: Kalish et al., 1993; pp. 2774–2779.

124.   A 6-year-old child is brought to the ED by his mother 15 minutes after having been stung in the forearm by a bee. On examination, a 2-cm circular lesion that is red, swollen, and tender is observed. The ED nurse knows that this is:
A.   probably an infection.
B.   an anaphylactic reaction.
C.   A NORMAL REACTION.
D.   an indication of serum sickness.

Rationale:

C.   Localized erythema at the site of a bee sting shortly after envenomation is a normal reaction.
A.   Infections generally become evident 48 to 72 hours after the sting. An infection would not be evident 15 minutes after the sting.
B.   Anaphylaxis is a generalized reaction that may include shock, airway obstruction, and skin manifestations.
D.   Serum sickness would not occur after a bee sting.

Content Category: Substance Abuse/Toxicology/Environment

Reference: Newberry, 1998.

125.   The Emergency Medical Treatment and Active Labor Act (EMTALA) includes which of the following situations?
A.   A visitor in the hospital lobby
B.   A hospital employee reporting for work
C.   A WOMAN IN LABOR ARRIVING AT THE HOSPITAL BY TAXICAB
D.   An injured lawn care worker whose condition the physician determines to be stable

Rationale:

C.   A patient in labor is discussed within the EMTALA legislation and defined as an emergency medical condition.
A.   A visitor in the hospital lobby may be included within EMTALA if he or she has been injured and is seen in the ED. EMTALA makes no provision for an uninjured visitor.
B.   A hospital employee without injury is not discussed within EMTALA legislation.
D.   A patient determined to be stable by a screening conducted by a physician may be determined nonemergent and transferred or referred if necessary. EMTALA is in effect until the patient has been screened, appropriate studies have been completed, and the determination that an emergency medical condition does not exist has been made.

Content Category: Professional Issues

Reference: Health Care Financing Administration, 1998.

126.   According to EMTALA, when a patient is transferred to another facility, the sending facility must provide:
A.   copies of a complete listing of charges from the sending facility.
B.   insurance information and worker's compensation information if the patient was injured on the job.
C.   A CERTIFICATE SIGNED BY THE PHYSICIAN CONFIRMING THAT BENEFITS OF THE TRANSFER OUTWEIGH THE RISK OF TRANSFER.
D.   a complete listing of the patient's valuables and personal belongings.

Rationale:

    C. The sending physician must sign a document or chart confirming that the benefits of the transfer outweigh the risk of transfer and that s/he is accepting the responsibility for the patient's safe and appropriate transfer.

    A. Complete fees charged by the sending facility are not part of the transfer packet and are not described in EMTALA.

    B. Insurance information and payment options are not part of EMTALA.

    D. Although a complete listing of valuables should be sent with the patient, EMTALA does not specifically address this issue.

Content Category: Professional Issues

Reference: Frank, 2001; p. 65.

127. In a negligence suit, the plaintiff must prove four key elements in a court of law: duty to the patient, breach of duty by the health care professional, injury resulting from the breach, and:
    A. inadequate education and training of the health care professional.
    B. BREACH OF DUTY IS THE PROXIMATE CAUSE OF INJURY.
    C. documentation inadequate to fully describe the situation that resulted in injury.
    D. incident report incomplete when retrieved by the plaintiff's attorney.

Rationale:

    B. In a negligence suit, breach of duty must be proven to be the proximate cause of the stated injury to the patient.

    A. Although appropriate education and training of the health care professional is necessary to maintain competence, it is not one of the key elements to be proven in a negligence suit.

    C. Complete and accurate documentation is described as the best defense, but is not described as a key component for proof of negligence.

    D. The incident report should be completed in a timely and accurate manner, but should be an internal document, not included as part of the patient care record.

Content Category: Professional Issues

Reference: ENA, 1998.

128. Hospitals that violate EMTALA provisions are subject to:
    A. FINES BY THE FEDERAL GOVERNMENT.
    B. a waiver of the CLIA (Clinical Laboratory Improvement Act) permit.
    C. a complete audit by OSHA.
    D. immediate closure until an investigation is completed.

Rationale:

    A. Under EMTALA, hospitals and physicians are subject to penalties by the federal government if EMTALA provisions are not observed.

    B. Although laboratory permits under CLIA are issued by a federal regulatory body, this permit would not be affected by an EMTALA violation.

    C. A potential EMTALA violation would not trigger a complete audit by OSHA.

    D. EMTALA violations are penalized with substantial fines to both the facility and the physician.

Content Category: Professional Issues

Reference: Frank, 2001; p. 65.

129.   When reviewing a medical record, you note the following documentation: "Patient condition deteriorated and physician notified at 1800." Which of the following statements about this documentation is correct?

    A. The notation is too short.

    B. Abbreviations should be used whenever possible.

    C. Military time is not acceptable in a patient chart.

    D. SPECIFICS ARE MISSING FROM THE DESCRIPTION.

Rationale:

    D. The chart notation should briefly describe the patient's condition and the basis for determining that the condition is deteriorating. Complete and accurate charting will be the best defense if the nurse's actions are questioned.

    A. Although the notation for the patient's chart does appear brief, the major concern is the lack of descriptions concerning the patient's condition. The content of the statement is much more important than its length.

    B. Accepted abbreviations may be used in charting, in accordance with accepted hospital policy, but that is not the important issue here.

    C. Military time is acceptable in charting.

Content Category: Professional Issues

Reference: ENA, Core Curriculum, 2000.

130.   Which of the following situations is considered an exception to required parental consent for treatment of a 14-year-old patient?

    A. Unemancipated minors

    B. Elevated alcohol level

    C. GONORRHEA

    D. Commission of a crime

Rationale:

    C. The age of consent varies in accordance with various state statutes. Most states have laws that allow minors of any age to consent to birth control counseling and the treatment of sexually transmitted diseases such as gonorrhea.

    A. If a minor is emancipated (economically independent or married), the minor may consent to treatment regardless of his or her age.

    B. An elevated alcohol level does not change the age of consent for treatment.

    D. The commission of a crime does not change the age of consent for treatment.

Content Category: Professional Issues

Reference: ENA, Core Curriculum, 2000.

Questions 131–134

A 17-year-old female presents to the ED with a chief complaint of left-sided pelvic pain. The patient states that the pain started suddenly 3 hours ago and has become constant, sharp, and very severe. Her last menstrual period was approximately 6 weeks ago, but she has been spotting for several days. The patient states that she is sexually active. Initial vital signs are BP 120/70 mmHg, pulse 128/min, respirations 22/min, and temperature 100° F (37.8° C). You suspect ectopic pregnancy.

131. Additional information that you should obtain includes the presence of any risk factors. Risk factors for the development of an ectopic pregnancy include:
    A. a history of pelvic inflammatory disease (PID).
    B. fertility drug use.
    C. previous tubal ligation.
    D. ALL OF THE ABOVE.

Rationale:

D. A history of PID, the use of fertility drugs, and a previous tubal ligation are among the risk factors for the development of an ectopic pregnancy. Other risk factors include previous surgical procedures on the fallopian tube, previous ectopic pregnancy, use of an intrauterine contraceptive device (IUD), induced abortion, peritubal adhesions, exposure in utero to diethyl stilbestrol (DES), and in vitro fertilization.

A. Pelvic inflammatory disease is the most common risk factor is the development of ectopic pregnancy. PID has been reported to increase the risk of ectopic pregnancy by sixfold to sevenfold. Each episode of PID increases the probability of the development of an ectopic pregnancy because of exacerbated damage to the mucosa of the fallopian tube. The end result is a mechanical and anatomic alteration in the tubal transport mechanism.

B. Fertility drugs lead to altered tubal motility from the effects of estrogen and progesterone.

C. The ligation procedure leads to tissue destruction in the fallopian tube, which in turn leads to an alteration in the tubal transport mechanism.

Content Category: GU/GYN/OB

References: ENA, Core Curriculum, 2000; Tintinalli et al., 2000; pp. 686–693.

132. What is the appropriate triage category for this patient?
    A. Urgent
    B. EMERGENT
    C. Nonurgent
    D. Referral to fast track

Rationale:

B. A suspected ectopic pregnancy in a patient with severe pain and tachycardia is an emergent situation. Spontaneous tubal rupture may occur, with resultant intraperitoneal hemorrhage and shock. Ectopic pregnancy is the leading cause of maternal death in the first trimester of pregnancy and the second leading cause of maternal mortality overall.

A. "Emergent" is not an appropriate triage category for this patient. A delay in diagnosis and definitive care would increase the risk for morbidity and mortality.

C. "Nonurgent" is not an appropriate triage category for this patient. A delay in diagnosis and definitive care would increase the risk for morbidity and mortality.

D. The patient should not be referred to the fast track. A delay in diagnosis and definitive care would increase the risk for morbidity and mortality.

Content Category: GU/GYN/OB

Reference: ENA, Core Curriculum, 2000.

133.   The most accurate diagnostic test for an ectopic pregnancy includes:
   A. quantitative urinary BhCG.
   B. TRANSVAGINAL ULTRASOUND.
   C. a complete blood count (CBC).
   D. serum electrolyte levels.

Rationale:

   B. Transvaginal ultrasound plays an essential role in the diagnosis of ectopic pregnancy. Use of transvaginal scanning allows earlier detection of an intrauterine or ectopic pregnancy. In a patient with a confirmed pregnancy that is suspected to be ectopic, the primary goal of ultrasound is to determine whether an intrauterine pregnancy is present. No further diagnostic tests are needed when sonographic findings confirm or are highly suggestive of ectopic pregnancy.
   A. Quantitative urinary BhCG is used as part of the overall diagnostic approach to raise or lower the suspicion for ectopic pregnancy but does not provide the information necessary to confirm an ectopic vs intrauterine pregnancy. A urinary pregnancy test is a quick and accurate diagnostic test used to confirm a pregnancy that is suspected to be ectopic. Urine pregnancy tests can be preformed rapidly at the bedside.
   C. A complete blood count would not provide the necessary information to diagnose an ectopic pregnancy. It is important, however, to assess the patient's baseline hemodynamic status as related to hemoglobin and hematocrit values in case the patient's uterus ruptures, resulting in an intraabdominal hemorrhage. Usually ectopic pregnancies do not produce significant anemia at the time of presentation. Orthostatic vital signs are an indicator of acute volume loss and should be performed in the ED. The white blood cell count is also an important clinical parameter in the overall differential diagnosis if infection is suspected.
   D. Serum electrolyte levels would not provide any of the essential information required to diagnose an ectopic pregnancy.

Content Category: GU/GYN/OB

References: ENA, Core Curriculum, 2000; Tintinalli et al., 2000; pp. 686–693.

134.   The most appropriate nursing diagnosis for this patient is:
   A. fear.
   B. pain.
   C. RISK FOR FLUID VOLUME DEFICIT.
   D. risk for injury.

Rationale:

   C. A ruptured ectopic pregnancy may lead to significant intraabdominal hemorrhage and shock. Therefore, risk for fluid volume deficit is the highest-priority nursing diagnosis for this patient.
   A. Fear is an important secondary nursing diagnosis for this patient, but not of the highest priority.
   B. Pain is an important secondary nursing diagnosis for this patient, but not of the highest priority.
   D. Risk for injury is an important secondary nursing diagnosis for this patient, but not of the highest priority.

Content Category: GU/GYN/OB

Reference: ENA, Core Curriculum, 2000.

Questions 135–137

A 39-year-old female presents to the ED with the chief complaints of vaginal bleeding, cramping pelvic pain, and low back pain for several hours. The patient states that she is 8 weeks pregnant by dates. Her pregnancy has been confirmed by a quantitative BhCG in her physician's office. This is her fourth pregnancy and she has 3 children. Her second pregnancy resulted in the birth of twins. She had a spontaneous abortion 1 year ago. She states that she has been using 1 pad per hour for the past several hours but has not passed any blood or tissue.

135.   When documenting the patient's pregnancy history, the ED nurse should write:
A.   GRAVIDA 4, PARA 3, ABORTION 1, LIVING 3.
B.   gravida 5, para 3, abortion 1, living 3.
C.   gravida 5, para 2, abortion 1, living 3.
D.   gravida 4, para 2, abortion 1, living 3.

Rationale:

A.   "Gravida" is the total number of pregnancies, including the current pregnancy. This patient has had 4 pregnancies, including the current one, and is therefore "gravida 4." "Para" refers to the number of deliveries of infants, whether born alive or dead, who have developed in utero past the point of viability. Viability is considered to be birthweight > 500 g or past 20 weeks of gestation. Multiple births are considered 1 parous event. This patient has delivered 3 children. Therefore, she is "para 3." "Abortion" refers to elective or spontaneous termination of a pregnancy before the point of viability. This patient has had 1 spontaneous abortion before the age of viability. Therefore, the correct term is "abortion 1." "Living" refers to the number of living children that the patient has at the present time. Since the patient has 3 children, the correct term is "living 3."
B.   The patient has been pregnant 4 times, not 5.
C.   The patient has been pregnant 4 times, not 5, and has delivered after 3, not 2, viable pregnancies.
D.   The patient has delivered after 3, not 2, viable pregnancies.

Content Category: GU/GYN/OB
Reference: ENA, 1996.

136.   The physical examination reveals a moderate amount of uterine bleeding without clots or tissue. The cervix is closed. Transvaginal ultrasound reveals an intrauterine pregnancy with a gestational age of approximately 7 weeks and with positive fetal cardiac motion. The patient's condition is classified as a(n):
A.   complete abortion.
B.   THREATENED ABORTION.
C.   incomplete abortion.
D.   missed abortion.

Rationale:

B.   Threatened abortion is characterized by mild to moderate vaginal bleeding and uterine cramping with a closed cervical os.
A.   A complete abortion is characterized by mild to moderate vaginal bleeding, mild uterine cramping with a closed cervical os, and complete expulsion of the products of conception.
C.   An incomplete abortion is characterized by heavy vaginal bleeding, severe uterine cramping with an open cervical os and tissue in the cervix, and incomplete expulsion of the products of conception.
D.   A missed abortion is characterized by slight vaginal bleeding and absent uterine contractions with a closed cervical os and prolonged retention of dead products of conception.

Content Category: GU/GYN/OB
Reference: ENA, Core Curriculum, 2000.

137. You are preparing the patient to be discharged to home, accompanied by her husband. Discharge teaching should include all of the following EXCEPT:
    A. MAINTAIN BED REST FOR THE REMAINDER OF THE PREGNANCY.
    B. Avoid the use of tampons. Use sanitary pads only.
    C. Pelvic rest until bleeding and cramping subside.
    D. Return to the ED or obstetrician if bleeding or pain increases.

Rationale:

    A. Bed rest is advised for the first 24 to 48 hours or until bleeding and cramping subside. However, low-level activity and bed rest have not been proven effective in preventing miscarriage.
    B. Tampons are to be avoided to minimize the development of an infection.
    C. Pelvic rest is advised to help prevent infection.
    D. The patient is advised to return to the ED or to follow up with her obstetrician if bleeding (more than 1 pad per hour), cramping, or both increase because the patient may be losing the pregnancy and is at risk for hemorrhage.

Content Category: GU/GYN/OB

References: ENA, Core Curriculum, 2000; Howell et al., 1998; pp. 1295–1305.

138. Which of the following nursing interventions would be a priority for the ED patient with hyperemesis gravidarum?
    A. INFUSION OF D5W AT A RATE OF 150 ML/HOUR.
    B. Evaluating baseline laboratory studies of serum electrolytes.
    C. Monitoring urinary output and dipstick urine for ketones.
    D. Administering antiemetics as ordered.

Rationale:

    A. Initial treatment consists of the rapid administration of an isotonic fluid such as lactated Ringer's solution or normal saline solution for volume replacement. Subsequent fluids should include the addition of glucose such as D5NS at a slower rate to reverse dehydration and ketonuria. Because D5W is a hypotonic solution, it is not the fluid of choice for the volume depletion and starvation that may be caused by hyperemesis gravidarum.
    B. The evaluation of baseline serum electrolytes is indicated to help determine whether the patient is acidotic, alkalotic, or dehydrated. Prolonged vomiting may lead to the loss of potassium, sodium, and chloride. In addition, blood urea nitrogen (BUN) levels may be elevated in the dehydrated patient.
    C. Monitoring urinary output is an important indicator of hydration status. The presence of ketonuria is an early sign of starvation. The increase or decrease in the amount of ketonuria is an important clinical parameter to assess the patient's response to treatment.
    D. Antiemetics may be administered if the patient remains nauseated or has persistent vomiting.

Content Category: GU/GYN/OB

Reference: Howell et al., 1998; pp. 1295–1305.

139. Risk factors for the development of hypertension during pregnancy include:
    A. maternal age greater than 40 years.
    B. African-American heritage.
    C. multiple gestation.
    D. ALL OF THE ABOVE.

Rationale:

D. Age over 40 years (A), African-American heritage (B), and multiple gestation (C) are all risk factors for the development of hypertension during pregnancy. Other such risk factors include nulliparity, prepregnancy hypertension, chronic renal disease, diabetes mellitus, gestational trophoblastic disease, personal or family history of hypertension during pregnancy, systemic lupus erythematosus, and vascular disease.

Content Category: GU/GYN/OB

Reference: ENA, Core Curriculum, 2000.

140. A 34-year-old female presents to the ED after having been involved in a motor vehicle collision. She is 34 weeks pregnant and has sustained blunt trauma to the chest and abdomen. All of the following interventions are appropriate EXCEPT:
    A. Initiate high-flow oxygen.
    B. Elevate the backboard 15 degrees in the left lateral position.
    C. Initiate 2 large-bore IVs with normal saline or Ringer's lactate solution.
    D. PERFORM A PELVIC EXAM TO ASSESS FOR POSSIBLE UTERINE BLEEDING.

Rationale:

D. A pelvic exam is not indicated in the immediate resuscitation phase of a pregnant trauma patient.

A. High-flow oxygen should be administered. A pregnant woman is likely to become hypoxic rapidly. Pregnant patients have a decreased functional residual capacity and therefore are less tolerant of hypoxia. The fetus is even more physiologically sensitive to hypoxia than the mother.

B. The backboard should be elevated 15 degrees in the left lateral position to displace the gravid uterus from compressing the inferior vena cava, possibly leading to a decrease in preload and a subsequent decrease in cardiac output. This condition is called supine hypotensive syndrome.

C. Fluid resuscitation should be more aggressive in the pregnant trauma patient than in one who is not pregnant. The physiologic change of maternal hypervolemia of pregnancy may delay the early recognition of shock. A pregnant patient may lose 30% of blood volume before showing any signs of shock.

Content Category: GU/GYN/OB

Reference: Hanlon & Duriseti, 2001; pp. 1–10.

141. The goals in treating all forms of shock include:
    A. restoration of anaerobic metabolism.
    B. RESTORATION OF OXYGENATION AND TISSUE PERFUSION.
    C. administration of dopamine (Intropin) to reverse acidosis.
    D. administration of D5W for fluid volume resuscitation.

Rationale:

B. Shock is reduced cellular perfusion that causes disruption of normal metabolic processes. The end result is cellular hypoxia, anaerobic metabolism, and cell death. Therefore, goals for treatment of any shock state include the restoration of oxygenation and perfusion to correct cellular hypoxia and stop anaerobic metabolism.

A. Shock *causes* anaerobic metabolism.

C. Dopamine is used at low doses as a renal protectant and at higher doses for vasoconstriction. It is not used to reverse acidosis but to increase blood pressure and support tissue perfusion.

D. Administration of isotonic crystalloid solutions to expand vascular volume includes such solutions as lactated Ringer's and 0.9% normal saline solution. D5W is a hypotonic solution that expands vascular volume.

Content Category: Shock/Trauma

References: ENA, Core Curriculum, 2000; American Association of Critical Care Nurses, 1998.

142.   Which stage of shock results in widespread cellular destruction and does not respond to any form of aggressive treatment?
   A.   Compensated (nonprogressive) shock
   B.   Uncompensated (progressive) shock
   C.   Irrefractory shock
   D.   IRREVERSIBLE (REFRACTORY) SHOCK

Rationale:

   D.   By definition, irreversible shock is the final stage of shock at which no treatment can reverse the process. The cellular destruction at this stage is so massively widespread that it is impossible to identify the different types of shock.
   A.   Compensated shock occurs when the body is initially responding to reduced cellular perfusion through vasoconstriction and activation of the sympathetic nervous system.
   B.   Uncompensated shock occurs after the compensatory mechanisms have begun to fail. Cellular perfusion to vital organs drops. Uncompensated shock may be reversed with aggressive treatment.
   C.   There is no such thing as irrefractory shock.

Content Category: Shock/Trauma

Reference: ENA, Core Curriculum, 2000.

143.   Assessment of the patient in shock should include which of the following in the primary survey?
   A.   Abdominal sounds
   B.   LEVEL OF CONSCIOUSNESS
   C.   Areas of deformity
   D.   Complete neurologic exam

Rationale:

   B.   Respiratory effort and efficacy of breathing should be assessed in the primary survey, as they determine the effectiveness of breathing. Administration of supplemental oxygen is included in the treatment of all forms of shock.
   A.   Bowel sounds are noted in the secondary assessment. The presence or absence of bowel sounds does not change the course of treatment with regard to life threats revealed in the primary survey.
   C.   Although noting areas of extremity deformity is an important aspect of assessment, such findings do not alter the course of treatment. The primary survey is geared to addressing life treats and intervening.
   D.   A complete neurologic exam may be important later in the exam if the patient has suffered a head or spinal cord injury, but only a limited neurologic exam should be completed in a primary survey.

Content Category: Shock/Trauma

Reference: ENA, Core Curriculum, 2000.

144.   Typical vital sign changes that occur in uncompensated (progressive) shock include:
   A.   a widening pulse pressure.
   B.   bradycardia.
   C.   decreased capillary refill time.
   D.   NARROWED PULSE PRESSURE.

Rationale:

 D. As the sympathetic nervous system is stimulated, catecholamines circulate and vasoconstriction occurs. Vasoconstriction raises the diastolic blood pressure, causing a narrowed pulse pressure.
 A. Widening pulse pressure is not a change that occurs in shock.
 B. Bradycardia does not typically occur in progressive shock because of the stimulation of the sympathetic nervous system.
 C. Capillary refill time is delayed in uncompensated shock.

Content Category: Shock/Trauma

Reference: ENA, Core Curriculum, 2000.

145. A 78-year-old patient who was involved in a major car crash was brought to your ED. The paramedics' report states that she was trapped in the vehicle and sustained a left femur fracture as well as closed fractures of the left forearm and pelvis. You expect this patient to be in hypovolemic shock because:
 A. older adults are normally anemic and the fractures have contributed to blood loss.
 B. closed forearm fractures can cause significant blood loss in any trauma patient.
 C. IMPAIRED RESPONSE TO PHYSIOLOGIC CHANGES CAUSES OLDER ADULTS TO TOLERATE BLOOD LOSS LESS WELL.
 D. the systemic body failure common in older adults makes them poor candidates for resuscitation.

Rationale:

 C. The losses of reserve volume and of catecholamine response prevent compensation mechanisms from aiding such patients. Typically, shock is poorly tolerated by older adults because of their lack of compensatory reserve.
 A. Older adults are not normally anemic.
 B. Closed forearm fractures are not commonly a cause of shock from blood loss.
 D. Older adults typically maintain good health and are active members of the community.

Content Category: Shock/Trauma

Reference: ENA, Core Curriculum, 2000.

146. A 42-year-old male patient presents via ambulance with a chief complaint of vomiting blood. Vital signs are BP 70/palpation, HR 128/min, and respirations 38/min. The patient's level of consciousness is confused. You conclude that your patient has which category of volume loss/hemorrhage?
 A. Class I
 B. Class II
 C. CLASS III
 D. Class IV

Rationale:

 C. In Class III volume loss/hemorrhage, blood loss typically is progressive and can be caused by significant and continued blood loss from solid organ injury. Class III volume loss typically involves hypotension associated with a heart rate > 120/min, a respiratory rate in the 30s/min, delayed capillary refill, and a decrease in sensorium.
 A. Class I volume loss/hemorrhage is compensated fluid loss. Signs of generalized failure of compensatory mechanisms (such as changes in vital signs, as noted in the scenario) do not occur.
 B. Class II volume loss/hemorrhage typically does not involve a significant drop in blood pressure or the drastic changes in sensorium as noted in this patient.
 D. Class IV volume loss/hemorrhage, the loss of more than 40% of blood volume, presents as irreversible (refractory) shock.

Content Category: Shock/Trauma

Reference: ENA, Core Curriculum, 2000.

147.   Your 36-year-old trauma patient has been diagnosed with a severe liver laceration. Initial vital signs are BP 82/palpation, pulse 126/min, and respirations 34/min. His level of consciousness is "confused." As the ED nurse, you anticipate that volume replacement will include:
   A. 0.3% normal saline.
   B. 0.9% normal saline.
   C. LACTATED RINGER'S SOLUTION AND BLOOD PRODUCTS.
   D. 3% normal saline.

Rationale:

   C. Lactated Ringer's solution and blood products expand vascular volume, replace hemoglobin losses, and restore oxygen-carrying capacity.
   A. This is incorrect because 0.3% normal saline is a hypotonic solution. It does not expand vascular volume, but contributes to tissue swelling.
   B. Although 0.9% normal saline is an isotonic crystalloid, it would not be sufficient to replace fluid losses in Class III volume loss/hemorrhage.
   D. This is incorrect because 3% normal saline does not aid in carrying oxygen to the cells, a primary goal of treatment for Class III volume loss/hemorrhage.

Content Category: Shock/Trauma

Reference: ENA, Core Curriculum, 2000.

148.   Blood products that are about to be administered to a patient with hemorrhagic shock should be warmed to prevent:
   A. a transfusion reaction.
   B. metabolic alkalosis.
   C. hypokalemia.
   D. HYPOTHERMIA.

Rationale:

   D. Patients receiving multiple transfusions are at risk for hypothermia, which impairs the coagulation cascade and exacerbates bleeding.
   A. Warming blood would not prevent a transfusion reaction.
   B. Patients receiving multiple transfusions are at risk for the development of metabolic acidosis, not metabolic alkalosis.
   C. Patients receiving multiple transfusions are at risk for hyperkalemia, not hypokalemia.

Content Category: Shock/Trauma

References: Kirkpatrick et al., 1999; pp. 333–343; Cinat et al., 1999; pp. 964–970.

149.   How much crystalloid should be given per bolus for the pediatric patient presenting in shock?
   A. 10 ml/kg
   B. 20 ML/KG
   C. 25 ml/kg
   D. 40 ml/kg

Rationale:

B. The appropriate amount of crystalloid bolus to replace fluid losses in shock is 20 ml/kg.
A. This (10 ml/kg) is the amount of bolus to be given when estimating blood replacement.
C. This (25 ml/kg) would constitute too great a volume per bolus.
D. This (40 ml/kg) is too great a volume of crystalloid to replace fluid losses in shock.

Content Category: Shock/Trauma

Reference: ENA, Core Curriculum, 2000.

150. Your trauma patient remains in shock despite aggressive fluid resuscitation. You note a distended abdomen and dropping blood pressure. Your patient is too unstable to be sent for a computed tomography (CT) scan. You anticipate that the physician will perform or order:
A. a flat plate x-ray of the abdomen.
B. DIAGNOSTIC PERITONEAL LAVAGE (DPL).
C. a peritoneal tap.
D. a pleural needle decompression.

Rationale:

B. If the patient is too unstable to be transported to a location for a CT scan and intraabdominal bleeding is suspected, DPL or bedside ultrasound (FAST scan) can assist in determining the need for surgical intervention.
A. Although x-rays of the abdomen may determine free air, the dropping blood pressure and continued distention of the abdomen should be clues to assess for intraabdominal bleeding.
C. A peritoneal tap consists of inserting a needle into the 4 abdominal quadrants and attempting to aspirate fluids. This is not a recommended therapy according to Advanced Trauma Life Support Guidelines.
D. The concern over possible intraabdominal bleeding without evidence of intrathoracic injury makes performing a pleural needle decompression inappropriate.

Content Category: Shock/Trauma

References: Ballard et al., 1999; pp. 145–151; American College of Surgeons, 1997.

Examination 1:
Self-Diagnostic Profile

Instructions

Step 1: Check your answers against the correct answers provided in Part 2 of this chapter. Then calculate your total score.

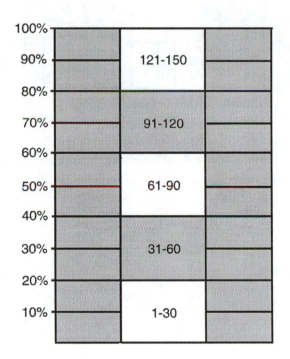

Figure 1: Total Score

Step 2: For each category of the practice examination, determine the number of items that you answered correctly and plot that number in Figure 2. The result will assist you in diagnosing your areas of knowledge strength and in determing which areas benefit from review.

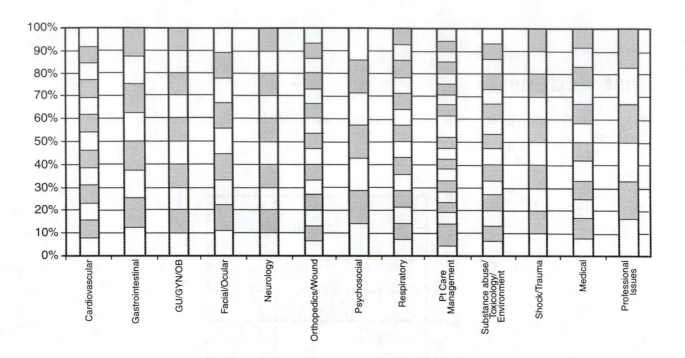

Figure 2: Practice Examination Content Areas

Practice Examination 2

• • • • • • • • • • • • • • • • • • Part 1 •

1. Intestinal perforation, hemorrhage, and toxic megacolon are all complications of:
    A. ulcerative colitis.
    B. Crohn's disease.
    C. gastritis.
    D. peritonitis.

2. Which of the following laboratory results would be important to consider in evaluating the patient with acute pancreatitis for complications?
    A. Serum calcium level
    B. Serum glutamate pyruvate transaminase (SGPT) level
    C. Stool for occult blood
    D. Serum blood urea nitrogen (BUN)/creatinine ratio

3. The parents of a 2-week-old breastfed infant present to the ED complaining that their infant has a "stomach bug" and needs treatment. The infant has been having 4 to 6 yellow mustard-colored stools per day for the past several days. The parents report these stools as loose. All serious causes for the reported problem are eliminated. The best response, based on an understanding of gastroenteritis, is:
    A. "Your child does not have a fever and therefore does not have gastroenteritis."
    B. "Gastroenteritis is very rare in infants less than 3 months of age."
    C. "We will need to start intravenous fluid therapy for your infant."
    D. "Breastfed infants usually have frequent loose, yellow stools."

4. The patient who is being discharged with a diagnosis of irritable bowel syndrome should be instructed to AVOID:
    A. sorbitol-containing foods.
    B. spicy foods.
    C. high-fiber foods.
    D. high-fat foods.

5. A 54-year-old male arrives in the ED complaining of anorexia and abdominal pain. Assessment reveals jaundice and a firm, lumpy area in the right upper quadrant upon palpation. The patient admits to a history of alcohol abuse. The ED nurse suspects that his diagnosis is:
    A. gallbladder attack.
    B. gastroenteritis.
    C. esophageal varices.
    D. cirrhosis.

6. You are caring for a 30-year-old female victim of a motor vehicle accident. Chest x-ray shows rib fractures of the right 8 to10 ribs and a right-sided pneumothorax. You are concerned that she may also have an injury of the:
   A. spleen.
   B. liver.
   C. kidney.
   D. stomach.

7. Upon receiving the results of diagnostic studies on the patient with bowel obstruction, the ED nurse is most likely to read which findings?
   A. Ultrasound examination shows thickened cecum.
   B. Radiographic examination shows dilated, fluid-filled loops of bowel.
   C. Barium swallow shows "string sign" or presence of narrow pylorus.
   D. Erect chest x-ray reveals free gas under the diaphragm.

8. A 32-year-old male comes into the ED at 12:00 a.m. complaining of vomiting and diarrhea. Additional history reveals that he ate shellfish earlier in the evening. He further complains of cramps and feeling weak. Vital signs are BP 100/70, HR 96/min, respirations 24/min, and temperature 100.4° F (38.0° C). When asked how many stools he has had, he replies, "Seven or eight." The priority nursing diagnosis for this patient is:
   A. pain related to abdominal cramping.
   B. fluid volume deficit related to vomiting/diarrhea.
   C. risk for fluid volume deficit.
   D. risk for fluid volume imbalance.

Questions 9 and 10

A 19-year-old male patient presents to the ED accompanied by his mother. He is disheveled and unshaven. He is wearing a sweatband with papers stuffed in it around his head. His mother states that he has become progressively disorganized and has been hearing voices. Upon questioning, he tells you that he is a Martian. In the middle of a sentence he begins to giggle, talk to himself, and pace. His mother states that he hasn't taken his thioridazine (Mellaril) for a few weeks.

9. You suspect a diagnosis of:
   A. conversion disorder.
   B. bipolar disorder.
   C. panic disorder.
   D. schizophrenia.

10. The most appropriate medication for this patient is:
    A. fluoxetine hydrochloride (Prozac).
    B. lithium carbonate (Eskalith).
    C. lorazepam (Ativan).
    D. haloperidol (Haldol).

11. A man who has just been fired from his job for drinking is brought to the ED by police after threatening to stab his wife with a knife. He is in handcuffs and admits to drinking a six-pack of beer today. The priority nursing diagnosis is:
    A. violence, risk for.
    B. ineffective coping.
    C. grieving, dysfunctional.
    D. family processes, altered: alcoholism.

12. A 48-year-old female presents with a chief complaint of intermittent palpitations, chest tightness, and choking sensations. She reports having had these symptoms for about 6 weeks and states that the episodes have become more frequent. Triage assessment reveals an intact airway and skin cool and slightly diaphoretic to touch. Vital signs are BP 168/72, HR 118/min, respirations 26/min, and temperature 99.2°F (37.3°C). The patient denies chest tightness, palpitations, and choking sensations. Diagnostic evaluation for cardiac disease is negative. Further assessment of this patient by the ED nurse reveals that she has recently been divorced and has relocated to this community, which is a substantial distance from her social support system. She has not been able to find employment that meets her career goals. Effectiveness of the plan of care for this patient will be demonstrated by:
    A. the patient's willingness to enter a cardiac rehabilitation program.
    B. A decrease in systolic blood pressure, pulse, and respiratory rate.
    C. An increase in the number of ED visits precipitated by palpitations and chest tightness.
    D. the patient's request for anxiolytic medications.

13. A 35-year-old woman has just been brought into the ED by the police after having been sexually assaulted. The patient is alert. Initial assessment reveals bruises and abrasions on her face, breasts, arms, and hands. She makes minimal eye contact with the ED nurse and speaks only in response to questions. The ED nurse should prepare the patient for which of the following diagnostic procedures in addition to the evidence collection examination?
    A. Pregnancy test, HIV test, hepatitis B screen, STD screen
    B. STD screen, pregnancy test, DNA testing, HIV test
    C. Hepatitis screen, CBC, routine chemistries
    D. HIV test, toxicology screen, CBC, DNA testing

14. A 25-year-old male is brought to the ED after a motor vehicle crash. He was a restrained driver whose vehicle ran out of control and struck a stone embankment. The front seat passenger, his girlfriend, was not restrained and was ejected through the windshield on impact. She was pronounced dead at the scene of the crash. As the ED nurse performs primary and secondary assessments on this patient, he insists that he must see his girlfriend and demands to know when the police will bring her to visit him. Primary and secondary assessments reveal minor contusions and abrasions. The patient has completed his evaluation process and the physician states that he is ready to be discharged. While the emergency nurse is reviewing the discharge instructions with this patient, he says, "Stop what you're doing and get this IV out of me! I need to find my girlfriend. The police and ambulance crew told me she didn't make it, but I know she's okay." The emergency nurse refers this patient to a crisis intervention team. Despite much effort, the team is unable to assist him. The ED nurse prepares for:
    A. inpatient admission.
    B. sedative hypnotic therapy.
    C. antidepressant therapy.
    D. referral to community resources.

15. Patients who experience panic attacks often complain of:
    A. palpitations, shortness of breath, and dizziness.
    B. irritability and anger and speak in a loud voice.
    C. headaches, irritability, and lack of energy.
    D. tiredness, worthlessness, and difficulty thinking.

16. Effective staffing of the ED is best defined as:
    A. a staffing plan with equal nursing staff on all shifts.
    B. variable staffing according to patient census flows.
    C. standard staffing, 7 days a week, without peaks.
    D. longer hours and fewer worked days per staff member

17.   The ED nurse educator develops competency-based orientation for experienced nurses in the ED. Determination of clinical competence is demonstrated when:
    A. the nurse preceptor validates the nurse's ability to perform skills safely.
    B. the nurse has a Certified Emergency Nurse (CEN) card.
    C. the nurse has attended a Pediatric Advanced Life Support (PALS) course and scored high on the exam.
    D. The nurse has attended an Emergency Nurse Pediatric Course (ENPC) and cared for a pediatric patient.

18.   Which of the following situations is reported to law enforcement in states with mandatory reporting laws?
    A. Animal bite
    B. Elder abuse
    C. Erratic behavior
    D. Homelessness

19.   Root cause analysis is a process for identifying basic or causal factors that underlie variation in performance, including sentinel events. A root cause analysis focuses on:
    A. processes and systems.
    B. individual performance.
    C. equipment function.
    D. policies and procedures.

20.   Current trends in assessing quality in health care are based on measuring the performance of the organization against:
    A. predetermined norms and standards of care.
    B. patient satisfaction results.
    C. outcomes of patient care.
    D. definitions from third-party payers.

21.   A nurse who attempts to render care without consent from the patient and inadvertently causes injury to the patient may be guilty of:
    A. assault.
    B. malpractice.
    C. negligence.
    D. battery.

22.   What is the case-fatality rate for persons infected with *Bacillus anthracis* (anthrax) acquired by inhalation?
    A. 25%
    B. 50%
    C. 75%
    D. $\geq 90\%$

23.   Botulism is a rare but serious paralytic illness caused by a nerve toxin that is produced by the bacterium *Clostridium botulinum*. Which of the following are the most common types of botulism?
    A. Infant, wound
    B. Foodborne
    C. Wound, infant, foodborne
    D. Foodborne, wound

24. How is Lyme disease treated?
    A. Antibiotic treatment with doxycycline or amoxicillin for 7 to 10 days
    B. Antibiotic treatment with cefuroxime axetil or erythromycin for 7 to 10 days
    C. There is no treatment; the disease must run its course.
    D. Antibiotic treatment with doxycycline or amoxicillin for 3 to 4 weeks

25. Plague is usually transmitted to humans by:
    A. indirect contact.
    B. respiratory contact
    C. direct contact.
    D. sexual contact.

26. A 79-year-old patient decides to stop taking digoxin (Lanoxin), prescribed for an irregularly irregular fast heart rate. Before the patient discontinued the medication, pulse was noted to be 92 and regular. The patient is at greatest risk for:
    A. cerebrovascular accident.
    B. pulmonary edema.
    C. renal failure.
    D. profound bradycardia.

27. A patient presents to the ED with a history of pesticide ingestion. Which of the following signs and symptoms should the ED nurse anticipate?
    A. Diarrhea, excessive salivation, vomiting, urinary incontinence
    B. Hot flushed skin, agitation, dilated pupils, dry mucous membranes
    C. Hallucinations, tachycardia, loss of control over sensory input
    D. Dizziness, headache, nausea and vomiting, red mucous membranes

28. A patient was admitted to the ED with subacute onset of progressive dizziness, blurred vision, slurred speech, difficulty swallowing, and nausea. Findings on examination included ptosis, extraocular palsies, facial paralysis, palatal weakness, and impaired gag reflex. The patient also had partially healed superficial knee wounds incurred while hunting 5 days earlier. The patient reported that during the 24 hours before onset of symptoms, he had eaten home-canned green beans and a stew containing roast beef and potatoes. Based on the clinical manifestations, you suspect:
    A. myasthenia gravis.
    B. organophosphate poisoning.
    C. Guillain-Barré syndrome.
    D. botulism.

29. The key antidote for acetaminophen poisoning is:
    A. naloxone (Narcan).
    B. glucagon.
    C. N-acetylcysteine (Mucomyst).
    D. atropine.

30. You are caring for a patient in the ED who has ingested 2000 mg (20 100-mg tablets) of amitriptyline (Elavil). While caring for this patient, you would expect which of the following?
    A. Hyperactive effect with increased excitability
    B. Premature ventricular contractions on the cardiac monitor
    C. Constricted pupils with slight variation in reactivity to light
    D. Oliguria and increased salivation

31.   A patient is exposed to a significant dose of radiation at work. He presents to the ED for treatment. He is immediately decontaminated with water and specimens are collected to determine any remaining radiation. The ED nurse would know that the patient had experienced significant exposure if:
A. he glowed when the lights were turned off.
B. he developed nausea, vomiting, and bloody diarrhea.
C. his blood pressure remained high after decontamination.
D. Geiger counters were unable to be calibrated.

32.   An adult patient takes an overdose of acetylsalicylic acid (aspirin). What is the average time for peak serum levels to occur?
A. 15 to 30 minutes
B. 1 hour
C. 90 minutes
D. 2 to 4 hours

33.   Host factors associated with severe or fatal Rocky Mountain spotted fever include:
A. advanced age, female sex, chronic alcohol abuse, Caucasian race.
B. male sex, glucose-6-phosphate dehydrogenase deficiency, chronic alcohol abuse, advanced age, African-American race.
C. glucose-6-phosphate dehydrogenase deficiency, male sex, advanced age.
D. African-American race, female sex, chronic alcohol abuse, advanced age.

34.   Which of the following is highest priority for a near-drowning victim brought to the ED?
A. Hypoxemia
A. Pneumonia
B. Cardiac dysrhythmias
C. Hypothermia

35.   What are the three principal routes of exposure for chemical hazardous materials?
A. Indirect contact, injection, direct contact
B. Rural, urban, suburban
C. Feet, hands, lungs
D. Inhalation, skin absorption, direct contact

36.   Information about any hazardous chemicals kept in the ED should be found in which of the following?
A. Poison control center
B. Material Safety Data Sheets
C. Joint Commission on Accreditation of Healthcare Organizations standards
D. Centers for Disease Control and Prevention (CDC)

37.   The key point for the ED nurse to remember in caring for a patient who is a phencyclidine (PCP) abuser is that the patient's:
A. increase in physical strength and ability.
B. decrease in pain sensation and judgment.
C. increase in insight into the drug abuse problem.
D. decrease in ability to metabolize the drug.

38. An 18-year-old basketball player has just suffered an inversion injury of the left ankle. The ankle is very swollen and the patient cannot weight bear. The 5 Ps are intact. In planning for the care of this patient, you know that this patient is at high risk for:
   A. avulsion fracture.
   B. impacted fracture.
   C. displaced fracture.
   D. segmental fracture.

39. When a nurse is planning care for an ED patient with chronic obstructive pulmonary disease (COPD), an understanding of which of the following is most important?
   A. Current vital signs
   B. Current peak flow
   C. Causes of the current illness
   D. Baseline respiratory function

40. A 68-year-old male, accompanied by his wife, presents to the ED with a history of Alzheimer's disease. His vital signs are stable. On examination, you determine that the patient has a positive snout test (tapping the face just below the nose causes the patient to grimace) and appears agitated. Your initial intervention would be to:
   A. obtain lab tests (CBC, electrolytes).
   B. place the patient in a quiet room.
   C. have the patient seen by the physician now.
   D. give the patient a sedative parentally.

41. Your 14-year-old patient presents with a sore throat (pain 7/10) and reports that it has been present for 2 days. Vital signs are BP 110/70, HR 88/min, respirations 18/min, oxygen saturation 95%, and temperature 102.4° F (39.1° C). A priority nursing intervention would be which of the following?
   A. Spray the throat with a local anesthetic to decrease the pain.
   B. Obtain a complete blood count (CBC).
   C. Have the patient do salt water gargles.
   D. Obtain a throat culture.

42. A 1-year-old patient presents with inconsolable crying and a 2-hour history of currant jelly stools. The physician diagnoses intussusception. Your immediate goal in the ED is to do which of the following?
   A. Obtain a surgical consult.
   B. Give an enema.
   C. Give narcotic analgesics.
   D. Console the patient and family.

43. A 6-month-old patient presents to the ED 4 hours after being diagnosed with respiratory syncytial virus (RSV) in the pediatrician's office. Which of the following would indicate the need for immediate intervention by the triage nurse?
   A. Respiratory rate of 44/min
   B. Oxygen saturation of 94%
   C. Nasal flaring
   D. Heart rate of 132 beats per minute

44. With the Glasgow Coma Scale (GCS), which of the following total scores indicates coma?
   A. 6
   B. 9
   C. 11
   D. 15

45.   In hemophilia, which lab test has abnormal results?
       A.   Hemoglobin
       B.   Partial thromboplastin time (PTT)
       C.   Prothrombin time (PT)
       D.   Platelet count

46.   Which of the following physical exam findings can indicate meningeal irritation?
       A.   Murphy's sign
       B.   Kehr's sign
       C.   Rovsing's sign
       D.   Kernig's sign

47.   A 58-year-old person presents to the ED with a 10-day history of copious vomiting and abdominal pain. Arterial blood gases are drawn and reveal a pH of 7.60, $PaCO_2$ of 48 mm Hg, and bicarbonate level of 52 mmol/L. What is your interpretation?
       A.   Metabolic acidosis with respiratory compensation
       B.   Metabolic alkalosis with respiratory compensation
       C.   Respiratory acidosis with metabolic compensation
       D.   Respiratory alkalosis with metabolic compensation

48.   A 24-year-old woman who is 26 weeks pregnant presents to the ED reporting right upper quadrant pain (rated at 7/10) for the past 6 hours. She describes the pain as constant and aching. She states that fetal movements are > 10 per hour. She is nauseated and has been constipated for 2 days. Urinalysis is negative. Liver function tests are within normal levels. WBC is slightly elevated. Vital signs are BP 120/84, HR 86/min, respirations 22/min, oxygen saturation 98%, temperature 99.4° F (37.5° C), and fetal heart rate (FHR) 134/min. Your assessment confirms that the plan of care should be directed toward which of the following conditions?
       A.   Appendicitis
       B.   Cholecystitis
       C.   Stretching of the broad ligament
       D.   Pyelonephritis

49.   The vasopressor of choice for tricyclic antidepressant (TCA) overdose is:
       A.   dopamine (Intropin).
       B.   norepinephrine (Levophed).
       C.   amrinone lactate (Inocor).
       D.   dobutamine (Dobutrex).

50.   The primary reason emergency staff do not always recognize potential organ donor patients is uncertainty about how to initiate:
       A.   conversation with the potential organ donor's family.
       B.   the donor referral process to an organ procurement organization.
       C.   a dialog with colleagues regarding the organ donation process.
       D.   brain death verification.

51.   Medical contraindications to organ donation include all of the following EXCEPT:
       A.   encephalitis of unknown cause.
       B.   hematologic malignant neoplasm.
       C.   disseminated tuberculosis.
       D.   seizure disorder.

52.   Potential organ donor variables that influence organ donation rates include which of the following?
    A. Race
    B. Sex
    C. Blood type
    D. Allergy status

53.   Common forms of emergency operations preparedness drills or exercises required by regulatory agencies include which of the following?
    A. On-site, hospital, ED
    B. Scene, in-house, departmental
    C. Tabletop, functional, full scale
    D. Written, acted, integrated

54.   The ED nurse is asked to administer the first dose of rifampin (Rifadin) prophylaxis to 3 young women who are roommates of a patient who has just been diagnosed with meningococcal meningitis. What advice should the ED nurse give to the roommates regarding this medication?
    A. "Taking this medication may turn your urine orange."
    B. "Take the medication with meals."
    C. "You may continue to wear your contact lenses."
    D. "There is no interaction between this medication and birth control pills."

55.   Appropriate interfacility transfer and transport of a medically unstable child must include which of the following?
    A. A screening exam by the triage nurse, consent to transfer, and copies of medical records related to the emergency medical condition to accompany the patient
    B. Parental request and consent to transfer to another facility by privately owned vehicle (POV)
    C. Physician certification that transfer is a medical necessity, consent, and an RN and a physician to accompany the patient to the referral hospital
    D. Acceptance by the receiving facility, copies of medical records related to the emergency medical condition to accompany the patient, and qualified personnel with adequate equipment to care for the patient en route

56.   A 4-year-old presents to the ED with an avulsed tooth. She was hit in the mouth with a toy thrown by another child at her day care center. The incident occurred approximately 45 minutes ago. Her day care attendant has the child's tooth wrapped in a clean cloth. Bleeding is minimal. Which of the following statements is correct?
    A. Treatment of the tooth should begin within 60 minutes of the avulsion.
    B. The avulsed tooth should be gently cleaned and placed in sterile water.
    C. The avulsed tooth should be scrubbed and gently replaced in the patient's gum.
    D. Baby teeth are seldom reimplanted.

57.   You are giving discharge instructions to the parents of a newborn. The parents brought the baby to your ED "to be checked out" because the family was involved in a motor vehicle accident. The baby, who was secured in an infant seat that his mother was holding, appears to be uninjured. Mom was the uninjured front seat passenger. You tell the parents that babies should be:
    A. placed in a rear-facing seat until they weigh 10 lb (4.5 kg)
    B. placed in a forward-facing seat in the rear seat of the car until they weigh 30 lb (13.6 kg).
    C. placed in a rear-facing seat in the rear seat of the car until they weigh 20 lb (9.0 kg).
    D. in a rear-facing seat unless they are in the back seat.

58.   An unrestrained driver is brought into the ED by EMS. Paramedics report that she was in an older car without airbags and the steering wheel was bent. The patient is drowsy, pale, and anxious and has labored respirations. A massive pulmonary contusion is suspected. She is being given 100% high-flow oxygen via nonrebreather mask. The priority intervention for this patient is:
   A. chest tube placement.
   B. arterial blood gases.
   C. diagnostic peritoneal lavage.
   D. administration of antianxiety medication.

59.   The priority nursing intervention for a patient suspected to have a massive hemothorax is which of the following?
   A. Preparation for diagnostic peritoneal lavage
   B. Send blood for type and crossmatch
   C. Prepare for pericardiocentesis
   D. Administer analgesic medication

60.   A victim of a stab wound to the epigastric area presents to the ED. Upon evaluation, he suddenly develops shortness of breath, chest pain, and decreased breath sounds. You suspect:
   A. diaphragmatic tear.
   B. myocardial contusion.
   C. flail chest.
   D. rib fractures.

61.   An anxious, panic-stricken patient arrives in the ED with a chief complaint of dyspnea, rapid respirations, and periorbital numbness. All serious causes for this breathing pattern are eliminated and the patient is diagnosed with hyperventilation. Which of the following findings do you anticipate?
   A. Respiratory alkalosis
   B. Dehydration
   C. Stroke
   D. Metabolic acidosis

62.   A 45-year-old patient presents to the ED with increased shortness of breath over the past 3 days. His history includes a chronic cough that has produced copious amounts of mucopurulent sputum for the past 5 years and smoking 2 packs of cigarettes per day for 30 years. Physical findings include scattered rhonchi, distended neck veins, polycythemia, and peripheral edema. The ED nurse knows that these findings are consistent with which of the following?
   A. Asthma
   B. Chronic bronchitis
   C. Emphysema
   D. Pneumonia

63.   An unrestrained passenger presents to the ED after having been involved in a high-speed motor vehicle crash (MVC) and having received multiple facial wounds. The primary assessment concern for this patient would be which of the following?
   A. Airway obstruction
   B. Infection
   C. Loss of sensation
   D. Skull fracture

64.   The most common cause of pleural effusion is:
       A. empyema.
       B. malignancy.
       C. congestive heart failure.
       D. asthma.

65.   Respiratory distress syndrome is most commonly associated with which of the following?
       A. Rib fracture
       B. Bronchitis
       C. Pulmonary contusion
       D. Spinal cord injury

66.   When you are teaching an asthma patient how to avoid potential triggers of the disease, which of
       the following should you be sure to discuss?
       A. Avoidance of spicy foods can help to reduce asthma attacks.
       B. Exacerbations of asthma can be reduced by decreasing physical activity.
       C. Chronic postnasal drip can contribute to recurrent asthma attacks.
       D. Most triggers of asthma cannot be avoided.

67.   A 53-year-old patient presents to the ED with repeated episodes of nocturnal asthma over several
       months. The condition has responded poorly to nebulized bronchodilators. Which of the following
       is a potential cause of these occurrences?
       A. Gastroesophageal reflux
       B. Bacterial pneumonia
       C. Medication allergy
       D. Diabetes mellitus

68.   A young patient comes into the ED with a rash that the mother suspects to be chickenpox. What
       precautions are appropriate?
       A. Contact and respiratory
       B. Respiratory and droplet
       C. Blood and body fluid
       D. Universal and respiratory

69.   A 4-year-old child presents to the ED with a barky cough, stridor, retractions, and hypoxia. This
       child is most likely to have:
       A. asthma.
       B. croup.
       C. pneumonia.
       D. epiglottitis.

70.   A child is brought to the ED after having eaten a cookie that contained peanuts. The child is audibly
       wheezing, has an oxygen saturation of 85%, and cannot talk. What is the priority medication for this
       child?
       A. Epinephrine (adrenalin)
       B. Diphenhydramine (Benadryl)
       C. Oxygen
       D. Lorazepam (Ativan)

71.   Respiratory syncytial virus (RSV) is responsible for which respiratory disease?
A. Bronchiolitis
B. Bacterial tracheitis
C. Epiglottitis
D. Tuberculosis

72.   A patient presents to the ED following a motorcycle collision with complete loss of sensation and movement below the clavicles. The priority in your assessment is which of the following?
A. Monitor the patient's inspiratory effort.
B. Monitor for resolution of spinal shock.
C. Monitor for signs of autonomic dysreflexia.
D. Monitor for signs of neurogenic shock.

73.   A female patient telephones the telephone triage nurse and describes a headache. She states that she is 55 years of age and has decreased vision with the headache. She emphasizes the location as the temporal region and tells the nurse that she has had this headache before, causing loss of sleep and jaw pain for several days. The telephone nurse advises the patient to report to the ED immediately. Based on her action, what do you think the telephone triage nurse suspects?
A. Meningitis
B. Cluster headache
C. Temporal arteritis
D. Cerebrovascular accident (CVA)

74.   A patient is brought to the ED from a motor vehicular crash. His initial Glasgow Coma Scale (GCS) score in the field was 5. Vital signs are BP 100/60, HR 106/min, and respirations 20/min, assisted via bag-valve mask. Pupils are 5 mm and equal and react sluggishly to light. The order of interventions for a patient with suspected head injury and increased intracranial pressure are:
A. hyperventilation, mannitol, fluid restriction, sedation, phenytoin (Dilantin).
B. hyperventilation, fluid resuscitation to maintain systolic BP > 90 mm Hg, sedation, phenytoin (Dilantin).
C. maintain oxygen saturation > 95%, mannitol (Osmitrol), fluid resuscitation, phenytoin (Dilantin).
D. maintain oxygen saturation >95%, fluid resuscitation to maintain systolic BP >90 mm Hg, sedation, mannitol (Osmitrol).

75.   A patient presents to the ED with facial muscle weakness, dysphagia, increasing fatigue, and respiratory distress. The provider orders an edrophonium (Tensilon) test for a differential diagnosis. The ED nurse suspects which of the following?
A. Multiple sclerosis
B. Myasthenia gravis
C. Cerebral aneurysm
D. Guillain-Barré syndrome

76.   Thiamine (vitamin B1) should be administered in addition to dextrose 50% when an unknown patient is seizing for which of the following reasons?
A. To prevent Wernicke-Korsakoff syndrome
B. To assure proper patient nutrition
C. To enhance the potency of the dextrose
D. To prevent hypoglycemia

77. The pupils of a patient are evaluated during an assessment after a motorcycle crash. The pupils are found to be 10 mm in diameter and very slow to react to light. The ED nurse considers these findings to be:
   A. normal pupil size but possible hypoxia as suggested by sluggish reaction of the pupils.
   B. dilated pupils, with possible injury or dysfunction of cranial nerves II and III.
   c. consistent with early tentorial herniation.
   D. related to an intracranial pressure of <15 mm Hg.

78. You are asked to administer fosphenytoin (Cerebyx) 750 mg IV to a patient in status epilepticus. Which of the following precautions should be taken in administering the medication?
   A. The blood pressure should be closely monitored, as hypertension may develop.
   B. The medication should be administered at 150 mg/min IV.
   C. Fosphenytoin should always be given in combination with phenytoin (Dilantin).
   D. The medication must be given through an inline filter.

79. What would be a priority nursing diagnosis for a patient with a diagnosis of Guillain- Barré syndrome?
   A. Ineffective breathing pattern
   B. Body image disturbance
   C. Impaired physical mobility
   D. Altered thought processes

80. A patient arrives in the ED by EMS following a fall from the stands at a high school football game. The patient is alert and oriented and able to answer questions, open his eyes as you speak, and lift his fingers and toes at your command. He is in full spinal protocol upon arrival. His initial Glasgow Coma Score is:
   A. eye movement 4, verbal 5, motor 6 = 15.
   B. eye movement 2, verbal 2, motor 2 = 6.
   C. eye movement 1, verbal 1, motor 1 = 3.
   D. eye movement 4, verbal 3, motor 4 = 11.

81. A 65-year-old patient arrives in the ED observation unit with a diagnosis of confusion. The family is concerned that their grandfather is becoming more confused. He apparently fell from a horse 2 weeks ago and was examined by a physician and discharged home with a diagnosis of concussion. The granddaughter states that her grandfather has a history of drinking several cocktails every evening, but has never acted this way before. As the ED nurse, which of the following interventions would you encourage?
   A. Skull x-ray to determine intracerebral bleeding
   B. Blood alcohol level evaluation
   C. Computed tomography (CT) scan of the head
   D. Metabolic evaluation for dementia

Questions 82 and 83

A 36-year-old female who is 32 weeks pregnant by dates presents to the ED with the chief complaint of a sudden onset of bright-red vaginal bleeding, severe low abdominal cramping, and low back pain for the past 6 hours. The patient has been saturating one pad per hour. She also reports decrease in fetal movement over the past few hours. The patient has had no prenatal care during this pregnancy. Vital signs are BP 100/60, HR 112/min, respirations 24/min, and temperature 101.2° F (38.4° C) orally.

82. You suspect that this patient has:
    A. placenta previa.
    B. pelvic inflammatory disease (PIV).
    C. abruptio placentae.
    D. threatened abortion.

83. In caring for this patient, you anticipate all of the following interventions EXCEPT:
    A. establishing 2 large-bore IVs for the administration of crystalloid fluids and possible blood products.
    B. obtaining laboratory tests to include a coagulation profile.
    C. administering a tocolytic agent such as oxytocin injection (Pitocin).
    D. pelvic ultrasound.

84. The most appropriate nursing diagnosis for the patient who is bleeding from abruptio placentae is:
    A. pain.
    B. fluid volume deficit.
    C. impaired gas exchange.
    D. altered tissue perfusion.

85. A 21-year-old female arrives at the ED via private vehicle after having delivered a term infant in the hospital parking lot. This is her third vaginal delivery. On arrival, the patient is experiencing heavy vaginal bleeding. Vital signs are BP 118/60, HR 112/min, respirations 18/min, and temperature 101° F (38.3° C). Your first intervention is to do which of the following?
    A. Obtain an order to administer 10 units of oxytocin (Pitocin) IVP
    B. Place the patient in the left lateral position
    C. Initiate 2 large-bore IVs with crystalloid fluid
    D. Palpate the abdomen and massage the uterus, if doughy, after confirming that the placenta has been delivered

86. A 36-year-old female at 38 weeks' gestation presents to the ED in active labor. On examination of the perineum, you observe that the umbilical cord is protruding. Interventions should include all of the following EXCEPT:
    A. gently elevating any presenting fetal parts off the cord.
    B. attempting to push the umbilical cord back into the vagina.
    c. assisting the mother into a left lateral decubitus (knee-chest) position.
    D. preparing the patient for an emergency cesarean section.

87. The objective signs included in the Apgar score include all of the following EXCEPT:
    A. heart rate.
    B. respiratory rate.
    C. muscle tone.
    D. reflex irritability.

Questions 88–90

A 17-year-old female presents to the ED with a chief complaint of low abdominal pain. The patient is crying and guarding her abdomen. Vital signs are BP 118/84, HR 116/min, and respirations 24/min.

88. Signs and symptoms that would indicate a possible ruptured ovarian cyst include which of the following?
    A. Fever > 101.2°F (38.5°C)
    B. The gradual onset of pelvic pain over the past week
    C. Severe diarrhea preceding crampy, generalized abdominal pain
    D. The sudden onset of severe pelvic pain during intercourse

89. Which of the following interventions should be implemented for this patient?
    A. Assist her in quantifying her level of pain using a pain scale.
    B. Anticipate an order for an IV for analgesia.
    C. Obtain laboratory specimens for a CBC, urinalysis, and pregnancy test.
    D. All of the above.

90. The highest-priority nursing diagnosis for this patient would be which of the following?
    A. Pain
    B. Knowledge deficit
    C. Risk for injury
    D. Fluid volume deficit

91. The most common infectious cause(s) of vulvovaginitis include which of the following?
    A. Bacterial vaginosis
    B. *Candida albicans*
    C. *Trichomonas*
    D. All of the above

92. A 68-year-old man presents with an acute onset of what he calls "excruciating back pain" and a history of hypertension. A widened mediastinum is present on chest radiograph. Shortly after arrival, the patient's BP drops to 67/48 mm Hg and his neck veins are flat. The most likely cause of this hypotension is:
    A. aortic rupture.
    B. myocardial infarction.
    C. cardiac tamponade.
    D. splenic rupture.

93. Before emergent repair, a patient with a dissecting aortic aneurysm has a BP of 142/82. Which of the following IV drip medications will the patient most likely receive while awaiting the vascular surgeon's arrival?
    A. Nitroprusside (Nipride)
    B. Dopamine (Intropin)
    C. Dobutamine (Dobutrex)
    D. Nitroglycerin (Tridil)

94. The primary nursing diagnosis for the patient with a dissecting thoracic aortic aneurysm is risk for:
    A. altered tissue perfusion related to decreased peripheral blood flow.
    B. fluid volume deficit related to a drop in renal perfusion.
    C. airway obstruction related to aneurysm pressure on the left main bronchus.
    D. impaired skin integrity related to decreased peripheral blood flow.

95.   A 57-year-old patient in excruciating pain is diagnosed with a descending thoracic aneurysm. The emergency physician has ordered a bolus and infusion of labetalol HCl (Normodyne). Which of the following items listed on the patient's past medical history would be cause for concern?
        A. Severe asthma
        B. Chronic hypertension
        C. Marfan's syndrome
        D. Coronary artery bypass graft surgery

96.   A patient is transported from a referral facility with hypotension, abdominal distention, renal failure, coagulopathies, and a pulsating abdominal mass. The ED nurse recognizes that these are all common findings associated with:
        A. sepsis.
        B. small bowel obstruction.
        C. hepatic laceration.
        D. aortic dissection.

97.   An unrestrained driver involved in a frontal motor vehicle collision presents with a flail sternum. Which of the following would the ED nurse expect to find on further assessment?
        A. Ventricular ectopy
        B. Priapism
        C. Borborygmi
        D. Ptosis

98.   Which of the following statements is most correct concerning premature ventricular contractions (PVCs) in the patient with blunt cardiac trauma?
        A. Aggressively eliminate PVCs by giving a bolus of amiodarone HCl (Cordarone).
        B. Drug therapy for PVCs is rarely indicated in blunt cardiac trauma.
        C. PVCs should be treated with procainamide (Pronestyl), but only if they exceed 6/min.
        D. PVCs can be avoided with the administration of a lidocaine (Xylocaine) drip prophylactically.

99.   Which of the following serum markers is the best indicator of blunt myocardial trauma?
        A. Lactate dehydrogenase (LDH)
        B. Creatine phosphokinase (CPK)
        C. Troponin I
        D. Alkaline phosphatase (AP)

100.   Which of the following studies best identifies wall motion abnormalities resulting from cardiac contusion?
        A. Thallium scan
        B. Echocardiogram
        C. Coronary arteriogram
        D. Electrocardiogram

101.   Which of the following mechanisms of injury is most likely to result in myocardial contusion?
        A. Blast injury in a confined space
        B. Kick to chest by a bull
        C. Stab wound to the left chest
        D. Fall from a changing table

102. Which of the following is the procedure of choice for the hypotensive patient with cardiac tamponade?
    A. Emergency thoracotomy
    B. Pericardial window
    C. Chest tube placement
    D. Pericardiocentesis

103. Classic signs of cardiac tamponade include distant heart sounds, hypotension, and which of the following?
    A. Absent breath sounds on the left side
    B. A crunching sound heard with each heartbeat
    C. Subcutaneous emphysema of the left chest
    D. Distended neck veins

104. Which of the following best describes blood removed from the pericardial sac in a trauma patient with cardiac tamponade?
    A. Platelet activation causes rapid clot formation in the syringe.
    B. The hematocrit will be low because of dilution with serous pericardial fluid.
    C. The blood will not clot in the syringe because of defibrination.
    D. The blood will appear frothy because of churning from cardiac motion.

105. Hyponatremia may be found in all of the following conditions EXCEPT:
    A. Addison's disease.
    B. diarrhea.
    C. acute uremia.
    D. excess water intake.

106. The effects of histamine release on the body include all of the following EXCEPT:
    A. increased capillary permeability.
    B. arteriolar dilation.
    C. muscular contraction.
    D. arteriolar constriction.

107. Common substances such as antibiotics, iodine, shellfish, and peanuts often cause an allergic reaction. The reason is that the body becomes sensitized to a substance through an antibody that it creates to recognize this substance. This substance is referred to as:
    A. an antibody.
    B. an antigen.
    C. a mast cell.
    D. an antinuclear antibody.

108. A 7-week-old infant presents to the ED with fever. Every child this age with fever should be evaluated for:
    A croup.
    B. Reye's syndrome.
    C. meningitis.
    D. rubeola.

109.   Two weeks after returning from traveling abroad, a patient presents with anorexia, a productive cough, fever, and night sweats. These signs and symptoms most likely indicate which of the following?
A. Hepatitis
B. Tuberculosis
C. Measles
D. Pertussis

110.   A 3-year-old boy is carried into the ED by his parents at 7 AM. He is unresponsive and has no obvious signs of trauma. He has pale, clammy skin and normal vital signs, although his respirations are shallow. He is described as a healthy child who was fine when put to bed last night. His parents found him on the living room floor this morning. They say there was no evidence that he had taken any pills or poisons. What assessment question may be most useful at this point?
A. "Are other children in the family sick?"
B. "Did your child have a baby-sitter last night?"
C. "Could your child have had access to alcohol?"
D. "Does anyone in the family have diabetes?"

111.   A 17-year-old girl comes to the ED on Sunday morning complaining of headache, weakness, and feeling ill. Her history is unremarkable, but she does admit to having attended a "rave"—a party designed to enhance a hallucinogenic experience through music and behavior—the previous evening and having taken Ecstasy there. Vital signs are BP 138/80, HR 102/min, respirations 22/min, and temperature 98° F (36.7° C). As the ED nurse finishes triaging, the patient has a grand mal seizure. What is the most likely cause of the seizure?
A. Hypoglycemia
B. Hyponatremia
C. Subdural hematoma
D. Acute drug intoxication

112.   The emergency physician orders tuberculin purified protein derivative (PPD) testing for family members of a patient in the ED with active TB disease. On the 3-year-girl, the PPD was placed subcutaneously. The next step is to do which of the following?
A. Place a second PPD at least 2 inches (5 cm) from the first attempt
B. Ask the patient to return in 24 hours for PPD placement
C. Ask the physician to order a chest x-ray
D. Apply a multiple puncture test (Mono-Vacc, Time Test PPD) to the opposite forearm.

113.   A 55-year-old female presents to the ED with a 2-day history of a diffuse (whole-head), dull, aching headache (rated at 6/10) that had a slow onset but cannot be relieved with her usual remedies. She denies trauma and demonstrates no neurologic deficits or nuchal rigidity. Vital signs are BP 134/70, HR 84/min, respirations 18/min, oxygen saturation 97%, and temperature 98.2° F (36.8° C). The patient has a history of chronic lymphocytic leukemia (CLL) that has been in remission for 2 years, migraine headaches, and a recent history of a mild upper respiratory infection. In addition to CT of the head, what other test must be done as a top priority?
A. Complete blood count (CBC)
B. Lumbar puncture
C. CT of sinuses
D. Angiogram (brain)

114. At what level does a patient classically demonstrate an altered level of consciousness related to hyponatremia?
    A. Serum Na^+ < 125 mEq/L
    B. Serum Na^+ = 125–130 mEq/L
    C. Serum Na^+ ≥ 131–135 mEq/L
    D. Serum Na^+ ≥ 150 mEq/L

115. A 64-year-old female presents to the ED with a 3-hour history of perioral numbness and tingling of the hands and feet. Her motor strength in all 4 extremities is normal. She has a history of a thyroidectomy and has been in remission from uterine cancer for 2 years. Vital signs are BP 100/50, HR 105/min, respirations 24/min, oxygen saturation 97%, and temperature 97.9° F (36.6° C). Your plan of care and urgency is related to the potential diagnosis of:
    A. hypernatremia.
    B. hypocalcemia.
    C. hypermagnesemia.
    D. hypokalemia.

116. Your patient has a serum potassium of 7.2 mEq/L. Initial treatment may include all of the following EXCEPT:
    A. calcium chloride.
    B. dextrose/insulin.
    C. sodium bicarbonate.
    D. sodium polystyrene sulfonate (Kayexalate).

117. A mother brings her 3-month-old infant to the ED with a fever and diarrhea. The mother states that the patient does not want to eat or drink and is difficult to arouse. You note sunken eyes and fontanelles. The mother states that her child has not wet a diaper today. Your two attempts at starting IVs have failed. IMMEDIATE priority for this patient is to:
    A. establish vascular access via cutdown.
    B. establish vascular access via external jugular vein.
    C. establish vascular access via intraosseous needle.
    D. establish vascular access via scalp vein.

118. A 55-year-old female enters your ED complaining of chest pain. Her long cardiac history includes anterior wall myocardial infarction and heart failure. She presents with chest pain and shortness of breath. You note crackles throughout both lungs; pale, mottled skin; and thready pulses. Your interventions to decrease preload include the administration of which of the following?
    A. Nitroglycerin (Tridil)
    B. Nitroprusside (Nipride)
    C. Amiodarone (Cordarone)
    D. Adrenalin (Epinephrine)

119. You are caring for a patient who was struck in the chest by a baseball thrown by a batting machine. Although initially your patient's vital signs were stable, you are noting muffled heart tones, distended neck veins, and rapidly dropping blood pressure. Which of the following conditions tells you that this patient is going into cardiogenic shock?
    A. Ventricular rupture
    B. Stunned myocardium
    C. Pericardial tamponade
    D. Myocardial infarction

120.   Your patient was an unrestrained driver who was involved in a car crash in which the steering wheel was bent. He initially complained of severe chest pain and shortness of breath at the scene, but has been deteriorating en route to your hospital. He arrives with distended neck veins, extreme dyspnea, and tachypnea and he is pale with circumoral cyanosis. His BP in the field was initially 140/90, but now you are having a difficult time palpating even a femoral pulse. Lungs sounds are diminished in the right lung fields and absent in the left lung fields. What is the cause of your patient's distress?
A. Multiple rib fractures
B. Pulmonary contusion
C. Pulmonary edema
D. Tension pneumothorax

121.   You are caring for a patient who has been diagnosed with an anterior wall myocardial infarction. Within 20 minutes after arrival in the ED, the patient is developing hypotension. Crackles are heard through all lung fields. The patient continues to have chest pain, is pale and diaphoretic, and does not have delayed capillary refill. While you wait for the intraaortic balloon pump team to arrive, what medications can be administered to reduce both preload and afterload?
A. Morphine sulfate, furosemide (Lasix)
B. Nitroprusside (Nipride), furosemide (Lasix)
C. Nitroglycerin (Tridil), high-dose dopamine (Intropin)
D. Nitroprusside (Nipride), captopril (Capoten)

122.   A 55-year-old female enters your ED complaining of severe chest pain that has lasted for 5 hours. She starts to complain of respiratory distress and is cool, pale, and diaphoretic. Her respiratory rate is 22/min and respirations appear to be slightly labored. Which of the following takes priority in your care for this patient?
A. Administration of 100% oxygen via nonrebreather mask and reassessing respiratory status
B. Obtaining a 12-lead electrocardiogram
C. Establishing an IV of 0.9% normal saline solution and administering a 500-ml fluid bolus
D. Performing endotracheal intubation

123.   Which of the following indicates stabilization of the patient in cardiogenic shock?
A. Urine output via Foley catheter of 1 ml/kg/hour
B. A systolic blood pressure of 88 mm Hg in an otherwise normotensive adult
C. Heart rate of 120/min
D. Respiratory rate of 26/min

124.   Your cardiogenic shock patient has been given morphine sulfate, furosemide (Lasix), and nitrates (e.g., nitroglycerin [Tridil]. His breathing continues to be labored even on 100% oxygen via nonrebreather mask. Blood gases show hypercarbia and hypoxia. You anticipate which of the following interventions to correct his blood gas abnormalities?
A. Give oxygen via bag-valve-mask device
B. Administer albuterol (Ventolin) nebulizer treatment
C. Begin a dopamine (Intropin) drip at 10 mcg/kg/min
D. Intubate and mechanically ventilate the patient with positive end-expiratory pressure (PEEP).

125.   A nursing home patient is brought to your ED with the complaints of fever and generalized weakness. Skin is warm, dry, and flushed. The patient is mildly agitated—an abnormal situation for this patient. Vital signs are HR 110/min, respirations 26/min, and temperature 101.8° F (38.8° C). A Foley catheter is draining cloudy yellow urine. You suspect this patient to have which of the following?

A. A urinary tract infection
B. Hyperdynamic sepsis
C. Hypodynamic sepsis
D. Toxic shock syndrome

126. A 10-year-old boy is brought to your ED after having injured himself while doing tricks on his bicycle. He was not wearing a helmet and landed on his head while trying to flip his bicycle. Upon your arrival, the patient is hypotensive and bradycardic. His respiratory rate is 30/min and respirations are shallow. He is most likely experiencing which of the following?
A. Respiratory failure
B. Neurogenic shock
C. Hysteria from his injuries
D. A severe head injury

127. A gradually enlarging lesion develops at the site of a brown recluse spider bite. If sufficient venom is injected, systemic features will also be found. Which of the following will reveal early evidence of systemic involvement?
A. Plain x-ray to locate osteomyelitis
B. Urinalysis to identify myoglobinuria
C. Arterial blood gases (ABGs) to seek perfusion/ventilation mismatch
D. Serum antibodies to quantify the venom injected

128. To minimize transmission of Lyme disease, an attached tick should be removed by:
A. grasping the body and removing it with a twisting motion.
B. smothering the tick in petroleum jelly, then wiping it off.
C. holding a hot matchstick near the tick until the tick falls off.
D. grasping the head and exerting a slow, steady pull.

129. After falling down 3 steps, a patient presents to the ED complaining of right ankle pain. He denies other injuries, but is unable to bear weight bear without pain. Besides examining the ankle, the nurse should:
A. assess the Babinski reflex of the foot.
B. evaluate ulnar and radial pulses.
C. palpate the head of the fibula.
D. examine the left ankle.

130. The nurse is preparing to discharge a patient with a diagnosis of cervical radiculopathy. Instructions should include which of the following?
A. Application of moist heat
B. Use of hard cervical collar
C. Massaging mild steroid cream into area
D. No use of pillow for sleep

131. A 36-year-old female complains of neck pain and stiffness upon waking. She spent the previous day "cleaning up the yard" and gardening. She noted a gradual onset of stiffness that evening, but states that the pain was much worse this morning. She has no fever and feels well otherwise. The ED nurse's assessment should focus on:
A. palpation of the skull.
B. evaluation of upper arm strength.
C. palpation of the trapezius.
D. evaluation of brachial nerve function.

132.   Discharge instructions for a patient with a rotator cuff injury of the arm should include:
A. use of a sling during the day and for sleep.
B. limiting use of the affected arm.
C. an ice massage twice a day for 30 minutes.
D. overhead exercises to strengthen the area.

Questions 133 and 134

A 3-year-old child is brought into triage by his mother. According to a 13-year-old cousin, they had been playing when the 3-year-old suddenly started crying and stopped using the right arm. There was no fall or blow to the arm.

133.   In triage, the child is quiet, gingerly holding the arm at his side and refusing to move it. As part of the history, the mother should be specifically asked if:
A. the child prefers to sleep on that side.
B. the child is right or left handed.
C. any older siblings have had similar conditions.
D. the arm was pulled during play.

134.   A radial head subluxation is successfully reduced. A short time later, the child is actively using the right arm to play in the waiting room. Discharge instructions should include the recommendation to:
A. use a sling during the day.
B. make sure the child avoids swinging by the arms.
C. apply moist heat to the elbow twice a day.
D. take the child to an orthopedist the next day.

135.   A 20-year-old male complains of pain in his right hand after being involved in an altercation. On exam the area over the fifth metacarpal is tender and swollen and the patient has difficulty moving his fingers. You suspect that he has:
A. avulsion fracture.
B. boxer fracture.
C. tendon rupture.
D. scaphoid fracture.

136.   A 21-year-old male returns to the ED complaining of severe pain that is unrelieved by oxycodone (Percocet). He was diagnosed with a distal tibia and fibula fracture after a fall from a ladder. On exam, the toes are swollen and tender to touch and capillary refill is > 3 seconds. You are concerned that the patient is developing which of the following?
A. Osteomyelitis
B. Thrombophlebitis
C. Cellulitis
D. Compartment syndrome

137.   A 19-year-old male arrives by ambulance from a motor vehicle collision. His knee hit the dashboard. He complains of severe pain in his right hip and the leg is internally rotated with flexion (pelican position). The ED nurse suspects which of the following?
A. Posterior hip dislocation
B. Anterior hip dislocation
C. Intertrochanteric hip fracture
D. Cervical neck hip fracture

138.   A 28-year-old female is in the ED with a finger laceration sustained while washing dishes. In a non-tetanus-prone wound such as this, tetanus/diphtheria (Td) immunization should be administered if the patient received her last vaccination:
   A. more than 10 years ago.
   B. within the past 7 years.
   C. within the past 5 years.
   D. within the past 2 years.

139.   Scapular fractures occur primarily as a result of:
   A. a fall on an outstretched hand.
   B. direct trauma.
   C. excessive use of the attached muscles.
   D. a fall on a flexed wrist.

Questions 140 and 141

An 82-year-old patient presents to the ED via EMS following a motor vehicle crash. The restrained driver was traveling slowly when his car was struck from behind by a high-velocity vehicle. The patient complains of severe pubic pain and pain upon palpation of the right iliac wing. There is no external rotation of the right lower extremity and the patient is pale and diaphoretic. Vital signs are BP 74/58, HR 118/min, and respirations 24/min.

140.   The nurse should suspect a:
   A. fractured hip.
   B. dislocated hip.
   C. fractured pelvis.
   D. dislocated pelvis.

141.   The patient demonstrates signs of shock. Which of the following types of shock is most likely?
   A. Hypovolemic
   B. Cardiogenic
   C. Distributive
   D. Obstructive

142.   A patient in triage complains of pain, tearing, and a foreign body sensation in both eyes. She states that she noticed a gradual onset of symptoms after dinner and now can't keep her eyes open. Photophobia is noted. Which of the following statements by the patient should be documented in the triage note?
   A. "I normally drive to work, but have taken the bus for 2 weeks now."
   B. "I was at the pool all day today."
   C. "I do a lot of computer work."
   D. "I was at an ice skating rink last night."

143.   A 76-year-old patient complains of headache with nausea and vomiting. The patient also complains of halos around lights and photophobia. Physical exam reveals a reddened left eye. The ED nurse should suspect which of the following?
   A. Migraine
   B. Conjunctivitis
   C. Acute angle-closure glaucoma
   D. Trauma

144.   Which of the following statements about epiglottitis is INCORRECT?
A. It is usually caused by *Haemophilus influenzae*.
B. It occurs only in children.
C. The usual symptoms include a sore throat, fever, and drooling.
D. It has a rapid onset.

145.   A patient with a nasal bone fracture is suspected to have cerebral spinal fluid draining from the nose. These findings suggest which of the following?
A. Septal hematoma
B. Cribriform fracture
C. Orbit fracture
D. Tripod fracture

146.   A college student presents with a history of facial fullness, dental pain, and purulent rhinorrhea. The nurse should suspect:
A. odontalgia.
B. upper respiratory infection.
C. acute sinusitis.
D. nasal foreign body.

147.   A patient diagnosed with hyphema is ready for discharge. Which of the following statements by the patient indicates successful patient discharge teaching?
A. "I will only use one pillow when I sleep."
B. "I can take 600 mg of ibuprofen if the pain is severe."
C. "I will return if the pain gets worse."
D. "I will see the ophthalmologist again in 3 days."

Questions 148 and 149

A 2-year-old child is brought to the ED by parents who state that he woke from sleep crying inconsolably. The mother reports he had a recent "cold" with fevers to 101°F (38.4°C). Assessment reveals a fussy child who is pulling and rubbing his right ear.

148.   To visualize the ear best during the otoscope exam, the ED nurse should:
A. gently pull the ear down and back.
B. gently pull the ear up and back.
C. maintain the head and ear in a neutral position.
D. have the child rotate his head to the right.

149.   Based on the parents' history and the child's behavior, the ED nurse should suspect:
A. otitis externa.
B. foreign body.
C. otitis media.
D. ruptured tympanic membrane.

150.   The most commonly found obstructive material of the ear canal is:
A. cerumen.
B. insects.
C. beads.
D. cotton swabs.

Practice Examination 2

1. Intestinal perforation, hemorrhage, and toxic megacolon are all complications of:
    A. ULCERATIVE COLITIS.
    B. Crohn's disease.
    C. gastritis.
    D. peritonitis.

Rationale:

   A. Intestinal perforation, hemorrhage, and toxic megacolon are all complications of ulcerative colitis.
   B. Complications of Crohn's disease include intestinal perforation and hemorrhage, but not toxic megacolon. Crohn's is usually manifested in the small intestine.
   C. Hemorrhage and perforation of the stomach are potential sequelae of gastritis.
   D. Complications of peritonitis include the spread of infection and fluid and electrolyte imbalance, which may lead to hemorrhage.

Content Category: Gastrointestinal

Reference: Black & Matassarin-Jacobs, 1997; pp. 1794–1801.

2. Which of the following laboratory results would be important to consider in evaluating the patient with acute pancreatitis for complications?
    A. SERUM CALCIUM LEVEL
    B. Serum glutamate pyruvate transaminase (SGPT) level
    C. Stool for occult blood
    D. Serum blood urea nitrogen (BUN)/creatinine ratio

Rationale:

   A. The nurse should anticipate serum calcium levels in the patient with acute pancreatitis. The common complication of acute pancreatitis is hypocalcemia. In that condition, calcium binds with the release of lipase into the soft tissue spaces, causing the decrease in ionized calcium.
   B. Serum glutamate pyruvate transaminase (SGPT) levels are more significant in the evaluation of complications from cholecystitis, whereas serum glutamic-oxaloacetic transaminase (SGOT) levels are elevated in acute pancreatitis.
   C. Stool for occult blood is an important indicator of the complications of diverticulitis.
   D. The serum BUN/creatinine ratio is an important indicator of the complication of dehydration; however, it is not specific to the diagnosis of pancreatitis.

Content Category: Gastrointestinal

References: Porth, 1998; pp. 769–771; ENA, Core Curriculum, 2000; pp. 29–45; Kidd et al., 2000; pp. 93–116; Newberry, 1998; pp. 550–552.

3.   The parents of a 2-week-old breastfed infant present to the ED complaining that their infant has a "stomach bug" and needs treatment. The infant has been having 4 to 6 yellow mustard-colored stools per day for the past several days. The parents report these stools as loose. All serious causes for the reported problem are eliminated. The best response, based on an understanding of gastroenteritis, is:
    A.   "Your child does not have a fever and therefore does not have gastroenteritis."
    B.   "Gastroenteritis is very rare in infants less than 3 months of age."
    C.   "We will need to start intravenous fluid therapy for your infant."
    D.   "BREASTFED INFANTS USUALLY HAVE FREQUENT LOOSE, YELLOW STOOLS."

Rationale:

    D.   Breastfed infants tend to have more frequent stools and of a looser consistency than those of bottlefed infants. The parents need some reassurance and education.
    A.   Children with gastroenteritis may have mild fever or no fever at all.
    B.   Gastroenteritis can occur at any age in a child, breastfed or not.
    C.   Intravenous fluid therapy is not indicated; the stools are normal for this situation.

Content Category: Gastrointestinal

References: Soud & Rogers, 1998; pp. 333–362; Wyatt et al., 1999; pp. 516–533.

4.   The patient who is being discharged with a diagnosis of irritable bowel syndrome should be instructed to AVOID:
    A.   SORBITOL-CONTAINING FOODS.
    B.   spicy foods.
    C.   high-fiber foods.
    D.   high-fat foods.

Rationale:

    A.   The patient is instructed to avoid sorbitol-containing foods because sorbitol can cause gas bubbles to form in the intestine, increasing motility.
    B.   Instructions to avoid spicy foods would be given to patients with esophagitis.
    C.   The patient would be instructed to eat foods that have high fiber content to alleviate the diarrhea.
    D.   Instructions to avoid high-fat foods are usually given to patients with cholecystitis.

Content Category: Gastrointestinal

Reference: ENA, Core Curriculum, 2000.

5.   A 54-year-old male arrives in the ED complaining of anorexia and abdominal pain. Assessment reveals jaundice and a firm, lumpy area in the right upper quadrant upon palpation. The patient admits to a history of alcohol abuse. The ED nurse suspects that his diagnosis is:
    A.   gallbladder attack.
    B.   gastroenteritis.
    C.   esophageal varices.
    D.   CIRRHOSIS.

Rationale:

    D.   Heavy alcohol ingestion is the most frequent cause of cirrhosis. Patients usually present with anorexia, nausea, and abdominal pain. Typically the assessment reveals splenomegaly, hepatomegaly, jaundice, and ascites. On physical exam the right upper quadrant feels firm (from scarring) and lumpy (from nodules).

A. A gallbladder attack usually produces nausea and vomiting, pain in the epigastric area that sometimes is referred to the right scapula, and a fever. Jaundice is present in 20% of people. Anorexia and splenomegaly are not usually part of the clinical picture.

B. Jaundice is not part of the clinical presentation of gastroenteritis.

C. Esophageal varices are a complication of cirrhosis.

Content Category: Gastrointestinal

Reference: Black & Matassarin-Jacobs, 1997; pp. 1872–1884.

6. You are caring for a 30-year-old female victim of a motor vehicle accident. Chest x-ray shows rib fractures of the right 8 to10 ribs and a right-sided pneumothorax. You are concerned that she may also have an injury of the:
    A. spleen.
    B. LIVER.
    C. kidney.
    D. stomach.

Rationale:

B. The liver is located on the right side of the abdomen. Liver injuries occur frequently with blunt trauma and are associated with lower-right-sided rib fractures.

A. The spleen is located in the upper left quadrant. Splenic injuries are associated with left-sided lower rib fractures.

C. Kidney injuries are associated with vertebral and flank injuries.

D. Most stomach injuries are caused by penetrating trauma and are not associated with rib fractures or pneumothorax.

Content Category: Gastrointestinal

References: ENA, Core Curriculum, 2000; pp. 45–55, 336–337; Newberry, 1998; p. 312.

7. Upon receiving the results of diagnostic studies on the patient with bowel obstruction, the ED nurse is most likely to read which findings?
    A. Ultrasound examination shows thickened cecum.
    B. RADIOGRAPHIC EXAMINATION SHOWS DILATED, FLUID-FILLED LOOPS OF BOWEL.
    C. Barium swallow shows "string sign" or presence of narrow pylorus.
    D. Erect chest x-ray reveals free gas under the diaphragm.

Rationale:

B. Dilated, fluid-filled loops of bowel will be present on the abdominal film, especially proximal to the area of obstruction.

A. Ultrasound scans are usually not performed in bowel obstruction, since a simple abdominal film can reveal the diagnosis in most cases. Thickened cecum is a finding in acute appendicitis.

C. "String sign" is the diagnostic indicator of pyloric stenosis when barium swallow is performed.

D. Erect chest x-ray films reveal free gas under the diaphragm in peptic ulcer disease, especially if a perforation is present.

Content Category: Gastrointestinal

References: Kidd et al., 2000; pp. 93–116; Wyatt et al., 1999; pp. 516–533; Huey, 1998; p. 554.

8.   A 32-year-old male comes into the ED at 12:00 a.m. complaining of vomiting and diarrhea. Additional history reveals that he ate shellfish earlier in the evening. He further complains of cramps and feeling weak. Vital signs are BP 100/70, HR 96/min, respirations 24/min, and temperature 100.4° F (38.0° C). When asked how many stools he has had, he replies, "Seven or eight." The priority nursing diagnosis for this patient is:
A.   pain related to abdominal cramping.
B.   FLUID VOLUME DEFICIT RELATED TO VOMITING/DIARRHEA.
C.   risk for fluid volume deficit.
D.   risk for fluid volume imbalance.

Rationale:

B.   After a person has eaten shellfish, an abrupt onset of vomiting and diarrhea can signal infectious diarrhea. A low-grade fever would support this. This patient's blood pressure is low; he is exhibiting tachycardia; and his respiratory rate is elevated—all signs of compensation for a fluid volume deficit related to vomiting and diarrhea.

A.   Although pain related to abdominal cramping is a nursing diagnosis related to this patient's condition, it is not the priority diagnosis.

C.   Risk for fluid volume deficit is not correct because there is actual fluid volume deficit.

D.   Risk for fluid volume imbalance is not correct because there is actual fluid volume imbalance.

Content Category: Gastrointestinal

References: ENA, Core Curriculum, 2000; pp. 27–36; Taptich et al., 1994; p. 775.

Questions 9 and 10

A 19-year-old male patient presents to the ED accompanied by his mother. He is disheveled and unshaven. He is wearing a sweatband with papers stuffed in it around his head. His mother states that he has become progressively disorganized and has been hearing voices. Upon questioning, he tells you that he is a Martian. In the middle of a sentence he begins to giggle, talk to himself, and pace. His mother states that he hasn't taken his thioridazine (Mellaril) for a few weeks.

9.   You suspect a diagnosis of:
A.   conversion disorder.
B.   bipolar disorder.
C.   panic disorder.
D.   SCHIZOPHRENIA.

Rationale:

D.   Patients with schizophrenia, a psychotic disorder, present with disorganized thinking, hallucinations, delusions, associative looseness (confused and haphazard thinking that is jumbled and illogical), and loss of ego boundaries.

A.   Conversion disorder is characterized by the presence of one or more symptoms that suggest the presence of a neurologic disorder that cannot be explained by a known medical or neurological problem. The symptoms are exacerbated by stress and conflict.

B.   Patients with bipolar disorder tend in the manic phase to be hyperactive, write lengthy letters, make long phone calls, spend large sums of money on frivolous items, and practice sexual indiscretion. They can be manipulative, profane, fault finding, and adept at exploiting others' vulnerabilities.

C.   Panic disorders are characterized by a sudden onset of intense, apprehensive dread and at least 4 of the following symptoms: dyspnea, palpitations, chest discomfort, syncope or dizziness, trembling or shaking, sweating, choking, nausea or abdominal distress, depersonalization, sensations of numbness or tingling, hot flashes or chills, and fear of dying, "going crazy," or losing control.

Content Category: Psychosocial

References: Newberry, 1998; pp. 771–781; Varacolis, 1998; pp. 486–495, 595–623, 627–675.

10.   The most appropriate medication for this patient is:
   A.   fluoxetine hydrochloride (Prozac).
   B.   lithium carbonate (Eskalith).
   C.   lorazepam (Ativan).
   D.   HALOPERIDOL (HALDOL).

Rationale:

   D.   This patient is psychotic and requires an antipsychotic medication such as haloperidol (Haldol).
   A.   Fluoxetine hydrochloride (Prozac) is an antidepressant. This patient requires an antipsychotic medication.
   B.   Lithium carbonate (Eskalith) is a antimanic drug used in bipolar disorder.
   C.   Lorazepam (Ativan) is an antianxiety medication used for anxiety disorders.

Content Category: Psychosocial

References: Copel, 1999; pp. 376–385; Varacolis, 1998; pp.1014–1018.

11.   A man who has just been fired from his job for drinking is brought to the ED by police after threatening to stab his wife with a knife. He is in handcuffs and admits to drinking a six-pack of beer today. The priority nursing diagnosis is:
   A.   VIOLENCE, RISK FOR.
   B.   ineffective coping.
   C.   grieving, dysfunctional.
   D.   family processes, altered: alcoholism.

Rationale:

   A.   The first priority must be safety. The patient's threat to hurt his wife must be taken seriously and care must be taken when dealing with him.
   B.   While it is true that the patient is coping ineffectively, but the *priority* must be risk of violence, to protect the safety of the patient, his wife, and ED staff.
   C.   Although the loss of the patient's job may warrant a nursing diagnosis of dysfunctional grieving, the priority must be safety and the risk for violence, especially since he has made threats.
   D.   The patient may be an alcoholic, but the priority is his risk for violence. Once that issue has been addressed, his possible alcoholism may be considered.

Content Category: Psychosocial

References: Carpenito, 1999; pp. 442–445; ENA, Core Curriculum, 2000; pp. 358–360.

12.   A 48-year-old female presents with a chief complaint of intermittent palpitations, chest tightness, and choking sensations. She reports having had these symptoms for about 6 weeks and states that the episodes have become more frequent. Triage assessment reveals an intact airway and skin cool and slightly diaphoretic to touch. Vital signs are BP 168/72, HR 118/min, respirations 26/min, and temperature 99.2° F (37.3° C). The patient denies chest tightness, palpitations, and choking sensations. Diagnostic evaluation for cardiac disease is negative. Further assessment of this patient by the ED nurse reveals that she has recently been divorced and has relocated to this community, which is a substantial distance from her social support system. She has not been able to find employment that meets her career goals. Effectiveness of the plan of care for this patient will be demonstrated by:
   A.   the patient's willingness to enter a cardiac rehabilitation program.
   B.   A DECREASE IN SYSTOLIC BLOOD PRESSURE, PULSE, AND RESPIRATORY RATE.
   C.   an increase in the number of ED visits precipitated by palpitations and chest tightness.
   D.   the patient's request for anxiolytic medications.

Rationale:

   B.   A decrease in pulse rate, respiratory rate, and blood pressure is indicative of a decrease in sympathetic stimulation as triggered by a decreased anxiety level.
   A.   This patient's cardiac complaints were the result of anxiety. Failure to recognize anxiety as a cause of these symptoms does not demonstrate effectiveness of the plan of care.
   C.   Recurring visits to the ED for chest tightness and palpitations would not demonstrate acceptance by the patient that her symptoms are the result of anxiety.
   D.   Chemical anxiolytic therapy is not the first line of treatment for anxiety disorders.

Content Category: Psychosocial

References: ENA, Core Curriculum, 2000; p. 351; Kitt et al., 1995; pp. 365–366.

13.   A 35-year-old woman has just been brought into the ED by the police after having been sexually assaulted. The patient is alert. Initial assessment reveals bruises and abrasions on her face, breasts, arms, and hands. She makes minimal eye contact with the ED nurse and speaks only in response to questions. The ED nurse should prepare the patient for which of the following diagnostic procedures in addition to the evidence collection examination?
   A.   PREGNANCY TEST, HIV TEST, HEPATITIS B SCREEN, STD SCREEN
   B.   STD screen, pregnancy test, DNA testing, HIV test
   C.   Hepatitis screen, CBC, routine chemistries
   D.   HIV test, toxicology screen, CBC, DNA testing

Rationale:

   A.   Pregnancy test, HIV test, hepatitis B screen, and screening for sexually transmitted diseases routinely are performed in addition to the evidence collection examination because of risks associated with the assault.
   B.   DNA testing is performed at the laboratory and used by local law enforcement agencies as a part of the evidence analysis process.
   C.   Complete blood counts and chemistries are performed if the patient's condition warrants.
   D.   DNA testing is performed at the law enforcement laboratory. Complete blood counts and chemistries are performed if the patient's condition warrants them.

Content Category: Psychosocial

References: ENA, Core Curriculum, 2000; pp. 463–464; Kitt et al., pp. 265–268.

14.   A 25-year-old male is brought to the ED after a motor vehicle crash.. He was a restrained driver whose vehicle ran out of control and struck a stone embankment. The front seat passenger, his girlfriend, was not restrained and was ejected through the windshield on impact. She was pronounced dead at the scene of the crash. As the ED nurse performs primary and secondary assessments on this patient, he insists that he must see his girlfriend and demands to know when the police will bring her to visit him. Primary and secondary assessments reveal minor contusions and abrasions. The patient has completed his evaluation process and the physician states that he is ready to be discharged. While the emergency nurse is reviewing the discharge instructions with this patient, he says, "Stop what you're doing and get this IV out of me! I need to find my girlfriend. The police and ambulance crew told me she didn't make it, but I know she's okay." The emergency nurse refers this patient to a crisis intervention team. Despite much effort, the team is unable to assist him. The ED nurse prepares for:

A. INPATIENT ADMISSION.
B. sedative hypnotic therapy.
C. antidepressant therapy.
D. referral to community resources.

Rationale:

A.   Inpatient admission to a mental health service is the next step in treating unresolved crisis. The rationale for the admission involves the possibility of violence directed at the self or others resulting from increased tension and frustration.
B.   Sedative hypnotic therapy will alter consciousness for a time but will not assist in the problem-solving process.
C.   Antidepressant therapy is not indicated in crisis therapy.
D.   Community support service referral is appropriate only if the patient demonstrates an ability to mobilize the coping mechanisms needed to resolve the crisis state.

Content Category: Psychosocial

Reference: Varcarolis, 1998; pp. 371–375.

15.   Patients who experience panic attacks often complain of:
A. PALPITATIONS, SHORTNESS OF BREATH, AND DIZZINESS.
B. irritability and anger and speak in a loud voice.
C. headaches, irritability, and lack of energy.
D. tiredness, worthlessness, and difficulty thinking.

Rationale:

A.   These symptoms as well as sweating, tremors, chest pain, nausea, and chills or hot flashes are all common complaints from patients who have panic attacks.
B.   During the triggering phase of the aggression cycle, the patient often exhibits irritability, anger, restlessness, muscle tension, rapid breathing, and sweating and speaks in a loud voice.
C.   A grieving client often exhibits palpitations, impaired appetite, and restlessness along with headaches, irritability, and lack of energy.
D.   Tiredness, a sense of worthlessness, and difficulty thinking are often exhibited by people experiencing depression.

Content Category: Psychosocial

Reference: Videbeck, 2001; pp. 192, 222, 267, 337.

16. Effective staffing of the ED is best defined as:
   A. a staffing plan with equal nursing staff on all shifts.
   B. VARIABLE STAFFING ACCORDING TO PATIENT CENSUS FLOWS.
   C. standard staffing, 7 days a week, without peaks.
   D. longer hours and fewer worked days per staff member

Rationale:

   B. Staffing should be planned to cover the department as well as possible with regard to variable hours and patient volumes. Patient census and peak flow should be major considerations.
   A. A staffing plan with equal nurses on all shifts may not meet the needs of a given institution's patient flow.
   C. Patient census should be a major determinant in the number of nurses scheduled for the 24-hour period. Creative shifts and variability may be indicated.
   D. Longer hours have been shown to be ineffective in areas of high stress such as EDs.

Content Category: Professional Issues

Reference: Newberry, 1998.

17. The ED nurse educator develops competency-based orientation for experienced nurses in the ED. Determination of clinical competence is demonstrated when:
   A. THE NURSE PRECEPTOR VALIDATES THE NURSE'S ABILITY TO PERFORM SKILLS SAFELY.
   B. the nurse has a Certified Emergency Nurse (CEN) card.
   C. the nurse has attended a Pediatric Advanced Life Support (PALS) course and scored high on the exam.
   D. The nurse has attended an Emergency Nurse Pediatric Course (ENPC) and cared for a pediatric patient.

Rationale:

   A. Competency-based orientation includes skill and knowledge assessment, competence standards, and demonstration of critical behaviors. The educator or preceptor may determine the success of that demonstration.
   B. Although the nurse is credentialed as a CEN, his or her competency evaluation must be validated.
   C. Even if a nurse has scored well on the PALS examination, competency skills must be validated in all aspects of emergency care.
   D. ENPC is only one component of emergency care.

Content Category: Professional Issues

Reference: ENA, Core Curriculum, 2000; p. 754.

18. Which of the following situations is reported to law enforcement in states with mandatory reporting laws?
   A. Animal bite
   B. ELDER ABUSE
   C. Erratic behavior
   D. Homelessness

Rationale:

    B. The laws of each state define situations that require reporting to a law enforcement agency. Examples include homicide, suicide (successful or attempted), child or elder abuse, rape, communicable disease, and death within 48 hours of admission to the hospital.

    A. Many states mandate that animal bites be reported to the animal control official, but not to law officials.

    C. Although erratic behavior may disrupt the ED to an extent that requires notification of law officials, there is no mandatory reporting requirement for this.

    D. No state includes homelessness as a criterion for reporting to law officials.

Content Category: Professional Issues

Reference: ENA, Core Curriculum, 2000.

19. Root cause analysis is a process for identifying basic or causal factors that underlie variation in performance, including sentinel events. A root cause analysis focuses on:
    A. PROCESSES AND SYSTEMS.
    B. individual performance.
    C. equipment function.
    D. policies and procedures.

Rationale:

    A. A root cause analysis focuses primarily on processes and systems, progressing from special causes in clinical processes to common causes in organizational processes. Potential improvements in processes or systems that might decrease the likelihood of such events in the future are identified.

    B. Individual performance is not the focus of root cause analysis.

    C. Equipment function may be a part of the root cause analysis, but is not the focus.

    D. Policies and procedures may be included in the root cause analysis, but are not the focus.

Content Category: Professional Issues

Reference: JCAHO, 2000.

20. Current trends in assessing quality in health care are based on measuring the performance of the organization against:
    A. predetermined norms and standards of care.
    B. patient satisfaction results.
    C. OUTCOMES OF PATIENT CARE.
    D. definitions from third-party payers.

Rationale:

    C. The results of care—patient outcomes—are being used more universally than before to define and measure the quality of patient care.

    A. Predetermined norms and standards of care were used as a measure of quality before patient outcomes were so closely scrutinized.

    B. Patient satisfaction surveys determine the perceptions of the health care experience and often share vital information.

    D. While third-party payers have many expectations of healthcare performance, the quality of health care is not based on their definitions.

Content Category: Professional Issues

Reference: Newberry, 1998.

21. A nurse who attempts to render care without consent from the patient and inadvertently causes injury to the patient may be guilty of:
    A. assault.
    B. malpractice.
    C. negligence.
    D. BATTERY.

Rationale:

    D. Battery is defined as nonconsensual touching of another person that results in injury to the person. Attempting, without receiving proper consent, to render care that resulted in injury to the patient would be considered battery.
    A. Assault is an intentional threat to inflict injury on another person by someone who has the ability to carry out that threat.
    B. Malpractice occurs when an individual fails to use the care that a reasonable and prudent person would use. The terms "malpractice" and "negligence" could be used interchangeably in this case.
    C. Proof of negligence usually incorporates 4 elements: duty to the patient, breach of duty by the health care professional, injury resulting from the breach, and breach of duty as the proximate cause of injury.

Content Category: Professional Issues

Reference: Newberry, 2000.

22. What is the case-fatality rate for persons infected with *Bacillus anthracis* (anthrax) acquired by inhalation?
    A. 25%
    B. 50%
    C. 75%
    D. $\geq$ 90%

Rationale:

    D. Case-fatality rates for inhalational anthrax are believed to approach 90% to 100%.
    A. The case-fatality rate for gastrointestinal anthrax is reported as = 25%.
    B. The case-fatality rate for gastrointestinal anthrax is reported to range from 25% to 75%.
    C. The case-fatality upper limit rate for gastrointestinal anthrax is 75%.

Content Category: Substance Abuse & Toxicological & Environmental

References: Smego et al., 1998; pp. 97–102; CDC, 1998; 4.

23. Botulism is a rare but serious paralytic illness caused by a nerve toxin that is produced by the bacterium *Clostridium botulinum*. Which of the following are the most common types of botulism?
    A. Infant, wound
    B. Foodborne
    C. WOUND, INFANT, FOODBORNE
    D. Foodborne, wound

Rationale:

    C. There are three main kinds of botulism. Foodborne botulism is caused by eating foods that contain the botulinum toxin. Wound botulism is caused by toxin produced from a wound infected with *C. botulinum*. Infant botulism is caused by an infant's consumption of the spores of the botulinum bacterium, which then grow in the intestines and release toxin. All forms of botulism can be fatal and are considered medical emergencies. Foodborne botulism can be especially dangerous because many people can be poisoned by eating contaminated foods.

A. The answer omits foodborne botulism.
B. The answer omits wound and infant botulism.
D. The answer omits infant botulism.

Content Category: Substance Abuse & Toxicological & Environmental

References: Shapiro et al., 1997; pp. 433–435; Shapiro et al., pp. 221–228.

24. How is Lyme disease treated?
   A. Antibiotic treatment with doxycycline or amoxicillin for 7 to 10 days
   B. Antibiotic treatment with cefuroxime axetil or erythromycin for 7 to 10 days
   C. There is no treatment; the disease must run its course.
   D. ANTIBIOTIC TREATMENT WITH DOXYCYCLINE OR AMOXCILLIN FOR 3 TO 4 WEEKS

Rationale:

   D. According to treatment experts, antibiotic treatment for 3 to 4 weeks with doxycycline or amoxicillin is generally effective in early disease. Cefuroxime axetil or erythromycin can be used for persons who are allergic to penicillin or who cannot take tetracyclines. Later disease, particularly with objective neurologic manifestations, may require treatment with intravenous ceftriaxone or penicillin for 4 weeks or more, depending on disease severity. In later disease, treatment failures may occur and retreatment may be necessary.
   A. Antibiotic treatment for 3 to 4 weeks with doxycycline or amoxicillin is generally effective in early disease.
   B. Cefuroxime axetil or erythromycin is in persons who are allergic to penicillin or who cannot take tetracyclines. However, treatment generally lasts 3 to 4 weeks, not 7 to 10 days.
   C. The proper antibiotic treatment of Lyme disease is an important strategy to avoid the morbidity and costs of complicated and late-stage illness.

Content Category: Substance Abuse & Toxicological & Environmental

Reference: Kalish et al., 1993; pp. 2774–2779.

25. Plague is usually transmitted to humans by:
   A. indirect contact.
   B. respiratory contact
   C. DIRECT CONTACT.
   D. sexual contact.

Rationale:

   C. Plague is usually transmitted to humans by the bites of infected rodent fleas. During rodent plague outbreaks, many animals die and their hungry fleas seek other sources of blood to survive. Persons and animals that visit places where rodents have recently died from plague risk contracting the disease from flea bites. People also can become directly infected from handling infected rodents, rabbits, or wild carnivores that prey on these animals, when plague bacteria enter through breaks in the skin. House cats also are susceptible to plague. Infected cats become sick and may directly transmit plague to persons who handle or care for them. Dogs and cats may carry plague-infected fleas into the home. Inhaling droplets expelled by the coughing of a plague-infected person or animal, especially house cats, can result in plague of the lungs (plague pneumonia). Transmission of plague pneumonia from person to person is uncommon but sometimes results in dangerous epidemics that can quickly spread.
   A. Plague is directly transmitted from the infected organism.

B. Inhaling droplets expelled by the coughing of a plague-infected person or animal (especially house cats) can result in plague of the lungs (plague pneumonia). Transmission of plague pneumonia from person to person is uncommon but sometimes results in dangerous epidemics that can quickly spread.

D. The most common mode of transmission of plague is direct contact. The potential for sexual contact does exist.

Content Category: Substance Abuse & Toxicological & Environmental

References: Campbell & Dennis, 1998; pp. 975–983; Gage, 1998; pp. 885–903.

26. A 79-year-old patient decides to stop taking digoxin (Lanoxin), prescribed for an irregularly irregular fast heart rate. Before the patient discontinued the medication, pulse was noted to be 92 and regular. The patient is at greatest risk for:
    A. CEREBROVASCULAR ACCIDENT.
    B. pulmonary edema.
    C. renal failure.
    D. profound bradycardia.

Rationale:

A. Patients with an irregularly irregular heart rate usually have atrial fibrillation. Digoxin (Lanoxin) is used to control the heart rate and atrial fibrillation. This patient is more than likely to have converted to atrial fibrillation by discontinuing the medication and is at risk for a cerebrovascular accident (CVA). Patients who have atrial fibrillation are more likely to have a CVA because of clot formations on the mitral valve.

B. Although any patient may experience pulmonary edema, the greatest risk for this patient is a CVA.

C. Renal failure is not the greatest risk for this patient.

D. Withholding digoxin (Lanoxin) would increase the heart rate, not cause bradycardia.

Content Category: Substance Abuse & Toxicological & Environmental

Reference: Newberry, 1998; pp. 533–534.

27. A patient presents to the ED with a history of pesticide ingestion. Which of the following signs and symptoms should the ED nurse anticipate?
    A. DIARRHEA, EXCESSIVE SALIVATION, VOMITING, URINARY INCONTINENCE
    B. Hot flushed skin, agitation, dilated pupils, dry mucous membranes
    C. Hallucinations, tachycardia, loss of control over sensory input
    D. Dizziness, headache, nausea and vomiting, red mucous membranes

Rationale:

A. Pesticides contain organophosphate, which have a cholinergic effect on the body. The mnemonic SLUDGE is used to describe these effects: salivation, lacrimation, urination, defecation, gastrointestinal (nausea), and emesis. Other cholinergic effects include bradycardia, CNS depression, and constricted pupils.

B. Hot, flushed skin, agitation, dilated pupils, and dry mucous membranes are consistent with anticholinergic overdoses.

A. Hallucinations, tachycardia, and loss of control over sensory input characterize psychedelic agent intoxication.

B. Dizziness, headache, nausea and vomiting, and red mucous membranes are consistent with carbon monoxide poisoning.

Content Category: Substance Abuse & Toxicological & Environmental

Reference: Rosen et al., 1999.

28.   A patient was admitted to the ED with subacute onset of progressive dizziness, blurred vision, slurred speech, difficulty swallowing, and nausea. Findings on examination included ptosis, extraocular palsies, facial paralysis, palatal weakness, and impaired gag reflex. The patient also had partially healed superficial knee wounds incurred while hunting 5 days earlier. The patient reported that during the 24 hours before onset of symptoms, he had eaten home-canned green beans and a stew containing roast beef and potatoes. Based on the clinical manifestations, you suspect:
      A.   myasthenia gravis.
      B.   organophosphate poisoning.
      C.   Guillain-Barré syndrome.
      D.   BOTULISM.

Rationale:

   D.   Botulism is suggested by clinical manifestations such as descending neuroparalysis, ptosis, and extraocular palsies. Physicians should obtain a thorough food history to assist in the diagnosis and in identifying and obtaining potentially contaminated leftover food. In the case described in this report, heat-resistant *Clostridium botulinum* spores either survived the initial cooking or were introduced afterwards; the spores subsequently germinated and produced toxin. The lid of the pot or the gravy of the stew most likely provided the anaerobic environment necessary for toxin production.
   A.   Electromyography (EMG) is helpful in distinguishing botulism from myasthenia gravis, a disease that botulism often mimics closely. A characteristic EMG pattern observed in adult patients with botulism has been well described. A normal edrophonium (Tensilon) test helps to differentiate botulism from MG.
   B.   RBC and serum cholinesterase levels will assist in ruling out organophosphate poisoning.
   C.   A normal cerebrospinal fluid (CSF) examination will help differentiate botulism from Guillain-Barré syndrome, although a slightly elevated CSF protein level is occasionally seen with botulism and the protein level may be initially normal in Guillain-Barré syndrome.

Content Category: Substance Abuse & Toxicological & Environmental

References: Shapiro et al, 1997; pp. 433–435; Shapiro et al., 1998; pp. 221–228.

29.   The key antidote for acetaminophen poisoning is:
      A.   naloxone (Narcan).
      B.   glucagon.
      C.   N-ACETYLCYSTEINE (MUCOMYST).
      D.   atropine.

Rationale:

   C.   N-acetylcysteine (Mucomyst) is the treatment for acetaminophen poisoning and may be given orally or via lavage tube. This medication prevents the toxic substances from binding to the liver cells and increases the body's ability to detoxify the acetaminophen byproducts.
   A.   Naloxone (Narcan) is used for narcotics overdose.
   B.   Glucagon is useful for calcium channel blocker toxicity.
   D.   Atropine is needed for overdoses of organophosphates.

Content Category: Substance Abuse & Toxicological & Environmental

References: ENA, Core Curriculum, 2000; p. 641; Oman et al., 2001; p. 117.

30.   You are caring for a patient in the ED who has ingested 2000 mg (20 100-mg tablets) of amitriptyline (Elavil). While caring for this patient, you would expect which of the following?
    A. Hyperactive effect with increased excitability
    B. PREMATURE VENTRICULAR CONTRACTIONS ON THE CARDIAC MONITOR
    C. Constricted pupils with slight variation in reactivity to light
    D. Oliguria and increased salivation

Rationale:

    B. Cardiac dysrhythmias are common after tricyclic antidepressant poisoning. Premature ventricular contractions and ventricular tachycardia along with cardiac depressant effects are most common. AV conduction disturbances may also be seen.
    A. Loss of consciousness or lethargy to comatose state with rapid progression is most common with a significant tricyclic antidepressant overdose.
    C. Mydriasis or dilated pupils are common.
    D. Oliguria is an anticholinergic effect. Increased salivation is a symptom associated with excessive cholinergic action.

Content Category: Substance Abuse & Toxicological & Environmental

Reference: ENA, Core Curriculum; 2000; pp. 641–642.

31.   A patient is exposed to a significant dose of radiation at work. He presents to the ED for treatment. He is immediately decontaminated with water and specimens are collected to determine any remaining radiation. The ED nurse would know that the patient had experienced significant exposure if:
    A. he glowed when the lights were turned off.
    B. HE DEVELOPED NAUSEA, VOMITING, AND BLOODY DIARRHEA.
    C. his blood pressure remained high after decontamination.
    D. Geiger counters were unable to be calibrated.

Rationale:

    B. Symptoms of nausea, vomiting, or bloody diarrhea within 3 hours of exposure to radiation indicate a significant dose of radiation.
    A. Although popular belief suggests that radiation causes a person to glow, no scientific proof of this exists.
    C. The vomiting and diarrhea may cause hypotension to develop.
    D. Geiger counters should be calibrated before use. Any Geiger counter that cannot be calibrated should not be used.

Content Category: Substance Abuse & Toxicological & Environmental

Reference: ENA, Core Curriculum, 2000; pp. 708–709.

32.   An adult patient takes an overdose of acetylsalicylic acid (aspirin). What is the average time for peak serum levels to occur?
    A. 15 to 30 minutes
    B. 1 hour
    C. 90 minutes
    D. 2 TO 4 HOURS

Rationale:

    D. Peak serum levels of salicylate occur 2 to 4 hours after an acute ingestion.
    A. Peak serum level is 2 to 4 hours, not 15 to 30 minutes.

B. Peak serum level is 2 to 4 hours, not 1 hour.
C. Peak serum level is 2 to 4 hours, not 90 minutes.

Content Category: Substance Abuse & Toxicological & Environmental
Reference: ENA, Core Curriculum, 2000; pp. 636–640.

33. Host factors associated with severe or fatal Rocky Mountain spotted fever include:
A. advanced age, female sex, chronic alcohol abuse, Caucasian race.
B. MALE SEX, GLUCOSE-6-PHOSPHATE DEHYDROGENASE DEFICIENCY, CHRONIC ALCOHOL ABUSE, ADVANCED AGE, AFRICAN-AMERICAN RACE.
C. Glucose-6-phosphate dehydrogenase deficiency, male sex, advanced age.
D. African-American race, female sex, chronic alcohol abuse, advanced age.

Rationale:

B. Host factors associated with severe or fatal Rocky Mountain spotted fever include advanced age, male sex, African-American race, chronic alcohol abuse, and glucose-6-phosphate dehydrogenase (G6PD) deficiency.
A. Female sex is not considered a primary host factor.
C. Caucasian race is not considered a primary host factor.
D. Female sex is not considered a primary host factor.

Content Category: Substance Abuse & Toxicological & Environmental
Reference: Abramson & Givner, 1999; pp. 539–540.

34. Which of the following is highest priority for a near-drowning victim brought to the ED?
A. HYPOXEMIA
B. Pneumonia
C. Cardiac dysrhythmias
D. Hypothermia

Rationale:

A. Hypoxemia, caused by laryngospasm and asphyxia, is the central clinical event for all near-drowning victims.
B. Pneumonia may be caused by aspiration in the recovery phase.
C. Dysrhythmias and cardiac decompensation may occur secondary to hypoxemia and acidosis.
D. Hypothermia secondary to cold-water submersion decreases metabolic demand, which may actually reduce potential hypoxia in prolonged submersion.

Content Category: Substance Abuse & Toxicological & Environmental
Reference: Tintinalli et al., 2000.

35. What are the three principal routes of exposure for chemical hazardous materials?
A. Indirect contact, injection, direct contact
B. Rural, urban, suburban
C. Feet, hands, lungs
D. INHALATION, SKIN ABSORPTION, DIRECT CONTACT

Rationale:

D. Inhalation, skin absorption, and direct contact are the most common routes of chemical exposure.
A. Indirect contact and injection are not common routes of exposure.

B. Rural, urban, and suburban are settings in which exposure may occur, not routes of exposure.

C. Feet, hands, and lungs may reflect the site of entrance to the body but are not routes of exposure.

Content Category: Substance Abuse & Toxicological & Environmental

Reference: ENA, Core Curriculum, 2000.

36.   Information about any hazardous chemicals kept in the ED should be found in which of the following?

A. Poison control center

B. MATERIAL SAFETY DATA SHEETS

C. Joint Commission on Accreditation of Healthcare Organizations standards

D. Centers for Disease Control and Prevention (CDC)

Rationale:

B. Material Safety Data Sheets (MSDS) are to be kept readily available to ED staff and should contain descriptions of any hazards that may be encountered while handling hazardous materials in the ED.

A. A poison control center may have information, but it may not be readily available to ED clinicians.

C. JCAHO standards do not contain specifics on hazardous materials.

D. The CDC is not a resource for hazardous materials information.

Content Category: Substance Abuse & Toxicological & Environmental

Reference: ENA, Core Curriculum, 2000.

37.   The key point for the ED nurse to remember in caring for a patient who is a phencyclidine (PCP) abuser is that the patient's:

A. increase in physical strength and ability.

B. DECREASE IN PAIN SENSATION AND JUDGMENT.

C. increase in insight into the drug abuse problem.

D. decrease in ability to metabolize the drug.

Rationale:

B. The PCP abuser has decreased pain sensation and judgment. Having altered sensory perception allows the PCP patient to believe that he or she can do things that a normal person cannot do.

A. The PCP abuser may mistakenly believe that he or she has increased physical strength and ability.

C. This type of patient tends to have little insight into his or her drug problem and its effect on their lives.

D. The PCP abuser does not necessarily have decreased hepatic function because of the use of PCP.

Content Category: Patient Care

Reference: ENA, Core Curriculum, 2000.

38.   An 18-year-old basketball player has just suffered an inversion injury of the left ankle. The ankle is very swollen and the patient cannot weight bear. The 5 Ps are intact. In planning for the care of this patient, you know that this patient is at high risk for:

A. AVULSION FRACTURE.

B. impacted fracture.

C. displaced fracture.

D. segmental fracture.

Rationale:

A. A patient with an inversion injury of the ankle is at highest risk for an avulsion fracture related to the twisting motion. The bone fragment is pulled out of place by a ligament.

B. An impacted fracture occurs when one bone fragment is forced into another and usually involves a great deal of force.

C. A displaced fracture occurs when the bone fragments are fractured, separated, and displaced.

D. In a segmental fracture, the fractured bone is in multiple pieces, usually a central portion with two adjacent portions.

Content Category: Patient Care

References: ENA, Core Curriculum, 2000; Moreau, 2001; p. 265.

39. When a nurse is planning care for an ED patient with chronic obstructive pulmonary disease (COPD), an understanding of which of the following is most important?
    A. Current vital signs
    B. Current peak flow
    C. Causes of the current illness
    D. BASELINE RESPIRATORY FUNCTION

Rationale:

D. It is most important for the nurse to know the patient's baseline respiratory function in order to determine the critical values based on optimal lung function.

A. Current vital signs are important to know, but must be based on the patient's normal status.

B. Current peak flow is vital information, but must be correlated to this patient's optimal lung function values.

C. Understanding the causes of the current illness are important, but this is not a priority for planning immediate patient care.

Content Category: Patient Care

References: ENA, Core Curriculum, 2000; Moreau, 2001; pp. 710–712.

40. A 68-year-old male, accompanied by his wife, presents to the ED with a history of Alzheimer's disease. His vital signs are stable. On examination, you determine that the patient has a positive snout test (tapping the face just below the nose causes the patient to grimace) and appears agitated. Your initial intervention would be to:
    A. obtain lab tests (CBC, electrolytes).
    B. PLACE THE PATIENT IN A QUIET ROOM.
    C. have the patient seen by the physician now.
    D. give the patient a sedative parentally.

Rationale:

B. This patient has become agitated and needs the quiet and calm of a private room with familiar family members to reduce agitation and stimulation. Grimacing or puckering the lips after stroking or tapping under the nose is a positive sign for Alzheimer's disease in the adult patient. (Infants normally have a positive snout test.)

A. Lab tests may be done on this patient during the course of the time he spends in the ED but are not a priority at present.

C. The patient does need to be seen by the physician in a timely fashion, but this is not an emergent situation.

D. Nonpharmacologic interventions such as reducing stimuli are more appropriate with Alzheimer's patients, who can easily become agitated.

Content Category: Patient Care

References: ENA, Core Curriculum, 2000; Moreau, 2001; p. 744.

41.   Your 14-year-old patient presents with a sore throat (pain 7/10) and reports that it has been present for 2 days. Vital signs are BP 110/70, HR 88/min, respirations 18/min, oxygen saturation 95%, and temperature 102.4° F (39.1° C). A priority nursing intervention would be which of the following?
      A. Spray the throat with a local anesthetic to decrease the pain.
      B. Obtain a complete blood count (CBC).
      C. Have the patient do salt water gargles.
      D. OBTAIN A THROAT CULTURE.

Rationale:

      D. Obtain a rapid strep throat swab as well as a regular throat culture. The rapid strep test may identify Streptococcus A but frequently misses the more common Strep C or G. It is most important to identify Strep A and treat it immediately to prevent serious complications such as rheumatic heart disease.
      A. The patient's throat may be sprayed with a local anesthetic by physician order, but not until after a throat culture had been obtained.
      B. CBC is not usually a priority for a patient with a sore throat.
      C. Salt water gargles are recommended as part of the treatment plan, but would not be a priority treatment and would be done after the throat culture had been obtained.

Content Category: Patient Care

References: ENA, Core Curriculum, 2000; Moreau, 2001; p. 1203.

42.   A 1-year-old patient presents with inconsolable crying and a 2-hour history of currant jelly stools. The physician diagnoses intussusception. Your immediate goal in the ED is to do which of the following?
      A. OBTAIN A SURGICAL CONSULT.
      B. Give an enema.
      C. Give narcotic analgesics.
      D. Console the patient and family.

Rationale:

      A. An intussusception is a pediatric emergency that requires an immediate surgical consult. In this condition, a portion of the bowel has telescoped into an adjacent bowel portion. Unless the area is reduced, it may become ischemic or gangrenous. The reduction can occur in the radiology department with the use of fluoroscopy or in the operating room.
      B. An enema would not be given unless the bowel could be visualized.
      C. A narcotic analgesic appropriate for the patient's age and weight may be given, typically after the surgeon has assessed the patient, but the priority is for the child to be assessed by a surgeon.
      D. The patient and family need reassurance and consolation, but this is not the priority intervention.

Content Category: Patient Care

References: ENA, Core Curriculum, 2000; Moreau, 2001; p. 943.

43.   A 6-month-old patient presents to the ED 4 hours after being diagnosed with respiratory syncytial virus (RSV) in the pediatrician's office. Which of the following would indicate the need for immediate intervention by the triage nurse?
      A. Respiratory rate of 44/min
      B. Oxygen saturation of 94%

C. NASAL FLARING
D. Heart rate of 132 beats per minute

Rationale:

C. Nasal flaring indicates acute respiratory distress and warrants immediate intervention.
A. A respiratory rate of 44/min is slightly elevated from the normal range of 20 to 40 per minute but is less worthy of concern than nasal flaring.
B. An O_2 sat of 94% is slightly below the expected rate for this infant but is not of immediate concern.
D. A heart rate of 132 bpm is within the normal range for a 6-month-old child. The normal range at this age is 80 to 160 bpm.

Content Category: Patient Care

References: ENA, Core Curriculum, 2000; Moreau, 2001; p.193.

44. With the Glasgow Coma Scale (GCS), which of the following total scores indicates coma?
A. 6
B. 9
C. 11
D. 15

Rationale:

A. Evaluating the 3 parameters of the Glasgow Coma Scale determines the patient's ability to respond to internal and external stimuli. A patient with a total score of 7 or less is considered comatose.
B. A score of 9 indicates some function across the 3 dimensions and indicates a higher level of intact cognitive function.
C. A score of 11 indicates a greater degree of function, although not full awareness and ability.
D. The highest score on the GCS is 15, which indicates an intact reticular activating system and adequate function of the cerebral hemispheres.

Content Category: Patient Care

Reference: ENA, Core Curriculum, 2000; pp. 303–307, 787.

45. In hemophilia, which lab test has abnormal results?
A. Hemoglobin
B. PARTIAL THROMBOPLASTIN TIME (PTT)
C. Prothrombin time (PT)
D. Platelet count

Rationale:

B. The PTT test assesses the intrinsic system and the common pathway of clot formation, evaluating factors I, II, V, VIII, IX, X, XI, and XII. In hemophilia with a deficiency of factor VIII or IX, PTT is prolonged.
A. Hemoglobin is normal; the disease impedes the clotting mechanism.
C. PT measures the extrinsic system and the common pathway. PT is prolonged in hepatitis, obstructive biliary disease, and hepatocellular liver disease. Taking coumadin also prolongs PT.
D. Platelet count is usually normal in patients with hemophilia.

Content Category: Patient Care

Reference: ENA, Core Curriculum, 2000; pp. 310–313.

46. Which of the following physical exam findings can indicate meningeal irritation?
    A. Murphy's sign
    B. Kehr's sign
    C. Rovsing's sign
    D. KERNIG'S SIGN

Rationale:

D. Meningeal irritation can be manifested as photophobia, nuchal rigidity, fever, headache, vomiting, a positive Brudzinski's sign, and a positive Kernig's sign. Flexing the leg at the hip and knee and then straightening the knee evaluate Kernig's sign. If resistance or pain is found, further evaluation of meningeal inflammation is required.

A. Murphy's sign—tenderness and limitation of deep inspiration—is evaluated for cholecystitis.

B. Free blood in the abdomen may present with referred pain to the left shoulder (Kehr's sign) because of irritation of the diaphragm.

C. Deep palpation of the left lower quadrant that causes pain in the right lower quadrant, an indicator of appendicitis, is a positive Rovsing's sign.

Content Category: Patient Care

References: Seidel et al., 1999; pp. 551, 790; Newberry, 1998; pp.312, 548–549; ENA, Core Curriculum, 2000; pp. 245–246.

47. A 58-year-old person presents to the ED with a 10-day history of copious vomiting and abdominal pain. Arterial blood gases are drawn and reveal a pH of 7.60, $PaCO_2$ of 48 mm Hg, and bicarbonate level of 52 mmol/L. What is your interpretation?
    A. Metabolic acidosis with respiratory compensation
    B. METABOLIC ALKALOSIS WITH RESPIRATORY COMPENSATION
    C. Respiratory acidosis with metabolic compensation
    D. Respiratory alkalosis with metabolic compensation

Rationale:

B. The patient's substantial amount of vomiting resulted in a loss of hydrogen ions, leading to metabolic alkalosis with dehydration and hypokalemia. Respiratory compensation is evident from the increased $PaCO_2$ level.

A. To indicate acidosis—reflecting more hydrogen ions, not fewer—the pH would have to be lower than the normal range of 7.35 to 7.45.

C. An increase in $PaCO_2$ would reflect a decrease in pH if this was a primary respiratory problem.

D. A decrease in $PaCO_2$ would result in an increase in pH, which is not reflected in the laboratory test findings.

Content Category: Patient Care

References: Guyton & Hall, 1996; pp. 385–388; Newberry, 1998; p. 172.

48. A 24-year-old woman who is 26 weeks pregnant presents to the ED reporting right upper quadrant pain (rated at 7/10) for the past 6 hours. She describes the pain as constant and aching. She states that fetal movements are > 10 per hour. She is nauseated and has been constipated for 2 days. Urinalysis is negative. Liver function tests are within normal levels. WBC is slightly elevated. Vital signs are BP 120/84, HR 86/min, respirations 22/min, oxygen saturation 98%, temperature 99.4° F (37.5° C), and fetal heart rate (FHR) 134/min. Your assessment confirms that the plan of care should be directed toward which of the following conditions?
    A. APPENDICITIS
    B. Cholecystitis

C. Stretching of the broad ligament
D. Pyelonephritis

Rationale:

A. The appendix is pushed upward as pregnancy advances. This is a classic presentation of a pregnant woman with appendicitis.

B. Liver function tests are within normal range and the patient has altered bowel function. These findings do not represent a classic presentation of cholecystitis, nor is that condition so common as appendicitis in pregnant women.

C. With stretching of the broad ligament, the pain is generally felt in the groin or low abdomen. This condition is not associated with an increased temperature or elevated WBC.

D. The urinalysis is negative and the woman has no genitourinary symptoms or pain over the kidney region. Therefore, pyelonephritis is ruled out.

Content Category: Patient Care

Reference: ENA, Core Curriculum, 2000.

49. The vasopressor of choice for tricyclic antidepressant (TCA) overdose is:
A. dopamine (Intropin).
B. NOREPINEPHRINE (LEVOPHED).
C. amrinone lactate (Inocor).
D. dobutamine (Dobutrex).

Rationale:

B. Norepinephrine is the pressor agent of choice for a TCA overdose because it does not compete at the receptor site and cause a rebound hypotension. In addition, the TCA overdose patient generally responds better to this direct-acting vasopressor.

A. Dopamine is a common vasopressor that is generally successful in the treatment of nonhypovolemic hypotension. Dopamine in moderate doses may not work well with TCA or cocaine overdoses because these drugs may block the pump and cause rebound hypotension.

C. Amrinone lactate is a positive inotropic drug that is used short term for refractory congestive heart failure.

D. Dobutamine is a positive inotropic drug that is used for refractory congestive heart failure.

Content Category: Patient Care

References: ENA, Core Curriculum, 2000; Newberry, 1998.

50. The primary reason emergency staff do not always recognize potential organ donor patients is uncertainty about how to initiate:
A. conversation with the potential organ donor's family.
B. THE DONOR REFERRAL PROCESS TO AN ORGAN PROCUREMENT ORGANIZATION.
C. a dialog with colleagues regarding the organ donation process.
D. brain death verification.

Rationale:

B. According to current estimates, 27% of the medically suitable organ donors in the United States are never recognized as potential donors. Several recent studies have indicated that hospital staff members and physicians consistently fail to recognize certain patients as potential organ donors and thus to notify the Organ Procurement Organization (OPO) so that a thorough evaluation can be done. Reasons that hospital staff do not recognize potential organ donors and therefore fail to refer these patients to the OPO include lack of knowledge about the criteria for organ donation, reluctance to spend the time to get the OPO involved, and uncertainty about how to initiate the donor referral process.

A. While some emergency nurses do feel uncomfortable discussing organ donation with families, studies have shown that this is not the primary reason too few potential donors are identified.

C. Hospital staff are most comfortable discussing issues surrounding organ donation with their colleagues.

D. The determination of brain death is usually made in the intensive care or critical care unit, not in the ED. Emergency nurses should be familiar with their institutions' definition and criteria for declaring a patient brain dead. It is recommended that the option of donation be offered to the family once the patient has been pronounced brain dead and the family has been given time to accept the death. Therefore, the presence or absence of brain death verification should not be a barrier against making at least the initial referral to the Organ Procurement Organization.

Content Category: Patient Care

Reference: Ehrle et al., 1999; pp. 21–33.

51.   Medical contraindications to organ donation include all of the following EXCEPT:
A. encephalitis of unknown cause.
B. hematologic malignant neoplasm.
C. disseminated tuberculosis.
D. SEIZURE DISORDER.

Rationale:

D. A seizure disorder does not signify that the patient's organs are unlikely to function. Seizure disorder is not on the list of medical contraindications to organ donation.

A. Encephalitis of unknown cause is a potentially transmissible infectious disease that would adversely affect an organ recipient.

B. Hematologic malignant neoplasm would adversely affect a recipient.

C. Disseminated tuberculosis is a transmissible infectious disease that would adversely affect a recipient.

Content Category: Patient Care

Reference: Ehrle et al., 1999; pp. 21–33.

52.   Potential organ donor variables that influence organ donation rates include which of the following?
A. RACE
B. Sex
C. Blood type
D. Allergy status

Rationale:

A. Racial and cultural demographics affect donation rates. African Americans are twice as likely not to donate because they are three times more likely not to be asked or because health care professionals do not request consent from them in an effective way. Organ Procurement Organizations (OPOs) are prepared to provide race-specific representatives and experts in dealing with such variables.

B. There is no evidence that families of males versus females have differences in consent rates for organ donation. There are more potential male donors when the cause of death is trauma because more patients who incur such injuries are male.

C. Once consent for organ donation has been given, a thorough evaluation is done. Blood is sent to the laboratory for typing if the patient's blood type has not already been documented on the chart. Potential organ donors are not screened and refused based on blood type. The blood and tissue types of the organ recipient must be compatible with those of the donor.

D. Donors are screened for a number of factors, including but not limited to any history or treatment of heart disease; hypertension; chest pain; diabetes; use of tobacco, drugs, or alcohol; and behavior that would place them at risk for transmitting human immunodeficiency and hepatitis viruses. The donor's allergy status is noted on the chart but is not a screening mechanism for potential donors.

Content Category: Patient Care

References: Ehrle et al., 1999; pp. 21–33; Holmquist et al., 1999; pp. 84–98.

53. Common forms of emergency operations preparedness drills or exercises required by regulatory agencies include which of the following?
    A. On-site, hospital, ED
    B. Scene, in-house, departmental
    C. TABLETOP, FUNCTIONAL, FULL SCALE
    D. Written, acted, integrated

Rationale:

C. Tabletop, functional, and full scale are types of drills that meet regulatory agency requirements.
A. Exercises may take place on site, in the hospital, and in the ED, but these locations are not required by regulatory agencies.
B. Exercises may take place at the scene, in-house, and in the department, but are not required by regulatory agencies.
D. Written, acted, and integrated are ways in which drills may be performed.

Content Category: Patient Care

Reference: Newberry, 1998; p. 205.

54. The ED nurse is asked to administer the first dose of rifampin (Rifadin) prophylaxis to 3 young women who are roommates of a patient who has just been diagnosed with meningococcal meningitis. What advice should the ED nurse give to the roommates regarding this medication?
    A. "TAKING THIS MEDICATION MAY TURN YOUR URINE ORANGE."
    B. "Take the medication with meals."
    C. "You may continue to wear your contact lenses."
    D. "There is no interaction between this medication and birth control pills."

Rationale:

A. Rifampin turns urine, stool, tears, sweat, saliva, and other bodily fluids a red-brown color.
B. If the medication causes GI upset, it may be taken with food. However, it is better absorbed and has better action if taken on an empty stomach.
C. Rifampin permanently stains soft contact lenses and clothing a red-brown color. Patients should wear soft contact lenses should not insert the lenses while they are taking rifampin and for several days afterward. The return of body fluids to normal colors indicates that the lenses will be safe from staining.
D. Taking rifampin decreases the effectiveness of birth control pills. Another form of birth control should be used in addition to oral contraceptives for the month of rifampin use.

Content Category: Patient Care

References: Peabody, 2000; pp. 227–274; Turkoski et al., 2000.

55.   Appropriate interfacility transfer and transport of a medically unstable child must include which of the following?
   A.   A screening exam by the triage nurse, consent to transfer, and copies of medical records related to the emergency medical condition to accompany the patient
   B.   Parental request and consent to transfer to another facility by privately owned vehicle (POV)
   C.   Physician certification that transfer is a medical necessity, consent, and an RN and a physician to accompany the patient to the referral hospital
   D.   ACCEPTANCE BY THE RECEIVING FACILITY, COPIES OF MEDICAL RECORDS RELATED TO THE EMERGENCY MEDICAL CONDITION TO ACCOMPANY THE PATIENT, AND QUALIFIED PERSONNEL WITH ADEQUATE EQUIPMENT TO CARE FOR THE PATIENT EN ROUTE

Rationale:

   D.   All these are essential components of an interfacility transfer of a patient with a medical emergency.
   A.   A screening exam by the triage nurse does not meet legal requirements for a screening exam before such a transfer.
   B.   These considerations do not address the legal requirement that another facility have the bed and resources to care for the patient. A privately owned vehicle would not be a suitable vehicle for the transport of a child with a medical emergency.
   C.   It is not always necessary for an RN or MD to accompany the patient. Many patients can be safely transported by emergency medical technician–paramedics (EMT-Ps) or other team configurations.

Content Category: Patient Care

Reference: ENA, 1999; pp. 355–356.

56.   A 4-year-old presents to the ED with an avulsed tooth. She was hit in the mouth with a toy thrown by another child at her day care center. The incident occurred approximately 45 minutes ago. Her day care attendant has the child's tooth wrapped in a clean cloth. Bleeding is minimal. Which of the following statements is correct?
   A.   Treatment of the tooth should begin within 60 minutes of the avulsion.
   B.   The avulsed tooth should be gently cleaned and placed in sterile water.
   C.   The avulsed tooth should be scrubbed and gently replaced in the patient's gum.
   D.   BABY TEETH ARE SELDOM REIMPLANTED.

Rationale:

   D.   Primary teeth are usually not reimplanted because of the risk of damage to the permanent tooth bud.
   A.   Because primary teeth are usually not reimplanted, there is no need to clean the tooth.
   B.   If a permanent tooth had been lost, the correct procedure would have been to rinse the tooth gently with water or saline and insert the tooth into the socket or place it in milk until the time of reimplantation.
   C.   Because primary teeth are usually not reimplanted, avulsed teeth should not be scrubbed.

Content Category: Patient Care

Reference: ENA, 1999; p.154.

57. You are giving discharge instructions to the parents of a newborn. The parents brought the baby to your ED "to be checked out" because the family was involved in a motor vehicle accident. The baby, who was secured in an infant seat that his mother was holding, appears to be uninjured. Mom was the uninjured front seat passenger. You tell the parents that babies should be:

A. placed in a rear-facing seat until they weigh 10 lb (4.5 kg)

B. placed in a forward-facing seat in the rear seat of the car until they weigh 30 lb (13.6 kg).

C. PLACED IN A REAR-FACING SEAT IN THE REAR SEAT OF THE CAR UNTIL THEY WEIGH 20 LB (9.0 KG).

D. in a rear-facing seat unless they are in the back seat.

Rationale:

C. From birth to at least 20 lb and at least 1 year of age, children riding in cars should be placed in rear-facing seats.

A. Incorrect.

B. Incorrect.

D. Incorrect.

Content Category: Patient Care

Reference: Wong, 1999; p. 610.

58. An unrestrained driver is brought into the ED by EMS. Paramedics report that she was in an older car without airbags and the steering wheel was bent. The patient is drowsy, pale, and anxious and has labored respirations. A massive pulmonary contusion is suspected. She is being given 100% high-flow oxygen via nonrebreather mask. The priority intervention for this patient is:

A. chest tube placement.

B. ARTERIAL BLOOD GASES.

C. diagnostic peritoneal lavage.

D. administration of antianxiety medication.

Rationale:

B. Pulmonary contusions can cause hypoxia related to a ventilation-perfusion mismatch. Arterial blood gases should be drawn to determine whether the patient requires intubation and mechanical ventilation.

A. Chest tube placement would be appropriate treatment for a pneumothorax or hemothorax to restore intrapleural pressure. There is no evidence that either of these conditions is present. The placement of a chest tube in this scenario would not repair the suspected ventilation-perfusion mismatch.

C. Diagnostic peritoneal lavage is used to determine the presence of peritoneal bleeding in the hemodynamically unstable patient.

D. Medication with an antianxiety agent may cause hypotension and respiratory depression, which could potentially worsen the hypoxia caused by a pulmonary contusion.

Content Category: Respiratory

References: ENA, Core Curriculum, 2000; pp. 385, 580–586; Newberry, 1998; pp. 298–302, 311, 782.

59. The priority nursing intervention for a patient suspected to have a massive hemothorax is which of the following?
    A. Preparation for diagnostic peritoneal lavage
    B. SEND BLOOD FOR TYPE AND CROSSMATCH
    C. Prepare for pericardiocentesis
    D. Administer analgesic medication

Rationale:

B. In massive hemothorax, cardiac output is decreased because of the high potential for hemorrhage and circulating blood volume. This intervention must be supported by the establishment of two large-bore IVs and the infusion of crystalloids, followed by blood replacement. Therefore, a type and crossmatch should be completed as soon as possible.

A. Diagnostic peritoneal lavage would be an appropriate diagnostic adjunct for abdominal trauma and occult abdominal hemorrhage.

C. Preparing for pericardiocentesis is not indicated for this patient, who exhibits no signs or symptoms of cardiac tamponade.

D. Although the administration of analgesic medication is an important consideration, airway, breathing, and circulation should be assessed and maintained first.

Content Category: Respiratory

References: Kidd et al., 2000; p. 688; ENA, Core Curriculum, 2000; pp. 8–11, 385, 600–603, 620–622; ENA, Trauma Nursing, 2000; pp. 43–46, 79–80, 154.

60. A victim of a stab wound to the epigastric area presents to the ED. Upon evaluation, he suddenly develops shortness of breath, chest pain, and decreased breath sounds. You suspect:
    A. DIAPHRAGMATIC TEAR.
    B. myocardial contusion.
    C. flail chest.
    D. rib fractures.

Rationale:

A. Any patient presenting with penetrating trauma below the nipple line is at risk for a diaphragmatic tear, which allows herniation of abdominal contents into the respiratory cavity, thus causing respiratory compromise.

B. A myocardial contusion is caused by blunt trauma. The patient presents with chest pain, ecchymosis to the chest wall, and ECG abnormalities. No evidence in the current case supports this diagnosis.

C. Blunt trauma, not penetrating trauma, causes flail chest. The patient presents with asymmetrical rise and fall of the chest, dyspnea, and chest wall pain. No evidence in the current case supports this diagnosis.

D. Rib fractures are unlikely to occur with penetrating trauma. The patient presents with localized pain, chest wall ecchymosis, and bony crepitus or deformity as well as dyspnea and chest wall pain. No evidence in the current case supports this diagnosis.

Content Category: Respiratory

References: ENA, Trauma Nursing, 2000; pp.122–125; Newberry, 1998; pp. 295–302; Blansfield et al., 1999; pp. 267–268.

61. An anxious, panic-stricken patient arrives in the ED with a chief complaint of dyspnea, rapid respirations, and periorbital numbness. All serious causes for this breathing pattern are eliminated and the patient is diagnosed with hyperventilation. Which of the following findings do you anticipate?
    A. RESPIRATORY ALKALOSIS

B. Dehydration
C. Stroke
D. Metabolic acidosis

Rationale:

A. Hyperventilation creates respiratory alkalosis with rapid respirations and a decrease in carbon dioxide levels.
B. Dehydration is not consistent with the signs and symptoms of hyperventilation.
C. There is no mention of the patient's level of consciousness, neurologic symptoms, or motor functions; therefore there is no evidence to support a diagnosis of stroke.
D. Metabolic acidosis is an acid-base imbalance that presents with diabetic ketoacidosis. Since there has been no mention of hyperglycemia, dehydration, or Kussmaul's respirations, there is no evidence to support the diagnosis of metabolic acidosis.

Content Category: Respiratory

References: ENA, Core Curriculum, 2000; pp. 569–570; Newberry, 1998; pp. 475–476.

62. A 45-year-old patient presents to the ED with increased shortness of breath over the past 3 days. His history includes a chronic cough that has produced copious amounts of mucopurulent sputum for the past 5 years and smoking 2 packs of cigarettes per day for 30 years. Physical findings include scattered rhonchi, distended neck veins, polycythemia, and peripheral edema. The ED nurse knows that these findings are consistent with which of the following?
A. Asthma
B. CHRONIC BRONCHITIS
C. Emphysema
D. Pneumonia

Rationale:

B. These changes are seen with the chronic inflammation of chronic bronchitis and the resulting cor pulmonale.
A. Asthma produces wheezes on auscultation and does not cause distended neck veins or peripheral edema.
C. While emphysema often occurs with chronic bronchitis, the symptoms it produces result from alveolar breakdown and inability to exhale normally and do not result in cor pulmonale.
D. Tuberculosis can cause a cough of long duration and scattered rhonchi, but it does not produce polycythemia or peripheral edema.

Content Category: Respiratory

References: Newberry, 1998; pp. 431–451; Kitt et al., 1995; pp. 188–200.

63. An unrestrained passenger presents to the ED after having been involved in a high-speed motor vehicle crash (MVC) and having received multiple facial wounds. The primary assessment concern for this patient would be which of the following?
A. AIRWAY OBSTRUCTION
B. Infection
C. Loss of sensation
D. Skull fracture

Rationale:

A. Because the patient has multiple facial wounds, airway obstruction must be considered. Potential proximate causes include facial fractures, edema, bleeding, accumulation of secretions, and debris.

B. Infection is likely, but prophylactic treatment can be initiated after the patient has been stabilized.

C. Loss of sensation may be present if the facial nerves have been damaged, but it is not the high priority initially.

D. Skull fracture may be present, but ABCs should be stabilized before this possibility is explored.

Content Category: Respiratory

References: ENA, Trauma Nursing, 2000; pp. 92–108; ENA, Core Curriculum, 2000; pp. 221–224.

64.   The most common cause of pleural effusion is:
A. empyema.
B. malignancy.
C. CONGESTIVE HEART FAILURE.
D. asthma.

Rationale:

C. Congestive heart failure is the most common cause of effusion.

A. Empyema is one type of an infective effusion.

B. Malignancy can cause effusion but is not as common as congestive heart failure.

D. Asthma does not cause pleural effusion.

Content Category: Respiratory

Reference: ENA, Core Curriculum, 2000; p. 570.

65.   Respiratory distress syndrome is most commonly associated with which of the following?
A. Rib fracture
B. Bronchitis
C. PULMONARY CONTUSION
D. Spinal cord injury

Rationale:

C. A pulmonary contusion is most likely to put a patient at risk for respiratory distress syndrome. Excess fluid intake can precipitate noncardiogenic pulmonary edema triggered by the fluid overload of the damaged alveolar-capillary membrane. ·

A. A simple rib fracture would not cause the severe damage to the lung tissue that can cause respiratory distress syndrome.

B. Bronchitis is an inflammatory process and not a likely cause of respiratory distress syndrome.

D. A spinal cord injury may interfere with the use of intercostal muscles or the diaphragm but does not cause damage to the lung tissue.

Content Category: Respiratory

References: Lombardi et al., 1995; pp. 239–240; Newberry, 1998; pp. 452–455, 522; O'Hanlon-Nichols, 1995; p. 42.

66.   When you are teaching an asthma patient how to avoid potential triggers of the disease, which of the following should you be sure to discuss?
A. Avoidance of spicy foods can help to reduce asthma attacks.
B. Exacerbations of asthma can be reduced by decreasing physical activity.
C. CHRONIC POSTNASAL DRIP CAN CONTRIBUTE TO RECURRENT ASTHMA ATTACKS.
D. Most triggers of asthma cannot be avoided.

Rationale:

    C. Sinusitis and allergic rhinitis with postnasal drip are common asthma triggers in adult patients.

    A. Food allergens are not common triggers. Spicy food in particular has not been found to induce asthma attacks.

    B. Developing a sedentary lifestyle will not improve the asthma condition. Exercise and physical activity should be included in the plan of care.

    D. A great majority of asthma triggers can be identified and lifestyle modifications made to reduce their impact on the patient's disease.

Content Category: Respiratory

References: Newberry, 1998; pp. 440–451; Kitt et al., 1995; pp. 194–197; ENA, Core Curriculum, 2000; pp. 559–561.

67.   A 53-year-old patient presents to the ED with repeated episodes of nocturnal asthma over several months. The condition has responded poorly to nebulized bronchodilators. Which of the following is a potential cause of these occurrences?
    A. GASTROESOPHAGEAL REFLUX
    B. Bacterial pneumonia
    C. Medication allergy
    D. Diabetes mellitus

Rationale:

    A. Nocturnal asthma that responds poorly to inhaled bronchodilators is frequently caused by gastroesophageal reflux, which the patient is experiencing after retiring to bed. Because the patient may not be aware of this condition, taking a history related to diet and time of meals is important.

    B. Bacterial pneumonia is an uncommon trigger of asthma and would not likely have a course of several months' duration without other symptoms.

    C. A medication allergy is unlikely to present as a recurring trigger at night and should respond to bronchodilator therapy.

    D. Diabetes mellitus does not have a causative relationship with asthma exacerbations.

Content Category: Respiratory

References: Newberry, 1998; pp. 440–451; Kitt et al., 1995; pp. 194–197; ENA, Core Curriculum, 2000; pp. 559–561.

68.   A young patient comes into the ED with a rash that the mother suspects to be chickenpox. What precautions are appropriate?
    A. CONTACT AND RESPIRATORY
    B. Respiratory and droplet
    C. Blood and body fluid
    D. Universal and respiratory

Rationale:

    A. Contact and respiratory precautions are appropriate. Chickenpox is spread via droplet and by contact with the draining lesions after the skin has broken out.

    B. Respiratory precautions include droplet precautions.

    C. Blood and body fluid precautions would not be sufficient.

    D. Universal precautions are appropriate, but not sufficient.

Content Category: Respiratory

References: Soud & Rogers, 1998; pp. 429–430; ENA, Core Curriculum, 2000; pp. 259–261.

69.   A 4-year-old child presents to the ED with a barky cough, stridor, retractions, and hypoxia. This
       child is most likely to have:
       A. asthma.
       B. CROUP.
       C. pneumonia.
       D. epiglottitis.

Rationale:

B. The signs and symptoms of croup are a barky, seallike cough; stridor; low-grade to no fever;
   retractions; tachycardia; and tachypnea.
A. The signs and symptoms of asthma are wheezing, hypoxia, dyspnea, and a dry, tight cough.
C. The signs and symptoms of pneumonia are cough, fever, chest pain, tachypnea, tachycardia, and
   fever.
D. The signs and symptoms of epiglottitis are high fever and sore throat, drooling, difficulty swallowing, and stridor.

Content Category: Respiratory

References: Soud, 1998; pp. 199–213; ENA, 1998; pp. 100–101.

70.   A child is brought to the ED after having eaten a cookie that contained peanuts. The child is audibly
       wheezing, has an oxygen saturation of 85%, and cannot talk. What is the priority medication for this
       child?
       A. EPINEPHRINE (ADRENALIN)
       B. Diphenhydramine (Benadryl)
       C. Oxygen
       D. Lorazepam (Ativan)

Rationale:

A. Epinephrine is the drug of choice for acute anaphylaxis to support the cardiovascular system and
   increase blood pressure.
B. Diphenhydramine will not open the airway quickly enough in a patient in acute anaphylaxis.
C. Oxygen will not help the patient if the airway is closing.
D. Lorazepam is used for seizures.

Content Category: Respiratory

References: Soud, 1998; p. 652; Newberry, 1998; p. 734.

71.   Respiratory syncytial virus (RSV) is responsible for which respiratory disease?
       A. BRONCHIOLITIS
       B. Bacterial tracheitis
       C. Epiglottitis
       D. Tuberculosis

Rationale:

A. Respiratory syncytial virus (RSV) most commonly causes bronchiolitis.
B. Some causes of bacterial tracheitis are *Staphylococcus aureus* and *Haemophilus influenzae*.
C. Epiglottitis is usually caused by *H. influenzae*.
D. Tuberculosis is caused by *Mycobacterium tuberculosis*.

Content Category: Respiratory

References: Soud, 1998; pp. 199–209; ENA, 1998; p. 107.

72. A patient presents to the ED following a motorcycle collision with complete loss of sensation and movement below the clavicles. The priority in your assessment is which of the following?
    A. MONITOR THE PATIENT'S INSPIRATORY EFFORT.
    B. Monitor for resolution of spinal shock.
    C. Monitor for signs of autonomic dysreflexia.
    D. Monitor for signs of neurogenic shock.

Rationale:

    A. Monitor the patient's inspiratory effort, respiratory rate and rhythm, and pulse oximetry. This patient's injury is at the C5 level. Innervation to the intercostal muscles is lost, resulting in potential ineffective airway clearance and impaired gas exchange.
    B. Spinal shock is an immediate response to acute injury that results in the loss of all motor, sensory, and reflex functions. Spinal shock may last hours to months.
    C. Autonomic dysreflexia is a potential problem only after spinal shock resolves, not in the immediate post injury phase.
    D. Neurogenic shock is a temporary loss of sympathetic vasomotor function resulting in orthostatic hypotension, bradycardia, and loss of the ability to sweat below the level of injury.

Content Category: Neurological

References: Hickey, 1997; pp. 419–465; ENA, Trauma Nursing, 2000; pp.161–183.

73. A female patient telephones the telephone triage nurse and describes a headache. She states that she is 55 years of age and has decreased vision with the headache. She emphasizes the location as the temporal region and tells the nurse that she has had this headache before, causing loss of sleep and jaw pain for several days. The telephone nurse advises the patient to report to the ED immediately. Based on her action, what do you think the telephone triage nurse suspects?
    A. Meningitis
    B. Cluster headache
    C. TEMPORAL ARTERITIS
    D. Cerebrovascular accident (CVA)

Rationale:

    C. Temporal arteritis (inflammation of branches of the carotid artery) usually occurs in patients over age 50, most often in females. Headache, the most common complaint, is described as severe and stabbing in one or both temporal regions. Patients report decreased visual acuity and pain in the jaw with mouth opening. Red nodules are sometimes noted over the temporal region. If untreated, the condition may lead to blindness.
    A. A patient with meningitis may describe a headache, but would have an accompanying fever.
    B. Males are 10 times more likely than females to have a cluster headache. Cluster headaches are described as frequently occurring headaches that may occur close together.
    D. Paralysis may be more likely to accompany a person who is having a CVA. The symptoms described seem more likely to indicate temporal arteritis.

Content Category: Neurological

Reference: ENA, 1998; p. 532.

74.   A patient is brought to the ED from a motor vehicular crash. His initial Glasgow Coma Scale (GCS) score in the field was 5. Vital signs are BP 100/60, HR 106/min, and respirations 20/min, assisted via bag-valve mask. Pupils are 5 mm and equal and react sluggishly to light. The order of interventions for a patient with suspected head injury and increased intracranial pressure are:
    A.   hyperventilation, mannitol, fluid restriction, sedation, phenytoin (Dilantin).
    B.   hyperventilation, fluid resuscitation to maintain systolic BP > 90 mm Hg, sedation, phenytoin (Dilantin).
    C.   maintain oxygen saturation > 95%, mannitol (Osmitrol), fluid resuscitation, phenytoin (Dilantin).
    D.   MAINTAIN OXYGEN SATURATION >95%, FLUID RESUSCITATION TO MAINTAIN SYSTOLIC BP >90 MM HG, SEDATION, MANNITOL (OSMITROL).

Rationale:

    D.   Hypoxia and hypotension are the two major causes of secondary brain injury; steps should be taken to prevent them. Maintaining adequate systemic blood pressure helps to ensure adequate cerebral perfusion pressure. Mannitol should be used only with evidence of neurologic deterioration.
    A.   Prophylactic hyperventilation and empiric use of mannitol are no longer indicated in the management of severe head injury. Fluid resuscitation to maintain systolic BP or MAP >90 mm Hg improves cerebral perfusion pressure. Dilantin does not affect intracranial pressure directly.
    B.   Prophylactic hyperventilation is no longer indicated in the management of severe head injury. Sedation may be used once oxygenation has been maximized.
    C.   Hypoxia and hypotension are the two major causes of secondary brain injury. Every effort must be made to maximize oxygenation and avoid hypotension. Dilantin does not directly affect intracranial pressure.

Content Category: Neurological

Reference: Conley, 1998; pp. 343–366.

75.   A patient presents to the ED with facial muscle weakness, dysphagia, increasing fatigue, and respiratory distress. The provider orders an edrophonium (Tensilon) test for a differential diagnosis. The ED nurse suspects which of the following?
    A.   Multiple sclerosis
    B.   MYASTHENIA GRAVIS
    C.   Cerebral aneurysm
    D.   Guillain-Barré syndrome

Rationale:

    B.   The symptoms described are consistent with myasthenia gravis. A Tensilon test is sometimes used for a differential diagnosis.
    A.   Although patients with multiple sclerosis may present with generalized weakness or weakness of an extremity, respiratory distress and dysphagia are not common.
    C.   Patients presenting with a cerebral aneurysm may initially complain of severe headache, followed by unconsciousness or severe neurologic compromise.
    D.   Patients with Guillain-Barré syndrome present with ascending weakness, usually beginning in the lower extremities.

Content Category: Neurological

References: ENA, 1998; p. 535; Tintinalli et al., 1995.

76.   Thiamine (vitamin B$_1$) should be administered in addition to dextrose 50% when an unknown patient is seizing for which of the following reasons?
   A. TO PREVENT WERNICKE-KORSAKOFF SYNDROME
   B. To assure proper patient nutrition
   C. To enhance the potency of the dextrose
   D. To prevent hypoglycemia

Rationale:

   A. Often an unknown patient with a seizure is a chronic alcohol abuser. Patients who are chronic alcohol abusers may be prone to sudden onset of Wernicke-Korsakoff syndrome, brought on by a thiamine deficiency that is exacerbated by the sudden administration of a large bolus of dextrose in the absence of adequate Vitamin B, a cofactor in glucose metabolism.
   B. Seizure is common in chronic alcohol abusers. It is evidenced by ataxia, nystagmus, or cranial nerve VI palsy and encephalopathy along with psychosis. Although nutritional support may be indicated, thiamine is not given to maintain adequate nutrition.
   C. Thiamine does not enhance the potency of dextrose and does not prevent hypoglycemia.
   D. Dextrose is given to prevent or treat hypoglycemia.

Content Category: Neurological

Reference: Sheehy & Lenehan, 1999.

77.   The pupils of a patient are evaluated during an assessment after a motorcycle crash. The pupils are found to be 10 mm in diameter and very slow to react to light. The ED nurse considers these findings to be:
   A. normal pupil size but possible hypoxia as suggested by sluggish reaction of the pupils.
   B. DILATED PUPILS, WITH POSSIBLE INJURY OR DYSFUNCTION OF CRANIAL NERVES II AND III.
   C. consistent with early tentorial herniation.
   D. related to an intracranial pressure of <15 mm Hg.

Rationale:

   B. Pupils normally range from 2 mm to 6mm in diameter and are round and reactive to light. Brisk constriction is a normal response to a bright light. Cranial nerves II (optic) and III (oculomotor) control the dilation and constriction of the pupil.
   A. A pupil size of 10 mm is considered dilated. The pupils are not examined to evaluate hypoxia.
   C. Early tentorial herniation typically demonstrates unequal pupils, since pressure is applied to cranial nerve III as a portion of the brain herniates over the tentorium. Later (complete) herniation may demonstrate bilateral, unreactive, dilated pupils.
   D. Normal intracranial pressure is <15 mm Hg.

Content Category: Neurological

Reference: Sheehy & Lenehan, 1999.

78. You are asked to administer fosphenytoin (Cerebyx) 750 mg IV to a patient in status epilepticus. Which of the following precautions should be taken in administering the medication?
     A. The blood pressure should be closely monitored, as hypertension may develop.
     B. THE MEDICATION SHOULD BE ADMINISTERED AT 150 MG/MIN IV.
     C. Fosphenytoin should always be given in combination with phenytoin (Dilantin).
     D. The medication must be given through an inline filter.

Rationale:

     B. Fosphenytoin (Cerebyx) must be administered IV slowly, at a rate not to exceed 150 mg/min.
     A. Blood pressure should be closely monitored because the medication may cause low blood pressure (hypotension), not hypertension.
     C. Fosphenytoin (Cerebyx), a newer medication for seizure control, is used in place of phenytoin (Dilantin) in many situations.
     D. The literature contains no reference concerning utilization of an inline filter for administration.

Content Category: Neurological

Reference: Skidmore-Roth, 2001; pp. 449–450.

79. What would be a priority nursing diagnosis for a patient with a diagnosis of Guillain- Barré syndrome?
     A. INEFFECTIVE BREATHING PATTERN
     B. Body image disturbance
     C. Impaired physical mobility
     D. Altered thought processes

Rationale:

     A. Because weakness of respiratory muscles may accompany Guillain-Barré syndrome, the priority nursing diagnosis would be ineffective breathing pattern. Patients with Guillain-Barré syndrome often require respiratory support.
     B. Body image disturbances may be of concern later; however, the immediate concern is respiratory distress.
     C. Impaired physical mobility is not of immediate concern. Once airway issues have been controlled, other considerations can be managed.
     D. Thought processes are not usually affected by Guillain-Barré syndrome.
     Content Classification: Neurological

Reference: Newberry, 1998; pp. 534–535.

80. A patient arrives in the ED by EMS following a fall from the stands at a high school football game. The patient is alert and oriented and able to answer questions, open his eyes as you speak, and lift his fingers and toes at your command. He is in full spinal protocol upon arrival. His initial Glasgow Coma Score is:
     A. EYE MOVEMENT 4, VERBAL 5, MOTOR 6 = 15.
     B. eye movement 2, verbal 2, motor 2 = 6.
     C. eye movement 1, verbal 1, motor 1 = 3.
     D. eye movement 4, verbal 3, motor 4 = 11.

Rationale:

A. The three components of the Glasgow Coma Scale for neurologic assessment are eye opening, verbal response, and motor response. This patient opens his eyes as the examiner begins to speak, scoring the maximum value of 4. The patient is alert and oriented, thus scoring the maximum score of 5 in the verbal category. His ability to lift the fingers and toes to verbal commands denotes a maximum score of 6 in the motor category. The maximum Glasgow Coma Scale score is 15.

B. The patient's responses do not match the given scores.

C. This (3) is the lowest score on the GCS.

D. The patient's responses do not match the given scores.

Content Category: Neurological

Reference: Dolan & Holt, 2000; p. 58.

81. A 65-year-old patient arrives in the ED observation unit with a diagnosis of confusion. The family is concerned that their grandfather is becoming more confused. He apparently fell from a horse 2 weeks ago and was examined by a physician and discharged home with a diagnosis of concussion. The granddaughter states that her grandfather has a history of drinking several cocktails every evening, but has never acted this way before. As the ED nurse, which of the following interventions would you encourage?
    A. Skull x-ray to determine intracerebral bleeding
    B. Blood alcohol level evaluation
    C. COMPUTED TOMOGRAPHY (CT) SCAN OF THE HEAD
    D. Metabolic evaluation for dementia

Rationale:

C. A 65-year-old patient with a history of possible recent head trauma and increasing confusion must be considered for a potential chronic subdural hematoma. A CAT scan would allow visualization inside the skull, thus allowing an evaluation for any intracerebral bleeding.

A. A skull x-ray would demonstrate only bone abnormalities, such as a skull fracture.

B. Although a blood alcohol determination may be part of the treatment plan for this patient, the described assessment finding should arouse suspicion for a chronic subdural hematoma.

D. A thorough assessment for dementia may be indicated for this patient, but if so, a more detailed evaluation than an ED assessment would be required. Any potentially life-threatening injury or illness should be evaluated first.

Content Category: Neurological

Reference: Newberry, 1998; pp. 271–272.

Questions 82 and 83

A 36-year-old female who is 32 weeks pregnant by dates presents to the ED with the chief complaint of a sudden onset of bright-red vaginal bleeding, severe low abdominal cramping, and low back pain for the past 6 hours. The patient has been saturating one pad per hour. She also reports decrease in fetal movement over the past few hours. The patient has had no prenatal care during this pregnancy. Vital signs are BP 100/60, HR 112/min, respirations 24/min, and temperature 101.2° F (38.4° C) orally.

82. You suspect that this patient has:
A. placenta previa.
B. pelvic inflammatory disease (PIV).
C. ABRUPTIO PLACENTAE.
D. threatened abortion.

Rationale:

C. Abruptio placentae is typically characterized by dark-red vaginal bleeding and is associated with low abdominal, pelvic, or back pain or a combination. The amount of bleeding in abruptio placentae is variable, as bleeding may be concealed in the uterus. Uterine tenderness is present in abruptio placentae.
A. Placenta previa is typically characterized by painless, bright-red vaginal bleeding. There is usually no report of a decrease in fetal movement.
B. Pelvic inflammatory disease does not cause the sudden onset of vaginal bleeding.
D. "Threatened abortion" is a term used for vaginal bleeding before viability of the fetus (20 to 24 weeks).

Content Category: Obstetrics & Genitourinary & Gynecology

References: ENA, Core Curriculum, 2000; Howell et al., 1998; pp. 1310–1312.

83. In caring for this patient, you anticipate all of the following interventions EXCEPT:
A. establishing 2 large-bore IVs for the administration of crystalloid fluids and possible blood products.
B. obtaining laboratory tests to include a coagulation profile.
C. ADMINISTERING A TOCOLYTIC AGENT SUCH AS OXYTOCIN INJECTION (PITOCIN).
D. pelvic ultrasound.

Rationale:

C. Tocolytic agents are contraindicated in abruptio placentae.
A. Two large-bore IVs must be established, as abruptio placentae may lead to maternal hemorrhage.
B. A coagulation profile should be sent to the laboratory with the initial blood work as abruptio placentae may lead to coagulopathy, which may progress to disseminated coagulation.
D. Pelvic ultrasound is indicated in abruptio placentae to monitor fetal well-being.

Content Category: Obstetrics & Genitourinary & Gynecology

Reference: ENA, Core Curriculum, 2000; pp. 437–439.

84. The most appropriate nursing diagnosis for the patient who is bleeding from abruptio placentae is:
A. pain.
B. FLUID VOLUME DEFICIT.
C. impaired gas exchange.
D. altered tissue perfusion.

Rationale:

B. Abruptio placentae may lead to significant intrauterine hemorrhage and shock. Therefore, fluid volume deficit is the highest priority nursing diagnosis for this patient.

A. Pain is an important secondary nursing diagnosis.

C. Impaired gas exchange is an important secondary nursing diagnosis.

D. Altered tissue perfusion is an important secondary nursing diagnosis.

Content Category: Obstetrics & Genitourinary & Gynecology

Reference: ENA, Core Curriculum, 2000.

85. A 21-year-old female arrives at the ED via private vehicle after having delivered a term infant in the hospital parking lot. This is her third vaginal delivery. On arrival, the patient is experiencing heavy vaginal bleeding. Vital signs are BP 118/60, HR 112/min, respirations 18/min, and temperature 101° F (38.3° C). Your first intervention is to do which of the following?

A. Obtain an order to administer 10 units of oxytocin (Pitocin) IVP

B. Place the patient in the left lateral position

C. Initiate 2 large-bore IVs with crystalloid fluid

D. PALPATE THE ABDOMEN AND MASSAGE THE UTERUS, IF DOUGHY, AFTER CONFIRMING THAT THE PLACENTA HAS BEEN DELIVERED

Rationale:

D. Uterine atony is the most common cause of bleeding in the first 24 hours after delivery. After delivery, the uterus should be firm, globular in shape, and palpable at or below the umbilicus. When uterine atony occurs, the fundus is doughy in consistency and possibly palpable above the umbilicus. The uterus should be massaged after it has been confirmed that the placenta has been delivered.

A. Oxytocin may be indicated if uterine atony is present and the uterus is large and doughy. The medication is administered as an IV infusion of 20 to 30 U in 1 L of normal saline or lactated Ringer's solution at 200 ml/hr.

B. The left lateral position is not indicated.

C. Two large-bore IVs may be indicated if bleeding cannot be controlled, but this is not the first intervention to take.

Content Category: Obstetrics & Genitourinary & Gynecology

Reference: ENA, Core Curriculum, 2000; p. 446.

86. A 36-year-old female at 38 weeks' gestation presents to the ED in active labor. On examination of the perineum, you observe that the umbilical cord is protruding. Interventions should include all of the following EXCEPT:

A. gently elevating any presenting fetal parts off the cord.

B. ATTEMPTING TO PUSH THE UMBILICAL CORD BACK INTO THE VAGINA.

C. assisting the mother into a left lateral decubitus (knee-chest) position.

D. preparing the patient for an emergency cesarean section.

Rationale:

B. No attempt should be made to manipulate the umbilical cord. Doing so could induce further cord compression and fetal compromise.

A. Elevating any fetal parts off the umbilical cord will prevent further compression of the cord.

C. These positions are recommended to prevent further cord compression.

D. The patient should be prepared for an emergency cesarean section.

Content Category: Obstetrics & Genitourinary & Gynecology

Reference: Tintinalli, et al., 2000; p. 713.

87. The objective signs included in the Apgar score include all of the following EXCEPT:
    A. heart rate.
    B. RESPIRATORY RATE.
    C. muscle tone.
    D. reflex irritability.

Rationale:

B. Respiratory rate is not included in the Apgar score. The second objective sign is respiratory effort.
A. Heart rate is included in the Apgar score.
C. Muscle tone is included in the Apgar score.
D. Reflex irritability is included in the Apgar score.

Content Category: Obstetrics & Genitourinary & Gynecology

Reference: ENA, Core Curriculum, 2000; Howell et al., 1998.

Questions 88–90

A 17-year-old female presents to the ED with a chief complaint of low abdominal pain. The patient is crying and guarding her abdomen. Vital signs are BP 118/84, HR 116/min, and respirations 24/min.

88. Signs and symptoms that would indicate a possible ruptured ovarian cyst include which of the following?
    A. Fever > 101.2°F (38.5°C)
    B. The gradual onset of pelvic pain over the past week
    C. Severe diarrhea preceding crampy, generalized abdominal pain
    D. THE SUDDEN ONSET OF SEVERE PELVIC PAIN DURING INTERCOURSE

Rationale:

D. The pain of a ruptured ovarian cyst is sudden in onset and frequently occurs during intercourse.
A. A fever greater than 101.2°F (38.5°C) in the presence of acute abdominal pain suggests an infectious etiology.
B. The pain of a ruptured ovarian cyst is not gradual in onset.
C. Diarrhea preceding crampy abdominal pain does not indicate a ruptured ovarian cyst.

Content Category: Obstetrics & Genitourinary & Gynecology

Reference: ENA, Core Curriculum, 2000; p. 454.

89. Which of the following interventions should be implemented for this patient?
    A. Assist her in quantifying her level of pain using a pain scale.
    B. Anticipate an order for an IV for analgesia.
    C. Obtain laboratory specimens for a CBC, urinalysis, and pregnancy test.
    D. ALL OF THE ABOVE.

Rationale:

D. The nursing interventions listed in A, B, and C are all appropriate for this patient.

A. Do assist the patient in quantifying her level of pain using a pain scale.

B. Do anticipate an order for an IV for analgesia.

C. Do obtain laboratory specimens for a CBC, urinalysis, and pregnancy test.

Content Category: Obstetrics & Genitourinary & Gynecology

Reference: ENA, Core Curriculum, 2000; p. 454.

90. The highest-priority nursing diagnosis for this patient would be which of the following?
   A. PAIN
   B. Knowledge deficit
   C. Risk for injury
   D. Fluid volume deficit

Rationale:

A. Pain is the highest priority nursing diagnosis at this time.

B. While knowledge deficit may be a secondary nursing diagnosis, it is not of the highest priority.

C. While risk for injury may be an important secondary nursing diagnosis, it is not of the highest priority.

D. While fluid volume deficit may be an important secondary nursing diagnosis, it is not of the highest priority.

Content Category: Obstetrics & Genitourinary & Gynecology

Reference: ENA, Core Curriculum, 2000; p. 456.

91. The most common infectious cause(s) of vulvovaginitis include which of the following?
   A. Bacterial vaginosis
   B. *Candida albicans*
   C. *Trichomonas*
   D. ALL OF THE ABOVE

Rationale:

D. All of the above conditions can cause vulvovaginitis.

A. Bacterial vaginosis, a common cause of vulvovaginitis, accounts for approximately 40% to 50% of all such infections.

B. *Candida albicans*, a common cause of vulvovaginitis, accounts for approximately 20% to 25% of all such infections.

C. *Trichomonas*, a common cause of vulvovaginitis, accounts for approximately 15% to 20% of all such infections.

Content Category: Obstetrics & Genitourinary & Gynecology

Reference: ENA, Core Curriculum, 2000; p. 456.

92.   A 68-year-old man presents with an acute onset of what he calls "excruciating back pain" and a history of hypertension. A widened mediastinum is present on chest radiograph. Shortly after arrival, the patient's BP drops to 67/48 mm Hg and his neck veins are flat. The most likely cause of this hypotension is:
A. AORTIC RUPTURE.
B. myocardial infarction.
C. cardiac tamponade.
D. splenic rupture.

Rationale:

A. While each of the conditions listed above is associated with hypotension, the patient's sex, age, hypertensive history, and acute pain onset point to myocardial infarction or aortic dissection. The presence of "excruciating back pain" and a widened mediastinum suggest aortic dissection.
B. The pain described is not typical of myocardial infarction. Mediastinal widening and flattened neck veins are also not characteristic of MI.
C. Cardiac tamponade is a potential complication of aortic dissection if retrograde dissection occurs. However, tamponade is associated with distended, not flattened, neck veins.
D. Splenic injury significant enough to produce profound hypotension involves abdominal rigidity, tenderness, and pain that radiates to the shoulder.

Content Category: Cardiovascular

Reference: Melander & Bucher, 1999.

93.   Before emergent repair, a patient with a dissecting aortic aneurysm has a BP of 142/82. Which of the following IV drip medications will the patient most likely receive while awaiting the vascular surgeon's arrival?
A. NITROPRUSSIDE (NIPRIDE)
B. Dopamine (Intropin)
C. Dobutamine (Dobutrex)
D. Nitroglycerin (Tridil)

Rationale:

A. It is essential to keep aortic pressure low in order to minimize dissection and prevent rupture. Vasodilators such as nitroprusside or beta blockers such as labetalol may be used.
B. The catecholamine effects of dopamine would raise intraarterial pressure.
C. Dobutamine increases cardiac contractility.
D. While nitroglycerin is a vasodilator, its greatest effect is on venous, not arterial, circulation.

Content Category: Cardiovascular

Reference: Barnason, 1998; pp. 459–513.

94.   The primary nursing diagnosis for the patient with a dissecting thoracic aortic aneurysm is risk for:
A. ALTERED TISSUE PERFUSION RELATED TO DECREASED PERIPHERAL BLOOD FLOW.
B. fluid volume deficit related to a drop in renal perfusion.
C. airway obstruction related to aneurysm pressure on the left main bronchus.
D. impaired skin integrity related to decreased peripheral blood flow.

Rationale:

A. Aneurysm dissection can cause obstruction of the aorta, thereby reducing peripheral blood flow. Additionally, if the aneurysm ruptures, hemorrhage will occur. Either way, peripheral blood flow is diminished and tissue perfusion will be altered.

    B. If the aneurysm ruptures, a fluid volume deficit will occur—but the reason is hemorrhage and is unrelated to a drop in renal perfusion.

    C. Aortic aneurysms do not significantly compress the airways.

    D. Skin integrity may be compromised by decreased peripheral blood flow, but this is not the primary diagnosis in the patient with a dissecting aortic aneurysm.

Content Category: Cardiovascular

Reference: Dennison, 2000.

95. A 57-year-old patient in excruciating pain is diagnosed with a descending thoracic aneurysm. The emergency physician has ordered a bolus and infusion of labetalol HCl (Normodyne). Which of the following items listed on the patient's past medical history would be cause for concern?
    A. SEVERE ASTHMA
    B. Chronic hypertension
    C. Marfan's syndrome
    D. Coronary artery bypass graft surgery

Rationale:

    A. Labetalol HCl (Normodyne) is commonly given to reduce blood pressure and slow the dissection process. However, it is a beta blocker. When given to a severe asthmatic, labetalol could initiate an exacerbation. A vasodilator may be a better choice in this patient.

    B. Most patients with aortic dissection have a longstanding history of hypertension.

    C. Because Marfan's syndrome is a connective tissue disorder, patients who have this syndrome are more likely to experience arterial dissection. However, this condition is congenital and is not affected by beta blocker administration.

    D. Since both coronary artery disease and aortic dissection commonly occur as a result of arteriosclerosis, it is not unusual to find them in combination. A history of bypass surgery will not influence immediate patient care.

Content Category: Cardiovascular

Reference: Dennison, 2000.

96. A patient is transported from a referral facility with hypotension, abdominal distention, renal failure, coagulopathies, and a pulsating abdominal mass. The ED nurse recognizes that these are all common findings associated with:
    A. sepsis.
    B. small bowel obstruction.
    C. hepatic laceration.
    D. AORTIC DISSECTION.

Rationale:

    D. Hypotension, renal failure, and coagulopathies may be found in conjunction with each of the conditions listed, but only aortic dissection is associated with a pulsating abdominal mass.

    A. Sepsis is not associated with a pulsating abdominal mass.

    B. Small bowel obstruction is not associated with a pulsating abdominal mass.

    C. Hepatic laceration is not associated with a pulsating abdominal mass.

Content Category: Cardiovascular

Reference: Dennison, 2000.

97. An unrestrained driver involved in a frontal motor vehicle collision presents with a flail sternum. Which of the following would the ED nurse expect to find on further assessment?
    A. VENTRICULAR ECTOPY
    B. Priapism
    C. Borborygmi
    D. Ptosis

Rationale:

    A. Blunt trauma sufficient to induce a flail sternum is usually associated with cardiac contusions. Contusions can cause myocardial irritability, in turn causing ventricular ectopy.
    B. Priapism can be a result of spinal cord injury.
    C. High-pitched bowel sounds (borborygmi) are associated with bowel obstruction.
    D. Drooping of the upper eyelids (ptosis) is caused by cranial nerve injury.

Content Category: Cardiovascular

Reference: Smith, 1998; pp. 107–123.

98. Which of the following statements is most correct concerning premature ventricular contractions (PVCs) in the patient with blunt cardiac trauma?
    A. Aggressively eliminate PVCs by giving a bolus of amiodarone HCl (Cordarone).
    B. DRUG THERAPY FOR PVCs IS RARELY INDICATED IN BLUNT CARDIAC TRAUMA.
    C. PVCs should be treated with procainamide (Pronestyl), but only if they exceed 6/min.
    D. PVCs can be avoided with the administration of a lidocaine (Xylocaine) drip prophylactically.

Rationale:

    B. Premature ventricular contractions in patients with blunt cardiac injury are a common phenomenon. Treatment is indicated only if cardiac output is significantly affected.
    A. Drug treatment is rarely indicated.
    C. Drug treatment is rarely indicated.
    D. Drug treatment is rarely indicated.

Content Category: Cardiovascular

Reference: Doherty, 2000; pp. 57–134.

99. Which of the following serum markers is the best indicator of blunt myocardial trauma?
    A. Lactate dehydrogenase (LDH)
    B. Creatine phosphokinase (CPK)
    C. TROPONIN I
    D. Alkaline phosphatase (AP)

Rationale:

    C. Troponin I is the only one of these four serum levels that is cardiospecific. CPK-MB may also be used.
    A. LDH is not specific to cardiac tissue.
    B. CPK is not specific to cardiac tissue.
    D. AP is not specific to cardiac tissue.

Content Category: Cardiovascular

Reference: Smith, 1998; pp. 107–123.

100.   Which of the following studies best identifies wall motion abnormalities resulting from cardiac contusion?
    A. Thallium scan
    B. ECHOCARDIOGRAM
    C. Coronary arteriogram
    D. Electrocardiogram

Rationale:

    B. Echocardiography, either noninvasive or transesophageal, provides visualization of wall motion abnormalities following blunt cardiac injury.
    A. A coronary arteriogram enables the clinician to visualize heart vessels, not specifically wall motion.
    C. Following myocardial contusion, the 12-lead electrocardiogram may demonstrate ischemic changes, ST-T wave changes, and dysrhythmias, but does not show wall motion abnormalities.
    D. Injected thallium becomes concentrated in normal tissue and permits the distinction between healthy and necrotic heart muscle in the patient with myocardial infarction.

Content Category: Cardiovascular

Reference: Smith, 1998; pp. 107–123.

101.   Which of the following mechanisms of injury is most likely to result in myocardial contusion?
    A. Blast injury in a confined space
    B. KICK TO CHEST BY A BULL
    C. Stab wound to the left chest
    D. Fall from a changing table

Rationale:

    B. Myocardial contusions, also called blunt cardiac trauma, result from any significant blow to the anterior chest. Common mechanisms include motor vehicle collisions, falls from a substantial height, and sports injuries. A kick by a large animal can also deliver a powerful direct force to the chest wall.
    A. Blast injury is usually associated with pneumothorax, not myocardial infarction.
    C. Stab wounds cause penetrating heart injuries, not contusions.
    D. A changing table is not high enough to deliver a high-energy blow to the chest in an infant who has fallen off the table.

Content Category: Cardiovascular

Reference: Doherty, 2000; pp. 57–134.

102.   Which of the following is the procedure of choice for the hypotensive patient with cardiac tamponade?

A. Emergency thoracotomy
B. Pericardial window
C. Chest tube placement
D. PERICARDIOCENTESIS

Rationale:

D. In the shocky patient with cardiac tamponade, pericardiocentesis is both a diagnostic and a therapeutic intervention that can provide the patient with immediate symptom relief.
A. If the pericardiocentesis is positive, the patient will most likely require emergent follow-up with a thoracotomy.
B. A pericardial window is an operative procedure used to drain fluid from around the heart. It is not indicated for the immediate treatment of tamponade.
C. A chest tube may be placed for management of hemothorax or pneumothorax, which frequently occur in conjunction with cardiac tamponade, but the placement has no effect on the tamponade itself.

Content Category: Cardiovascular
Reference: Smith, 1998; pp. 107–123.

103.   Classic signs of cardiac tamponade include distant heart sounds, hypotension, and which of the following?

A. Absent breath sounds on the left side
B. A crunching sound heard with each heartbeat
C. Subcutaneous emphysema of the left chest
D. DISTENDED NECK VEINS

Rationale:

D. Distant or muffled heart sounds, hypotension, and distended neck veins comprise the classic signs of cardiac tamponade known as Beck's triad.
A. Cardiac tamponade has no effect on breath sounds, although pneumothorax and hemothorax are commonly associated conditions.
B. A crunching sound heard on heart auscultation is caused by pneumopericardium resulting from communication between the pericardial space and the lungs, the mainstem bronchus, or the esophagus.
C. Subcutaneous emphysema of the chest is the result of an air leak, from tears in the lungs or bronchi, into the soft tissues of the chest wall.

Content Category: Cardiovascular
Reference: Mullins, 2000; pp. 195–232.

104.   Which of the following best describes blood removed from the pericardial sac in a trauma patient with cardiac tamponade?

A. Platelet activation causes rapid clot formation in the syringe.
B. The hematocrit will be low because of dilution with serous pericardial fluid.
C. THE BLOOD WILL NOT CLOT IN THE SYRINGE BECAUSE OF DEFIBRINATION.
D. The blood will appear frothy because of churning from cardiac motion.

Rationale:

C. Blood that has been in contact with pleura rarely clots, because fibrin adheres to pleural tissue. This is the reason chest tube blood, intraabdominal blood, and pericardial blood usually remain liquid. However, in the event of very rapid bleeding, blood may not have sufficient opportunity to defibrinate.

A. Blood withdrawn on pericardiocentesis that clots in the syringe suggests that the blood was removed not from the pericardium but rather from the ventricle itself. Blood that has already clotted within the pericardium cannot be removed with syringe aspiration.

B. Inflammatory conditions cause serous fluid to accumulate in the pericardium. This fluid may or may not be mixed with blood. Since the accumulation is slow, the pericardium stretches and true tamponade is rare.

D. Since there is no air in the pericardial sac, cardiac wall motion does not cause pericardial blood to become frothy.

Content Category: Cardiovascular

Reference: Mullins, 2000; pp. 195–232.

105. Hyponatremia may be found in all of the following conditions EXCEPT:
    A. Addison's disease.
    B. diarrhea.
    C. ACUTE UREMIA.
    D. excess water intake.

Rationale:

C. The kidney loses the ability to conserve sodium and calcium while retaining potassium and phosphate.

A. Addison's disease causes inadequate secretion of aldosterone, resulting in decreased resorption of sodium by the tubules.

B. Diarrhea impairs absorption from the GI tract of dietary sodium and of sodium from the pancreatic juices, causing an excessive amount to be excreted in the feces.

D. Excess water intake results in a dilutional effect that leads to hyponatremia.

Content Category: General Medical

References: ENA, Core Curriculum, 2000; pp. 289, 322–325; Newberry, 1998; pp.562–565.

106. The effects of histamine release on the body include all of the following EXCEPT:
    A. increased capillary permeability.
    B. arteriolar dilation.
    C. muscular contraction.
    D. ARTERIOLAR CONSTRICTION.

Rationale:

D. Arteriolar constriction is the goal of intervention and administration of epinephrine.

A. Histamine effect includes a change in the permeability of the capillary membrane, leading to a shift of fluid in the interstitial space and capillary leakage.

B. Vasodilation is one of the expected results of histamine release.

C. Histamine is one of many circulating hormones that cause smooth muscle contraction.

Content Category: General Medical

References: Newberry, 1998; p. 522; Guyton & Hall, 1996; pp. 101, 454.

107.   Common substances such as antibiotics, iodine, shellfish, and peanuts often cause an allergic reaction. The reason is that the body becomes sensitized to a substance through an antibody that it creates to recognize this substance. This substance is referred to as:
A. an antibody.
B. AN ANTIGEN.
C. a mast cell.
D. an antinuclear antibody.

Rationale:

B. Antigens are the body's mechanism to recognize self from foreign chemical compounds that may be harmful.
A. Antibodies are made by the body in response to initial exposure of a foreign protein or polysaccharide that sensitizes the body for future response to an agent.
C. Mast cells release substances to help destroy the antigen.
D. Antinuclear antibodies are found in autoimmune disorders, in which the body damages its own cell structure.

Content Category: General Medical

Reference: Guyton & Hall, 1996; pp. 445–451.

108.   A 7-week-old infant presents to the ED with fever. Every child this age with fever should be evaluated for:
A croup.
B. Reye's syndrome.
C. MENINGITIS.
D. rubeola.

Rationale:

C. Bacterial meningitis in particular has high mortality and morbidity rates in children and must be considered.
A. Croup tends to be seen in children aged 6 months to 3 years.
B. Reye's syndrome typically occurs after recovery from a viral illness, often influenza B or varicella.
D. Measles (rubeola) may occur at any age. It is more serious in infants than in older children, but is not so life threatening as meningitis.

Content Category: General Medical

Reference: ENA, Core Curriculum, 2000; pp. 243–247.

109.   Two weeks after returning from traveling abroad, a patient presents with anorexia, a productive cough, fever, and night sweats. These signs and symptoms most likely indicate which of the following?
A. Hepatitis
B. TUBERCULOSIS
C. Measles
D. Pertussis

Rationale:

B. These signs and symptoms represent a classic presentation of tuberculosis. Weight loss, hemoptysis, and fatigue are also common.
A. Hepatitis presents with anorexia, fatigue, fever, and abdominal pain. Jaundice often occurs at some point in the illness.

C. The combination of fever, anorexia, cough, Koplik spots on the buccal membrane, and a red, blotchy rash that progresses from the face downward is the common presentation of measles.

D. Patients with pertussis present with fever, rhinorrhea, fatigue, and a dry, nonproductive cough that becomes paroxysmal at times.

Content Category: General Medical

References: Newberry, 1998; pp. 612–617, 731; ENA, Core Curriculum, 2000; p. 257.

110.   A 3-year-old boy is carried into the ED by his parents at 7 AM. He is unresponsive and has no obvious signs of trauma. He has pale, clammy skin and normal vital signs, although his respirations are shallow. He is described as a healthy child who was fine when put to bed last night. His parents found him on the living room floor this morning. They say there was no evidence that he had taken any pills or poisons. What assessment question may be most useful at this point?

A. "Are other children in the family sick?"

B. "Did your child have a baby-sitter last night?"

C. "COULD YOUR CHILD HAVE HAD ACCESS TO ALCOHOL?"

D. "Does anyone in the family have diabetes?"

Rationale:

C. Although the history is minimal, this story is suspicious for alcohol intoxication, which in a child can cause profound hypoglycemia. The typical scenario is that the parents had a party and went to bed without cleaning up. The child awakens in the morning, finds glasses with alcoholic beverages within easy reach, and drinks them because he is curious and thirsty. It takes very little alcohol to cause unresponsiveness and hypoglycemia in a 3-year-old.

A. One would ask whether other children in the family are ill, but even if other children are ill, all the nurse has learned is that the problem may be infectious in nature.

B. A baby-sitter may have inflicted trauma or failed to report it. The fact that this child has normal vital signs tends to make unresponsiveness caused by trauma unlikely.

D. As part of a comprehensive history, the nurse would ask whether anyone in the family had diabetes. Young children can develop type I (insulin-dependent) diabetes, an autoimmune process. Type II diabetes is hereditary but not seen in children this young. Since the situation is potentially life threatening, it is more important to ask questions that are situational in nature because toddlers are more at risk for acute than for chronic illness or injury.

Content Category: General Medical

References: Peabody, 2000; pp. 227–274; Ragland, 1996; pp. 939–972.

111.   A 17-year-old girl comes to the ED on Sunday morning complaining of headache, weakness, and feeling ill. Her history is unremarkable, but she does admit to having attended a "rave"—a party designed to enhance a hallucinogenic experience through music and behavior—the previous evening and having taken Ecstasy there. Vital signs are BP 138/80, HR 102/min, respirations 22/min, and temperature 98° F (36.7° C). As the ED nurse finishes triaging, the patient has a grand mal seizure. What is the most likely cause of the seizure?

A. Hypoglycemia

B. HYPONATREMIA

C. Subdural hematoma

D. Acute drug intoxication

Rationale:

B. Hyponatremia is a common problem with Ecstasy use. Those who are about to take the drug are often told to drink a substantial amount of water when they take the drug and the following morning to avoid hyperthermia and hangover. Ecstasy stimulates the secretion of vasopressin, the antidiuretic hormone (ADH). The kidneys resorb water, leading to increased extracellular fluid volume, which dilutes serum sodium. Coupled with increased water intake, serum sodium levels drop rapidly, and the patient has a seizure. This patient's sodium level was 110 mEq/L.

A. Hypoglycemia can cause seizures and should always be considered, but glucose levels typically are very low. One would have expected to find signs and symptoms of hypoglycemia, including altered level of consciousness, in this patient before her seizure.

C. Unknown or unremembered trauma is always possible with drug intoxication. One would expect some change in level of consciousness before the seizure. A CT scan would be indicated if other more likely causes of her seizure are ruled out.

D. Since the half-life of Ecstasy is 3 to 7 hours, the drug has probably been metabolized by time of admission. It is possible that this patient took other drugs; however, the fact that she talked about being at a "Rave," admits to taking Ecstasy, and has normal mental status and behavior lessen the likelihood that she has acute drug intoxication.

Content Category: General Medical

Reference: Holmes et al., 1999; pp. 32–33.

112. The emergency physician orders tuberculin purified protein derivative (PPD) testing for family members of a patient in the ED with active TB disease. On the 3-year-girl, the PPD was placed subcutaneously. The next step is to do which of the following?
A. PLACE A SECOND PPD AT LEAST 2 INCHES (5 CM) FROM THE FIRST ATTEMPT
B. Ask the patient to return in 24 hours for PPD placement
C. Ask the physician to order a chest x-ray
D. Apply a multiple puncture test (Mono-Vacc, Time Test PPD) to the opposite forearm.

Rationale:

A. If the first attempt to place a PPD is missed, a second try can be made at least 2 inches (5 cm) from the first. The patient is not sensitized by the first injection.

B. Since a second PPD can be placed immediately, there is no reason to have the patient return.

C. A missed attempt to place a PPD is not sufficient reason to order a chest x-ray. The physician may order a chest x-ray as a baseline in the nonsymptomatic patient.

D. Mono-Vacc is used for mass screening only. It is not appropriate for patients, even children, with known exposure to TB. A positive Mono-Vacc is followed up with a PPD.

Content Category: General Medical

References: Peabody, 2000; pp. 227–274; Welsh, 1996; pp. 422–425.

113. A 55-year-old female presents to the ED with a 2-day history of a diffuse (whole-head), dull, aching headache (rated at 6/10) that had a slow onset but cannot be relieved with her usual remedies. She denies trauma and demonstrates no neurologic deficits or nuchal rigidity. Vital signs are BP 134/70, HR 84/min, respirations 18/min, oxygen saturation 97%, and temperature 98.2° F (36.8° C). The patient has a history of chronic lymphocytic leukemia (CLL) that has been in remission for 2 years, migraine headaches, and a recent history of a mild upper respiratory infection. In addition to CT of the head, what other test must be done as a top priority?
A. COMPLETE BLOOD COUNT (CBC)
B. Lumbar puncture
C. CT of sinuses
D. Angiogram (brain)

Rationale:

A. Because this patient has a history of CLL, the WBC must be evaluated. The WBC is significantly elevated with CLL. This patient's WBC was 245,000/ml.

B. The patient is afebrile and demonstrates no indicators for infection or trauma. An LP may be done, but not as a priority.

C. This patient would not be likely to have a CT of the sinuses because the whole head is involved, not just the sinus area.

D. An angiogram of the brain may be done in the ED but would not be ordered for this stable patient as an initial test.

Content Category: General Medical

Reference: ENA, Core Curriculum, 2000.

114. At what level does a patient classically demonstrate an altered level of consciousness related to hyponatremia?
    A. SERUM NA$^+$ < 125 MEQ/L
    B. Serum Na$^+$ = 125–130 mEq/L
    C. Serum Na$^+$ ≥ 131–135 mEq/L
    D. Serum Na$^+$ ≥ 150 mEq/L

Rationale:

A. The patient's ability to maintain an appropriate level of consciousness (LOC) relates to the sodium level as well as to the speed with which the level drops. If the sodium quickly drops from 135 mEq/L to 125 mEq/L, the patient may display an acutely altered LOC. If the sodium level falls gradually, however, the patient may tolerate a lower level before demonstrating an altered LOC.

B. Incorrect.

C. Incorrect.

D. Incorrect.

Content Category: General Medical

References: ENA, Core Curriculum, 2000; Goodfellow, 1995.

115. A 64-year-old female presents to the ED with a 3-hour history of perioral numbness and tingling of the hands and feet. Her motor strength in all 4 extremities is normal. She has a history of a thyroidectomy and has been in remission from uterine cancer for 2 years. Vital signs are BP 100/50, HR 105/min, respirations 24/min, oxygen saturation 97%, and temperature 97.9° F (36.6° C). Your plan of care and urgency is related to the potential diagnosis of:
    A. hypernatremia.
    B. HYPOCALCEMIA.
    C. hypermagnesemia.
    D. hypokalemia.

Rationale:

B. Hypocalcemia is often an outcome of a thyroidectomy secondary to trauma of the parathyroid glands during surgery. The hypocalcemic patient may have subjective complaints of paresthesias, numbness, muscle cramps, tetany, and carpopedal spasm.

A. The function of sodium is not affected by the thyroid/parathyroid glands.

C. The function of magnesium is not affected by the thyroid/parathyroid glands.

D. The function of potassium is not affected by the thyroid/parathyroid glands.

Content Category: General Medical

Reference: ENA, Core Curriculum, 2000.

116.   Your patient has a serum potassium of 7.2 mEq/L. Initial treatment may include all of the following EXCEPT:
   A.   calcium chloride.
   B.   dextrose/insulin.
   C.   sodium bicarbonate.
   D.   SODIUM POLYSTYRENE SULFONATE (KAYEXALATE).

Rationale:

   D.   Kayexalate is a drug that is used to remove potassium from the body. Its action is to exchange the potassium and sodium in the gut, bind with the potassium, and eliminate it via the gut. Use of this drug is a slow-acting treatment modality.
   A.   Calcium chloride quickly stabilizes the cell membrane to prevent the leakage of potassium.
   B.   Dextrose and insulin quickly drive the potassium back into the cell.
   C.   Sodium bicarbonate also quickly drives the potassium back into the cell and stabilizes the pH.

Content Category: General Medical

References: ENA, Core Curriculum, 2000; Roth-Skidmore, 2000.

117.   A mother brings her 3-month-old infant to the ED with a fever and diarrhea. The mother states that the patient does not want to eat or drink and is difficult to arouse. You note sunken eyes and fontanelles. The mother states that her child has not wet a diaper today. Your two attempts at starting IVs have failed. IMMEDIATE priority for this patient is to:
   A.   establish vascular access via cutdown.
   B.   establish vascular access via external jugular vein.
   C.   ESTABLISH VASCULAR ACCESS VIA INTRAOSSEOUS NEEDLE.
   D.   establish vascular access via scalp vein.

Rationale:

   C.   Emergency vascular access for the pediatric patient presenting in shock includes attempting intravenous access. If multiple attempts are unsuccessful, initiate vascular access via intraosseous needle.
   A.   Establishing emergency vascular access after two unsuccessful attempts does not include venous cutdown.
   B.   Establishing emergency vascular access after two unsuccessful attempts does not include external jugular vein access, as pediatric neck anatomy (e.g., a short neck) makes this intervention difficult, if not impossible.
   D.   Establishing emergency vascular access after two unsuccessful attempts does not include scalp vein; this is not a large-bore site.

Content Category: Shock & Trauma

Reference: American Heart Association, 1994.

118.   A 55-year-old female enters your ED complaining of chest pain. Her long cardiac history includes anterior wall myocardial infarction and heart failure. She presents with chest pain and shortness of breath. You note crackles throughout both lungs; pale, mottled skin; and thready pulses. Your interventions to decrease preload include the administration of which of the following?
   A.   NITROGLYCERIN (TRIDIL)
   B.   Nitroprusside (Nipride)
   C.   Amiodarone (Cordarone)
   D.   Adrenalin (Epinephrine)

Rationale:

    A. Nitroglycerin is a vasodilator that reduces venous return, thereby reducing preload.

    B. Nitroprusside is an arterial dilatory medication that assists in reducing afterload.

    C. Amiodarone is a medication that increases the contractility of the heart but is not a preload reducer.

    D. Epinephrine is a sympathetic drug that increases vasoconstriction, thus increasing afterload.

Content Category: Shock & Trauma

References: ENA, Core Curriculum, 2000; American Association of Critical Care Nurses, 1998; pp. 239–240, 262.

119. You are caring for a patient who was struck in the chest by a baseball thrown by a batting machine. Although initially your patient's vital signs were stable, you are noting muffled heart tones, distended neck veins, and rapidly dropping blood pressure. Which of the following conditions tells you that this patient is going into cardiogenic shock?

    A. Ventricular rupture

    B. Stunned myocardium

    C. PERICARDIAL TAMPONADE

    D. Myocardial infarction

Rationale:

    C. Pericardial tamponade is characterized by Beck's triad: muffled heart tones, distended neck veins, and narrowing pulse pressure. The rapidly dropping blood pressure is related to the heart's inability to pump blood out of the ventricles because of increased pressure in the pericardial sac.

    A. A patient in ventricular standstill has no blood pressure or pulse.

    B. Stunned myocardium can cause cardiogenic shock, but does not do so with the triad of symptoms listed above.

    D. Although myocardial infarction can cause cardiogenic shock, it is not a likely cause of this patient's deterioration. In addition, MI is not associated with the triad of symptoms listed above.

Content Category: Shock & Trauma

References: ENA, Core Curriculum, 2000; American Association of Critical Care Nurses, 1998; pp. 239–240, 262.

120. Your patient was an unrestrained driver who was involved in a car crash in which the steering wheel was bent. He initially complained of severe chest pain and shortness of breath at the scene, but has been deteriorating en route to your hospital. He arrives with distended neck veins, extreme dyspnea, and tachypnea and he is pale with circumoral cyanosis. His BP in the field was initially 140/90, but now you are having a difficult time palpating even a femoral pulse. Lung sounds are diminished in the right lung fields and absent in the left lung fields. What is the cause of your patient's distress?

    A. Multiple rib fractures

    B. Pulmonary contusion

    C. Pulmonary edema

    D. TENSION PNEUMOTHORAX

Rationale:

    D. Absent breath sounds along with distended neck veins and clinical signs of shock are hallmark for tension pneumothorax.

    A. Although rib fractures can cause dyspnea and tachypnea, rib fractures alone do not cause severe hypotension.

B. Although pulmonary contusion can cause respiratory distress, it takes time to develop the signs and symptoms of pulmonary contusion.

C. There is no clinical evidence in the above scenario to support the diagnosis of pulmonary edema.

Content Category: Shock & Trauma

References: ENA, Core Curriculum, 2000; Holleran, 1996.

121. You are caring for a patient who has been diagnosed with an anterior wall myocardial infarction. Within 20 minutes after arrival in the ED, the patient is developing hypotension. Crackles are heard through all lung fields. The patient continues to have chest pain, is pale and diaphoretic, and does not have delayed capillary refill. While you wait for the intraaortic balloon pump team to arrive, what medications can be administered to reduce both preload and afterload?

A. Morphine sulfate, furosemide (Lasix)
B. NITROPRUSSIDE (NIPRIDE), FUROSEMIDE (LASIX)
C. Nitroglycerin (Tridil), high-dose dopamine (Intropin)
D. Nitroprusside (Nipride), captopril (Capoten)

Rationale:

B. Nitroprusside and furosemide together reduce both preload and afterload.
A. Morphine sulfate and furosemide both work on preload reduction.
C. Nitroglycerin reduces preload, but high-dose dopamine increases afterload.
D. Nipride and captopril reduce afterload.

Content Category: Shock & Trauma

Reference: ENA, Core Curriculum, 2000.

122. A 55-year-old female enters your ED complaining of severe chest pain that has lasted for 5 hours. She starts to complain of respiratory distress and is cool, pale, and diaphoretic. Her respiratory rate is 22/min and respirations appear to be slightly labored. Which of the following takes priority in your care for this patient?

A. ADMINISTRATION OF 100% OXYGEN VIA NONREBREATHER MASK AND REAS-SESSING RESPIRATORY STATUS
B. Obtaining a 12-lead electrocardiogram
C. Establishing an IV of 0.9% normal saline solution and administering a 500-ml fluid bolus
D. Performing endotracheal intubation

Rationale:

A. Administration of 100% oxygen via nonrebreather mask can increase oxygen delivery to the cells and reduce the workload of the heart. Reassessment is important to determine adequacy of treatment.

B. Obtaining a 12-lead electrocardiogram, although a priority, does not take priority over increasing oxygen delivery.

C. Establishing an IV of 0.9% NSS is important so that medications can be delivered, but since the patient is currently in respiratory distress, clearing the airway takes precedence over establishing an IV.

D. Performing endotracheal intubation would be overly aggressive in treating this patient's respiratory problem.

Content Category: Shock & Trauma

Reference: ENA, Core Curriculum, 2000.

123.   Which of the following indicates stabilization of the patient in cardiogenic shock?
   A. URINE OUTPUT VIA FOLEY CATHETER OF 1 ML/KG/HOUR
   B. A systolic blood pressure of 88 mm Hg in an otherwise normotensive adult
   C. Heart rate of 120/min
   D. Respiratory rate of 26/min

Rationale:

   A. Normal urine output, an indication of restored cardiac output, is 0.5–1.0 ml/kg/hour for adults
       and 1–2 ml/kg/hour in a pediatric patient.
   B. Systolic pressures < 90 mm Hg in a normotensive patient with cardiogenic shock are an indica-
       tor of uncompensated shock.
   C. Tachycardia indicates continued sympathetic nervous system discharge in an attempt to com-
       pensate for low cardiac output/perfusion.
   D. Tachypnea indicates continued attempts for lactic acidosis due to hypoperfusion.

Content Category: Shock & Trauma

Reference: ENA, Core Curriculum, 2000.

124.   Your cardiogenic shock patient has been given morphine sulfate, furosemide (Lasix), and nitrates
       (e.g., nitroglycerin [Tridil]. His breathing continues to be labored even on 100% oxygen via nonre-
       breather mask. Blood gases show hypercarbia and hypoxia. You anticipate which of the following
       interventions to correct his blood gas abnormalities?
   A. Give oxygen via bag-valve-mask device
   B. Administer albuterol (Ventolin) nebulizer treatment
   C. Begin a dopamine (Intropin) drip at 10 mcg/kg/min
   D. INTUBATE AND MECHANICALLY VENTILATE THE PATIENT WITH POSITIVE END-
       EXPIRATORY PRESSURE (PEEP).

Rationale:

   D. The patient described above is in respiratory failure. Intubation and mechanical ventilation will
       increase the patient's oxygen saturations and decrease the work of breathing. Adding PEEP to
       the ventilator settings can decrease preload by reducing venous return to the heart.
   A. Giving oxygen via bag-valve-mask device will initially help build up oxygen reserves, but will
       not be done as a continuous measure to correct the blood gas problems described.
   B. An albuterol nebulizer treatment is not appropriate for cardiogenic shock.
   C. Although furosemide may reduce preload further, patients presenting with hypercarbia and
       hypoxia are also in respiratory failure. Their respiratory problem must be addressed.

Content Category: Shock & Trauma

References: ENA, Core Curriculum, 2000; American Association of Critical Care Nurses, 1998.

125.   A nursing home patient is brought to your ED with the complaints of fever and generalized weakness. Skin is warm, dry, and flushed. The patient is mildly agitated—an abnormal situation for this patient. Vital signs are HR 110/min, respirations 26/min, and temperature 101.8°F (38.8°C). A Foley catheter is draining cloudy yellow urine. You suspect this patient to have which of the following?
   A.   A urinary tract infection
   B.   HYPERDYNAMIC SEPSIS
   C.   Hypodynamic sepsis
   D.   Toxic shock syndrome

Rationale:

   B.   Hyperdynamic sepsis is characterized by tachycardia, tachypnea, and moderate changes in sensation. Fever is a common finding in patients with hyperdynamic sepsis.
   A.   Although the cloudy urine could be a sign of a urinary tract infection, the presence of tachycardia, fever, tachypnea, and changes in mentation are not symptoms of UTI.
   C.   Hypodynamic sepsis presents as decompensating shock. Mentation changes are usually more severe, leading to coma. The skin is cool and clammy because of intense vasoconstriction and sympathetic activation.
   D.   Toxic shock syndrome is most commonly caused by Group A streptococcus. This syndrome most commonly affects otherwise healthy adults. The presentation of this patient does not mimic that of a patient with toxic shock syndrome.

Content Category: Shock & Trauma

References: ENA, Core Curriculum, 2000; Stevens, 1995.

126.   A 10-year-old boy is brought to your ED after having injured himself while doing tricks on his bicycle. He was not wearing a helmet and landed on his head while trying to flip his bicycle. Upon your arrival, the patient is hypotensive and bradycardic. His respiratory rate is 30/min and respirations are shallow. He is most likely experiencing which of the following?
   A.   Respiratory failure
   B.   NEUROGENIC SHOCK
   C.   Hysteria from his injuries
   D.   A severe head injury

Rationale:

   B.   Hypotension and bradycardia are hallmark signs of neurogenic shock. An elevated respiratory rate suggests severe inefficiency of the diaphragm, necessitating immediate inline intubation.
   A.   Although the patient's respiratory rate is rapid and respirations are shallow, the mechanism of injury suggests more than respiratory failure.
   C.   The presentation warrants assessment for spinal cord injury.
   D.   Although severe head injuries are common with this type of injury, they do not cause hypotension, tachypnea, and bradycardia.

Content Category: Shock & Trauma

References: ENA, Core Curriculum, 2000; American Association of Critical Care Nurses, 1998; pp. 441–448, 399–408.

127.   A gradually enlarging lesion develops at the site of a brown recluse spider bite. If sufficient venom is injected, systemic features will also be found. Which of the following will reveal early evidence of systemic involvement?
   A. Plain x-ray to locate osteomyelitis
   B. URINALYSIS TO IDENTIFY MYOGLOBINURIA
   C. Arterial blood gases (ABGs) to seek perfusion/ventilation mismatch
   D. Serum antibodies to quantify the venom injected

Rationale:

   B. Venom causes hemolysis, which can be identified early by the presence of myoglobin in the urine.
   A. Osteomyelitis would be unlikely to occur unless a concurrent fracture were present.
   C. ABGs would identify a mismatch, but brown recluse venom has an initial effect of hemolysis.
   D. Serum antibodies would not reflect the amount of venom injected.

Content Category: Orthopedics & Wound Care
Reference: Barkin et al., 1999.

128.   To minimize transmission of Lyme disease, an attached tick should be removed by:
   A. grasping the body and removing it with a twisting motion.
   B. smothering the tick in petroleum jelly, then wiping it off.
   C. holding a hot matchstick near the tick until the tick falls off.
   D. GRASPING THE HEAD AND EXERTING A SLOW, STEADY PULL.

Rationale:

   D. By grasping the head, you are less likely to cause regurgitation. Exerting a slow, steady pull will eventually cause the tick to release the skin.
   A. Grasping the tick's body would enhance regurgitation by pressure. Transmission occurs with regurgitation.
   B. Smothering the tick would cause the tick to experience distress, which results in regurgitation.
   C. Applying a hot matchstick would also cause the tick to become distressed.

Content Category: Orthopedics & Wound Care
Reference: Barkin et al., 1999.

129.   After falling down 3 steps, a patient presents to the ED complaining of right ankle pain. He denies other injuries, but is unable to bear weight without pain. Besides examining the ankle, the nurse should:
   A. assess the Babinski reflex of the foot.
   B. evaluate ulnar and radial pulses.
   C. PALPATE THE HEAD OF THE FIBULA.
   D. examine the left ankle.

Rationale:

   C. A Maisonneuve fracture (fracture of the proximal fibula) can be a concomitant fracture arising from the forces of a severe inversion of the ankle.
   A. Assessing the Babinski reflex would be appropriate as part of a central neurologic exam.
   B. The dorsalis pedis and posterior tibialis pulses, not the ulnar and radial pulses, should be palpated.
   D. The left ankle may be compared to the right, but a complete exam does not need to be performed.

Content Category: Orthopedic & Wound

Reference: Pfeffer, 1999; pp. 368–489.

130. The nurse is preparing to discharge a patient with a diagnosis of cervical radiculopathy. Instructions should include which of the following?
    A. APPLICATION OF MOIST HEAT
    B. Use of hard cervical collar
    C. Massaging mild steroid cream into area
    D. No use of pillow for sleep

Rationale:

    A. Moist heat is indicated to ease muscle spasm and enhance circulation to the area.
    B. Use of a hard cervical collar is not indicated in cervical disc syndrome.
    C. Steroid creams can be used for topical inflammations but are not appropriate for inflammations of underlying structures.
    D. A pillow should be used during sleep to prevent malalignment of the cervical spine.

Content Category: Orthopedics& Wound Care

Reference: Merceir et al., 1995.

131. A 36-year-old female complains of neck pain and stiffness upon waking. She spent the previous day "cleaning up the yard" and gardening. She noted a gradual onset of stiffness that evening, but states that the pain was much worse this morning. She has no fever and feels well otherwise. The ED nurse's assessment should focus on:
    A. palpation of the skull.
    B. evaluation of upper arm strength.
    C. PALPATION OF THE TRAPEZIUS.
    D. evaluation of brachial nerve function.

Rationale:

    C. Neck pain that begins at a time remote from overuse is likely muscular in nature. Therefore, assessment should focus on muscles of the neck.
    A. The patient did not strike her head; therefore, skull injury is unlikely.
    B. Evaluation of upper arm strength would be indicated if cervical nerve damage were suspected; however, cervical spine injury is unlikely in this scenario.
    D. Evaluation of brachial nerve function would be indicated if there were evidence of upper arm injury.

Content Category: Orthopedics & Wound Care

Reference: Merceir et al., 1995.

132. Discharge instructions for a patient with a rotator cuff injury of the arm should include:
    A. use of a sling during the day and for sleep.
    B. LIMITING USE OF THE AFFECTED ARM.
    C. an ice massage twice a day for 30 minutes.
    D. overhead exercises to strengthen the area.

Rationale:

    B. Use of the affected arm should be limited to permit the injury to heal. The patient should follow up with a health care provider who can determine when full use of the arm may resume.
    A. While a sling may be appropriate for use during the day, use during sleep could result in neck injury or strangulation.

C. Application of ice is useful; however, it should be applied in a covered bag, not as a massage directly to the skin.

D. Since the rotator cuff is used for overhead motions, exercises of this type are not appropriate in the period immediately after the injury. When to begin exercise should be determined at follow-up.

Content Category: Orthopedics & Wound Care

Reference: Johnson, 1997; pp. 71–123.

Questions 133 and 134

A 3-year-old child is brought into triage by his mother. According to a 13-year-old cousin, they had been playing when the 3-year-old suddenly started crying and stopped using the right arm. There was no fall or blow to the arm.

133. In triage, the child is quiet, gingerly holding the arm at his side and refusing to move it. As part of the history, the mother should be specifically asked if:
   A. the child prefers to sleep on that side.
   B. the child is right or left handed.
   C. any older siblings have had similar conditions.
   D. THE ARM WAS PULLED DURING PLAY.

Rationale:

D. Subluxation of the radial head (nursemaid's elbow) commonly occurs in this age group. It occurs when the arm is pulled along a longitudinal axis. There is immediate onset of pain and the child refuses to use the extremity. The mother needs to determine specifically what was happening right before the onset of arm pain.

A. No preferred sleeping position would cause an acute onset of this scenario.

B. The dominant hand is not yet evident in a 3-year-old child.

C. There is no familial component to subluxation of the radial head.

Content Category: Orthopedics & Wound Care

Reference: Greene & Luck, 1997; pp. 550–668.

134. A radial head subluxation is successfully reduced. A short time later, the child is actively using the right arm to play in the waiting room. Discharge instructions should include the recommendation to:
   A. use a sling during the day.
   B. MAKE SURE THE CHILD AVOIDS SWINGING BY THE ARMS.
   C. apply moist heat to the elbow twice a day.
   D. take the child to an orthopedist the next day.

Rationale:

B. Radial head subluxation may recur if the arm is pulled again. This injury generally does not occur after age 6 or 7.

A. There is no need to restrict activity if the child is comfortable using the arm.

C. No physical therapy is necessary after reduction of the subluxation.

D. Orthopedic evaluation is not needed if the child is actively using the arm after reduction.

Content Category: Orthopedics & Wound Care

Reference: Greene & Luck, 1997; pp. 550–668.

135.   A 20-year-old male complains of pain in his right hand after being involved in an altercation. On exam the area over the fifth metacarpal is tender and swollen and the patient has difficulty moving his fingers. You suspect that he has:
A. avulsion fracture.
B. BOXER FRACTURE.
C. tendon rupture.
D. scaphoid fracture.

Rationale:

B. Boxer fracture is a fracture of the fifth metacarpal. This type of fracture frequently occurs with activities such as fighting.

A. Avulsion fracture occurs when distal attachments of the extensor tendons tear loose, bringing with them a piece of the bone. Catching a baseball can cause this type of fracture.

C. Tendon rupture usually results from a laceration, bite, or puncture wound but can be caused by closed injury with superficial lacerations.

D. Scaphoid fracture, the most common carpal bone fracture, usually presents with tenderness over the anatomic snuffbox.

Content Category: Orthopedics & Wound Care

Reference: Sokolove, 1998; pp. 805–817; Sheehy, 1997; pp. 351–382.

136.   A 21-year-old male returns to the ED complaining of severe pain that is unrelieved by oxycodone (Percocet). He was diagnosed with a distal tibia and fibula fracture after a fall from a ladder. On exam, the toes are swollen and tender to touch and capillary refill is > 3 seconds. You are concerned that the patient is developing which of the following?
A. Osteomyelitis
B. Thrombophlebitis
C. Cellulitis
D. COMPARTMENT SYNDROME

Rationale:

D. Compartment syndrome results from an increasing pressure within a limited space that results in compromised tissue perfusion and ultimate dysfunction of neural and vascular structures contained in the space. The patient develops pain out of proportion to the injury, decreased capillary refill, decreased sensation, and decreased function.

A. Osteomyelitis is an infection in the bone. Predisposing factors include recent orthopedic procedure, open fracture, poor nutrition, chronic debilitating disease, intravenous drug abuse, and immunocompromise.

B. Thrombophlebitis is a venous obstruction usually caused by stasis, mechanical injury, and hypercoagulability. Signs and symptoms include edema, warmth, erythema, pain, tenderness of calf, and positive Homén's sign.

C. Cellulitis is a localized bacterial infection of the skin with soft tissue inflammation. Signs and symptoms include local tenderness, induration, and erythema. Cellulitis can be caused by lacerations, abrasions, crush injuries, and puncture wounds.

Content Category: Orthopedics & Wound Care

References: Stack, 1998; pp. 932–946; Strauss, 1999; pp. 487–536.

137.   A 19-year-old male arrives by ambulance from a motor vehicle collision. His knee hit the dashboard. He complains of severe pain in his right hip and the leg is internally rotated with flexion (pelican position). The ED nurse suspects which of the following?
A.   POSTERIOR HIP DISLOCATION
B.   Anterior hip dislocation
C.   Intertrochanteric hip fracture
D.   Cervical neck hip fracture

Rationale:

A.   The impact of the knee against the dashboard transmits the energy down the line to the hip. In a patient this age, a dislocation is more common than a fracture. As the ball of this ball-and-socket joint is forced out posteriorly, it can cause a fracture to the acetabulum.

B.   Anterior hip dislocation is uncommon, particularly with his legs crossed. To force the femoral head out, the anterior legs would have to have been apart at the time of the collision. In additional, the presentation would be external rotation.

C.   Intertrochanteric hip fracture occurs in older individuals. The presentation includes adduction, external rotation, and shortening.

D.   Cervical neck hip fracture occurs in older individuals. The presentation includes external rotation.

Content Category: Orthopedic & Wound Care

References: Bailey, 1998; pp. 415–447; Yarnold, 1999; pp. 36–41.

138.   A 28-year-old female is in the ED with a finger laceration sustained while washing dishes. In a non-tetanus-prone wound such as this, tetanus/diphtheria (Td) immunization should be administered if the patient received her last vaccination:
A.   MORE THAN 10 YEARS AGO.
B.   within the past 7 years.
C.   within the past 5 years.
D.   within the past 2 years.

Rationale:

A.   Td vaccine need not be administered in a nontetanus-prone wound (less than 6 hours old, linear, without contaminants or devitalized tissue) if the patient was vaccinated within 10 years. However, the patient's last vaccination was more than 10 years ago; therefore, she should be vaccinated now.

B.   Seven years is within the time frame for a nontetanus-prone wound; therefore, vaccination would not be needed in this case.

C.   If the wound were tetanus prone and the patient was last vaccinated more than 5 years earlier, Td vaccine should be administered. This is not a tetanus-prone wound, however.

D.   Td would not be needed if the patient's last vaccination took place within 2 years.

Content Category: Orthopedics & Wound Care

Reference: Gilbert et al., 2001; Boyles et al., 1998; pp. 44–49.

139.   Scapular fractures occur primarily as a result of:
   A. a fall on an outstretched hand.
   B. DIRECT TRAUMA.
   C. excessive use of the attached muscles.
   D. a fall on a flexed wrist.

Rationale:

   B. The scapula is one of the most difficult bones to break. Fracturing it usually requires direct, forceful trauma, such as a blow from a baseball bat.
   A. A fall on an outstretched hand represents an indirect force, which would be more likely to fracture bones in the upper extremity.
   C. Excessive use of attached muscles may result in an avulsion fracture. This types of fracture is more likely to occur in the lower than in the upper extremities.
   D. A fall on a flexed wrist is more likely to injure the wrist than to break the scapula.

Content Category: Orthopedics & Wound Care

Reference: Bailey, 1998; pp.415–447.

Questions 140 and 141

An 82-year-old patient presents to the ED via EMS following a motor vehicle crash. The restrained driver was traveling slowly when his car was struck from behind by a high-velocity vehicle. The patient complains of severe pubic pain and pain upon palpation of the right iliac wing. There is no external rotation of the right lower extremity and the patient is pale and diaphoretic. Vital signs are BP 74/58, HR 118/min, and respirations 24/min.

140.   The nurse should suspect a:
   A. fractured hip.
   B. dislocated hip.
   C. FRACTURED PELVIS.
   D. dislocated pelvis.

Rationale:

   C. Fractured pelvis generally occurs in the elderly from a fall or motor vehicle crash at low speed. Upon examination, the patient experiences pubic pain and pain with iliac compression. The dependent limb will not appear to be rotated or shortened.
   A. Fractured hip does occur in the elderly from falls or other trauma as well. Patients demonstrate external rotation and may or may not demonstrate shortening of the involved leg.
   B. Dislocated hip occurs in the elderly from falls or other trauma. Patients usually demonstrate internal rotation and severe pain at hip site and may or may not demonstrate shortening of the involved leg.
   D. The pelvis cannot be dislocated without spinal cord injury or other massive trauma to the body. Dislocated pelvis is highly unlikely in this case.

Content Category: Orthopedics & Wound Care

Reference: Walker, 2000; pp. 501–535.

141.   The patient demonstrates signs of shock. Which of the following types of shock is most likely?
   A. HYPOVOLEMIC
   B. Cardiogenic
   C. Distributive
   D. Obstructive

Rationale:

    A. A pelvic fracture can rapidly lead to hypovolemic shock. Hypovolemic shock results in loss of blood, plasma, or fluids, resulting predominately from trauma. The pelvis, a highly vascular region, can account for massive blood loss. The retroperitoneal cavity can hold up to 4 L of blood.

    B. Cardiogenic shock occurs in MI, cardiac tamponade, pulmonary emboli, and other events in which the heart cannot pump sufficiently.

    C. Distributive shock occurs in the presence of maldistribution of blood volume induced by changes in vascular resistance and permeability. This type of shock includes septic, anaphylactic, and neurogenic shock.

    D. Obstructive shock occurs in the presence of an obstruction to the outflow of blood from the heart. Common causes include pulmonary embolism, tension pneumothorax, and pericardial tamponade.

Content Category: Orthopedics & Wound Care

Reference: Walker, 2000; pp. 501–535.

142. A patient in triage complains of pain, tearing, and a foreign body sensation in both eyes. She states that she noticed a gradual onset of symptoms after dinner and now can't keep her eyes open. Photophobia is noted. Which of the following statements by the patient should be documented in the triage note?
    A. "I normally drive to work, but have taken the bus for 2 weeks now."
    B. "I WAS AT THE POOL ALL DAY TODAY."
    C. "I do a lot of computer work."
    D. "I was at an ice skating rink last night."

Rationale:

    B. The patient is demonstrating signs of ultraviolet keratitis, which can follow prolonged exposure to ultraviolet light. Prolonged exposure to sun, especially when there is water nearby, can cause keratitis.

    A. Using public transportation would not cause eye changes.

    C. Computer work might lead to eyestrain, but the above symptoms do not suggest eyestrain.

    D. Spending time in an ice skating rink would not cause keratitis.

Content Category: Maxillofacial & Ocular

Reference: Rosen et al., 1999.

143. A 76-year-old patient complains of headache with nausea and vomiting. The patient also complains of halos around lights and photophobia. Physical exam reveals a reddened left eye. The ED nurse should suspect which of the following?
    A. Migraine
    B. Conjunctivitis
    C. ACUTE ANGLE-CLOSURE GLAUCOMA
    D. Trauma

Rationale:

    C. The symptoms of acute angle-closure glaucoma include headache in the brow arch, eye pain, and a red, inflamed eye. Additional associated symptoms include nausea, vomiting, seeing halos around objects, photophobia, and tearing.

    A. Migraine headaches usually present with a unilateral headache, photophobia, nausea, and vomiting.

B. Conjunctivitis usually presents as a red, tearing, itching eye.

D. Trauma patients usually describe some mechanism of injury. Although their symptoms can be very similar to those in this patient's case, they usually do not describe seeing halos around objects.

Content Category: Maxillofacial & Ocular

Reference: Birinyi & Mauger, 1997; pp. 26–65.

144. Which of the following statements about epiglottitis is INCORRECT?
   A. It is usually caused by *Haemophilus influenzae*.
   B. IT OCCURS ONLY IN CHILDREN.
   C. The usual symptoms include a sore throat, fever, and drooling.
   D. It has a rapid onset.

Rationale:

B. Epiglottitis is more common in adults than children. It usually occurs during the fifth decade of life.

A. The most common cause of epiglottitis is *Haemophilus influenzae*, which can also be caused by mycobacteria, herpes simplex, candidal organisms, and thermal and caustic causes.

C. The usual symptoms of epiglottitis include sore throat, fever, drooling, cervical adenopathy, stridor, muffled voice, respiratory distress, hypoxia, and a toxic-appearing patient.

D. Epiglottitis has a rapid onset.

Content Category: Maxillofacial & Ocular

References: Cosby, 1998; pp. 721–741; Jauch et al., 1997; pp. 108–140.

145. A patient with a nasal bone fracture is suspected to have cerebral spinal fluid draining from the nose. These findings suggest which of the following?
   A. Septal hematoma
   B. CRIBRIFORM FRACTURE
   C. Orbit fracture
   D. Tripod fracture

Rationale:

B. Cribriform fracture, a fracture through the cribriform plate of the ethmoid bone, can be a complication of nasal bone fractures. A cerebral spinal fluid leak may occur because of a torn meningea.

A. Septal hematoma is a complication of nasal fracture. It is rare but can cause a serious nasal deformity called saddle nose.

C. Although an orbit fracture can be a part of facial trauma, its complication is nerve entrapment.

D. Tripod fracture can be another complication of a nasal fracture and should be ruled out when a patient presents with facial fracture.

Content Category: Maxillofacial & Ocular

References: Waters & Peacock, 2000; pp.1532–1539; Munter & McGuirk, 1997; pp. 4–23.

146. A college student presents with a history of facial fullness, dental pain, and purulent rhinorrhea. The nurse should suspect:
   A. odontalgia.
   B. upper respiratory infection.
   C. ACUTE SINUSITIS.
   D. nasal foreign body.

Rationale:

    C. Acute sinusitis usually presents with facial fullness, purulent nasal discharge, and dental pain.

    A. Odontalgia (tooth pain) is one symptom of sinusitis but can also occur with other conditions.

    B. Upper respiratory infection often precedes sinusitis. The presence of purulent rhinorrhea is more suggestive of sinusitis.

    D. Nasal foreign body is possible, but this situation would normally be found in a pediatric population.

Content Category: Maxillofacial & Ocular

References: Jauch et al., 1997; pp. 108–140; Waters & Peacock, 2000; pp.1532–1539.

147.   A patient diagnosed with hyphema is ready for discharge. Which of the following statements by the patient indicates successful patient discharge teaching?
    A. "I will only use one pillow when I sleep."
    B. "I can take 600 mg of ibuprofen if the pain is severe."
    C. "I WILL RETURN IF THE PAIN GETS WORSE."
    D. "I will see the ophthalmologist again in 3 days."

Rationale:

    C. Rebleed is associated with increased incidence of glaucoma, traumatic cataracts, loss of vision, and loss of the eye. If rebleeding occurs, immediate hospitalization is required. Signs of a rebleed are sudden increase in pain and decrease in vision.

    A. The patient should be instructed to sleep with the head elevated approximately 30 degrees to decrease intraocular pressure. That may require the use of more than one pillow.

    B. Nonsteroidal anti-inflammatory drugs and aspirin are contraindicated after hyphema, as they may cause more bleeding.

    D. Patients who are discharged with hyphema should be reevaluated by an ophthalmologist daily.

Content Category: Maxillofacial & Ocular

References: Birinyi & Mauger, 1997; pp. 26–65; Rhee & Pyfer, 1999; pp. 366–369.

Questions 148 and 149

A 2-year-old child is brought to the ED by parents who state that he woke from sleep crying inconsolably. The mother reports he had a recent "cold" with fevers to 101°F (38.4°C). Assessment reveals a fussy child who is pulling and rubbing his right ear.

148.   To visualize the ear best during the otoscope exam, the ED nurse should:
    A. GENTLY PULL THE EAR DOWN AND BACK.
    B. gently pull the ear up and back.
    C. maintain the head and ear in a neutral position.
    D. have the child rotate his head to the right.

Rationale:

    A. The ear should be pulled down and back to straighten the ear canal in children.

    B. The ear should be pulled up and back in adults.

    C. Maintaining a neutral position has no relevance.

    D. Rotating the head to the right would make it more difficult for the nurse to access the ear.

Content Category: Maxillofacial & Ocular

Reference: Olson, 1998; pp. 673–688.

149.   Based on the parents' history and the child's behavior, the ED nurse should suspect:
   A. otitis externa.
   B. foreign body.
   C. OTITIS MEDIA.
   D. ruptured tympanic membrane.

Rationale:

   C. Crying, fever, and tugging the ears are common signs of otitis media, which tends to occur in toddlers and often follows an upper respiratory infection.
   A. Otitis externa is an inflammation of the external ear canal that causes pain when the ear is pulled. A toddler with otitis externa would avoid touching the ear.
   B. Children with a foreign body of the ear present with a foul-smelling ear and discharge.
   D. Ruptured tympanic membrane occurs most frequently in children with chronic ear infections or trauma.

Content Category: Maxillofacial & Ocular

Reference: Olson, 1998; pp. 673–688.

150.   The most commonly found obstructive material of the ear canal is:
   A. CERUMEN.
   B. insects.
   C. beads.
   D. cotton swabs.

Rationale:

   A. Cerumen (wax) is the most commonly found obstructive material of the ear canal. Children often present with this problem after pushing wax into the canal with cotton swabs. Hearing aids contribute to this problem in adults.
   B. Insects are foreign bodies, but not the most common.
   C. Beads are foreign bodies, but not the most common.
   D. Cotton swabs are foreign bodies, but not the most common.

Content Category: Maxillofacial & Ocular

Reference: Olson, 1998; pp. 673–688.

Examination 2:
Self-Diagnostic Profile

Instructions

Step 1: Check your answers against the correct answers provided in Part 2 of this chapter. Then calculate your total score.

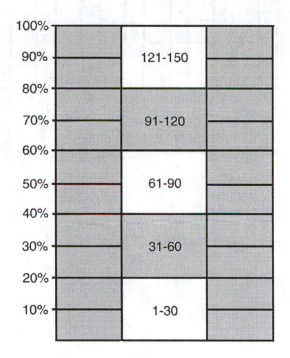

Figure 1: Total Score

Step 2: For each category of the practice examination, determine the number of items that you answered correctly and plot that number in Figure 2. The result will assist you in diagnosing your areas of knowledge strength and in determing which areas benefit from review.

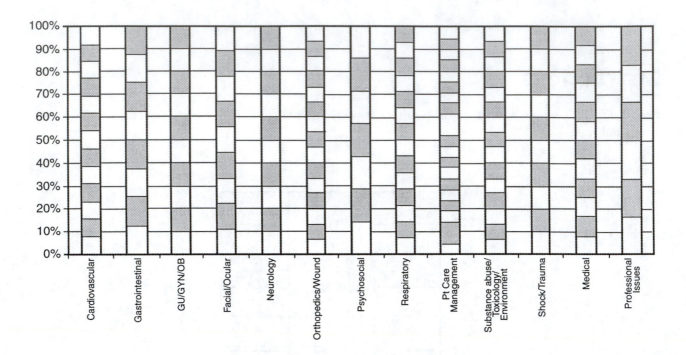

Figure 2: Practice Examination Content Areas

Practice Examination 3

Part I

1. A front-seat passenger involved in a motor vehicle crash (MVC) arrives via a Basic Life Support (BLS) ambulance complaining of right-sided chest pain. He is pale, tachypneic, and dyspneic. Decreased breath sounds are auscultated on the right side and a hemothorax is suspected. A patent airway has been assured; c-spine precautions are in effect; and a chest tube has been inserted. Your next priority intervention would be to:
   A. insert a nasogastric tube.
   B. determine the patient's Glasgow Coma Scale (GCS) score.
   C. insert 2 large-bore IV lines for crystalloid infusion.
   D. prepare autotransfuser.

2. You are caring for an unrestrained driver of a motor vehicle crash (MVC). He is severely dyspneic and cyanotic, has labored respirations, absent breath sounds on the right, unilateral chest rise and fall, and jugular venous distention You suspect which of the following?
   A. Aspiration
   B. Flail chest
   C. Tension pneumothorax
   D. Cardiac tamponade

3. What potential problem would a patient with a tracheobronchial injury be at risk for immediately after the insertion of a chest tube?
   A. Pneumonia
   B. Local cellulitis
   C. Bronchospasm
   D. Continuous air leak

4. A victim of a stab wound to the epigastric area presents to the ED. Upon evaluation he suddenly develops shortness of breath, chest pain, and decreased breath sounds. What is the priority nursing diagnosis for this patient?
   A. Ineffective airway clearance
   B. Ineffective breathing pattern
   C. Decreased cardiac output
   D. Fluid volume deficit

5. The first-line pharmacologic treatment used to improve air exchange for the chronic obstructive pulmonary disease (COPD) patient who is experiencing an acute exacerbation is which of the following?
   A. Intravenous theophylline (Aminophyllin)
   B. Nebulized ipratropium (Albuterol)
   C. Subcutaneous epinephrine (Adrenalin)
   D. Oral zileuton (Zyflo)

6. A motorcyclist presents to the ED after a clothesline accident in which he sustained multiple face and neck fractures. He is unable to speak and has hemoptysis and inspiratory stridor. A high-priority nursing diagnosis for this patient is:
    A. alteration in skin integrity.
    B. altered body image.
    C. ineffective airway clearance.
    D. altered mental status.

7. In caring for the patient with Ludwig's angina, the nurse should first assess for:
    A. pain, leukocytosis, and hypotension.
    B. chest pain, diaphoresis, and nausea.
    C. airway obstruction, shortness of breath, and fever.
    D. dysrhythmias, chest pain, and numbness down the arm.

8. One priority to consider while caring for a patient with respiratory distress syndrome is to monitor which of the following?
    A. Pneumonia
    B. Urine output
    C. Infection
    D. Fluid intake

9. When teaching an asthma patient about his/her disease, it is important for the emergency nurse to explain which of the following?
    A. Asthma is primarily caused by airway inflammation and hyperresponsiveness to stimuli.
    B. Physiologic changes seen in asthma exacerbation are often irreversible.
    C. Asthma exacerbations are most frequently a result of a respiratory infection.
    D. Most asthma attacks occur suddenly and without warning in the early morning.

10. When teaching an asthma patient about medication usage, it is important for the emergency nurse to discuss which of the following?
    A. Inhaled steroids are addictive and their use should be limited to acute exacerbations.
    B. Patients often develop a tolerance to daily asthma medications and require increased doses.
    C. Inhaled bronchodilators should not be used with inhaled corticosteroids.
    D. Oral corticosteroids are often used for short-term treatment of exacerbations.

11. A 6-year-old child is being treated for asthma in the ED. In teaching the patient's caregiver about medication administration, the nurse should include which of the following statements?
    A. Liquid asthma medications have a quicker onset of effects than inhaled medications.
    B. Children under 12 years old do not have sufficient coordination to use metered-dose inhalers.
    C. A spacer attached to a metered-dose inhaler can increase medication effectiveness.
    D. Oral steroids should not be given to children under the age of 5 years.

12. A patient experiencing an acute asthma exacerbation states that his routine medications include use of a cromolyn (Intal) inhaler. This medication is given to:
    A. relieve acute bronchospasm on an as-needed basis.
    B. block the release of chemical mediators from mast cells.
    C. inhibit cough receptors in the bronchial lining.
    D. block the uptake of calcium in the bronchial smooth muscle.

13. The nurse is obtaining a history from a 23-year-old patient with shortness of breath, bilateral wheezing on expiration in all fields, and a pulse oximetry reading of 92% on room air. Which of the following is the most significant history finding?
    A. Three to four visits to the ED in the past year for similar episodes
    B. Previous episode requiring admission to ICU and intubation 2 years ago
    C. Increased episodes occurring in the spring months of the year
    D. Limitation of normal daily activities for the past 2 days

14. Measurement of peak expiratory flow rate is a useful tool in the management of asthma because:
    A. rising values can indicate an impending exacerbation of asthma.
    B. it helps clear airway passages of mucus plugs.
    C. measurement does not rely on patient effort.
    D. it can document reversibility of airway narrowing.

15. The Joint Commission on Accreditation of Healthcare Organizations (JCAHO) defines a sentinel event as:
    A. any incident that occurs within the hospital environment at least once each year.
    B. any incident that results in lost work time for a hospital employee.
    C. an unexpected occurrence involving death or serious physical or psychological injury or risk.
    D. a patient outcome that exceeds expected hospital days as outlined by the clinical pathway.

16. A manager in an urban ED considers benchmarking to establish staffing levels. If this were done, the manager would incorporate which of the following?
    A. Database from EDs of varying volume and size
    B. Database capturing trends in emergency as well as ambulatory care
    C. Database being current and reflective of similar volume and practice
    D. Database from rural hospital EDs across the U.S.

17. An emergency nurse receives special recognition as a role model for customer service. Which of the following actions demonstrates this nurse's dedication to customer service?
    A. Informs the patient that the social worker will explain the visitation policies in the ED
    B. Describes the events of the day leading to the patient's visit to the ED
    C. Informs the family in the waiting room that the patient is in the radiology department
    D. Complains that a coworker has left the otoscope tip holder empty during a patient examination.

18. Which of the following would be considered appropriate for constructive criticism of an employee?
    A. Always have another employee present during any conversations involving criticism.
    B. Do not offer any positive feedback, as it may overshadow the reason for the criticism.
    C. State the facts to the employee and do not focus on the employee's opinion.
    D. Explain the rationale for the error action as part of the criticism.

19. Which of the following is the rationale for an ED nurse to take the Advanced Cardiac Life Support Provider course?
    A. Taking the course will help the ED nurse to memorize the algorithms and protocols.
    B. Taking the course will helps the ED nurse to memorize the drug dosages.
    C. The hospital requires that all nurses take the course.
    D. Taking the course will help the ED nurse learn a systematic approach to cardiopulmonary emergencies.

20. The emergency nurse manager wishes to evaluate staffing as part of a continuous improvement plan. The manager would benchmark information such as which of the following?
    A. A sense by the staff that patients are staying longer while awaiting in house beds
    B. Actual staffing, wait times, and length of stay by patient triage classification
    C. Chief Financial Officer statement that ED is overstaffed by full-time equivalents for unit of service
    D. Patient complaint letter stating ED is understaffed

21. A 21-year-old male is brought to the ED with a history of having skated head first into the boards while playing hockey. He was immediately flaccid but has been able to maintain his own respirations. He never lost consciousness. One of the first medications you would anticipate administering is which of the following?
    A. Mannitol (Osmitrol)
    B. Dexamethasone (Decadron)
    C. Furosemide (Lasix)
    D. Antibiotics

22. A patient presents to triage with a sudden onset of what she calls "the worse headache in my life." She describes the onset as being "like a thunderclap." What triage decision would you make for this patient?
    A. Have someone escort the patient to an acute bed immediately.
    B. Send her to the waiting room to wait for an available bed.
    C. Give her directions to the neurology clinic.
    D. Send her to the Fast Track/Walk-In Clinic, as the ED is currently very busy.

23. The most common cause of nontraumatic subarachnoid hemorrhage is which of the following?
    A. Old age
    B. Drug abuse
    C. Ruptured aneurysm
    D. Preeclampsia

24. Nimodipine (Nimotop) is given to a patient with a subarachnoid hemorrhage to:
    A. prevent vasospasm.
    B. control bleeding.
    C. control blood pressure.
    D. assist with airway management.

25. A trauma patient is evaluated and treated in the ED. The initial diagnosis is diffuse axonal injury: many nonfocal deficits, in contrast to mass lesions, hemorrhage, or focal contusions). The main goal of care for this patient is to do which of the following?
    A. Prevent contractures and foot drop
    B. Prevent hemorrhage by administering specific antihemorrhagic medications
    C. Control intracranial hypertension and prevent secondary brain injury
    D. Reduce body core temperature to preserve brain tissue

26. A 19-year-old soldier is brought to your ED after experiencing a syncopal episode during inspection. Upon further investigation, you learn that the air temperature at the training facility was 104° F (40.0° C) and that the soldier had been standing at attention for several minutes immediately after participating in a 3-mile run. The EMTs tell you that the patient's systolic blood pressure, which was 86 mm Hg when they first arrived, quickly rose to 110 mm Hg when they elevated his legs. The most likely cause of this syncopal episode is which of the following?
    A. Neurogenic disease
    B. Fatigue

C. Congenital disposition

D. Autonomic dysfunction

27. Priapism (sustained erection) may be indicative of which of the following?

A. Prostate cancer

B. High spinal cord lesion

C. Migraine headache

D. Sexual dysfunction

28. You are discharging a patient who sustained a concussion following a motor vehicle crash. It is important to tell the patient which of the following?

A. "You may have difficulty concentrating at work."

B. "You do not need to have anyone stay with you."

C. "Call your private physician if you develop vomiting."

D. "It is OK to drink coffee today."

29. You are preparing to administer mannitol (Osmitrol) 130 g to a 150-lb (68.2-kg) patient with a closed head injury. Which of the following nursing interventions should be considered?

A. Notify the physician concerning a possible incorrect dose.

B. An inline IV filter should be used.

C. The medication should be administered over 8 hours.

D. An intracranial pressure monitor should be in place.

30. The goal of interventions for an adult patient with seizures is to:

A. sedate the patient so rest can occur.

B. reduce fever.

C. prevent prolonged/recurrent seizures.

D. prevent injuries to the limbs.

31. Pediatric victims of a MVC (motor vehicle crash) with an improper application of the lap belt safety restraint are at a high risk for injury to the:

A. kidney.

B. spleen.

C. bowel.

D. liver.

32. With which of the following presentations would a patient with a small-bowel obstruction present?

A. Rapid onset of colicky, cramplike, intermittent pain in the abdomen

B. Gradual onset of low-grade crampy pain in the abdomen, with constipation

C. Rapid onset of vomiting, fever, and crampy abdominal pain followed by diarrhea

D. Sudden acute abdominal pain with bloody stools mixed with mucus ("currant jelly" stools)

33. Which of the following statements is helpful in excluding cardiac origin as the differentiating diagnosis of a patient presenting with chest discomfort?

A. "The pain is in my midabdominal area and chest, feeling like a pressure."

B. "Nitroglycerine relieved the chest discomfort."

C. "The antacid I took helped to relieve the discomfort somewhat."

D. "I have pain that is in my upper midback area."

34.   Many gastrointestinal diseases incorporate similar patient education strategies. One teaching point that is unique to hiatal hernia is which of the following?
A.   "Stop smoking."
B.   "Eat small, frequent, bland meals."
C.   "Avoid highly seasoned foods and alcoholic beverages."
D.   "Wear loose, nonconstricting clothing."

35.   A patient presents to the ED with a chief complaint of sudden onset of colicky abdominal pain and nausea after eating a meal of fried chicken and French fries. Vital signs are BP 140/80 mm Hg, HR 116/min, respirations 18/min, and temperature 100.4° F (38.0° C). The priority intervention is which of the following?
A.   Administration of pain control
B.   Immediate preparation for the operating room
C.   Nasogastric intubation
D.   Administration of a stool softener

36.   In the presentation of acute pancreatitis, the MOST COMMON causes are which of the following?
A.   Gastroesophageal reflux disorder and injury
B.   Hyperlipidemia and aging
C.   Infection and carcinoma
D.   Alcoholism and gallstones

37.   A 23-year-old male patient presents to the ED complaining of right testicular pain, nausea, and vomiting for 2 hours. He has a mild fever on exam and generalized tenderness in the abdomen. The nurse must consider which of the following diagnoses?
A.   Appendicitis
B.   Small-bowel obstruction
C.   Acute cholecystitis
D.   Urinary tract infection

38.   A 75-year-old female arrives in the ED complaining of a 2-day history of gastroenteritis. Which of the following additional past medical history findings would put the patient at an increased risk for this disease?
A.   Recent depression
B.   Recent antibiotic use
C.   Obesity or weight gain
D.   Taking anticholinergics

39.   An 18-year-old college student is brought to the ED by her boyfriend after he noticed that she had superficially cut herself on her forearm numerous times with a razor. After caring for the wounds, your next intervention would be to:
A.   question the patient about any suicidal thoughts, plans, means, or actions.
B.   contract with the patient not to harm herself while in the ED.
C.   give the patient the phone number of a 24-hour hot line to call if she should feel like hurting herself again.
D.   reduce the external stimuli by placing her in a seclusion room.

40.   A 48-year-old female presents to the ED with complaints of intermittent palpitations, chest tightness, and choking sensations. The patient reports having had these symptoms for about 6 weeks and states that the episodes are becoming more frequent. Triage assessment reveals an intact airway and skin cool and slightly diaphoretic to touch. Vital signs are BP 168/72 mm Hg, HR 118/min, respirations 26/min, and temperature 99.2° F (37.4° C). The patient does not report any chest tightness, palpitations, or choking sensations at this time. Further assessment of this patient by the emergency

nurse reveals that she has recently divorced and has relocated to this community, which is a great distance from her support system. The patient has not been able to find employment that meets career goals she has set for herself. Which of the following nursing diagnoses are most appropriate to guide the plan of care for this patient?

A. Impaired verbal communication
B. Knowledge deficit related to problem solving
C. Altered thought processes related to physical manifestations
D. Anxiety/fear related to etiology as determined through assessment

41. A 35-year-old woman has just been brought into the ED by the police after having been sexually assaulted. The patient is alert. Initial assessment reveals bruises and abrasions on her face, breasts, arms, and hands. She makes minimal eye contact with the nurse and responds only when asked a question. During her ED evaluation, the patient expresses concern that the assault may have occurred during ovulation and that she may become pregnant. A treatment modality available that may relieve her concerns is:

A. azithromycin (Zithromax) 1 g PO stat.
B. doxycycline (Vibramycin) 100 mg bid for 10 days.
C. oxytocin (Pitocin) 10 U IM.
D. ethinyl estradiol/norgestrel (Ovral) 2 tablets initially followed by 2 tablets 12 hours later.

42. What is the first step in crisis intervention?

A. Assist the person is gaining an intellectual understanding of the problem
B. Explore coping mechanisms
C. Include support system to review the event
D. Assess the precipitating event and its impact on the person

43. Depressed patients with suicidal ideation who are being evaluated are at greatest risk for committing suicide:

A. during the winter months.
B. before starting antidepressants.
C. after the depression lifts.
D. when they are agitated and unfocused.

44. A 16-year-old female arrives in the ED accompanied by her parents. She appears cachectic. Vital signs are BP 86/50 mm Hg, HR 60/min and irregular, and respirations 20/min. Her lips are dry and cracked; skin turgor is tented. As an intravenous line is being started, she states, "There's no sugar in the IV, is there?" You suspect that this patient has which of the following?

A. Influenza
B. Diabetes
C. Anorexia
D. Heat stroke

45. A young woman is brought to the ED with the history of seizures. Soon after arrival, she has a "seizure." There is no loss of consciousness and she is not incontinent. Afterward, she is alert and oriented and seems to enjoy the attention she receives. The neurologist is notified. He states that he is familiar with this patient's case as she had just completed a complete neurologic workup that failed to reveal any neurologic cause. He suggests that this patient be seen by a psychiatrist. The patient agrees. You suspect which of the following?

A. Conversion disorder
B. Bipolar disorder
C. Panic disorder
D. Schizophrenia

46.   A patient with a suspected corneal abrasion is in a treatment room awaiting evaluation by the doc-
      tor. While waiting, the ED nurse can enhance patient comfort by:
      A. giving the patient the dropperette of topical anesthesia to be applied ad lib.
      B. irrigating the involved eye with cooled saline.
      C. keeping the lights dimmed.
      D. applying an occlusive eye patch.

47.   Signs and symptoms of croup include which of the following?
      A. Stridor, intercostal retractions, unequal breath sounds
      B. Stridor, barking cough, intercostal retraction
      C. Tachypnea, barking cough, difficulty swallowing
      D. Fever, hoarse voice, difficulty swallowing

48.   The expected results of the fluorescein stain of the cornea in a patient with suspected bacterial con-
      junctivitis are which of the following?
      A. Cornea clear
      B. Dendritic ulcerations seen
      C. Occasional punctate staining
      D. Corneal ulcerations

49.   Common symptoms in a patient with otitis media include:
      A. otalgia and fever.
      B. otorrhea and nystagmus.
      C. hearing loss and vertigo.
      D. fever and tinnitus.

50.   A patient who has sustained a splash of lye into both eyes is undergoing irrigation. Irrigation should
      continue until:
      A. the pH reaches 8.4.
      B. 1,000 ml of fluid has been instilled.
      C. 500 ml of fluid has been instilled.
      D. the pH reaches 7.4.

51.   Discharge instructions for a patient with otitis media will most likely include:
      A. application of warm compresses every 2 hours.
      B. bed rest for 24 hours.
      C. aggressive cleansing of the ear canal.
      D. reevaluation in 10 days to confirm resolution.

52.   A patient with an orbital blowout fracture should have a thorough evaluation of:
      A. hearing.
      B. extraocular movements.
      C. tongue movement.
      D. swallowing.

53.   A 4-year-old child is found to have a tender, red nodule on the upper eyelid. Discharge instructions
      include antibiotic ophthalmic ointment and direction to:
      A. wash eyelashes daily with baby shampoo.
      B. flush with eye wash three times a day.
      C. instill over-the-counter vasoconstricting drops twice a day.
      D. apply cool compresses four times a day.

54. A 30-year-old male presents with a 5-day history of unilateral sore throat. He is also complaining of ear pain, fever, and difficulty swallowing. If you consider these symptoms, the patient most likely has which of the following conditions?
   A. Mononucleosis
   B. Epiglottitis
   C. Peritonsillar abscess
   D. Pharyngitis

55. A 21-year-old female presents to the ED with complaints of weakness and leg cramps. She appears to be underweight for her height. Vital signs are BP 90/60 mm Hg and HR 55/min. All other vital signs are within normal parameters. During the general survey, you would be likely to observe, as a potential behavior that a patient with anorexia nervosa, would display, the wearing of:
   A. tight-fitting clothing.
   B. loose-fitting clothing.
   C. seasonally appropriate clothing.
   D. fitted clothing.

56. Your patient presents at triage with shortness of breath and chest pain with inspiration. Past history reveals that this patient is HIV positive. Vital signs are BP 124/64 mm Hg, HR 96/min, respirations 24/min, and temperature 99.8° F (37.7° C). Which of the following is a priority for the ED nurse?
   A. Airborne precautions
   B. Contact precautions
   C. Isolation precautions
   D. Standard precautions

57. Your patient has a 6-month history of fibromyalgia. She presents in the ED with complaints of dull, aching, unprovoked back pain (rated at 3/10) for the past several days. Her vital signs are all within normal limits. What is a priority in the management of a patient with fibromyalgia?
   A. Narcotic pain management
   B. Patient education about fibromyalgia
   C. Physical therapy
   D. NSAID pain management

58. A 34-year-old female comes to the ED complaining of muscle cramps in her legs and numbness of her fingers for the past several days. She has a history of gallbladder disease and pancreatitis. This patient is demonstrating signs and symptoms of:
   A. hypermagnesemia.
   B. hypocalcemia.
   C. hyperkalemia.
   D. hyponatremia.

59. Which of the following complications is of most concern with rapid reduction of circulating glucose and administration of fluids?
   A. Seizures
   B. Congestive heart failure
   C. Cerebral edema
   D. Hyperthermia

60.   Suspended droplets that carry tuberculosis (TB) infection may remain in still air for days. This route of disease transmission is prevented by the use of which of the following?
A. Surgical mask
B. Nonlatex gloves
C. Impervious gown
D. HEPA mask

61.   A 20-year-old presents with a 2-week history of fatigue, thirst, nausea, and polyuria. Lab analysis shows a glucose level of 654 mg/dl and a potassium level of 5.4 mEq/dl. IV fluids and insulin are begun. Which of the following orders should the ED nurse anticipate?
A. Administration of bicarbonate with a pH of 7.3
B. Potassium added to IV fluid
C. IV fluid changed from normal saline (NS) solution to 5% dextrose and 0.5% normal saline
D. Administration of low-dose heparin

62.   On arrival at the ED, a patient is confused. The skin is hot and dry with poor turgor. Glucometer findings come up as "high." A history of infection, thirst, and polyuria is gathered from the family. Vital signs are BP 96/50 mm Hg, HR 142/min, and respirations 18/min and normal, with no odor. What is the likely problem?
A. Hyperglycemic hyperosmolar nonketotic coma
B. Diabetic ketoacidosis
C. Thyroid storm
D. Myxedema coma

63.   Which of the following electrolyte deficiencies can cause tetany?
A. Decreased chloride
B. Decreased potassium
C. Decreased sodium
D. Decreased phosphate

64.   Identification of rashes leads to clues about the causative agent. Measles presents with which type of rash?
A. Vesicular
B. Petechial
C. Pustular
D. Maculopapular

65.   Although children are immunized against this disease, by age 12 or so the inoculation is no longer protective. Which disease is it?
A. Polio
B. Pertussis
C. Diphtheria
D. Mumps

66.   Which of the following diseases is transmitted through the bloodborne pathway?
A. Hepatitis A
B. Hepatitis C
C. Encephalitis
D. Rocky Mountain spotted fever

67.   The common pathologic processes leading to brain death do NOT include which of the following?
      A. Massive head trauma
      B. Myxedema coma
      C. Intracranial hemorrhage
      D. Hypoxic ischemic brain damage suffered during cardiopulmonary arrest

68.   According to the American College of Surgeons Committee on Trauma standards, which one of the following patients should be transported to a designated trauma center?
      A. A 72-year-old female with a fractured clavicle after automobile crash
      B. A 26-year-old male with a Glasgow Coma Scale score of 16 after motorcycle crash
      C. A 15-year-old female with a systolic blood pressure of 148 after automobile crash
      D. A 7-year-old male who fell 15 feet out of a tree

69.   When the nurse is treating victims of a weapon of mass destruction, which of the following are considered personal protective equipment?
      A. Respirator, gown, bottled water
      B. Oxygen mask, gown, hair covering
      C. Respirator, gown, eye protection
      D. Portable oxygen tank, gown, eye protection

70.   A disease agent that may be used as a biological weapon is which of the following?
      A. Rubella
      B. Smallpox
      C. Viral influenza
      D. Chlamydia

71.   When a patient agrees to a procedure after having been made aware of the procedure to be performed, the alternatives available, and the risks of the procedure, the patient's consent is said to be:
      A. implied.
      B. involuntary.
      C. express.
      D. informed.

72.   In the event of a major catastrophe, the National Disaster Medical System can:
      A. take over state operations for a 2-week period of recovery.
      B. be activated only in response to a request from the governor of the state.
      C. send federal personnel to the state within 8 hours.
      D. exert federal control over a hospital.

73.   Justin is a 2-year-old with HR 264/minute, respirations 32/min, and a peripheral capillary refill of 2 seconds, with fast but strong peripheral pulses. He is sitting in his mother's lap and cries at your approach. Crying causes no change in the rhythm on the monitor. His skin is pale pink and warm.

      His tympanic temperature is 98.2°F (36.8°C). Your interventions would include:
      A. oxygen by face mask, IV access, sedation, and vagal maneuvers.
      B. sedation and synchronized cardioversion at 2 joules/kg.
      C. IV access and administration of adenosine phosphate (Adenocard) IV.
      D. IV access, sedation, and cardioversion at 0.5 joules/kg.

74.   Parents bring their 5-day-old infant to the ED for "poor feeding." Mom reports the baby was breast-feeding well until yesterday evening. Your triage exam reveals a term female infant who is pale, slightly mottled, and listless, with poor muscle tone. Vital signs are HR 160/min, respirations 44/min with mild retractions, and temperature 100.8° F (38.2° C) rectally. Capillary refill time is 3 seconds centrally and 4 seconds peripherally. Based on your assessment, you would do which of the following?
   A. Send the family to the registration desk.
   B. Triage the infant as emergent and send the infant directly to the treatment area.
   C. Place mother and baby behind the curtain at triage so you can see if the infant will breastfeed.
   D. Triage the infant as urgent and send the family to the waiting room.

75.   In most situations, the maximum volume of a medication that should be administered IM in a single site to small children and older infants is:
   A. 0.5 ml.
   B. 1.0 ml.
   C. 2.0 ml.
   D. 3.0 ml.

76.   The initial priority in the treatment of a pediatric patient with an avulsed tooth is:
   A. airway management.
   B. to control hemorrhage.
   C. to assess neurologic status.
   D. preservation of the tooth for reimplantation.

77.   A 4-year-old male fell from a moving all-terrain vehicle (ATV) and has multiple injuries. He has been stabilized in your ED and will be transported to a regional pediatric hospital for ongoing evaluation and treatment. A pediatric transport team is flying in to pick up and transport the patient. Which of the following interventions is NOT appropriate in preparing the patient for air medical transport?
   A. Initiate IV access and secure lines
   B. Splint suspected fractures with air splints
   C. Secure and maintain a patent airway
   D. Insert a gastric tube

78.   The emergency nurse knows that infants and small children have anatomic and physiologic differences from older children and adults. Which of the following is NOT an important difference?
   A. Infants and children have lower oxygen requirements than adults.
   B. Infants and children have greater amounts of soft tissue surrounding the airway.
   C. The heads of infants and children are larger and heavier in relation to the body than are adults'.
   D. Infants and children have poorly developed intercostal accessory muscles.

79.   A hypotensive patient with multiple trauma is to be transferred from a small rural facility to a level I trauma center. Prior to departure, it is imperative that which of the following be done for the patient?
   A. Diagnostic peritoneal lavage (DPL)
   B. Thoracotomy
   C. Computed tomography (CT) scan
   D. Boluses of normal saline

Questions 80 and 81

A patient with chest pain has 3-mm to 5-mm ST segment elevations in leads II, III, and AVF on electrocardiogram (ECG). Vital signs are BP 128/62 mm Hg, HR 96/min, and respirations 22/min. After sublingual nitroglycerin has been administered, vital signs are BP 88/50 mm Hg, HR 108/min, and respirations 22/min.

80. The diagnostic test that would be most useful in determining the specific problem is:
    A. right-sided ECG.
    B. cardiac enzymes and isoenzymes.
    C. chest x-ray.
    D. stress test.

81. This patient will probably need large doses of:
    A. morphine sulfate.
    B. nitroglycerin.
    C. furosemide (Lasix).
    D. normal saline.

82. A patient with a large flail segment to the anterior chest is to be transported from a rural facility to a level I trauma center. It is most important to:
    A. transport the patient on oxygen by nonrebreather mask.
    B. intubate the patient before departure and provide controlled mechanical ventilation.
    C. stabilize the flail segment with a large sandbag.
    D. transport the patient on the uninjured side.

83. A 35-year-old man comes to the ED complaining of nausea, pain in the left upper quadrant, and malaise. History includes a liver transplant 3 months ago. The ED nurse should anticipate the possibility of:
    A. gallstones.
    B. transplant rejection.
    C. alcohol use and possible pancreatitis.
    D. infection masked by immunosuppressive therapy.

84. A vasopressin (Pitressin) infusion of 30 units/hour is ordered for an adult patient with bleeding esophageal varices. Fifty units of vasopressin is added to 200 ml of normal saline solution. The drip factor is 15 gtt/ml. Flow should be adjusted to:
    A. 10 gtt/min.
    B. 15 gtt/min.
    C. 25 gtt/min.
    D. 30 gtt/min.

85. When evaluating the medication regimen of an older adult, the ED nurse should expect the prescribed dose to be:
    A. increased due to decreased absorption.
    B. increased due to decreased serum albumin.
    C. decreased due to diminished hepatic blood flow.
    D. decreased due to reduced gastrointestinal motility.

86.   Which of the following dressings should be applied to a patient with burns over 40% of the body surface area (BSA) before transfer to a regional burn center?
A. Silver sulfadiazine (Silvadene) dressings
B. Mafenide (Sulfamylon) dressings
C. Sterile, saline-soaked dressings
D. Dry, sterile dressings

87.   An elderly woman taken to a small rural hospital after a motor vehicle crash has a fractured femur, multiple pelvic fractures, and numerous lacerations and abrasions. Initial assessment reveals weak, thready pulses and cool, clammy skin. The patient is awake, oriented, and asking for water. Ketorolac tromethamine (Toradol) is given for pain and transfer to a regional trauma center is arranged. Copies of the patient's medical records and x-ray films are prepared. This transfer violates EMTALA because:
A. the risks of the transfer outweigh the benefits.
B. appropriate acceptance has not been obtained.
C. the patient has not been adequately stabilized.
D. adequate documentation has not been prepared.

88.   Complications associated with pelvic inflammatory disease (PID) may include:
A. tubo-ovarian abscess.
B. pelvic peritonitis.
C. perihepatitis (Fitz-Hugh–Curtis syndrome).
D. all of the above.

89.   Discharge teaching for a female with a urinary tract infection should include all of the following EXCEPT:
A. Void frequently and completely.
B. Decrease consumption of fruit juice.
C. Void immediately after sexual intercourse.
D. Increase fluid intake.

90.   Risk factors associated with the development of pelvic inflammatory disease include all of the following EXCEPT:
A. multiple sexual partners.
B. younger age.
C. IUD use.
D. pregnancy.

Questions 91–95

A 36-year-old female presents to the ED with the complaint of nausea and vomiting for 3 days and reports that she "can't keep anything down." She states that her menses are 3 weeks late. As part of your initial assessment, you obtain a reproductive history. She tells you that she has 3 living children, including a pair of twins, and had one ectopic pregnancy at 10 weeks' gestation and one spontaneous abortion at 12 weeks' gestation.

91.   You would document her reproductive history as:
A. Gravida 6, Para 3, Abortion 1, Living 3.
B. Gravida 3, Para 3, Abortion 2, Living 3.
C. Gravida 4, Para 2, Abortion 2, Living 3.
D. Gravida 5, Para 2, Abortion 1, Living 3.

92.   Your initial documented assessment of this patient would include all of the following EXCEPT:
      A. fetal heart tones.
      B. orthostatic vital signs.
      C. temperature.
      D. respiratory rate.

93.   The nursing diagnosis with the highest priority for this patient would be which of the following?
      A. Alteration in comfort related to nausea
      B. Fluid volume deficit related to persistent vomiting
      C. Knowledge deficit related to disease process
      D. Anxiety related to disease process

94.   The Emergency Nurse Practitioner (ENP) orders a serum beta human chorionic gonadotrophin (HCG) level. What is the rationale for this blood test?
      A. To determine whether the patient is pregnant
      B. To determine approximately how many at weeks of gestation her pregnancy has advanced
      C. To obtain a baseline value in order to determine whether the patient has another ectopic pregnancy or is threatening an abortion
      D. All of the above

95.   The ENP performs a bimanual exam on the patient and notes fullness and tenderness to the left adnexal area. The serum beta-HCG test is positive. You would expect the next order to be which of the following?
      A. Radiographic abdominal series
      B. Computed tomography (CT) of the abdomen
      C. Pelvic ultrasound
      D. Abdominal ultrasound

Questions 96 and 97

A female who is at 36 weeks' gestation has been involved in a motor vehicle crash (MVC). She was the driver and was not wearing safety restraints. The air bag did not deploy. The patient is brought to your ED via EMS on a backboard with a hard cervical collar and 2 large-bore IVs in place. Oxygen is being delivered via 100% nonrebreather mask (NRM). Vital signs are BP 80/40 mm Hg; HR 138/min, respirations 34/min, and oxygen saturation 98%.

96.   Your first priority when caring for this patient and her unborn child is to ensure which of the following?
      A. That fetal heart tones are present
      B. To maintain a patent airway
      C. To increase fluid resuscitation in order to decrease heart rate and increase blood pressure
      D. To place the patient on her left side to relieve pressure on the inferior vena cava

97.   During your secondary survey, you note that the patient's abdomen is misshapen and lacks uterine tone. She states that was having contractions prior to the MVC. Immediately following the MVC, she had an episode of intense abdominal pain. She denies having had any contractions since the MVC, but continues to experience diffuse abdominal pain. You determine that the patient most likely has:
      A. abruptio placentae.
      B. placenta previa.
      C. ruptured uterus.
      D. a normal pregnant uterus.

98.   Rabies prophylaxis should be considered for patients bitten by any of the following EXCEPT:
       A. bats.
       B. raccoons.
       C. dogs.
       D. hamsters.

99.   A patient presents to the ED with a laceration of the left eyebrow. Wound preparation includes all of the following EXCEPT:
       A. wound irrigation.
       B. tetanus prophylaxis.
       C. local anesthesia.
       D. shaving the eyebrow.

100.   Treatment for carpal tunnel syndrome includes anti-inflammatory medication and:
       A. elastic compression bandage.
       B. sling.
       C. volar cockup splint.
       D. thumb spica splint.

101.   Initial treatment for a scaphoid fracture is:
       A. ulnar gutter splint.
       B. volar splint.
       C. sugar tong splint.
       D. thumb spica splint.

102.   The organism responsible for early cellulitis (less than 24 hours) after a cat bite is most likely which of the following?
       A. *Staphylococcus aureus*
       B. *Moraxella catarrhalis*
       C. *Pasteurella multocida*
       D. *Rochalimaea henselae*

103.   Correct crutch walking includes instruction to:
       A. avoid axillary pressure on the crutch.
       B. wear sandals.
       C. keep the elbows flexed to 90 degrees.
       D. keep the crutch tips 12 inches to the side and front of the foot.

104.   An orthopedic emergency that usually requires surgical intervention is:
       A. talus fracture.
       B. elbow dislocation.
       C. bimalleolar fracture.
       D. knee dislocation.

105.   A 21-year-old male is receiving care for a plantar puncture wound after stepping on a nail. The footwear that carries the greatest risk for serious infections from this type of injury is:
       A. plastic sandals.
       B. sneakers.
       C. leather work boots.
       D. leather dress shoes.

Questions 106-108

A 54-year-old male patient is transferred to the ED from the scene after his right hand and forearm were crushed in a cardboard bailing machine. There is severe tissue damage with unknown bony involvement to the right hand and forearm. The patient fainted briefly after the accident but is currently awake, alert, and oriented. Vital signs are BP 156/98 mm Hg, HR 112/min, and respirations 24/min. The patient is moaning in extreme pain. EMS personnel established an IV of Ringer's lactate and administered IV meperidine (Demerol).

106. Upon the patient's arrival at the ED, the ED nurse should *first*:
   A. establish a second large-bore IV.
   B. prepare the patient for immediate surgery.
   C. perform primary and secondary surveys.
   D. administer more pain medication.

107. The patient's right hand is splinted and appears to be swollen, discolored, and deformed. The patient is not moving the extremity. The nurse should assess the extremity for pallor and:
   A. pain, paresthesia, paralysis, and pulse.
   B. previous injury, pulse, paresthesia, and paralysis.
   C. pain, paralysis, paresthesia, and projectiles.
   D. position, pain, paralysis, and pulse.

108. The patient's right hand is splinted and appears to be swollen, discolored, and deformed. The patient complains that the pain is becoming more intense and he can no longer feel his fingers. The nurse notes that the fingers are pale and dusky and more swollen than before. The splint is loosened, but there is no change in the hand. The nurse should suspect that the patient has developed:
   A. a blood clot that is occluding the blood flow to the hand.
   B. a fatty embolism.
   C. compartment syndrome.
   D. venous thrombus.

109. A 48-year-old man is on call for operative repair of an angulated femur fracture sustained in a skiing accident. During reassessment, the nurse notes that he is pale, diaphoretic, and complaining of shortness of breath. Vital signs are HR 124/min, respirations 34/min, and oxygen saturation 84%. The ED nurse should suspect that the patient is experiencing:
   A. an anxiety attack.
   B. a myocardial infarction.
   C. a panic disorder.
   D. fat embolism syndrome.

110. An elderly female is brought to the ED complaining of right hip pain and inability to walk after a fall. Which of the following places her at risk for osteoporosis?
   A. Lacto-ovarian vegetarian diet
   B. Large skeletal frame
   C. African-American ethnicity
   D. Smoking

111. A 5-year-old child is carried into the ED by her father with a toothpick impaled in the plantar aspect of her foot. Which of the interventions below should be implemented by the ED nurse?
   A. Soak the foot in iodine/saline solution.
   B. Assess distal neurovascular status.
   C. Cleanse the area with hydrogen peroxide.
   D. Obtain an x-ray.

112.   An elderly female is brought to the ED complaining of right hip pain and inability to walk following a fall. Approaching the bed, the nurse notes that the patient's right leg is shortened and externally rotated. Formal assessment of the leg should begin with:
    A. inspection of the leg for any bruising, swelling, or breaks in the skin.
    B. palpation of the leg for areas of tenderness.
    C. evaluation of restrictions by moving the leg through range of motion.
    D. auscultation over the femoral area to search for bruits.

113.   Which of the following heart sounds would you expect to hear in a patient with pericardial tamponade?
    A. Muffled heart tones
    B. Pericardial friction rub
    C. Systolic ejection murmur
    D. S_3 gallop

114.   Which of the following cardiovascular assessment findings is associated with cardiac tamponade?
    A. Pulsus magnus
    B. Pulsus paradoxus
    C. Pulsus alternans
    D. Pulsus parvus

115.   Which of the following is the initial diagnostic study of choice for the patient with suspected traumatic aortic injury?
    A. Chest radiography
    B. Computed tomography
    C. Aortography
    D. Transesophageal echocardiography

116.   A blunt trauma patient with a descending thoracic aortic tear has been rapidly transfused with 12 units of packed red blood cells. Based on the following information, the ED nurse should anticipate infusion of which blood product?

BP 92/64 mm Hg	PT 38 sec	Hct 30%
HR 132/min	PTT 105 sec	
Respirations 19/min	PLT 88,000/mm^3	
	Hgb 11 g/dl	

    A. Fresh frozen plasma
    B. Cryoprecipitate
    C. Platelets
    D. Packed red blood cells

117.   On physical assessment of a blunt trauma patient, which of the following findings would lead the ED nurse to suspect a thoracic aortic injury?
    A. Subxiphoid tenderness to palpation
    B. Crushing back pain between the scapulae
    C. Tearing back pain between the scapulae
    D. Squeezing pain radiating down the left arm

118.   In a patient who has sustained chest trauma from a motor vehicle collision, which of the following findings on a chest radiograph would be consistent with aortic injury?
    A. Calcified aortic knob
    B. Widened mediastinum
    C. Hilar infiltrates
    D. Pneumomediastinum

119. Which of the following is the most common site of fatal aortic tearing after blunt trauma?
    A. Descending thoracic aorta
    B. Abdominal aorta
    C. Ascending thoracic aorta
    D. Aortic arch

120. Which of the following cardiovascular assessment findings is indicative of an aortic arch injury after blunt trauma?
    A. Blood pressure in the left arm is lower than in the right.
    B. Femoral pulse is weaker on the left than on the right.
    C. Pulsus paradoxus is present on inspiration.
    D. Carotid bruit is palpable on the left but absent on the right.

121. Which of the following is indicative of arterial trauma?
    A. Bounding pulse
    B. Bruit
    C. Murmur
    D. Pulsus paradoxus

122. Which of the following mechanisms of arterial trauma is generally the most difficult to repair?
    A. Stab wound
    B. Crush injury
    C. Blunt trauma
    D. Partial-thickness burn

123. Which of the following is a complication of peripheral arterial injury?
    A. Deep-vein thrombosis
    B. Compartment syndrome
    C. Fat embolism syndrome
    D. Intimal disruption

124. Which of the following arterial injuries commonly results in the greatest amount of blood loss?
    A. Complete vessel transection
    B. Intimal flap tear
    C. Arterial crush injury
    D. Arterial wall laceration

125. In a patient with significant hemorrhage from penetrating trauma to the iliac artery, which of the following interventions would be contraindicated?
    A. Tourniquet application
    B. Direct pressure to the site of injury
    C. Surgical exploration of the wound
    D. Reverse Trendelenburg positioning

126. Envenomation from a jellyfish, Portuguese man-of-war, or sea wasp can produce which the following symptoms?
    A. Swelling
    B. Hallucinations
    C. Cardiac dysrhythmias
    D. Dermatitis

127.   As the evening charge nurse in the ED, you have been notified that you will be receiving patients who were exposed to the chemical agent sarin. Signs and symptoms of cholinergic toxicity include which of the following?
A. Pulmonary congestion
B. Miosis
C. Dry mouth
D. Diarrhea

128.   The most likely nursing diagnosis for a patient with a hydrocarbon inhalation would be:
A. impaired gas exchange
B. body image disturbance.
C. impaired physical mobility.
D. decreased cardiac output.

129.   An ice skater does not follow the rules of the rink and skates on the ice during the cleaning procedure. As the large Zamboni machine crosses the ice, the skater collapses. What is the most likely cause?
A. Hydrocarbon exposure
B. Carbon monoxide toxicity
C. Cyanide inhalation
D. Nitrogen narcosis

130.   An elderly patient is brought to the ED by EMS. S/he states that chest pain started about 1 hour ago. The patient states that the problem was indigestion and admits to having ingested an entire full bottle of Rolaids antacid. You note an empty bottle whose label reads, "100 Fruit-flavored Rolaids, Extra Strength." You would be concerned about an overdose of:
A. sodium.
B. calcium.
C. phosphorus.
D. potassium.

131.   An adult patient has taken more than 40 mg/kg of acetaminophen (Tylenol). What is the only reliable indicator of the potential hepatic damage?
A. Serum acetaminophen level
B. Potassium level
C. Arterial blood gases (ABGs)
D. Urine toxicology screen

132.   One possible intervention needed for an inhaled hydrocarbon is:
A. activated charcoal.
B. syrup of ipecac.
C. to increase the administration of intravenous fluids.
D. sodium bicarbonate.

133.   You are caring for a patient who has a fractured hip. As you prepare the patient for surgery, you learn that s/he Echinacea daily to prevent colds. Based on your knowledge of Echinacea, you would be concerned about an unfavorable reaction if the patient were to receive:
A. anticoagulants.
B. immunosuppressants.
C. anesthetics.
D. anticonvulsants.

134.   A child is brought to the ED screaming. The mother states that the child has chewed several leaves of a dieffenbachia plant. You note some bloody emesis on the child's shirt, increased salivation, and a swollen tongue. Treatment for this type of ingestion should include:
   A. ice to lips and milk to flush out the mouth.
   B. warm compresses to lips and IV atropine.
   C. charcoal to the lips and physostigmine (Antilirium) IV.
   D. lubricant to lips and hydrogen peroxide mouthwash.

135.   A bus driver is brought to the ED following a crash. S/he has several minor abrasions and edema to the left ankle. Vital signs are BP 140/80 mm Hg, HR 80/min, and respirations 18/min. Because of a Department of Transportation requirement, the patient is given a breath alcohol test. S/he gives permission and the test is administered. The results are positive for alcohol (0.04). The patient denies the use of alcohol. Which of the following over-the-counter products might be the source of the positive alcohol test?
   A. Scope mouthwash
   B. Alka-Seltzer cold tablets
   C. Nyquil cold medication
   D. Arrid Extra Dry Deodorant

136.   A drug of choice for treatment of suspected organophosphate poisoning would be:
   A. naloxone (Narcan).
   B. physostigmine (Antilirium).
   C. pralidoxime (2-PAM).
   D. flumazenil (Romazicon).

137.   A patient is discharged from the ED following an evaluation for dizziness. Upon evaluation, the patient is found to have mild hypertension. The provider has prescribed verapamil (Calan). In addition to returning to the family physician for follow-up and monitoring of blood pressure, what additional teaching point should be stressed with the patient and family?
   A. Decrease fluid intake and discontinue any fiber.
   B. Continue to drink 3–4 cups of regular coffee daily.
   C. MONITOR AND RECORD HEART RATE PRIOR TO TAKING MEDICATION.
   D. May take over-the-counter drugs except aspirin and acetaminophen (Tylenol).

138.   A patient in the hospital becomes confused and disoriented. S/he pulls leaves from a lily-of-the-valley plant and eats several of them. The floor nurse brings the patient to the ED for treatment. As the triage nurse, you would choose the following triage category:
   A. Emergent
   B. Urgent
   C. Nonurgent
   D. Refer back to medical floor

139.   A patient presents to the Urgent Care Center for treatment following an injury at work. The patient has a laceration to the left hand. The company protocol mandates that a urine drug screen be performed on all worker's compensation injuries. After you assess the wound and perform vital signs, you ask the patient to sign a permit for the urine drug screen. The patient refuses to sign the permit. You should:
   A. collect a urine specimen as part of your assessment and send for drug screen.
   B. note the refusal on the permit and continue to collect the specimen.
   C. discontinue the drug screen process and notify the employer.
   D. omit the drug screen and continue treating the patient.

140.   The drug of choice used for the reversal effects of opiates is:
        A. N-acetylcysteine (Mucomyst).
        B. flumazenil (Romazicon).
        C. syrup of ipecac.
        D. naloxone (Narcan).

141.   Upon assessing a victim of a head-on motor vehicle crash, you note that the patient has moderate respiratory difficulty. He is tachycardic and anxious and has jugular vein distention as well as decreased capillary refill. There is equal lung expansion, but on auscultation you note distant lung sounds in the left lower lobe and dullness to percussion. You would suspect what injury?
        A. Tension pneumothorax
        B. Hemothorax
        C. Pneumothorax
        D. Pulmonary contusion

142.   How is the Glasgow Coma Scale (GCS) related to the Trauma Score?
        A. The Glasgow Coma Scale is part of the trauma score.
        B. The Glasgow Coma Scale provides a survival percentage equivalency.
        C. A Glasgow Coma Scale score of less than 5 invalidates the Trauma Scale.
        D. The Trauma Score is part of the Glasgow Coma Scale.

143.   An elderly patient who is a frequent visitor to your ED is being treated for injuries he sustained in a fall yesterday. His daughter has been providing all of the information and the patient appears reluctant to speak. You must screen for:
        A. lead contamination.
        B. elder abuse.
        C. alcohol poisoning.
        D. nutritional status.

144.   After an indwelling urinary catheter and a nasogastric tube have been inserted, a peritoneal catheter is inserted. If no gross blood is obtained from the catheter, what action would the ED nurse expect?
        A. Instilling a liter of normal saline, then allowing gravity drainage and checking for return of gross blood
        B. Instilling 1 L of room temperature D5W, then sending a drainage specimen for electrolytes and cell count
        C. Further action is not indicated if gross blood is not seen after the tap.
        D. Lavaging the peritoneum with warmed Ringer's lactate and sending the specimen to a laboratory to be tested for red and white blood cells.

145.   In what way does a level I trauma center differ from centers at other levels?
        A. A level II trauma center is a regional trauma resource center.
        B. A level I center has highly sophisticated trauma equipment.
        C. A level III trauma center is located in near proximity to other major trauma centers.
        D. A level II trauma center focuses on patient care and research.

146.   Within the last decade, firearms have become the weapons of choice in penetrating trauma. What do the assailants and victims of penetrating injuries have in common?
        A. Both have become progressively younger.
        B. More than 50% have handled a handgun.
        C. Both come from a household in which both parents work.
        D. None of the above.

147. Trauma has become the third leading cause of death in the United States. Which of the following is also TRUE of this national crisis?
      A. The largest age range of trauma deaths is 16–25 years.
      B. Although males are victims more frequently, there has been no correlation with race.
      C. The greater frequency of male deaths has been attributed to increased risk taking.
      D. Homicides continue to outpace suicide as a leading cause of death.

148. What type of force occurs when a body in motion comes to a sudden stop?
      A. External forces
      B. Velocity force
      C. Acceleration force
      D. Deceleration force

149. What body system in an unrestrained passenger is most likely to be injured regardless of the direction from which a vehicle was struck?
      A. Head and neck
      B. Abdomen
      C. Extremities
      D. Face

150. During your nursing assessment of the patient's airway, what would you address before proceeding to the next step?
      A. Any uncontrolled abdominal bleeding
      B. An angulated fractured femur
      C. Distended external jugular veins
      D. Loose teeth or foreign objects in the mouth.

1. A front-seat passenger involved in a motor vehicle crash (MVC) arrives via a Basic Life Support (BLS) ambulance complaining of right-sided chest pain. He is pale, tachypneic, and dyspneic. Decreased breath sounds are auscultated on the right side and a hemothorax is suspected. A patent airway has been assured; c-spine precautions are in effect; and a chest tube has been inserted. Your next priority intervention would be to:
   A. insert a nasogastric tube.
   B. determine the patient's Glasgow Coma Scale (GCS) score.
   C. INSERT 2 LARGE-BORE IV LINES FOR CRYSTALLOID INFUSION.
   D. prepare autotransfuser.

Rationale:

   C. Insertion of 2 large-bore IVs is necessary to support the circulation of this patient, who is bleeding into the pulmonary cavity and developing a hemothorax.
   A. Insertion of a nasogastric tube in a trauma patient can be very important; however, breathing and circulation must be supported first.
   B. Performing a GCS is a necessary step in the assessment of the trauma patient, but airway, breathing, and circulation should be assessed and maintained first.
   D. Preparation of an autotransfuser device is an appropriate intervention for a patient with a hemothorax; however, IV access with 2 large-bore catheters and infusion of crystalloid solution must be in place first in order to support the patient's circulation.

Content Category: Respiratory

References: ENA, Core Curriculum, 2000; pp. 7–14, 385; ENA, Trauma Nursing, 2000; pp. 134–137.

2. You are caring for an unrestrained driver of a motor vehicle crash (MVC). He is severely dyspneic and cyanotic, has labored respirations, absent breath sounds on the right, unilateral chest rise and fall, and jugular venous distention You suspect which of the following?
   A. Aspiration
   B. Flail chest
   C. TENSION PNEUMOTHORAX
   D. Cardiac tamponade

Rationale:

   C. Dyspnea, labored respirations, decreased or absent breath sounds on affected side, unilateral chest rise and fall, cyanosis, and jugular venous distention are the most common signs and symptoms of a tension pneumothorax.
   A. Patients who have aspirated can demonstrate fever, cough, hypoxia, chest pain, and tachypnea; breath sounds are present but diminished. There is no evidence that this patient has aspirated.

B. A patient with a flail chest segment exhibit dyspnea, labored respirations, paradoxical chest wall movement, and chest pain. Patients sustaining a flail chest would not have jugular venous distention.

D. The patient with a cardiac tamponade can demonstrate Beck's triad: hypotension, muffled heart tones, and jugular venous distention, anxiety, dyspnea, and duskiness. Patients sustaining a cardiac tamponade would not have absent breath sounds and there would not be unilateral chest rise and fall.

Content Category: Respiratory

References: Kidd et al., 2000; pp. 668–669, 690; Newberry, 1998; p. 437.

3. What potential problem would a patient with a tracheobronchial injury be at risk for immediately after the insertion of a chest tube?
   A. Pneumonia
   B. Local cellulitis
   C. Bronchospasm
   D. CONTINUOUS AIR LEAK

Rationale:

D. A continuous air leak can occur if the site of injury in the large airway is not repaired surgically.

A. Pneumonia is an acute infection caused by bacteria, a virus, or a fungus and may occur later.

B. Local cellulitis can occur at the tube insertion site, but not immediately.

C. Bronchospasm is a spasmodic contraction of the smooth muscles found in conditions such as asthma. There would be no relationship with a chest tube complication.

Content Category: Respiratory

References: Newberry, 1998; pp. 297–298; Blansfield et al., 1999; pp. 265–266.

4. A victim of a stab wound to the epigastric area presents to the ED. Upon evaluation he suddenly develops shortness of breath, chest pain, and decreased breath sounds. What is the priority nursing diagnosis for this patient?
   A. Ineffective airway clearance
   B. INEFFECTIVE BREATHING PATTERN
   C. Decreased cardiac output
   D. Fluid volume deficit

Rationale:

B. This patient's symptoms are consistent with a diaphragmatic tear, in which the integrity of the major respiratory muscle or diaphragm is lost and the abdominal contents invade the respiratory compartment. Results include respiratory compromise and impairment of lung capacity. Therefore, the patient is at risk for ineffective breathing pattern.

A. Maintenance of the patient's airway is important, but there is no evidence that his airway is compromised. This patient's symptoms relate to increased work of breathing.

C. There is a potential that this patient will have decreased cardiac output, as venous return can be diminished; however, the patient's breathing must be stabilized first.

D. There is a potential for fluid volume deficit if major bleeding occurs. This patient's breathing must first be stabilized.

Content Category: Respiratory

References: ENA, Trauma Nursing, 2000; pp.122–125; Newberry, 1998; pp. 295–302; Blansfield et al., 1999; pp. 267–268.

5. The first-line pharmacologic treatment used to improve air exchange for the chronic obstructive pulmonary disease (COPD) patient who is experiencing an acute exacerbation is which of the following?
    A. Intravenous theophylline (Aminophyllin)
    B. NEBULIZED IPRATROPIUM (ALBUTEROL)
    C. Subcutaneous epinephrine (Adrenalin)
    D. Oral zileuton (Zyflo)

Rationale:

B. Nebulized albuterol and ipratropium are used to treat bronchospasm associated with COPD. Ipratropium augments the beta agonist effect of albuterol.
A. Theophylline use is controversial in the treatment of COPD and is not considered first-line treatment.
C. Subcutaneous epinephrine may aggravate the cardiac status of the COPD patient and lead to cardiac arrhythmias.
D. Zileuton is a leukotriene modifier used in the treatment of asthma.

Content Category: Respiratory

References: Newberry, 1998; pp. 431–451; Kitt et al., 1995; pp. 188–200; ENA, Core Curriculum, 2000; pp. 559–566.

6. A motorcyclist presents to the ED after a clothesline accident in which he sustained multiple face and neck fractures. He is unable to speak and has hemoptysis and inspiratory stridor. A high-priority nursing diagnosis for this patient is:
    A. alteration in skin integrity.
    B. altered body image.
    C. INEFFECTIVE AIRWAY CLEARANCE.
    D. altered mental status.

Rationale:

C. This patient is at high risk for ineffective airway clearance because he presents with symptoms of airway obstruction that need immediate attention.
A. Alteration in skin integrity will need to be addressed, as wound care needs to be done, but his airway concerns are more critical.
B. Altered body image will need to be addressed later, since he has multiple facial and neck fractures and will be a candidate for possible plastics/cosmetic repair; however, the priority is his airway.
D. There is no evidence that this patient is at risk for altered mental status. Maintenance of a patent airway is the first priority.

Content Category: Respiratory

References: ENA, Trauma Nursing, 2000; pp. 41–60, 92–108; ENA, Core Curriculum, 2000; pp. 165, 218.

7. In caring for the patient with Ludwig's angina, the nurse should first assess for:
    A. pain, leukocytosis, and hypotension.
    B. chest pain, diaphoresis, and nausea.
    C. AIRWAY OBSTRUCTION, SHORTNESS OF BREATH, AND FEVER.
    D. dysrhythmias, chest pain, and numbness down the arm.

Rationale:

    C. Assess for airway obstruction, shortness of breath, and fever. Ludwig's angina is a disease caused by extension of dental infections, resulting in swelling. The tongue is pushed upward, causing partial airway obstruction.

    A. Pain, leukocytosis, and hypotension are nonspecific signs of severe infection; however, the priority is the patient's airway and breathing status.

    B. Chest pain, diaphoresis, and nausea are clinical signs of coronary artery disease (angina or myocardial infarction). The priority is the patient's airway and breathing status.

    D. Dysrhythmias, chest pain, and numbness down the arm are more likely symptoms of coronary artery disease.

Content Category: Respiratory

References: Newberry, 1998; pp. 679–680; Aghababian, 1998; p. 341.

8. One priority to consider while caring for a patient with respiratory distress syndrome is to monitor which of the following?
    A. Pneumonia
    B. Urine output
    C. Infection
    D. FLUID INTAKE

Rationale:

    D. Fluid restriction is the key to help minimize noncardiogenic pulmonary edema and to prevent fluid overload to the already damaged alveolar–capillary membrane.

    A. Pneumonia would be a late complication of respiratory distress syndrome.

    B. Urine output measurement is important to measure the success of diuretics, but fluid restriction is the priority.

    C. Infection is always a risk but does not play any role in treating respiratory distress syndrome.

Content Category: Respiratory

References: Newberry, 1998; pp. 452–455, 522; O'Hanlon-Nichols, 1995; p. 42.

9. When teaching an asthma patient about his/her disease, it is important for the emergency nurse to explain which of the following?
    A. ASTHMA IS PRIMARILY CAUSED BY AIRWAY INFLAMMATION AND HYPER-RESPONSIVENESS TO STIMULI.
    B. Physiologic changes seen in asthma exacerbation are often irreversible.
    C. Asthma exacerbations are most frequently a result of a respiratory infection.
    D. Most asthma attacks occur suddenly and without warning in the early morning.

Rationale:

    A. The patient needs to understand that inflammation and response to stimuli are key factors in the treatment and prevention of asthma.

    B. Asthma changes are episodic and reversible with treatment and medication.

    C. While infection can trigger an asthma exacerbation, most patients have specific triggers that can be identified and avoided.

    D. Asthma attacks do not occur without warning and can be predicted through the identification of triggers and by using peak flow rate measurements.

Content Category: Respiratory

References: Newberry, 1998; pp. 440–451; Kitt et al., 1995; pp. 194–197; ENA, Core Curriculum, 2000; pp. 559–561.

10.   When teaching an asthma patient about medication usage, it is important for the emergency nurse to discuss which of the following?
   A. Inhaled steroids are addictive and their use should be limited to acute exacerbations.
   B. Patients often develop a tolerance to daily asthma medications and require increased doses.
   C. Inhaled bronchodilators should not be used with inhaled corticosteroids.
   D. ORAL CORTICOSTEROIDS ARE OFTEN USED FOR SHORT-TERM TREATMENT OF EXACERBATIONS.

Rationale:

   D. Oral corticosteroids are frequently given for acute exacerbation to gain control of the inflammatory process.
   A. Inhaled steroids are not the same as anabolic steroids and are not addictive.
   B. Asthma patients are frequently maintained on the same dosages for many years and do not experience tolerance to medication with continued use.
   C. Inhaled bronchodilators and inhaled corticosteroids are common treatments for asthma and can safely be administered together.

Content Category: Respiratory

References: Newberry, 1998; pp. 440–451; Kitt et al., 1995; pp. 194–197; ENA, Core Curriculum, 2000; pp. 559–561.

11.   A 6-year-old child is being treated for asthma in the ED. In teaching the patient's caregiver about medication administration, the nurse should include which of the following statements?
   A. Liquid asthma medications have a quicker onset of effects than inhaled medications.
   B. Children under 12 years old do not have sufficient coordination to use metered-dose inhalers.
   C. A SPACER ATTACHED TO A METERED-DOSE INHALER CAN INCREASE MEDICATION EFFECTIVENESS.
   D. Oral steroids should not be given to children under the age of 5 years.

Rationale:

   C. A spacer can help a patient to get a full inhaled dose of the medication instead of hitting the mouth with the spray and therefore can increase the effectiveness of the medication.
   A. Inhaled asthma medications have a 5- to 10-minute onset of action. Liquid medications can take up to 1 to 3 hours to take effect.
   B. Children over 5 years of age can generally learn to use inhalers.
   D. Oral steroids can be given to children of any age.

Content Category: Respiratory

References: Newberry, 1998; pp. 440–451; Kitt et al., 1995; pp. 194–197; ENA, Core Curriculum, 2000; pp. 559–561.

12.   A patient experiencing an acute asthma exacerbation states that his routine medications include use of a cromolyn (Intal) inhaler. This medication is given to:
   A. relieve acute bronchospasm on an as-needed basis.
   B. BLOCK THE RELEASE OF CHEMICAL MEDIATORS FROM MAST CELLS.
   C. inhibit cough receptors in the bronchial lining.
   D. block the uptake of calcium in the bronchial smooth muscle.

Rationale:

   B. Cromolyn inhibits mast cell degranulation and blocks the late-phase reaction of asthma by blocking release of chemical mediators. It is used as a prophylactic treatment for patients who are prone to frequent exacerbations.

A. Cromolyn is not given on an as-needed basis. The powdered form can cause, not alleviate, bronchospasm.
C. Ipratropium (Atrovent) blocks cough receptors; cromolyn has no such effect.
D. Cromolyn does not affect calcium uptake in muscle.

Content Category: Respiratory

References: Newberry, 1998; pp. 440–451; Kitt et al., 1995; pp. 194–197; ENA, Core Curriculum, 2000; pp. 559–561.

13. The nurse is obtaining a history from a 23-year-old patient with shortness of breath, bilateral wheezing on expiration in all fields, and a pulse oximetry reading of 92% on room air. Which of the following is the most significant history finding?
    A. Three to four visits to the ED in the past year for similar episodes
    B. PREVIOUS EPISODE REQUIRING ADMISSION TO ICU AND INTUBATION 2 YEARS AGO
    C. Increased episodes occurring in the spring months of the year
    D. Limitation of normal daily activities for the past 2 days

Rationale:

B. An episode that resulted in intubation indicates that the patient's exacerbations can progress to a severe stage and should warrant careful monitoring and aggressive treatment.
A. Three to four visits to the ED over a year's time may be a sign that the disease process is not well controlled, but it is not the most significant finding at this time.
C. Many asthma patients suffer increased numbers of attacks during the pollen-prone spring months of the year.
D. Gradual limitation of activities over a 2-day period would be an expected finding in a patient experiencing an asthma attack.

Content Category: Respiratory

References: Newberry, 1998; pp. 440–451; Kitt et al., 1995; pp. 194–197; ENA, Core Curriculum, 2000; pp. 559–561.

14. Measurement of peak expiratory flow rate is a useful tool in the management of asthma because:
    A. rising values can indicate an impending exacerbation of asthma.
    B. it helps clear airway passages of mucus plugs.
    C. measurement does not rely on patient effort.
    D. IT CAN DOCUMENT REVERSIBILITY OF AIRWAY NARROWING.

Rationale:

D. When used before and after a bronchodilator treatment, an increase in peak flow rate can demonstrate that the airway obstruction has been reduced or reversed and the patient can move more air in the respiratory effort.
A. Decreasing peak flow rates indicate impending asthma attacks. Inflammation causes airways to narrow.
B. While the forced air movement of peak flow measurement could potentially move some loose secretions, significant airway clearing is not found and is not a rationale for its use.
C. Accurate measurement requires a cooperative patient who will perform the measurement correctly.

Content Category: Respiratory

References: Newberry, 1998; pp. 440–451; Kitt et al., 1995; pp. 194–197; ENA, Core Curriculum, 2000; pp. 559–561.

15. The Joint Commission on Accreditation of Healthcare Organizations (JCAHO) defines a sentinel event as:
    A. any incident that occurs within the hospital environment at least once each year.
    B. any incident that results in lost work time for a hospital employee.
    C. AN UNEXPECTED OCCURRENCE INVOLVING DEATH OR SERIOUS PHYSICAL OR PSYCHOLOGICAL INJURY OR RISK.
    D. a patient outcome that exceeds expected hospital days as outlined by the clinical pathway.

Rationale:

    C. By JCAHO definition, a sentinel event is an unexpected occurrence involving death or serious physical or psychological injury or risk. The definition of a sentinel event describes occurrences that require attention.
    A. Sentinel events are not defined by frequency.
    B. Sentinel events may include hospital employees and patients.
    D. A sentinel event may extend hospital days, but the definition is unrelated to a clinical pathway.

Content Category: Professional Issues

Reference: JCAHO, 2000.

16. A manager in an urban ED considers benchmarking to establish staffing levels. If this were done, the manager would incorporate which of the following?
    A. Database from EDs of varying volume and size
    B. Database capturing trends in emergency as well as ambulatory care
    C. DATABASE BEING CURRENT AND REFLECTIVE OF SIMILAR VOLUME AND PRACTICE
    D. Database from rural hospital EDs across the U.S.

Rationale:

    C. In order to benchmark staffing data adequately, the database must be current and must capture trends of similar volume and practice.
    A. An adequate analysis could not be accomplished with data from variously sized EDs.
    B. A comparison must occur with similar EDs exclusive of other hospital departments.
    D. The comparison should be from similar facilities, not urban to rural.

Content Category: Professional Issues

Reference: ENA 1999; Benchmark and Staffing Database Guide; pp. 1–3.

17. An emergency nurse receives special recognition as a role model for customer service. Which of the following actions demonstrates this nurse's dedication to customer service?
    A. Informs the patient that the social worker will explain the visitation policies in the ED.
    B. Describes the events of the day leading to the patient's visit to the ED.
    C. INFORMS THE FAMILY IN THE WAITING ROOM THAT THE PATIENT IS IN THE RADIOLOGY DEPARTMENT.
    D. Complains that a coworker has left the otoscope tip holder empty during a patient examination.

Rationale:

    C. Customer service skills in the ED should include the family as well as the patient. Keeping a family informed in the waiting room would be an excellent example of demonstrating positive customer service skills.
    A. This action would only delay a patient's being given necessary information and defer simple information delivery to another individual.

    B. Discussing the daily happenings of the ED with a patient would not be a demonstration of positive customer service.

    D. A discussion about a coworker would not be appropriate during a patient examination.

Content Category: Professional Issues

Reference: Salluzzo, 1997.

18. Which of the following would be considered appropriate for constructive criticism of an employee?
    A. Always have another employee present during any conversations involving criticism.
    B. Do not offer any positive feedback, as it may overshadow the reason for the criticism.
    C. State the facts to the employee and do not focus on the employee's opinion.
    D. EXPLAIN THE RATIONALE FOR THE ERROR ACTION AS PART OF THE CRITICISM.

Rationale:

    D. An explanation as to why the action was an error should always occur. Employees will remember a correction if they understand the rationale behind it.
    A. An employee should never be criticized or reprimanded in the presence of another employee.
    B. Positive feedback should be shared with the employee even while constructive criticism is being offered. Both good and bad aspects of the situation should be discussed.
    C. The manager should always ask for the employee's version of the story.

Content Category: Professional Issues

Reference: Newberry, 1998.

19. Which of the following is the rationale for an ED nurse to take the Advanced Cardiac Life Support Provider course?
    A. Taking the course will help the ED nurse to memorize the algorithms and protocols.
    B. Taking the course will helps the ED nurse to memorize the drug dosages.
    C. The hospital requires that all nurses take the course.
    D. TAKING THE COURSE WILL HELP THE ED NURSE LEARN A SYSTEMATIC APPROACH TO CARDIOPULMONARY EMERGENCIES.

Rationale:

    D. Advanced Cardiac Life Support presents a way of thinking—a systematic approach to dealing with people who are experiencing a cardiopulmonary emergency or sudden death.
    A. Memorization of algorithms should be avoided, since each cardiac emergency may have different methods of presentation and require individualized treatment options. The algorithms are presented as a suggested treatment plan.
    B. Although a familiarity with drug dosages is essential, reference material is presented in the Advanced Cardiac Life Support Provider course for participants to use as needed.
    C. Although Advanced Cardiac Life Support may be a requirement for most nurses in many facilities, some facilities do not require all nurses to participate in the course.

Content Category: Professional Issues

Reference: American Heart Association, 2000; I-1– I-384.

20.   The emergency nurse manager wishes to evaluate staffing as part of a continuous improvement plan. The manager would benchmark information such as which of the following?
A. A sense by the staff that patients are staying longer while awaiting in house beds
B. ACTUAL STAFFING, WAIT TIMES, AND LENGTH OF STAY BY PATIENT TRIAGE CLASSIFICATION
C. Chief Financial Officer statement that ED is overstaffed by full-time equivalents for unit of service
D. Patient complaint letter stating ED is understaffed

Rationale:

B. Using objective data such as actual staffing ratios, wait times, and length of stay by triage is the appropriate method to benchmark against other EDs.
A. To be used as benchmarking information, a sense of patient length of stay needs to be validated by objective data.
C. Overstaffing information is an internal issue. To support the need for staffing ratios better, the ED manager needs benchmark data to demonstrate appropriate staffing ratios in the ED.
D. Patient complaints need to be collated in the aggregate to demonstrate trends of patient perceptions of care rather than to react to a single letter.

Content Category: Professional Issues

Reference: Salluzzo et al., 1997.

21.   A 21-year-old male is brought to the ED with a history of having skated head first into the boards while playing hockey. He was immediately flaccid but has been able to maintain his own respirations. He never lost consciousness. One of the first medications you would anticipate administering is which of the following?
A. Mannitol (Osmitrol)
B. DEXAMETHASONE (DECADRON)
C. Furosemide (Lasix)
D. Antibiotics

Rationale:

B. Dexamethasone (Decadron) is a corticosteroid. The purpose for administration is to attempt to prevent edema of the spinal cord, which may occur after a spinal cord injury. As the cord becomes edematous, the space between the spinal cord and the spinal canal is decreased. If the edema is severe, the spinal cord may receive additional damage. Methylprednisolone (Depo-Medrol) may also be administered.
A. Mannitol (Osmitrol) would be used in a severe head injury to assist with decreasing intracranial pressure.
C. Furosemide (Lasix) is a diuretic and would not have an effect on reducing edema to the spinal cord.
D. Antibiotics would not have an effect on reducing edema to the spinal cord.

Content Category: Neurological

Reference: Sheehy & Lenehan, 1999.

22.   A patient presents to triage with a sudden onset of what she calls "the worse headache in my life." She describes the onset as being "like a thunderclap." What triage decision would you make for this patient?
A. HAVE SOMEONE ESCORT THE PATIENT TO AN ACUTE BED IMMEDIATELY.
B. Send her to the waiting room to wait for an available bed.

C. Give her directions to the neurology clinic.

D. Send her to the Fast Track/Walk-In Clinic, as the ED is currently very busy.

Rationale:

A. Although sudden onset of "the worse headache in my life" may be a symptom of many diagnoses, the first thing that should come to mind is the possibility of a subarachnoid hemorrhage, which is often characterized by this specific description. A patient with a subarachnoid hemorrhage should be immediately taken to an acute bed for evaluation.

B. A patient with this presenting complaint should not be sent to the waiting room.

C. The presenting symptoms would classify this patient as emergent and would require immediate attention.

D. This patient should be seen in the ED in rapid fashion.

Content Category: Neurological

Reference: Sheehy & Lenehan, 1999.

23. The most common cause of nontraumatic subarachnoid hemorrhage is which of the following?

A. Old age

B. Drug abuse

C. RUPTURED ANEURYSM

D. Preeclampsia

Rationale:

C. Aneurysms are present in 0.5% to 1% of the population. Of these, 1–2% rupture per year. A large majority of aneurysms are located at the circle of Willis, near bifurcations of vessels.

A. Although aging may demonstrate blood vessel disease, the most common cause of subarachnoid hemorrhage is an aneurysm.

B. Various drugs may have serious effects on blood vessels, but the most common cause for intracerebral bleeds is aneurysm.

D. Preeclampsia is generally characterized by edema and hypertension, not by subarachnoid bleeding.

Content Category: Neurological

Reference: Sheehy & Lenehan, 1999.

24. Nimodipine (Nimotop) is given to a patient with a subarachnoid hemorrhage to:

A. PREVENT VASOSPASM.

B. control bleeding.

C. control blood pressure.

D. assist with airway management.

Rationale:

A. Frequently, when a subarachnoid hemorrhage occurs, vasospasm occurs as well. Vasospasm may cause a lack of blood flow to noninjured areas of the brain, causing hypoxia, which will result in cerebral edema. Nimodipine (Nimotop) is used to control vasospasm.

B. Nimodipine (Nimotop) is used to control vasospasm, not control bleeding.

C. Nimodipine (Nimotop) is not used to control blood pressure.

D. Nimodipine (Nimotop) is not used in assisting with airway control.

Content Category: Neurological

Reference: Sheehy & Lenehan, 1999.

25.   A trauma patient is evaluated and treated in the ED. The initial diagnosis is diffuse axonal injury: many nonfocal deficits, in contrast to mass lesions, hemorrhage, or focal contusions). The main goal of care for this patient is to do which of the following?

A.   Prevent contractures and foot drop

B.   Prevent hemorrhage by administering specific antihemorrhagic medications

C.   CONTROL INTRACRANIAL HYPERTENSION AND PREVENT SECONDARY BRAIN INJURY

D.   Reduce body core temperature to preserve brain tissue

Rationale:

C.   Diffuse axonal injury usually causes prolonged coma or death. The cause is changes that occur in brain tissue after severe head trauma that lead to separation because of shearing or tearing of axons. The deficits are usually found to be diffuse. The goal of therapeutic interventions is to reduce hypoxia (oxygen supplementation, slight elevation of the head of the bed, pharmacologic intervention) that will prevent secondary brain injury.

A.   The primary goal would be to prevent hypoxia, although positioning issues should be addressed as well.

B.   If hemorrhaging is present, efforts should be made to control bleeding.

D.   The patient's temperature should be monitored and measures taken to maintain normal body temperature.

Content Category: Neurological

Reference: Newberry, 1998.

26.   A 19-year-old soldier is brought to your ED after experiencing a syncopal episode during inspection. Upon further investigation, you learn that the air temperature at the training facility was 104° F (40.0° C) and that the soldier had been standing at attention for several minutes immediately after participating in a 3-mile run. The EMTs tell you that the patient's systolic blood pressure, which was 86 mm Hg when they first arrived, quickly rose to 110 mm Hg when they elevated his legs. The most likely cause of this syncopal episode is which of the following?

A.   Neurogenic disease

B.   Fatigue

C.   Congenital disposition

D.   AUTONOMIC DYSFUNCTION

Rationale:

D.   Autonomic dysfunction, also known as vasovagal syncope, may occur as a response to stress, excitement, or anxiety that usually occurs in conjunction with prolonged periods of standing upright, fatigue, hunger, poor physical condition, a hot environment, or anemia. The treatment of choice is to place the patient in a supine position and elevate the legs to increase venous return to the heart.

A.   Although neurogenic disease may present with syncopal episodes, the above symptoms more closely relate to an autonomic dysfunction.

B.   Fatigue may indeed cause syncope, but the change in blood pressure as noted would not.

C.   The cause of the described symptoms would be autonomic dysfunction.

Content Category: Neurological

Reference: Newberry, 1998.

27. Priapism (sustained erection) may be indicative of which of the following?
    A. Prostate cancer
    B. HIGH SPINAL CORD LESION
    C. Migraine headache
    D. Sexual dysfunction

Rationale:

   B. Priapism (sustained erection) is common among male patients with high spinal cord lesions. The cause may be the severe vasodilation that occurs in spinal shock.
   A. Priapism is not present with prostate cancer.
   C. Priapism is not a characteristic symptom of a migraine headache.
   D. Although penile erection dysfunction may be a characteristic of sexual dysfunction, priapism would not be noted.
   Content Classification: Neurological

Reference: Rosen et al., 1998.

28. You are discharging a patient who sustained a concussion following a motor vehicle crash. It is important to tell the patient which of the following?
    A. "YOU MAY HAVE DIFFICULTY CONCENTRATING AT WORK."
    B. "You do not need to have anyone stay with you."
    C. "Call your private physician if you develop vomiting."
    D. "It is OK to drink coffee today."

Rationale:

   A. Headaches, dizziness, memory problems, and difficulty concentrating are symptoms of postconcussive syndrome. This is a nonemergent syndrome that may last from days to weeks following a concussion. Treatment consists of education and supportive counseling.
   B. Changes in level of consciousness, pupil changes, vomiting, and seizures are all signs of increasing intracranial pressure and require immediate intervention; the patient should be able to note these changes and does not require another individual to monitor the condition.
   C. Vomiting may indicate increasing intracranial pressure and an evolving lesion. Patients should be instructed to return to a medical facility that is capable of diagnosing and treating traumatic brain injury.
   D. Caffeine may act as a stimulant and mask possible signs of a worsening condition. Because of this potential, caffeine should be avoided.

Content Category: Neurological

References: ENA, Core Curriculum, 2000; Hickey, 1997; pp. 385–417.

29. You are preparing to administer mannitol (Osmitrol) 130 g to a 150-lb (68.2-kg) patient with a closed head injury. Which of the following nursing interventions should be considered?
    A. Notify the physician concerning a possible incorrect dose.
    B. AN INLINE IV FILTER SHOULD BE USED.
    C. The medication should be administered over 8 hours.
    D. An intracranial pressure monitor should be in place.

Rationale:

   B. Because of the possibility that there are crystals in the fluid, mannitol should be administered using an inline IV filter.
   A. The dose of mannitol for decreasing intracranial pressure is 1.5 to 2.0 g/kg of a 15–25% solution over 0.5 1 hour. The dose listed, 130 g, would be correct for this patient.

C. The medication infusion should be given over 0.5 to 1 hour, not 8 hours.

D. Although an intracranial pressure monitor (ICP) would be ideal for monitoring the patient's condition, it is not needed for the administration of mannitol.

Content Category: Neurological

Reference: Skidmore-Roth, 2001; pp. 586–587.

30.   The goal of interventions for an adult patient with seizures is to:
   A. sedate the patient so rest can occur.
   B. reduce fever.
   C. PREVENT PROLONGED/RECURRENT SEIZURES.
   D. prevent injuries to the limbs.

Rationale:

C. Frequent, recurrent, or prolonged seizures may result in cerebral hypoxia, which leads to permanent central nervous system (CNS) damage because the CNS is highly dependent on oxygen to function adequately.

A. Sedation may be indicated to assist in terminating the seizure activity.

B. Fever control may be indicated, but is not a goal of a nursing intervention.

D. The patient should be protected from potential injury, but the primary goal of any intervention should be aimed toward stopping the seizure activity and preventing further seizures.

Content Category: Neurological

Reference: Sheehy & Lenehan, 1999.

31.   Pediatric victims of a MVC (motor vehicle crash) with an improper application of the lap belt safety restraint are at a high risk for injury to the:
   A. kidney.
   B. spleen.
   C. BOWEL.
   D. liver.

Rationale:

C. Children are at high risk for gastrointestinal injuries because of their protuberant abdomens, proclivity to swallow a large amount of air, and thin abdominal muscle wall. Inappropriate placed lap belt safety restraints commonly result in bowel trauma.

A. Renal trauma in children is usually caused by falls, sports, and motor vehicle crashes. Trauma to the kidneys from inappropriately placed seat belts is very rare because of the position of the kidneys in the abdomen.

B. The majority of splenic injuries are caused by high-speed motor vehicle crashes. They can also be caused by sports, particularly the handlebars of bicycles, and child abuse. Because of the position of the spleen in the abdomen, a splenic injury from a seat belt is not common.

D. The liver is commonly injured by blunt trauma, usually a rapid acceleration–deceleration mechanism. The liver may also be injured by penetrating trauma.

Content Category: Gastrointestinal

References: Soud & Rogers, 1998; pp. 530–531; ENA, Trauma Nursing, 2000; p. 250.

32. With which of the following presentations would a patient with a small-bowel obstruction present?
   A. RAPID ONSET OF COLICKY, CRAMPLIKE, INTERMITTENT PAIN IN THE ABDOMEN
   B. Gradual onset of low-grade crampy pain in the abdomen, with constipation
   C. Rapid onset of vomiting, fever, and crampy abdominal pain followed by diarrhea
   D. Sudden acute abdominal pain with bloody stools mixed with mucus ("currant jelly" stools)

Rationale:

   A. Rapid onset of colicky, cramplike, intermittent pain in the abdomen most likely represents the signs and symptoms of small-bowel obstruction.
   B. A gradual onset of low-grade crampy pain is commonly indicative of large-bowel obstruction, with absolute constipation as a chief complaint.
   C. Gastroenteritis is more likely to present with fever, vomiting, and diarrhea.
   D. Intussusception (the telescoping of one loop of bowel into the next, more distal segment) is marked by "currant jelly" stools.

Content Category: Gastrointestinal

References: Newberry, 1998; pp. 537–555; Soud & Rogers, 1998; pp. 333–362.

33. Which of the following statements is helpful in excluding cardiac origin as the differentiating diagnosis of a patient presenting with chest discomfort?
   A. "The pain is in my midabdominal area and chest, feeling like a pressure."
   B. "Nitroglycerine relieved the chest discomfort."
   C. "THE ANTACID I TOOK HELPED TO RELIEVE THE DISCOMFORT SOMEWHAT."
   D. "I have pain that is in my upper midback area."

Rationale:

   C. The problem of a patient who describes relief of chest discomfort with antacids can be considered to be gastrointestinal in origin. Although atypical presentations of cardiac origin exist, cardiac origin can be more likely excluded in the patient presenting with relief of discomfort from antacids.
   A. Pain located in the midabdominal area and chest may be of gastrointestinal or cardiac origin.
   B. Nitroglycerine usually relieves the chest discomfort associated with angina; therefore, it is not helpful in excluding pain of cardiac origin.
   D. Upper midback pain is usually associated with disease of the spine or of the mediastinum, especially the aorta, esophagus, or heart. Therefore, this statement cannot exclude cardiac origin as well as can the symptoms of the patient who presents with relief of discomfort by antacids.

Content Category: Gastrointestinal

References: Newberry, 1998; pp. 474–478; Kidd et al., 2000; pp. 215–218.

34. Many gastrointestinal diseases incorporate similar patient education strategies. One teaching point that is unique to hiatal hernia is which of the following?
   A. "Stop smoking."
   B. "Eat small, frequent, bland meals."
   C. "Avoid highly seasoned foods and alcoholic beverages."
   D. "WEAR LOOSE, NONCONSTRICTING CLOTHING."

Rationale:

   D. All the listed patient education strategies apply to hiatal hernia. The one point that is unique to hiatal hernia is to wear loose, nonconstrictive clothing.
   A. To stop smoking is a teaching point used not only for hiatal hernia but also for gastroesophageal reflux disorder, Crohn's disease, ulcerative colitis, and esophagitis.

B. Advice to eat small, frequent, bland meals is an education strategy used for esophageal reflux and ulcers as well as for hiatal hernia.

C. To avoid highly seasoned foods and alcoholic beverages is a teaching point used for gastroesophageal reflux, gastritis, and ulcers as well as for hiatal hernia.

Content Category: Gastrointestinal

References: ENA, Core Curriculum, 2000; pp 38–39; Black & Matassarin-Jacobs, 1997; pp. 1734, 1738–1741.

35. A patient presents to the ED with a chief complaint of sudden onset of colicky abdominal pain and nausea after eating a meal of fried chicken and French fries. Vital signs are BP 140/80 mm Hg, HR 116/min, respirations 18/min, and temperature 100.4°F (38.0°C). The priority intervention is which of the following?
A. ADMINISTRATION OF PAIN CONTROL
B. Immediate preparation for the operating room
C. Nasogastric intubation
D. Administration of a stool softener

Rationale:

A. Pain control is the priority for this patient with suspected cholecystitis. Treatment is conservative and consists of IV hydration, pain control, and antibiotic and antiemetic therapy.

B. Medical management is tried for 24 to 48 hours before surgery. The patient would have been taken to the operating room earlier if it had been anticipated that medical management would not be successful. There is no evidence of this.

C. Nasogastric intubation would be necessary for a patient who is vomiting or who has gastric distention or ileus. There is no evidence of these.

D. A stool softener would be administered to patients suffering from diverticulitis. There is no evidence that this patient has diverticulitis.

Content Category: Gastrointestinal

References: Kidd et al., 2000; p. 107; Newberry, 1998; pp. 549–550; ENA, Core Curriculum, 2000; pp. 44–45.

36. In the presentation of acute pancreatitis, the MOST COMMON causes are which of the following?
A. Gastroesophageal reflux disorder and injury
B. Hyperlipidemia and aging
C. Infection and carcinoma
D. ALCOHOLISM AND GALLSTONES

Rationale:

D. Alcoholism and gallstones are noted as the two most common causes of acute pancreatitis and account for 90% of these cases.

A. Gastroesophageal reflux disorder does not cause pancreatitis. Although pancreatic injury is a cause of pancreatitis, this injury is seen in only 2% of all cases of abdominal trauma.

B. Hyperlipidemia is another less-common cause of pancreatitis. Although the disease process is rare in children, the obstruction of the duct and the abuse of alcohol are still considered to be the most common causes of pancreatitis.

C. Infection and cancer are less-common causes of acute pancreatitis.

Content Category: Gastrointestinal

References: Porth, 1998; pp 769–771; Kidd et al., 2000; pp. 93–116; Wyatt et al., 1999; pp. 516–533.

37. A 23-year-old male patient presents to the ED complaining of right testicular pain, nausea, and vomiting for 2 hours. He has a mild fever on exam and generalized tenderness in the abdomen. The nurse must consider which of the following diagnoses?
    A. APPENDICITIS
    B. Small-bowel obstruction
    C. Acute cholecystitis
    D. Urinary tract infection

Rationale:

A. Appendicitis can present in males as right testicular pain and must be considered a possible diagnosis in this patient, especially given the other signs and symptoms.
B. Small-bowel obstruction does not usually cause testicular pain. Nausea, vomiting, and abdominal pain, however, are common.
C. Cholecystitis presents as right upper quadrant abdominal pain with nausea and vomiting. Testicular pain is rare.
D. Urinary tract infections present with dysuria, hematuria, and suprapubic tenderness. Testicular pain does not usually suggest a urinary tract infection and is more commonly associated with appendicitis, testicular torsion, and hernias.

Content Category: Gastrointestinal

References: Kidd et al., 2000; pp. 93–116, 438–445; Porth, 1998; pp 769–771.

38. A 75-year-old female arrives in the ED complaining of a 2-day history of gastroenteritis. Which of the following additional past medical history findings would put the patient at an increased risk for this disease?
    A. Recent depression
    B. RECENT ANTIBIOTIC USE
    C. Obesity or weight gain
    D. Taking anticholinergics

Rationale:

B. Gastroenteritis is caused by an imbalance of the normal flora in the gut. This imbalance can be caused by antibiotic use.
A. Depression is often associated with such chronic physiologic conditions as irritable bowel syndrome.
C. Obesity and weight gain are more commonly seen in patients complaining of gastroesophageal reflux disorder.
D. Anticholinergics decrease the tone of the lower esophageal sphincter. Their use is seen in patients with gastroesophageal reflux disorder.

Content Category: Gastrointestinal

References: ENA, Core Curriculum, 2000; Newberry, 1998; p. 552.

39.   An 18-year-old college student is brought to the ED by her boyfriend after he noticed that she had superficially cut herself on her forearm numerous times with a razor. After caring for the wounds, your next intervention would be to:

A. QUESTION THE PATIENT ABOUT ANY SUICIDAL THOUGHTS, PLANS, MEANS, OR ACTIONS.

B. contract with the patient not to harm herself while in the ED.

C. give the patient the phone number of a 24-hour hot line to call if she should feel like hurting herself again.

D. reduce the external stimuli by placing her in a seclusion room.

Rationale:

A. The patient's actions may be self-mutilation, often defined as self-injury with low lethality and performed as a way to relieve stress; a suicide gesture, an action designed to receive attention; or a suicide threat, in which the patient is considering suicide. The nurse needs to assess the patient before any determination can be made.

B. A contract for safety is helpful for many patients who exhibit self-harming behaviors, but an assessment must be done before any contract is made between the patient and the nurse.

C. Giving the patient a 24-hour emergency hot line or the phone number of a mental health professional is recommended when planning for support systems upon discharge. First, however, the nurse needs to assess the patient. Treatment, including psychiatric evaluation, should be obtained before planning discharge.

D. A seclusion room may not be necessary. An assessment should be done before the patient is placed in seclusion.

Content Category: Psychosocial

Reference: Carpenito, 1999; pp. 366–376.

40.   A 48-year-old female presents to the ED with complaints of intermittent palpitations, chest tightness, and choking sensations. The patient reports having had these symptoms for about 6 weeks and states that the episodes are becoming more frequent. Triage assessment reveals an intact airway and skin cool and slightly diaphoretic to touch. Vital signs are BP 168/72 mm Hg, HR 118/min, respirations 26/min, and temperature 99.2° F (37.4° C). The patient does not report any chest tightness, palpitations, or choking sensations at this time. Further assessment of this patient by the emergency nurse reveals that she has recently divorced and has relocated to this community, which is a great distance from her support system. The patient has not been able to find employment that meets career goals she has set for herself. Which of the following nursing diagnoses are most appropriate to guide the plan of care for this patient?

A. Impaired verbal communication

B. Knowledge deficit related to problem solving

C. Altered thought processes related to physical manifestations

D. ANXIETY/FEAR RELATED TO ETIOLOGY AS DETERMINED THROUGH ASSESSMENT

Rationale:

D. Anxiety is often the result of situational crisis in the adult population. Anxiety is physically manifested by ailments that cause pain or impairment in function. In this case, the patient has recently been divorced and has moved away from her social support system. Physiologically, anxiety produces such symptoms as tachycardia, tachypnea, and diaphoresis due to stimulation of the CNS and subsequent catecholamine release.

A. This patient has not demonstrated impaired verbal communication.
B. This patient has not verbalized an inability to solve problems. She has stated her problems, both physical and social.
C. This patient has not demonstrated any alteration in her thought processes.

Content Category: Psychosocial

Reference: ENA, Core Curriculum, 2000; pp. 349–350.

41. A 35-year-old woman has just been brought into the ED by the police after having been sexually assaulted. The patient is alert. Initial assessment reveals bruises and abrasions on her face, breasts, arms, and hands. She makes minimal eye contact with the nurse and responds only when asked a question. During her ED evaluation, the patient expresses concern that the assault may have occurred during ovulation and that she may become pregnant. A treatment modality available that may relieve her concerns is:
A. azithromycin (Zithromax) 1 g PO stat.
B. doxycycline (Vibramycin) 100 mg bid for 10 days.
C. oxytocin (Pitocin) 10 U IM.
D. ETHINYL ESTRADIOL/NORGESTREL (OVRAL) 2 TABLETS INITIALLY FOLLOWED BY 2 TABLETS 12 HOURS LATER.

Rationale:

D. Ovral 2 tablets followed by another 2 tablets 12 hours later is the recommended pregnancy prophylaxis following sexual assault.
A. Azithromycin is the treatment of choice for most sexually transmitted diseases.
B. Doxycycline is a treatment for some sexually transmitted diseases.
C. Pitocin is a hormone used to stimulate labor or to enhance uterine contraction in the postpartum period or in miscarriage.

Content Category: Psychosocial

References: ENA, Core Curriculum, 2000; pp. 463–464; Kitt et al., 1995; pp. 265–268.

42. What is the first step in crisis intervention?
A. Assist the person is gaining an intellectual understanding of the problem
B. Explore coping mechanisms
C. Include support system to review the event
D. ASSESS THE PRECIPITATING EVENT AND ITS IMPACT ON THE PERSON

Rationale:

D. Assessing the actual event, the patient's perception of the event, and the impact on the patient's ability to solve problems is the first step in crisis intervention.
A. Assisting the patient in gaining an understanding of the problem is the second step in crisis intervention.
B. Exploring available coping mechanisms is the third step in crisis intervention.
C. Including support systems is the fourth step in crisis intervention.

Content Category: Psychosocial

References: ENA, Core Curriculum, 2000; p. 352; Kitt et al., 1995; p. 457; Varcarolis, 1998; pp. 371–375.

43.   Depressed patients with suicidal ideation who are being evaluated are at greatest risk for committing suicide:
A.   during the winter months.
B.   before starting antidepressants.
C.   AFTER THE DEPRESSION LIFTS.
D.   when they are agitated and unfocused.

Rationale:

C.   After the depression lifts, the patient with suicidal ideation often is able to carry out the plans made while depressed but that s/he was unable to carry out.
A.   The suicide rate increases during the spring as the amount of daylight increases.
B.   After taking antidepressants for a few weeks, a depressed patient may have the energy to commit suicide that s/he did not have before starting treatment.
D.   A depressed patient who has made the decision to commit suicide may appear serene and goal directed.

Content Category: Psychosocial

Reference: Videbeck, 2001; p. 371.

44.   A 16-year-old female arrives in the ED accompanied by her parents. She appears cachectic. Vital signs are BP 86/50 mm Hg, HR 60/min and irregular, and respirations 20/min. Her lips are dry and cracked; skin turgor is tented. As an intravenous line is being started, she states, "There's no sugar in the IV, is there?" You suspect that this patient has which of the following?
A.   Influenza
B.   Diabetes
C.   ANOREXIA
D.   Heat stroke

Rationale:

C.   This patient is malnourished and dehydrated and has expressed concern that sugar might be an ingredient in her intravenous line. Anorexics manifest an extreme fear of becoming fat and have a distorted body image. The fine hair growth (lanugo) of these patients is a result of malnutrition. Absence of at least 3 consecutive menstrual cycles is often the first physiologic manifestation. The patient's blood pressure, pulse, and temperature are low because of dehydration. The pulse is usually irregular because of an electrolyte imbalance.
A.   Flu is an acute viral respiratory tract infection. Assessment findings would include fever myalgias and cough. There is no evidence to support this diagnosis.
B.   A person with diabetes could present as dehydrated from excessive thirst and urination. However, this patient's overall symptoms are more consistent with anorexia.
D.   Patients presenting with heat stroke tend to have a high fever, not a low one, which needs to be rapidly reduced, along with possible dehydration from perspiration. There is not enough evidence to support this diagnosis.

Content Category: Psychosocial

References: Varcarolis, 1998; pp. 801–815; Copel, 1999; pp. 235–245; Black & Matassarin-Jacobs, 1997; pp. 1133, 1955–1963, 2535.

45. A young woman is brought to the ED with the history of seizures. Soon after arrival, she has a "seizure." There is no loss of consciousness and she is not incontinent. Afterward, she is alert and oriented and seems to enjoy the attention she receives. The neurologist is notified. He states that he is familiar with this patient's case as she had just completed a complete neurologic workup that failed to reveal any neurologic cause. He suggests that this patient be seen by a psychiatrist. The patient agrees. You suspect which of the following?
A. CONVERSION DISORDER
B. Bipolar disorder
C. Panic disorder
D. Schizophrenia

Rationale:

A. Conversion disorder is characterized by the presence of one or more symptoms that suggest the presence of a neurologic disorder that cannot be explained by a known medical or neurologic problem. The symptoms are exacerbated by stress and conflict.
B. Patients with bipolar disorder tend to be hyperactive, write lengthy letters, make long phone calls, spend large sums of money on frivolous items, and engage in sexual indiscretion. They can be manipulative, profane, fault finding, and adept at exploiting others' vulnerabilities.
C. Panic disorders are characterized by a sudden onset of intense, apprehensive dread and at least 4 of the following symptoms: dyspnea, palpitations, chest discomfort, syncope or dizziness, trembling or shaking, sweating, choking, nausea or abdominal distress, depersonalization, sensations of numbness or tingling, hot flashes or chills, and fear of dying, "going crazy," or losing control.
D. Patients with schizophrenia, a psychotic disorder, present with disorganized thinking, hallucinations, delusions, associative looseness (confused and haphazard thinking that is jumbled and illogical), and loss of ego boundaries.

Content Category: Psychosocial
Reference: Varacolis, 1998; pp. 486–495, 595–623, 627–675.

46. A patient with a suspected corneal abrasion is in a treatment room awaiting evaluation by the doctor. While waiting, the ED nurse can enhance patient comfort by:
A. giving the patient the dropperette of topical anesthesia to be applied ad lib.
B. irrigating the involved eye with cooled saline.
C. KEEPING THE LIGHTS DIMMED.
D. applying an occlusive eye patch.

Rationale:

C. Patients with corneal abrasions frequently have intense photophobia. Dimming the lights often diminishes symptoms.
A. Repeated and excessive administration of ocular topical anesthesia delays healing. Medications should be administered only by staff following appropriate orders.
B. Irrigation is indicated in chemical exposures, not in corneal abrasions.
D. Occlusive patching is generally no longer favored for corneal abrasions.

Content Category: Maxillofacial & Ocular
Reference: Rhee & Pyfer, 1999; pp. 19–52.

47.   Signs and symptoms of croup include which of the following?
    A. Stridor, intercostal retractions, unequal breath sounds
    B. STRIDOR, BARKING COUGH, INTERCOSTAL RETRACTION
    C. Tachypnea, barking cough, difficulty swallowing
    D. Fever, hoarse voice, difficulty swallowing

Rationale:

    B. Viral croup is responsible for more than 90% of cases of stridor outside the neonatal period. Stridor is unaffected by position but increases with crying or agitation. The child often has a barking cough that typically worsens in the late evening and at night. Intercostal retractions and tachypnea are common signs.
    A. Viral croup is classically associated with biphasic stridor, although often the inspiratory component is much greater than the expiratory component. Stridor is unaffected by position, but increases with crying or agitation. The child often has a barking cough that typically worsens in the late evening and at night. The child with croup may have diminished breath sounds, but they should be equal on both sides of the chest.
    C. Tachypnea is a common sign in croup. The barking cough is common in croup and is typically worse in the late evening and at night. There should not be any difficulty swallowing in this illness.
    D. Children with croup may have a low-grade fever. The voice of the child with croup is often hoarse, but not muffled. There should be no difficulty swallowing.

Content Category: Maxillofacial & Ocular

Reference: Tintinalli et al., 2000; pp. 879–890.

48.   The expected results of the fluorescein stain of the cornea in a patient with suspected bacterial conjunctivitis are which of the following?
    A. CORNEA CLEAR
    B. Dendritic ulcerations seen
    C. Occasional punctate staining
    D. Corneal ulcerations

Rationale:

    A. The expectation with a fluorescein stain of the cornea in a patient with bacterial conjunctivitis is no uptake of the stain. The cornea should be clear of stain.
    B. Dendritic ulcerations are characteristic of herpetic disease.
    C. Punctate staining (multiple tiny dots of stain uptake) may be seen with viral conjunctivitis or ultraviolet burns of the cornea.
    D. Corneal ulcerations are not seen with conjunctivitis; they are often seen with overuse syndrome related to extended-wear disposable contact lenses.

Content Category: Maxillofacial & Ocular

Reference: Tintinalli et al., 2000; pp. 1501–1518.

49.   Common symptoms in a patient with otitis media include:
    A. OTALGIA AND FEVER.
    B. otorrhea and nystagmus.
    C. hearing loss and vertigo.
    D. fever and tinnitus.

Rationale:

    A. Ear pain, otalgia, and fever are frequently present with otitis media.

    B. Otorrhea may be present with otitis media, but nystagmus is uncommon.

    C. Hearing loss may be present in some cases with otitis media, but vertigo is uncommon.

    D. Fever is often present in otitis media, but tinnitus is uncommon.

Content Category: Maxillofacial & Ocular

Reference: Tintinalli et al., 2000; pp. 1518–1526.

50. A patient who has sustained a splash of lye into both eyes is undergoing irrigation. Irrigation should continue until:

    A. the pH reaches 8.4.

    B. 1,000 ml of fluid has been instilled.

    C. 500 ml of fluid has been instilled.

    D. THE pH REACHES 7.4.

Rationale:

    D. Acid burns cause immediate damage, but alkaline substances continue to damage the cornea until the substance is removed. Therefore, irrigation is pH dependent rather than volume dependent. A pH of 7.4 is recommended.

    A. A pH of 8.4 remains too alkaline.

    B. 1,000 ml of fluid may not be adequate.

    C. 500 ml of volume may not be adequate.

Content Category: Maxillofacial & Ocular

Reference: Newberry, 1998; pp. 689–706.

51. Discharge instructions for a patient with otitis media will most likely include:

    A. application of warm compresses every 2 hours.

    B. bed rest for 24 hours.

    C. aggressive cleansing of the ear canal.

    D. REEVALUATION IN 10 DAYS TO CONFIRM RESOLUTION.

Rationale:

    D. Children with otitis media require reevaluation to confirm resolution or persistence of effusion. Chronic otitis media or effusion may require referral for specialized care.

    A. Warm compresses offer no benefit to the patient with otitis media.

    B. Bed rest is not indicated for otitis media.

    C. Aggressive cleaning of the ear offers no benefit and is not indicated.

Content Category: Maxillofacial & Ocular

Reference: Newberry, 1998; pp. 673–688.

52. A patient with an orbital blowout fracture should have a thorough evaluation of:
    A. hearing.
    B. EXTRAOCULAR MOVEMENTS.
    C. tongue movement.
    D. swallowing.

Rationale:

    B. If there is nerve, tissue, and extraocular muscle entrapment, the exam of extraocular movements will be abnormal.
    A. Hearing is not affected with a blowout fracture.
    C. Tongue movement is not affected with a blowout fracture.
    D. Swallowing is not affected with a blowout fracture.

Content Category: Maxillofacial & Ocular

Reference: Newberry, 1998; pp. 373–387.

53. A 4-year-old child is found to have a tender, red nodule on the upper eyelid. Discharge instructions include antibiotic ophthalmic ointment and direction to:
    A. WASH EYELASHES DAILY WITH BABY SHAMPOO.
    B. flush with eye wash three times a day.
    C. instill over-the-counter vasoconstricting drops twice a day.
    D. apply cool compresses four times a day.

Rationale:

    A. Eyelids should be washed daily as a hygiene measure to minimize recurrence.
    B. Eye flushing will not enhance resolution of hordeolum.
    C. Vasoconstrictive drops act on the conjunctiva, not the lid.
    D. Warm compresses should be applied to the eye.

Content Category: Maxillofacial & Ocular

Reference: Palay & Krachmer, 1997; pp. 169–207.

54. A 30-year-old male presents with a 5-day history of unilateral sore throat. He is also complaining of ear pain, fever, and difficulty swallowing. If you consider these symptoms, the patient most likely has which of the following conditions?
    A. Mononucleosis
    B. Epiglottitis
    C. PERITONSILLAR ABSCESS
    D. Pharyngitis

Rationale:

    C. The classic symptoms of peritonsillar abscess include a sore throat that becomes more severe and is unilateral, headache, dysphasia, difficulty opening the mouth wide, neck pain, and referred ear pain.
    A. Mononucleosis usually can be distinguished from peritonsillar abscess because in the former, the adenopathy is bilateral and anterior and posterior cervical nodes are noted.
    B. Epiglottitis has similar symptoms, but the cervical adenopathy is bilateral.
    D. Pharyngitis has similar symptoms, except adenopathy is bilateral.

Content Category: Maxillofacial & Ocular

Reference: ENA, Core Curriculum, 2000; pp. 227–274.

55. A 21-year-old female presents to the ED with complaints of weakness and leg cramps. She appears to be underweight for her height. Vital signs are BP 90/60 mm Hg and HR 55/min. All other vital signs are within normal parameters. During the general survey, you would be likely to observe, as a potential behavior that a patient with anorexia nervosa, would display, the wearing of:
   A. tight-fitting clothing.
   B. LOOSE-FITTING CLOTHING.
   C. seasonally appropriate clothing.
   D. fitted clothing.

Rationale:

   B. The anorexic patient may wear loose or oversize clothing to hide actual body size. These patients usually dress warmly and in layers, as they are often cold due to a deceased amount of adipose tissue and have cold intolerance.
   A. Generally not worn by patients with anorexia.
   C. Anorexia patients generally wear warm, layered clothing regardless of the season.
   D. Generally not worn by patients with anorexia

Content Category: General Medical

Reference: Moreau, 2001; p. 9.

56. Your patient presents at triage with shortness of breath and chest pain with inspiration. Past history reveals that this patient is HIV positive. Vital signs are BP 124/64 mm Hg, HR 96/min, respirations 24/min, and temperature 99.8° F (37.7° C). Which of the following is a priority for the ED nurse?
   A. Airborne precautions
   B. Contact precautions
   C. Isolation precautions
   D. STANDARD PRECAUTIONS

Rationale:

   D. Standard precautions are to be used by all health care workers in providing care for all patients. The precautions involve information and actions to be carried out when exposure to blood, bodily fluids, mucous membranes, or nonintact skin is likely in providing care to the patient. This term replaces the previous "universal precautions."
   A. Airborne precautions are part of the second level of precautions related to transmission-based precautions. A nurse caring for a patient who is at high risk for transmitting by airborne droplet such diseases as measles and tuberculosis must use standard precautions and wear a mask.
   B. Contact precautions are part of the second level of precautions related to transmission-based precautions. These precautions involve direct or indirect patient contact and the use of gowns, gloves, and masks. Contact precautions are used in addition to standard precautions.
   C. "Isolation precautions" is a nonspecific term that indicates a need to take more than standard precautions. The term is generally not used today, as it not specific in terms of the type of precaution to use.

Content Category: General Medical

References: ENA, Core Curriculum, 2000; Moreau, 2001; p. 101.

57.   Your patient has a 6-month history of fibromyalgia. She presents in the ED with complaints of dull, aching, unprovoked back pain (rated at 3/10) for the past several days. Her vital signs are all within normal limits. What is a priority in the management of a patient with fibromyalgia?
      A. Narcotic pain management
      B. PATIENT EDUCATION ABOUT FIBROMYALGIA
      C. Physical therapy
      D. NSAID pain management

Rationale:

      B. Patients with fibromyalgia need to understand the course of their illness; that it is a chronic illness; the plan of care (especially in dealing with the pain); and that the consequences of the disease are not life threatening.
      A. While narcotic pain management may be needed on occasion, it should not be a priority in the management of this chronic type of pain. Pain treatment should be guided by a pain management clinic.
      C. Physical therapy assists in improving muscle conditioning and mobility, but it is not a priority for management of fibromyalgia.
      D. NSAIDs are typically not helpful in treating the pain of fibromyalgia.

Content Category: General Medical

Reference: Moreau, 2001; p.424.

58.   A 34-year-old female comes to the ED complaining of muscle cramps in her legs and numbness of her fingers for the past several days. She has a history of gallbladder disease and pancreatitis. This patient is demonstrating signs and symptoms of:
      A. hypermagnesemia.
      B. HYPOCALCEMIA.
      C. hyperkalemia.
      D. hyponatremia.

Rationale:

      B. This patient is exhibiting signs of hypocalcemia. Pancreatitis can cause malabsorption of calcium and loss of calcium in the stools. Hypocalcemia patients complain of digital and perioral paresthesia and muscle cramps as well as tetany and seizures.
      A. Hypermagnesemia is related to renal failure, severe dehydration, or overdose of magnesium salts. These patients present with muscle weakness and decreased tendon reflexes.
      C. Hyperkalemia is usually caused by renal failure. Patients present with muscle weakness, ECG changes, nausea, and abdominal cramping.
      D. Hyponatremia is caused by excessive loss of sodium or excessive water gains. The patient complains of anorexia, headache, nausea, and fatigue.

Content Category: General Medical

References: ENA, Core Curriculum, 2000; Moreau, 2001; pp.1020–1035.

59.   Which of the following complications is of most concern with rapid reduction of circulating glucose and administration of fluids?
      A. Seizures
      B. Congestive heart failure
      C. CEREBRAL EDEMA
      D. Hyperthermia

Rationale:

C. Cerebral edema is the most dangerous of the complications listed above. Fluid shifts are probably caused by a decrease in serum osmolality, which allows excess fluid to enter the brain cells. Although significant amounts occur in only a small number of cases, cerebral edema has severe neurologic effects.

A. Low glucose levels make less glucose available to cross the barrier into brain cells. Without having sufficient glucose available for energy, the brain becomes increasingly irritable, especially at levels below 45 mg/dl. Close monitoring is essential when reducing glucose levels.

B. Circulatory overload—although a risk with the large volume replacement necessary in hyperglycemic states—is able to be more easily corrected than cerebral edema. Accurate intake and output data are vital to obtain.

D. In hypoglycemia, the skin becomes cool, pale, and diaphoretic.

Content Category: General Medical

References: Newberry, 1998; pp. 603–604; ENA, Core Curriculum, 2000; pp. 263–268.

60. Suspended droplets that carry tuberculosis (TB) infection may remain in still air for days. This route of disease transmission is prevented by the use of which of the following?
    A. Surgical mask
    B. Nonlatex gloves
    C. Impervious gown
    D. HEPA MASK

Rationale:

D. Since tuberculosis particles are smaller than 5 microns, a high-efficiency particulate respirator mask is essential for filtering out smaller particles, such as *Mycobacterium tuberculosis*, measles, and varicella.

A. A surgical mask does not block particles this small or offer protection to the health care worker.

B. Nonlatex gloves are an essential part of standard precautions for preventing skin contact with patients' body substances.

C. The barrier protection offered by a gown is valuable for reducing contact with patients' body substances but does nothing for respiratory protection.

Content Category: General Medical

References: ENA, Core Curriculum, 2000; pp. 257–259; Moss & Arbogast, 1997; pp. 26–31.

61. A 20-year-old presents with a 2-week history of fatigue, thirst, nausea, and polyuria. Lab analysis shows a glucose level of 654 mg/dl and a potassium level of 5.4 mEq/dl. IV fluids and insulin are begun. Which of the following orders should the ED nurse anticipate?
    A. Administration of bicarbonate with a pH of 7.3
    B. POTASSIUM ADDED TO IV FLUID
    C. IV fluid changed from normal saline (NS) solution to 5% dextrose and 0.5% normal saline
    D. Administration of low-dose heparin

Rationale:

B. The process of increased glyconeogenesis creates hyperglycemia, which leads to excessive water, sodium, and potassium loss. Fluid replacement further dilutes potassium. The administration of insulin pushes potassium out of the vascular system into the cell. After the initial liter of NS, potassium needs to be replaced.

A. Bicarbonate would not be appropriate for this patient with a pH of 7.3, since it would cause rebound alkalosis, thus worsening hypokalemia.

C. Initial replacement fluid is NS and continues to be NS until the glucose level reaches 250–300 mg/dl. Hypovolemia may require 8–10 L of replacement. After the glucose level has reached this point, the fluid is changed to 5% dextrose and 0.5% normal saline to provide an energy source until the patient can resume adequate intake.

D. Thromboses are very rare in diabetic ketoacidosis but occur frequently in hyperglycemic hyperosmolar nonketotic coma (HHNC). This would be an appropriate order for a patient with HHNC.

Content Category: General Medical

References: Newberry, 1998; pp.601–604; ENA, Core Curriculum, 2000; pp. 263–267.

62. On arrival at the ED, a patient is confused. The skin is hot and dry with poor turgor. Glucometer findings come up as "high." A history of infection, thirst, and polyuria is gathered from the family. Vital signs are BP 96/50 mm Hg, HR 142/min, and respirations 18/min and normal, with no odor. What is the likely problem?
A. HYPERGLYCEMIC HYPEROSMOLAR NONKETOTIC COMA
B. Diabetic ketoacidosis
C. Thyroid storm
D. Myxedema coma

Rationale:

A. Classic findings of hyperglycemic hyperosmolar nonketotic coma (HHNC) are confusion, dehydration, glucose levels often above 800, hypovolemia, tachycardia, and respirations normal or increased but with no ketone odor. Ketones are not formed because the type II diabetic produces some insulin, thereby avoiding ketoacidosis.

B. Although the same stressors can lead to diabetic ketoacidosis, the body is not producing enough insulin to balance gluconeogenesis. Once the body become unable to metabolize glucose, fat and muscle are used for energy, resulting in a buildup of fatty acids, leading in turn to ketoacidosis.

C. The patient experiencing rapid elevation of thyroid hormones, leading to thyroid storm, may present with fever, poor skin turgor, confusion, tachycardia, and hypertension. Elevated thyroid hormones, not glucose, are the problem.

D. Myxedema coma due to hypothyroidism presents very differently. The skin is usually cool and pale; respiratory effort is poor; glucose levels may be low; and metabolism slows. Fatigue, weight gain, and bradycardia are common.

Content Category: General Medical

References: Newberry, 1998; pp.601–608; ENA, Core Curriculum, 2000; pp. 263–272.

63. Which of the following electrolyte deficiencies can cause tetany?
A. DECREASED CHLORIDE
B. Decreased potassium
C. Decreased sodium
D. Decreased phosphate

Rationale:

A. Hypochloremia occurs with hyponatremia, manifesting with the additional symptoms of muscle weakness; twitching; tetany; shallow, slow respirations; and respiratory arrest.

B. Hypokalemia presents with muscle weakness, often in the lower extremities and proximal muscle groups. Respiratory muscle weakness may occur, leading to respiratory failure. ECG changes include a flattened or inverted T wave, depressed ST segment, U waves, and ventricular ectopy.

C. Hyponatremia, difficult to recognize because of a vague presentation, includes anorexia, nausea, weakness, confusion, agitation, and disorientation. Continued loss of electrolytes can lead to seizures, coma, and death.

D. Hypophosphatemia may present with no symptoms or with anorexia, muscle weakness, respiratory failure, rhabdomyolysis, hemolysis, and changes in mental status.

Content Category: General Medical

Reference: Newberry, 1998; pp. 582–591.

64. Identification of rashes leads to clues about the causative agent. Measles presents with which type of rash?
   A. Vesicular
   B. Petechial
   C. Pustular
   D. MACULOPAPULAR

Rationale:

D. The classic measles rash begins after 3 to 7 days as maculopapular, small, red, elevated areas, then progresses to confluent or joined areas.

A. Vesicular areas as seen in chickenpox are fluid-filled blisters that dry, forming a yellow crust.

B. Petechiae are small, round, flat, deep-red or purplish spots, often found in meningitis.

C. Pustules are raised areas filled with a purulent fluid and found in impetigo or acne.

Content Category: General Medical

References: ENA, Core Curriculum, 2000; pp. 243–261; Seidel et al., 1999; pp.175–177.

65. Although children are immunized against this disease, by age 12 or so the inoculation is no longer protective. Which disease is it?
   A. Polio
   B. PERTUSSIS
   C. Diphtheria
   D. Mumps

Rationale:

B. Pertussis or whooping cough is a bacterial infection that is highly contagious in infants and in children presenting with more severe cases. Immunization given as part of the DPT series lasts for less than 12 years. Adults usually have minor respiratory symptoms and a persistent cough. Most cases in the adult population are undiagnosed.

A. Polio, on its way to being eradicated through strong immunization programs, appears stable in the immunized population. Repeat doses are recommended only if an adult has not received prior immunization or is working in a high-risk area.

C. Diphtheria, a devastating disease, is less severe if immunization has occurred.

D. Immunity is long lasting when the MMR series is administered or the mumps vaccine is given individually.

Content Category: General Medical

References: ENA, Core Curriculum, 2000; Chin, 2000; pp. 375, 398–405.

66.   Which of the following diseases is transmitted through the bloodborne pathway?
       A. Hepatitis A
       B. HEPATITIS C
       C. Encephalitis
       D. Rocky Mountain spotted fever

Rationale:

       B. Hepatitis C, parenterally transmitted, is the most common form of posttransfusion hepatitis identified. Found in blood or blood products, it often becomes chronic.
       A. Hepatitis A is transmitted through the fecal-oral route, contaminated water or food, or sexual contact with an infected person.
       C. Encephalitis is caused by one of the following: arbovirus, herpes simplex type I, varicella zoster virus, Epstein-Barr virus, and rabies. Transmission may be through an animal bite, vector, or airborne droplet contaminate.
       D. Ticks act as the vector in Rocky Mountain spotted fever.

Content Category: General Medical

References: ENA, Core Curriculum, 2000; pp. 243–261; Moss & Arbogast, 1997; pp.131–140, 228–230.

67.   The common pathologic processes leading to brain death do NOT include which of the following?
       A. Massive head trauma
       B. MYXEDEMA COMA
       C. Intracranial hemorrhage
       D. Hypoxic ischemic brain damage suffered during cardiopulmonary arrest

Rationale:

       B. Untreated hypothyroidism progresses over months to years before culminating in myxedema coma. Neurologic changes include confusion, lethargy, and coma. Survival rates increase when patients receive prompt hormone replacement with intensive supportive care. Although mortality can approach 50%, myxedema coma is not so common a cause of brain death as traumatic head injuries, gunshot wounds to the head, ruptured cerebral aneurysms, arteriovenous malformations, severe strokes, and severe anoxic events resulting from prolonged cardiac arrest.
       A. Massive head trauma, intracranial hemorrhage, and hypoxic ischemic damage suffered during cardiopulmonary arrest are conditions that rapidly produce marked brain edema, which increases brain volume. Because of the skull's fixed capacity, the increase in brain volume produces an inevitable increase in intracranial pressure, causing two morbid events to occur: 1) herniation and infarction of the brainstem as it is forcibly displaced from its original location; and 2) loss of cerebral perfusion pressure as intracranial pressure exceeds mean arterial blood pressure.
       C. See above (A).
       D. See above (A).

Content Category: Patient Care

References: Newberry, 1998; pp. 593–610; Sullivan et al., 1999; pp. 37–46.

68.   According to the American College of Surgeons Committee on Trauma standards, which one of the following patients should be transported to a designated trauma center?
       A. A 72-YEAR-OLD FEMALE WITH A FRACTURED CLAVICLE AFTER AUTOMOBILE CRASH
       B. A 26-year-old male with a Glasgow Coma Scale score of 16 after motorcycle crash
       C. A 15-year-old female with a systolic blood pressure of 148 after automobile crash
       D. A 7-year-old male who fell 15 feet out of a tree

Rationale:

    A. The American College of Surgeons Committee on Trauma recommends that patients less than 5 years of age or more than 55 years of age who have incurred trauma be transported to a designated trauma center.

    B. Patients with a Glasgow Coma Scale score of 14 or more should go directly to a designated trauma center.

    C. Systolic blood pressure of less than 90 mm Hg indicates a need for direct transport to a trauma center.

    D. The criterion for direct transport to a designated trauma center for fall victims is a fall from a height greater than 20 feet.

Content Category: Patient Care

Reference: American College of Surgeons, 1997.

69. When the nurse is treating victims of a weapon of mass destruction, which of the following are considered personal protective equipment?
    A. Respirator, gown, bottled water
    B. Oxygen mask, gown, hair covering
    C. RESPIRATOR, GOWN, EYE PROTECTION
    D. Portable oxygen tank, gown, eye protection

Rationale:

    C. Respirators, gowns, and eye protection are among the items used for personal protection in treating victims of a weapon of mass destruction.

    A. Bottled water is not considered personal protection against a weapon of mass destruction.

    B. An oxygen mask is not considered personal protection against a weapon of mass destruction.

    D. A portable oxygen tank is not considered personal protection against a weapon of mass destruction.

Content Category: Patient Care

Reference: ENA, Core Curriculum, 2000; p. 706.

70. A disease agent that may be used as a biological weapon is which of the following?
    A. Rubella
    B. SMALLPOX
    C. Viral influenza
    D. Chlamydia

Rationale:

    B. Smallpox, often considered an extinct disease, is one of the biologicals that may be used by a terrorist.

    A. Rubella can be a serious disease in some people, but is not deadly enough to be considered a terrorist weapon.

    C. Viral influenza often causes widespread epidemics, but is not deadly enough to be considered a terrorist weapon.

    D. Chlamydia is a very contagious sexually transmitted disease, but is not a candidate for the terrorist's arsenal.

Content Category: Patient Care

Reference: ENA, Core Curriculum, 2000; p. 715.

71.   When a patient agrees to a procedure after having been made aware of the procedure to be performed, the alternatives available, and the risks of the procedure, the patient's consent is said to be:
    A. implied.
    B. involuntary.
    C. express.
    D. INFORMED.

Rationale:

    D. Meeting all elements of informed consent is required before surgery or other procedures.
    A. Consent to treat is implied when an individual is unable to provide consent and is in a life- or limb-threatening situation.
    B. Involuntary consent is obtained when an individual refuses needed medical treatment and someone else, usually a psychiatrist, signs papers that hold the patient for treatment.
    C. A competent person who voluntarily consents to medical treatment is said to have given express consent.

Content Category: Patient Care

Reference: ENA, Core Curriculum, 2000; p. 726.

72.   In the event of a major catastrophe, the National Disaster Medical System can:
    A. take over state operations for a 2-week period of recovery.
    B. BE ACTIVATED ONLY IN RESPONSE TO A REQUEST FROM THE GOVERNOR OF THE STATE.
    C. send federal personnel to the state within 8 hours.
    D. exert federal control over a hospital.

Rationale:

    B. Only the governor of a state can request activation of the National Disaster Medical System.
    A. The National Disaster Medical System has no authority to take over state operations. No definitive time frame for on-site operations is specified.
    C. Normal response time to a state for National Disaster Medical System personnel is at least 48 hours.
    D. The National Disaster Medical System cannot supply major medical equipment to the scene of a disaster.

Content Category: Patient Care

Reference: Newberry, 1998; p. 204.

73.   Justin is a 2-year-old with HR 264/minute, respirations 32/min, and a peripheral capillary refill of 2 seconds, with fast but strong peripheral pulses. He is sitting in his mother's lap and cries at your approach. Crying causes no change in the rhythm on the monitor. His skin is pale pink and warm. His tympanic temperature is 98.2° F (36.8° C). Your interventions would include:
    A. oxygen by face mask, IV access, sedation, and vagal maneuvers.
    B. sedation and synchronized cardioversion at 2 joules/kg.
    C. IV ACCESS AND ADMINISTRATION OF ADENOSINE PHOSPHATE (ADENOCARD) IV.
    D. IV access, sedation, and cardioversion at 0.5 joules/kg.

Rationale:

> C. Adenosine is the drug of choice for conversion of supraventricular tachycardia in stable children.
>
> A. Sedation is required only for cardioversion of a hemodynamically unstable child. Justin is still alert; his skin is warm and pink; his capillary refill time is 2 seconds; and his peripheral pulses are strong.
>
> B. Cardioversion is delivered at 0.5 joule/kg initially. Repeat doses are delivered at 1.0 joule/kg.
>
> D. The patient is stable and does not require cardioversion.

Content Category: Patient Care

Reference: ENA, Pediatric Course, 1999; pp.192–193.

74. Parents bring their 5-day-old infant to the ED for "poor feeding." Mom reports the baby was breast-feeding well until yesterday evening. Your triage exam reveals a term female infant who is pale, slightly mottled, and listless, with poor muscle tone. Vital signs are HR 160/min, respirations 44/min with mild retractions, and temperature 100.8° F (38.2° C) rectally. Capillary refill time is 3 seconds centrally and 4 seconds peripherally. Based on your assessment, you would do which of the following?
    A. Send the family to the registration desk.
    B. TRIAGE THE INFANT AS EMERGENT AND SEND THE INFANT DIRECTLY TO THE TREATMENT AREA.
    C. Place mother and baby behind the curtain at triage so you can see if the infant will breastfeed.
    D. Triage the infant as urgent and send the family to the waiting room.

Rationale:

> B. A sick/symptomatic neonate is classified as "emergent" and is sent immediately to the treatment area.
>
> A. A sick/symptomatic neonate is classified as "emergent" and is sent immediately to the treatment room.
>
> C. Incorrect answer.
>
> D. Incorrect answer.

Content Category: Patient Care

Reference: ENA, Pediatric Course, 1999; p. 253.

75. In most situations, the maximum volume of a medication that should be administered IM in a single site to small children and older infants is:
    A. 0.5 ml.
    B. 1.0 ML.
    C. 2.0 ml.
    D. 3.0 ml.

Rationale:

> B. Usually 1 ml is the maximum volume that should be administered in a single site to small children and older infants.
>
> A. Incorrect answer.
>
> C. Incorrect answer.
>
> D. Incorrect answer.

Content Category: Patient Care

Reference: Wong, 1999; p. 1264.

76.   The initial priority in the treatment of a pediatric patient with an avulsed tooth is:
      A. AIRWAY MANAGEMENT.
      B. to control hemorrhage.
      C. to assess neurologic status.
      D. preservation of the tooth for reimplantation.

Rationale:

      A. Correct answer: the tooth may cause airway compromise or be aspirated.
      B. Incorrect answer. Airway management is the first priority.
      C. Incorrect answer. Airway management is the first priority.
      D. Incorrect answer. Airway management is the first priority.

Content Category: Patient Care

Reference: ENA, Pediatric Course, 1999; p. 154.

77.   A 4-year-old male fell from a moving all-terrain vehicle (ATV) and has multiple injuries. He has
      been stabilized in your ED and will be transported to a regional pediatric hospital for ongoing evalu-
      ation and treatment. A pediatric transport team is flying in to pick up and transport the patient.
      Which of the following interventions is NOT appropriate in preparing the patient for air medical
      transport?
      A. Initiate IV access and secure lines
      B. SPLINT SUSPECTED FRACTURES WITH AIR SPLINTS
      C. Secure and maintain a patent airway
      D. Insert a gastric tube

Rationale:

      B. Air splints are NOT used in air medical transports because gases expand at higher altitudes and
          can result in compression of the affected extremity as air expands in air splints.
      A. Incorrect. This intervention would be performed.
      C. Incorrect. This intervention would be performed.
      D. Incorrect. This intervention would be performed.

Content Category: Patient Care

Reference: ENA, Trauma Nursing, 2000; p. 356.

78.   The emergency nurse knows that infants and small children have anatomic and physiologic differ-
      ences from older children and adults. Which of the following is NOT an important difference?
      A. INFANTS AND CHILDREN HAVE LOWER OXYGEN REQUIREMENTS THAN ADULTS.
      B. Infants and children have greater amounts of soft tissue surrounding the airway.
      C. The heads of infants and children are larger and heavier in relation to the body than are adults'.
      D. Infants and children have poorly developed intercostal accessory muscles.

Rationale:

      A. Infants and children have higher oxygen requirements than adults.
      B. The statement is true and important because the greater amount of soft tissue in the airways of
          infants and children make the airway more susceptible to obstruction from edema than in adults.
      C. The statement is true and important because an infant's or a child's proportionately larger head
          poses a greater risk for injury.
      D. The statement is true and important because infants and children rely more on their abdominal
          muscles for effective breathing than adults do.

Content Category: Patient Care

Reference: ENA, Core Curriculum, 2000; pp. 22–23, 464.

79. A hypotensive patient with multiple trauma is to be transferred from a small rural facility to a level I trauma center. Prior to departure, it is imperative that which of the following be done for the patient?
    A. Diagnostic peritoneal lavage (DPL)
    B. Thoracotomy
    C. Computed tomography (CT) scan
    D. BOLUSES OF NORMAL SALINE

Rationale:

D. COBRA/OBRA/EMTALA mandate that sending facilities stabilize patients within the capabilities of those facilities. For a hypotensive trauma patient, boluses of normal saline would be the minimum treatment expected of the sending facility before transfer.

A. COBRA/OBRA/EMTALA mandate that sending facilities stabilize patients within the capabilities of those facilities. An emergency physician in the rural setting may not be familiar with performing a DPL. If it is done and the test is positive, the patient should be sent for operative intervention immediately. A small rural facility transferring the patient does not have the resources to deal with this kind of surgical emergency.

B. Same justification as answer A for a thoracotomy procedure.

C. Most small rural facilities do not have CT scanners.

Content Category: Patient Care

Reference: Moy, 2000; pp. 94–95, 268.

Questions 80 and 81

A patient with chest pain has 3-mm to 5-mm ST segment elevations in leads II, III, and AVF on electrocardiogram (ECG). Vital signs are BP 128/62 mm Hg, HR 96/min, and respirations 22/min. After sublingual nitroglycerin has been administered, vital signs are BP 88/50 mm Hg, HR 108/min, and respirations 22/min.

80. The diagnostic test that would be most useful in determining the specific problem is:
    A. RIGHT-SIDED ECG.
    B. cardiac enzymes and isoenzymes.
    C. chest x-ray.
    D. stress test.

Rationale:

A. Significant ST segment elevation in leads II, III, and AVF indicates an inferior wall infarction. Right ventricular infarctions (RVIs) are found in 30–40% of patients with inferior wall infarction. Patients with RVI are often hypotensive or blood pressure drops significantly with nitroglycerine. To determine whether a patient has an RVI, a right-sided ECG is done. Lead V4r (V4 on the right-sided ECG) will be the most diagnostic.

B. Cardiac and isoenzymes are elevated in all patients with myocardial infarction, regardless of the part of the heart affected.

C. Chest x-ray would not be helpful in distinguishing between an inferior wall infarction and a right ventricular infarction.

D. Although stress tests are frequently done in cardiac patients, they are not done when the patient is acutely infarcting or in the early stages of recovery.

Content Category: Patient Care

Reference: American Heart Association, 1997; pp. 9-26–9-31.

81.   This patient will probably need large doses of:
   A. morphine sulfate.
   B. nitroglycerin.
   C. furosemide (Lasix).
   D. NORMAL SALINE.

Rationale:

   D. Patients with a right ventricular infarct (RVI) are often hypotensive or blood pressure drops sig-
       nificantly with nitroglycerine. The patient with an RVI needs intravenous fluid infused to
       increase the circulating volume.
   A. Morphine causes central circulatory dilation and triggers hypotension. If morphine is to be used
       in the patient with an RVI, the patient must first have adequate circulating volume. Meperidine
       (Demerol) is often a better choice for pain control in RVI patients, since it does not have the
       effect of central unloading.
   B. Nitroglycerin causes peripheral circulatory dilation and triggers hypotension. If nitroglycerine is
       to be used in the patient with an RVI, the patient must first have adequate circulating volume.
   C. The patient with RVI needs intravenous fluid infused to increase circulating volume. Furo-
       semide (Lasix) is a diuretic, which would remove fluid.

Content Category: Patient Care

Reference: American Heart Association, 2000; I-1–I-384.

82.   A patient with a large flail segment to the anterior chest is to be transported from a rural facility to a
       level I trauma center. It is most important to:
   A. transport the patient on oxygen by nonrebreather mask.
   B. INTUBATE THE PATIENT BEFORE DEPARTURE AND PROVIDE CONTROLLED
       MECHANICAL VENTILATION.
   C. stabilize the flail segment with a large sandbag.
   D. transport the patient on the uninjured side.

Rationale:

   B. Intubation and controlled positive pressure ventilation are optimal for the patient with flail
       chest and provide internal stabilization of the flail segment. Intubation should occur in the con-
       trolled environment of the sending facility, where space is ample and multiple personnel are
       available for assistance.
   A. Oxygen by nonrebreather mask would probably not suffice, considering the cumulative effects of
       poor lung expansion, pulmonary contusion, pain, and altitude.
   C. Sandbags are not usually used in current practice, since they tend to decrease alveolar ventila-
       tion and trigger alveolar collapse.
   D. When patient conditions allow, transporting the patient on the injured side stabilizes the flail
       segment.

Content Category: Patient Care

References: Holleran, 1994; p. 250; Holleran, 1996; pp. 120–122.

83. A 35-year-old man comes to the ED complaining of nausea, pain in the left upper quadrant, and malaise. History includes a liver transplant 3 months ago. The ED nurse should anticipate the possibility of:
    A. gallstones.
    B. TRANSPLANT REJECTION.
    C. alcohol use and possible pancreatitis.
    D. infection masked by immunosuppressive therapy.

Rationale:

 B. Acute rejection is seen early, whereas chronic rejection is seen within the first 6 months of transplantation.

 A. In a liver transplant, the gallbladder is removed from both the liver donor and the recipient. Therefore, gallstones do not occur in liver transplant patients.

 C. All potential transplant recipients are screened to determine whether they are good candidates. Patients who need the transplant because of cirrhosis must be undergoing rehabilitation for alcohol abuse and provide evidence that they are improving their lifestyle. This does not mean alcohol abuse does not occur, but that it does not occur frequently.

 D. Prednisone and medications such as cyclosporin can mask infectious processes; however, this usually does not occur early in the posttransplant period.

Content Category: Patient Care

Reference: ENA, Core Curriculum, 2000; pp. 495–496.

84. A vasopressin (Pitressin) infusion of 30 units/hour is ordered for an adult patient with bleeding esophageal varices. Fifty units of vasopressin is added to 200 ml of normal saline solution. The drip factor is 15 gtt/ml. Flow should be adjusted to:
    A. 10 gtt/min.
    B. 15 gtt/min.
    C. 25 gtt/min.
    D. 30 GTT/MIN.

Rationale:

 D. Convert dilution of 200 ml to drops; 200 ml x 15 drops = 3000 drops. Determine number of units per minute; 30 units per hour = 0.5 units per minute. Calculate as follows: 50 units: 3,000 = 0.5 units: X50 units X =1,500; X = 30 drops/minute.

 A. This flow rate delivers 10 units per hour.

 B. This flow rate delivers 15 units per hour.

 C. This flow rate delivers 25 units per hour.

Content Category: Patient Care

References: ENA, Core Curriculum, 2000; pp. 789–799; Skidmore-Roth, 2001.

85.   When evaluating the medication regimen of an older adult, the ED nurse should expect the pre-
       scribed dose to be:
       A. increased due to decreased absorption.
       B. increased due to decreased serum albumin.
       C. DECREASED DUE TO DIMINISHED HEPATIC BLOOD FLOW.
       D. decreased due to reduced gastrointestinal motility.

Rationale:

       C. Medication dosing should be decreased in the geriatric population because drug metabolism,
            especially first-pass metabolism, is decreased. Changes associated with aging, such as decreased
            hepatic blood flow, decrease the amount of drug delivered to the liver. As hepatic function is
            decreased, the presence of the drug in the circulatory system increases. Therefore, doses should
            be decreased in elderly patients.
       A. Drug absorption is one of the pharmacokinetic factors least affected by aging.
       B. Decreased serum albumin increases circulating levels of drugs that are protein bound. In addi-
            tion, polypharmacy provides competition for protein binding sites and increases drug-active
            metabolite levels. Therefore, dosing must be decreased.
       D. Decreased gastric motility does occur with aging; however, it is not a factor in dosing.

Content Category: Patient Care

References: ENA, Core Curriculum, 2000; p. 232; Newberry, 1998.

86.   Which of the following dressings should be applied to a patient with burns over 40% of the body sur-
       face area (BSA) before transfer to a regional burn center?
       A. Silver sulfadiazine (Silvadene) dressings
       B. Mafenide (Sulfamylon) dressings
       C. Sterile, saline-soaked dressings
       D. DRY, STERILE DRESSINGS

Rationale:

       D. Major burns should be covered with dry, sterile dressings before transport. These dressings pro-
            tect damaged tissue without increasing the risk for hypothermia.
       A. Silvadene dressings are appropriate once the burns have been fully evaluated. Application before
            transfer may delay the transfer and definitive treatment once the patient arrives at the burn cen-
            ter, as these dressings must be removed before the burns can be adequately assessed.
       B. Application of topical ointments would delay transfer to the regional burn center and assess-
            ment once the patient arrived there.
       C. A patient with burns is at risk for infection and hypothermia. Wet dressings increase the likeli-
            hood of both.

Content Category: Patient Care

Reference: ENA, Core Curriculum, 2000; p. 189.

87.   An elderly woman taken to a small rural hospital after a motor vehicle crash has a fractured femur,
       multiple pelvic fractures, and numerous lacerations and abrasions. Initial assessment reveals weak,
       thready pulses and cool, clammy skin. The patient is awake, oriented, and asking for water. Ketoro-
       lac tromethamine (Toradol) is given for pain and transfer to a regional trauma center is arranged.
       Copies of the patient's medical records and x-ray films are prepared. This transfer violates EMTALA
       because:

A. the risks of the transfer outweigh the benefits.
B. appropriate acceptance has not been obtained.
C. THE PATIENT HAS NOT BEEN ADEQUATELY STABILIZED.
D. adequate documentation has not been prepared.

Rationale:

C. The clinical presentation of this patient suggests hypovolemic shock. This patient does not have an IV line in place, nor has she received fluids. This places the transferring facility at risk for an EMTALA violation.
A. The benefits of transfer of a major trauma patient from a small rural hospital to a regional trauma center outweigh the risks.
B. Appropriate acceptance has been obtained from the trauma center.
D. Copies of the medical records and x-rays are adequate documentation of care.

Content Category: Patient Care

Reference: ENA, Core Curriculum, 2000; p. 728.

88. Complications associated with pelvic inflammatory disease (PID) may include:
A. tubo-ovarian abscess.
B. pelvic peritonitis.
C. perihepatitis (Fitz-Hugh–Curtis syndrome).
D. ALL OF THE ABOVE.

Rationale:

D. All of the above is the correct answer.
A. Tubo-ovarian abscess is reported in up to one-third of all patients hospitalized with pelvic inflammatory disease.
B. Pelvic peritonitis is a possible complication of PID.
C. Perihepatitis is a possible complication of PID.

Content Category: Genitourinary & Obstetrics & Gynecology

Reference: Tintinalli et al., 2000; p. 720.

89. Discharge teaching for a female with a urinary tract infection should include all of the following EXCEPT:
A. Void frequently and completely.
B. DECREASE CONSUMPTION OF FRUIT JUICE.
C. Void immediately after sexual intercourse.
D. Increase fluid intake.

Rationale:

B. Fruit juice has been shown to increase the acidity of the urine, which may decrease the frequency of urinary tract infections.
A. The bladder should be emptied frequently and completely in an attempt to decrease the frequency of urinary tract infections.
C. A woman who tends to get urinary tract infections should void immediately after sexual intercourse.
D. Fluid intake should be increased.

Content Category: Genitourinary & Obstetrics & Gynecology

Reference: ENA, Core Curriculum, 2000.

90.   Risk factors associated with the development of pelvic inflammatory disease include all of the following EXCEPT:
       A. multiple sexual partners.
       B. younger age.
       C. IUD use.
       D. PREGNANCY.

Rationale:

       D. Pregnancy is not a risk factor for the development of PID. The cervical os is protected by a mucus plug.
       A. Having multiple sexual partners is a risk factor for the development of PID.
       B. Younger age is a risk factor for the development of PID.
       C. IUD use is a risk factor for the development of PID.

Content Category: Genitourinary & Obstetrics & Gynecology

Reference: Tintinalli et al., 2000; p. 720.

Questions 91–95

A 36-year-old female presents to the ED with the complaint of nausea and vomiting for 3 days and reports that she "can't keep anything down." She states that her menses are 3 weeks late. As part of your initial assessment, you obtain a reproductive history. She tells you that she has 3 living children, including a pair of twins, and had one ectopic pregnancy at 10 weeks' gestation and one spontaneous abortion at 12 weeks' gestation.

91.   You would document her reproductive history as:
       A. Gravida 6, Para 3, Abortion 1, Living 3.
       B. Gravida 3, Para 3, Abortion 2, Living 3.
       C. GRAVIDA 4, PARA 2, ABORTION 2, LIVING 3.
       D. Gravida 5, Para 2, Abortion 1, Living 3.

Rationale:

       C. The patient has been pregnant four times. She has not been diagnosed with a pregnancy at this time. Two pregnancies (including one set of twins) have progressed to viability and two others, one of them ectopic, were aborted before viability. "Gravida" represents the total number of pregnancies. "Para" represents the total number of pregnancies that have reached viability (> 500 g). That number is 2, not 3, because of the twins. "Abortions" signifies the number of pregnancies that have been interrupted by either elective or spontaneous abortion before attaining viability.
       A. Incorrect.
       B. Incorrect.
       D. Incorrect.

Content Category: Genitourinary & Obstetrics & Gynecology

Reference: Jarvis, 1996.

92.   Your initial documented assessment of this patient would include all of the following EXCEPT:
       A. FETAL HEART TONES.
       B. orthostatic vital signs.
       C. temperature.
       D. respiratory rate.

Rationale:

> A. Fetal heart tones are detectable by Doppler methods at 10–12 weeks' gestation. Based on the patient's last menstrual cycle, if she were found to be pregnant, she would be at approximately 7 weeks' gestation.
>
> B. These would be assessed for and documented.
>
> C. This would be assessed for and documented.
>
> D. This would be assessed for and documented.

Content Category: Genitourinary & Obstetrics & Gynecology

Reference: Seidel et al., 1999.

93. The nursing diagnosis with the highest priority for this patient would be which of the following?
    A. Alteration in comfort related to nausea
    B. FLUID VOLUME DEFICIT RELATED TO PERSISTENT VOMITING
    C. Knowledge deficit related to disease process
    D. Anxiety related to disease process

Rationale:

> B. The patient is at high risk for dehydration. Therefore, fluid volume deficit is the highest priority at this time.
>
> A. An important diagnosis, but not a priority at this time.
>
> C. An important diagnosis, but not a priority at this time.
>
> D. An important diagnosis, but not a priority at this time.

Content Category: Genitourinary & Obstetrics & Gynecology

Reference: ENA, Core Curriculum, 2000.

94. The Emergency Nurse Practitioner (ENP) orders a serum beta human chorionic gonadotrophin (HCG) level. What is the rationale for this blood test?
    A. To determine whether the patient is pregnant
    B. To determine approximately how many at weeks of gestation her pregnancy has advanced
    C. To obtain a baseline value in order to determine whether the patient has another ectopic pregnancy or is threatening an abortion
    D. ALL OF THE ABOVE

Rationale:

> D. Beta-HCG production occurs in normal and pathologic pregnancy. Beta-HCG rises rapidly early in pregnancy. If the pregnancy is nonviable, the beta-HCG level will fall. Because of the variability in beta-HCG levels, serial quantitative levels are obtained to determine whether the serum level is rising (viable pregnancy) or falling (nonviable pregnancy).
>
> A. Incorrect.
>
> B. Incorrect
>
> C. Incorrect.

Content Category: Genitourinary & Obstetrics & Gynecology

Reference: Tintinalli et al., 2000; pp. 694–702.

95. The ENP performs a bimanual exam on the patient and notes fullness and tenderness to the left adnexal area. The serum beta-HCG test is positive. You would expect the next order to be which of the following?
    A. Radiographic abdominal series
    B. Computed tomography (CT) of the abdomen
    C. PELVIC ULTRASOUND
    D. Abdominal ultrasound

Rationale:

    C. A transvaginal pelvic ultrasound scan can detect a gestational sac at 4 to 5 weeks' gestation. With a positive beta-HCG test and left adnexal tenderness, it is important to rule out an ectopic pregnancy.
    A. Radiation for imaging should be avoided during pregnancy.
    B. Radiation for imaging should be avoided during pregnancy.
    D. An abdominal ultrasound scan cannot be used to evaluate the uterus, ovaries, or fallopian tubes.

Content Category: Genitourinary & Obstetrics & Gynecology

Reference: Tintinalli et al., 2000; pp. 680–686.

Questions 96 and 97

A female who is at 36 weeks' gestation has been involved in a motor vehicle crash (MVC). She was the driver and was not wearing safety restraints. The air bag did not deploy. The patient is brought to your ED via EMS on a backboard with a hard cervical collar and 2 large-bore IVs in place. Oxygen is being delivered via 100% nonrebreather mask (NRM). Vital signs are BP 80/40 mm Hg; HR 138/min, respirations 34/min, and oxygen saturation 98%.

96. Your first priority when caring for this patient and her unborn child is to ensure which of the following?
    A. That fetal heart tones are present
    B. TO MAINTAIN A PATENT AIRWAY
    C. To increase fluid resuscitation in order to decrease heart rate and increase blood pressure
    D. To place the patient on her left side to relieve pressure on the inferior vena cava

Rationale:

    B. Survival of the fetus is wholly dependent on maternal survival. During the initial phase of care, care should be focused entirely on the mother. Maintaining the airway is of highest priority in all trauma care.
    A. Important, but the first priority is to maintain adequate airway.
    C. Important, but the first priority is to maintain adequate airway.
    D. Important, but the first priority is to maintain adequate airway.

Content Category: Genitourinary & Obstetrics & Gynecology

Reference: Tintinalli et al., 2000.

97. During your secondary survey, you note that the patient's abdomen is misshapen and lacks uterine tone. She states that was having contractions prior to the MVC. Immediately following the MVC, she had an episode of intense abdominal pain. She denies having had any contractions since the MVC, but continues to experience diffuse abdominal pain. You determine that the patient most likely has:
    A. abruptio placentae.
    B. placenta previa.

C. RUPTURED UTERUS.

D. a normal pregnant uterus.

Rationale:

C. Ruptured uterus classically presents with a sudden onset of intense abdominal pain. The abdomen has an abnormal contour and may assume the shape of the fetus. A ruptured uterus is associated with a 32% rate of fetal mortality, but less than 1% maternal mortality with rapid intervention.

A. Abruptio placentae is the premature separation of a normally implanted placenta. Abruptio placentae presents with painful vaginal bleeding and uterine tenderness, increased uterine tone, and hyperactivity.

B. Placenta previa is associated with a low-lying placenta. The placenta may either completely or partial cover the cervical os. The patient usually presents with painless vaginal bleeding in a previously normal pregnancy.

D. A normal pregnant uterus is smooth and round.

Content Category: Genitourinary & Obstetrics & Gynecology

Reference: Hacker & Moore, 1998.

98. Rabies prophylaxis should be considered for patients bitten by any of the following EXCEPT:

A. bats.

B. raccoons.

C. dogs.

D. HAMSTERS.

Rationale:

D. Hamsters and other rodents such as squirrels, mice, rats, chipmunks, gerbils, guinea pigs, and rabbits have not caused rabies in the United States.

A. Rabies is carried by bats.

B. Rabies is carried by raccoons.

C. Humans can be indirectly infected by dogs, cats, and other domestic animals. Pets with an uncertain vaccination history can be quarantined for 10 days in lieu of initiating rabies prophylaxis.

Content Category: Orthopedics & Wound Care

References: Sheehy, 1997; pp. 251–261; Garcia, 1999; pp. 91–107.

99. A patient presents to the ED with a laceration of the left eyebrow. Wound preparation includes all of the following EXCEPT:

A. wound irrigation.

B. tetanus prophylaxis.

C. local anesthesia.

D. SHAVING THE EYEBROW.

Rationale:

D. Shaving the eyebrow can cause difficulty with alignment when suturing. In addition, it may prevent complete regrowth.

A. All lacerations should be irrigated.

B. Tetanus prophylaxis should be administered if needed.

C. Local anesthesia should be administered before wound repair.

Content Category: Orthopedics& Wound Care

Reference: Proehl, 1999; pp. 446–449.

100.   Treatment for carpal tunnel syndrome includes anti-inflammatory medication and:
    A. elastic compression bandage.
    B. sling.
    C. VOLAR COCKUP SPLINT.
    D. thumb spica splint.

Rationale:

   C. A volar cockup splint keeps the wrist in a neutral position that lessens pressure on the median nerve.
   A. An elastic compression bandage would support the wrist but would not keep the wrist immobilized in the neutral position.
   B. A sling would elevate the arm but would not immobilize the wrist in the neutral position.
   D. A thumb spica splint would immobilize the thumb, but not necessarily the wrist.

Content Category: Orthopedics & Wound Care

Reference: Sheehy & Lenehan, 1999; pp. 487–536.

101.   Initial treatment for a scaphoid fracture is:
    A. ulnar gutter splint.
    B. volar splint.
    C. sugar tong splint.
    D. THUMB SPICA SPLINT.

Rationale:

   D. The thumb spica splint provides immobilization of the scaphoid bone, fractures of the first metacarpal, and soft-tissue injuries.
   A. Ulnar gutter splints are used for fractures or soft-tissue injuries of the fourth and fifth metacarpals.
   B. Volar splints are used for fractures of the wrist or other carpal bones.
   C. Sugar tong splints are used for fractures of the radius and ulna.

Content Category: Orthopedics & Wound Care

Reference: Proehl, 1999; pp. 410–417.

102.   The organism responsible for early cellulitis (less than 24 hours) after a cat bite is most likely which of the following?
    A. *Staphylococcus aureus*
    B. *Moraxella catarrhalis*
    C. *PASTEURELLA MULTOCIDA*
    D. *Rochalimaea henselae*

Rationale:

   C. *Pasteurella multocida* is most often the cause of early cellulitis following a cat bite.
   A. *Staphylococcus aureus* cellulitis generally occurs more than 24 hours after injury.
   B. *Moraxella catarrhalis* is not an organism found in the cat mouth.
   D. *Rochalimaea henselae* is the organism responsible for cat scratch fever, not cellulitis.

Content Category: Orthopedics & Wound Care

References: Sheehy, 1997; pp. 255–261; Sheehy & Lenehan, 1999; pp. 369–381.

103.   Correct crutch walking includes instruction to:
   A. AVOID AXILLARY PRESSURE ON THE CRUTCH.
   B. wear sandals.
   C. keep the elbows flexed to 90 degrees.
   D. keep the crutch tips 12 inches to the side and front of the foot.

Rationale:

   A. Pressure on the axilla may cause damage to the brachial plexus.
   B. The patient should wear sturdy, supportive shoes to prevent falls. Sandals could cause falls.
   C. The arms should be flexed at 30 degrees, not 90 degrees.
   D. The tips of crutches should be held 6 to 8 inches to the side and front, not 12 inches.

Content Category: Orthopedics & Wound Care

References: Sheehy, 1997; pp. 255–261; Proehl, 1999; pp. 437–442.

104.   An orthopedic emergency that usually requires surgical intervention is:
   A. talus fracture.
   B. elbow dislocation.
   C. bimalleolar fracture.
   D. KNEE DISLOCATION.

Rationale:

   D. A knee dislocation threatens the popliteal artery and therefore the limb.
   A. A talus fracture may need intraoperative repair but seldom threatens the limb.
   B. Elbow dislocations may need surgical intervention but seldom threaten the limb.
   C. Bimalleolar fractures need operative intervention but do not generally threaten the limb.

Content Category: Orthopedics & Wound Care

Reference: Bayley & Turcke, 1998; pp. 415–447.

105.   A 21-year-old male is receiving care for a plantar puncture wound after stepping on a nail. The footwear that carries the greatest risk for serious infections from this type of injury is:
   A. plastic sandals.
   B. SNEAKERS.
   C. leather work boots.
   D. leather dress shoes.

Rationale:

   B. The risk of osteomyelitis from *Pseudomonas aeruginosa* is greatest after puncture wounds through the rubber found in sneakers and tennis shoes.
   A. *Pseudomonas* and other virulent organisms are not found in plastic shoes.
   C. Leather does not hoard *Pseudomonas*. Antibiotics that cover normal skin flora may be needed.
   D. Leather does not hoard *Pseudomonas*.

Content Category: Orthopedics & Wound Care

Reference: Trott, 1997; pp. 285–314.

Questions 106–108

A 54-year-old male patient is transferred to the ED from the scene after his right hand and forearm were crushed in a cardboard bailing machine. There is severe tissue damage with unknown bony involvement to the right hand and forearm. The patient fainted briefly after the accident but is currently awake, alert, and oriented. Vital signs are BP 156/98 mm Hg, HR 112/min, and respirations 24/min. The patient is moaning in extreme pain. EMS personnel established an IV of Ringer's lactate and administered IV meperidine (Demerol).

106.   Upon the patient's arrival at the ED, the ED nurse should *first*:
   A. establish a second large-bore IV.
   B. prepare the patient for immediate surgery.
   C. PERFORM PRIMARY AND SECONDARY SURVEYS.
   D. administer more pain medication.

Rationale:

   C. The first duty of the ED nurse is to perform primary and secondary surveys on the patient. This is done to establish a baseline and comparative assessment with EMS findings and determine whether any other life-threatening injuries are present.
   A. All patients with significant injury need a second large-bore IV; however, initiating it should not be the nurse's first action.
   B. Eventually this patient will need surgery, but it is not the priority. The neurovascular assessment and the physician's plan will determine when this patient will have surgery.
   D. Pain medication is important but can be administered only with a physician's order and after an initial assessment has been completed.

Content Category: Orthopedics & Wound Care

References: ENA, Core Curriculum, 2000; pp. 501–535; ENA, Trauma Nursing, 2000.

107.   The patient's right hand is splinted and appears to be swollen, discolored, and deformed. The patient is not moving the extremity. The nurse should assess the extremity for pallor and:
   A. PAIN, PARESTHESIA, PARALYSIS, AND PULSE.
   B. previous injury, pulse, paresthesia, and paralysis.
   C. pain, paralysis, paresthesia, and projectiles.
   D. position, pain, paralysis, and pulse.

Rationale:

   A. Crush injuries need to be assessed on multiple levels, including cellular destruction, vessel and nerve damage, and tissue involvement. The 5 P's allow the ED nurse to assess all of the above.
   B. Previous injury is important in the patient's history and should be assessed during the primary and secondary assessment. In addition, the pain assessment of the 5 P's is missing.
   C. The adequacy of circulation is not completely evaluated unless the pulse is assessed. The search for projectiles is important and could be a priority, depending on the mechanism, but that is not likely with this patient's crush injury.
   D. While position of the extremity is important, it is assessed in the overall circulation, motion, and sensation (CMS) check. Should the ED nurse suspect a decrease in CMS, the splint should be removed and the position of the affected extremity checked and possibly repositioned.

Content Category: Orthopedics & Wound Care

Reference: ENA, Core Curriculum, 2000; pp. 501–535.

108. The patient's right hand is splinted and appears to be swollen, discolored, and deformed. The patient complains that the pain is becoming more intense and he can no longer feel his fingers. The nurse notes that the fingers are pale and dusky and more swollen than before. The splint is loosened, but there is no change in the hand. The nurse should suspect that the patient has developed:

    A. a blood clot that is occluding the blood flow to the hand.

    B. a fatty embolism.

    C. COMPARTMENT SYNDROME.

    D. venous thrombus.

Rationale:

    C. Compartment syndrome tends to occur most often in the distal aspect of an extremity. It is common with fractures and crush injuries and develops when there is increased internal pressure as a result of soft-tissue swelling and bleeding. Elevated internal pressure causes vascular and neurologic structures to be compromised.

    A. The patient may develop a blood clot, but this is more common with a large-bone fracture.

    B. It is highly unlikely for a fatty embolus to develop from a fracture distal to the humerus. Fatty emboli are associated with fractures of the large bones, such as the femur.

    D. The findings above are suggestive of arterial rather than venous occlusion.

Content Category: Orthopedics & Wound Care

Reference: ENA, Core Curriculum, 2000; pp. 501–535.

109. A 48-year-old man is on call for operative repair of an angulated femur fracture sustained in a skiing accident. During reassessment, the nurse notes that he is pale, diaphoretic, and complaining of shortness of breath. Vital signs are HR 124/min, respirations 34/min, and oxygen saturation 84%. The ED nurse should suspect that the patient is experiencing:

    A. an anxiety attack.

    B. a myocardial infarction.

    C. a panic disorder.

    D. FAT EMBOLISM SYNDROME.

Rationale:

    D. Patients may experience fat embolism syndrome after fracturing or undergoing long-bone surgery. The patient may experience tachypnea, tachycardia, hypoxemia, and fever. Fatty emboli are released from the fractured long bone and released into the blood system.

    A. This is a possibility, but unlikely, since the oxygen saturation is low.

    B. This is also a possibility, but the patient is relatively young and no other clinical evidence has been presented that suggests MI.

    C. This is a possibility, but unlikely, since oxygen saturation would be expected to be elevated.

Content Category: Orthopedics & Wound Care

Reference: ENA, Core Curriculum, 2000; pp. 501–535.

110.   An elderly female is brought to the ED complaining of right hip pain and inability to walk after a fall. Which of the following places her at risk for osteoporosis?
    A. Lacto-ovarian vegetarian diet
    B. Large skeletal frame
    C. African-American ethnicity
    D. SMOKING

Rationale:

    D. A smoking history is associated with increased risk for osteoporosis.
    A. Milk products are permissible in the lacto-ovarian vegetarian diet; therefore, acceptable calcium intake can be achieved.
    B. Individuals with small frames are predisposed to osteoporosis.
    C. There is a higher incidence of osteoporosis in Asian and Caucasian backgrounds.

Content Category: Orthopedics & Wound Care
Reference: Snider, 1997; pp. 2–69.

111.   A 5-year-old child is carried into the ED by her father with a toothpick impaled in the plantar aspect of her foot. Which of the interventions below should be implemented by the ED nurse?
    A. Soak the foot in iodine/saline solution.
    B. ASSESS DISTAL NEUROVASCULAR STATUS.
    C. Cleanse the area with hydrogen peroxide.
    D. Obtain an x-ray.

Rationale:

    B. Distal neurovascular status should be assessed to determine whether there is damage to underlying structures.
    A. Soaking should be avoided, since the wooden toothpick would absorb the solution and swell.
    C. Hydrogen peroxide is a poor bacteriocidal solution; there are more effective solutions for cleaning the area after the foreign body has been removed.
    D. Wood objects are not radiopaque; therefore, an x-ray would not provide any useful information.

Content Category: Orthopedics & Wound Care
Reference: Trott, 1997; pp. 1–11.

112.   An elderly female is brought to the ED complaining of right hip pain and inability to walk following a fall. Approaching the bed, the nurse notes that the patient's right leg is shortened and externally rotated. Formal assessment of the leg should begin with:
    A. INSPECTION OF THE LEG FOR ANY BRUISING, SWELLING, OR BREAKS IN THE SKIN.
    B. palpation of the leg for areas of tenderness.
    C. evaluation of restrictions by moving the leg through range of motion.
    D. auscultation over the femoral area to search for bruits.

Rationale:

    A. All physical assessments should begin with inspection. This can help identify potential areas of underlying injury.
    B. Palpation for tenderness is essential, but should not be the first maneuver.
    C. The shortened, externally rotated leg should raise the suspicion of hip fracture; therefore, the leg should not be placed through range of motion evaluation.
    D. Auscultation for bruits is performed to search for vascular injury, not orthopedic injuries.

Content Category: Orthopedics & Wound Care

Reference: ENA, Core Curriculum, 2000; pp. 501–535.

113. Which of the following heart sounds would you expect to hear in a patient with pericardial tamponade?
   A. MUFFLED HEART TONES
   B. Pericardial friction rub
   C. Systolic ejection murmur
   D. S_3 gallop

Rationale:

   A. Because of the surrounding layer of pericardial fluid, heart sounds are muffled, distant, or inaudible.
   B. A pericardial friction rub is heard in patients with an inflamed pericardium.
   C. A systolic ejection murmur occurs in the presence of heart valve defects.
   D. An S_3 gallop is heard when the heart is overfull, as in congestive heart failure.

Content Category: Cardiovascular

Reference: Oman et al., 2001; pp. 151–160.

114. Which of the following cardiovascular assessment findings is associated with cardiac tamponade?
   A. Pulsus magnus
   B. PULSUS PARADOXUS
   C. Pulsus alternans
   D. Pulsus parvus

Rationale:

   A. Pulsus paradoxus is an exaggerated decrease in systolic blood pressure with inspiration. In the patient with pericardial tamponade, even the normal increase in intrathoracic pressure associated with inspiration is enough to drop cardiac output.
   B. Pulsus magnus is a readily palpable pulse that is not easily obliterated and does not fade.
   C. In patients with pulsus alternans, pulse amplitude varies from beat to beat.
   D. Pulsus parvus is a pulse that is difficult to palpate and that can easily be obliterated by finger pressure.

Content Category: Cardiovascular

Reference: Dennison, 2000.

115. Which of the following is the initial diagnostic study of choice for the patient with suspected traumatic aortic injury?
   A. CHEST RADIOGRAPHY
   B. Computed tomography
   C. Aortography
   D. Transesophageal echocardiography

Rationale:

   A. Chest radiography is the best initial screening exam for aortic injury. Look for the presence of a widened (>8 mm) mediastinum.
   B. Helical CT is very useful for detecting aortic injury but is not an initial screening exam.
   C. Although not 100% accurate, aortic angiography remains the gold standard for diagnosis of aortic injuries. However, this study cannot be performed as part of the initial resuscitation.
   D. Transesophageal echocardiography may be used in the ED but takes several minutes to perform and requires the presence of a skilled operator.

Content Category: Cardiovascular

Reference: Mattox et al., 2000; pp. 559–582.

116. A blunt trauma patient with a descending thoracic aortic tear has been rapidly transfused with 12 units of packed red blood cells. Based on the following information, the ED nurse should anticipate infusion of which blood product?

BP 92/64 mm Hg	PT 38 sec	Hct 30%
HR 132/min	PTT 105 sec	
Respirations 19/min	PLT 88,000/mm^3	
	Hgb 11 g/dl	

   A. FRESH FROZEN PLASMA
   B. Cryoprecipitate
   C. Platelets
   D. Packed red blood cells

Rationale:

   A. Fresh frozen plasma expands vascular volume and restores a wide variety of clotting factors to correct the PT/PTT.
   B. Cryoprecipitate restores some clotting factors but is more expensive and more complicated to prepare and administer than fresh frozen plasma. It does not expand vascular volume and is not used as an initial treatment for prolonged PT/PTT.
   C. This patient's platelet count is adequate.
   D. Packed red blood cells contain no clotting factors and would not correct PT/PTT.

Content Category: Cardiovascular

Reference: Dennison, 2000.

117. On physical assessment of a blunt trauma patient, which of the following findings would lead the ED nurse to suspect a thoracic aortic injury?
   A. Subxiphoid tenderness to palpation
   B. Crushing back pain between the scapulae
   C. TEARING BACK PAIN BETWEEN THE SCAPULAE
   D. Squeezing pain radiating down the left arm

Rationale:

   C. The pain associated with a thoracic aortic injury radiates to the back and is described as excruciating and tearing in quality.
   A. Chest tenderness to palpation is characteristic of injury to or inflammation of the chest wall.
   B. Crushing substernal chest pain is classically associated with acute myocardial infarction.
   D. Squeezing pain radiating down the left arm is characteristic of angina or acute myocardial infarction.

Content Category: Cardiovascular

Reference: Oman et al., 2001; pp. 151–160.

118. In a patient who has sustained chest trauma from a motor vehicle collision, which of the following findings on a chest radiograph would be consistent with aortic injury?
    A. Calcified aortic knob
    B. WIDENED MEDIASTINUM
    C. Hilar infiltrates
    D. Pneumomediastinum

Rationale:

B. A widened mediastinum (>8 mm at the level of the aortic knob) is grossly suggestive of aortic injury and requires further investigation.
A. A calcified aortic knob is an indicator of aortic vascular disease.
C. Hilar infiltrates are associated with early pulmonary edema.
D. Pneumomediastinum indicates a tear to the lungs or bronchial system.

Content Category: Cardiovascular

Reference: Oman et al., 2001; pp. 151–160.

119. Which of the following is the most common site of fatal aortic tearing after blunt trauma?
    A. DESCENDING THORACIC AORTA
    B. Abdominal aorta
    C. Ascending thoracic aorta
    D. Aortic arch

Rationale:

A. Because of its proximity to the fixed ligamentum arteriosum, the descending thoracic aorta is the site of approximately 60% of fatal tears.
B. The abdominal aorta is uncommonly injured in blunt trauma.
C. Injuries to the ascending thoracic aorta are much less common than are those to the descending aorta.
D. Injuries to the aortic arch are much less common than are those to the descending aorta.

Content Category: Cardiovascular

Reference: Mattox et al., 2000; pp. 559–582.

120. Which of the following cardiovascular assessment findings is indicative of an aortic arch injury after blunt trauma?
    A. BLOOD PRESSURE IN THE LEFT ARM IS LOWER THAN IN THE RIGHT.
    B. Femoral pulse is weaker on the left than on the right.
    C. Pulsus paradoxus is present on inspiration.
    D. Carotid bruit is palpable on the left but absent on the right.

Rationale:

A. Injury to the aortic arch can cause complete or partial obstruction of the innominate or subclavian vessels, reducing blood pressure and pulse amplitude in the left arm.
B. An aortic injury may cause diminution of both femoral pulses, but they should be equal in strength.
C. Pulsus paradoxus is associated with pericardial tamponade.
D. Bruits result from increased turbulence in a vessel.

Content Category: Cardiovascular

Reference: Mattox et al., 2000; pp. 559–582.

121. Which of the following is indicative of arterial trauma?
A. Bounding pulse
B. BRUIT
C. Murmur
D. Pulsus paradoxus

Rationale:

B. Bruits occur as a result of turbulent flow at the site of vessel injury. Their presence indicates disruption, but not complete separation.
A. In the presence of arterial injury, pulse intensity is diminished.
C. A murmur is heard only in the heart.
D. Pulsus paradoxus is associated with cardiac tamponade.

Content Category: Cardiovascular

Reference: Bayley & Turcke, 1998; pp. 501–514.

122. Which of the following mechanisms of arterial trauma is generally the most difficult to repair?
A. Stab wound
B. CRUSH INJURY
C. Blunt trauma
D. Partial-thickness burn

Rationale:

B. Crush injuries destroy large portions of arteries and their surrounding tissues, making repair very difficult.
A. An artery that has been cleanly cut is the easiest to repair.
C. Blunt arterial trauma is associated with contusions and partial vessel tears that are prone to thrombus formation.
D. Partial-thickness burns are limited to the dermal tissues that do not contain major arteries.

Content Category: Cardiovascular

Reference: Bayley & Turcke, 1998; pp. 501–514.

123. Which of the following is a complication of peripheral arterial injury?
A. Deep-vein thrombosis
B. Compartment syndrome
C. Fat embolism syndrome
D. INTIMAL DISRUPTION

Rationale:

D. Injuries to the arteries may involve all vascular layers or only the intima.
A. Deep-vein thrombosis is associated with venous, not arterial, injury.
B. Compartment syndrome may occur in conjunction with arterial injury but is not a direct result of it.
C. Fat embolism syndrome is a sequela of long-bone fracture.

Content Category: Cardiovascular

Reference: Bayley & Turcke, 1998; pp. 501–514.

124. Which of the following arterial injuries commonly results in the greatest amount of blood loss?
A. Complete vessel transection
B. Intimal flap tear

C. Arterial crush injury

D. ARTERIAL WALL LACERATION

Rationale:

D. Incomplete tears of the arterial wall are associated with significant hemorrhage.

A. Complete transaction of the artery causes the muscular ends of the cut vessel to curl inward, thereby limiting hemorrhage.

B. An intimal flap tear occludes only the vessel lumen and is associated with thrombosis, not bleeding.

C. Arterial crush injuries tend to thrombose or ooze blood.

Content Category: Cardiovascular

Reference: Bayley & Turcke, 1998; pp. 501–514.

125.   In a patient with significant hemorrhage from penetrating trauma to the iliac artery, which of the following interventions would be contraindicated?

A. TOURNIQUET APPLICATION

B. Direct pressure to the site of injury

C. Surgical exploration of the wound

D. Reverse Trendelenburg positioning

Rationale:

A. Since the iliac artery is in the pelvis, tourniquet application would be impractical.

B. Direct pressure to the site of injury would be the first intervention to control hemorrhage to this site.

C. Surgical exploration of the wound and vascular repair are probably indicated.

D. Reverse Trendelenburg positioning may be of short-term benefit if the patient is significantly hypovolemic.

Content Category: Cardiovascular

Reference: Bayley & Turcke, 1998; pp. 501–514.

126.   Envenomation from a jellyfish, Portuguese man-of-war, or sea wasp can produce which the following symptoms?

A. Swelling

B. Hallucinations

C. Cardiac dysrhythmias

D. DERMATITIS

Rationale:

D. Dermatitis may be caused by envenomation of marine animals, especially those listed in the above question.

A. Severe swelling is caused by spiny creatures, such as sting rays and sea urchins, that cause puncture wounds and lacerations.

B. Envenomation by none of the listed animals would cause hallucinations.

C. Envenomation by none of the listed animals would cause cardiac dysrhythmias.

Content Category: Substance Abuse & Toxicological & Environmental

References: Newberry, 1998; p. 634; Oman et al., 2001; p. 102.

127.   As the evening charge nurse in the ED, you have been notified that you will be receiving patients who were exposed to the chemical agent sarin. Signs and symptoms of cholinergic toxicity include which of the following?
A. Pulmonary congestion
B. MIOSIS
C. Dry mouth
D. Diarrhea

Rationale:

B. Miosis (pupil constriction) is a common sign and symptom of cholinergic toxicity.
A. Although pulmonary congestion may be present, it is not a common sign of cholinergic toxicity.
C. Increased salivation rather than dry mouth is noted.
D. Diarrhea is not a common sign of cholinergic toxicity.

Content Category: Substance Abuse & Toxicological & Environmental
Reference: Oman et al., 2001; p. 115.

128.   The most likely nursing diagnosis for a patient with a hydrocarbon inhalation would be:
A. IMPAIRED GAS EXCHANGE
B. body image disturbance.
C. impaired physical mobility.
D. decreased cardiac output.

Rationale:

A. Inhalation of hydrocarbons may lead to chemical pneumonitis. Pulmonary edema is a common finding.
B. Body image disturbance is not a common issue with hydrocarbon inhalation.
C. Although impaired physical mobility may develop, this is not a primary nursing diagnosis.
D. Decreased cardiac output may also be a consideration, but impaired gas exchange is of top priority.

Content Category: Substance Abuse & Toxicological & Environmental
Reference: ENA, Core Curriculum, 2000; pp. 651–653.

129.   An ice skater does not follow the rules of the rink and skates on the ice during the cleaning procedure. As the large Zamboni machine crosses the ice, the skater collapses. What is the most likely cause?
A. Hydrocarbon exposure
B. CARBON MONOXIDE TOXICITY
C. Cyanide inhalation
D. Nitrogen narcosis

Rationale:

B. The Zamboni, an ice rink cleaning machine, emits carbon monoxide as it operates. For this reason, the rink is to be cleared during its operation. Since the carbon monoxide is odorless and colorless, a person may not realize the exposure level and may suddenly lose consciousness.
A. Not associated with this type of emergency.
C. Not associated with this type of emergency.
D. Not associated with this type of emergency.

Content Category: Substance Abuse & Toxicological & Environmental
Reference: Herington & Morse, 1995.

130. An elderly patient is brought to the ED by EMS. S/he states that chest pain started about 1 hour ago. The patient states that the problem was indigestion and admits to having ingested an entire full bottle of Rolaids antacid. You note an empty bottle whose label reads, "100 Fruit-flavored Rolaids, Extra Strength." You would be concerned about an overdose of:
    A. sodium.
    B. CALCIUM.
    C. phosphorus.
    D. potassium.

Rationale:

    B. Rolaids Antacid, Extra Strength, contain 675 mg of calcium carbonate and 135 mg of magnesium hydroxide per tablet. Ingesting 100 tablets would constitute a primary overdose of calcium.

    A. Sodium is not a component of Rolaids.

    C. Phosphorus is not a component of Rolaids.

    D. Potassium is not a component of Rolaids.

Content Category: Substance Abuse & Toxicological & Environmental

Reference: Skidmore-Roth, 2001.

131. An adult patient has taken more than 40 mg/kg of acetaminophen (Tylenol). What is the only reliable indicator of the potential hepatic damage?
    A. SERUM ACETAMINOPHEN LEVEL
    B. Potassium level
    C. Arterial blood gases (ABGs)
    D. Urine toxicology screen

Rationale:

    A. Serum acetaminophen levels that are indicative of the potential hepatic damage must be obtained at 4 hours after the ingestion.

    B. It is important to obtain a potassium level if there is inhalant toxicity.

    C. ABGs should be checked to measure acidosis in salicylate poisoning.

    D. A urine toxicology screen cannot be used to measure hepatic damage because acetaminophen is excreted in the liver, not in the kidneys.

Content Category: Substance Abuse & Toxicological & Environmental

Reference: ENA, Core Curriculum, 2000; pp. 640–641.

132. One possible intervention needed for an inhaled hydrocarbon is:
    A. activated charcoal.
    B. syrup of ipecac.
    C. to increase the administration of intravenous fluids.
    D. SODIUM BICARBONATE.

Rationale:

    D. Sodium bicarbonate will help alleviate the metabolic acidosis.

    A. Activated charcoal does not effectively bind with hydrocarbons.

    B. Syrup of ipecac is contraindicated because of the risk of aspiration.

    C. Increasing intravenous fluids increases the risk of fluid overload and pulmonary edema.

Content Category: Substance Abuse & Toxicological & Environmental

Reference: ENA, Core Curriculum, 2000; p. 636.

133.   You are caring for a patient who has a fractured hip. As you prepare the patient for surgery, you learn that s/he Echinacea daily to prevent colds. Based on your knowledge of Echinacea, you would be concerned about an unfavorable reaction if the patient were to receive:
   A.   anticoagulants.
   B.   IMMUNOSUPPRESSANTS.
   C.   anesthetics.
   D.   anticonvulsants.

Rationale:

   B.   Echinacea is an herbal medication that is used to stimulate the immune system. Some believe it can be effective in symptom reduction and for prophylaxis of colds, flu, and other upper respiratory infections. Echinacea may interfere with immunosuppressive therapy.
   A.   Although some herbal medications may alter anticoagulants, this is not described for Echinacea.
   C.   There have been no documented issues with anesthetics.
   D.   No interaction has been described with anticonvulsants.

Content Category: Substance Abuse & Toxicological & Environmental

Reference: ENA, Core Curriculum, 2000.

134.   A child is brought to the ED screaming. The mother states that the child has chewed several leaves of a dieffenbachia plant. You note some bloody emesis on the child's shirt, increased salivation, and a swollen tongue. Treatment for this type of ingestion should include:
   A.   ICE TO LIPS AND MILK TO FLUSH OUT THE MOUTH.
   B.   warm compresses to lips and IV atropine.
   C.   charcoal to the lips and physostigmine (Antilirium) IV.
   D.   lubricant to lips and hydrogen peroxide mouthwash.

Rationale:

   A.   Dieffenbachia contains oxalic acids. The crystal needles of the calcium oxalate produce severe pain when ingested. Symptoms include bloody emesis, diarrhea, pain, and a burning sensation. Treatment includes applying ice to the lips and oral area to decrease swelling and administration of milk or water to flush out oxalic crystals from the oral cavity.
   B.   Warm compresses may further enhance the swelling. Atropine would not be indicated.
   C.   Charcoal to the lips would accomplish no purpose. Physostigmine (Antilirium) is given for an anticholinergic overdose.
   D.   A lubricant to the lips after ice may be appropriate, but hydrogen peroxide to the mouth would not be indicated.

Content Category: Substance Abuse & Toxicological & Environmental

Reference: ENA, Core Curriculum, 2000; p. 658.

135.   A bus driver is brought to the ED following a crash. S/he has several minor abrasions and edema to the left ankle. Vital signs are BP 140/80 mm Hg, HR 80/min, and respirations 18/min. Because of a Department of Transportation requirement, the patient is given a breath alcohol test. S/he gives permission and the test is administered. The results are positive for alcohol (0.04). The patient denies the use of alcohol. Which of the following over-the-counter products might be the source of the positive alcohol test?
   A.   Scope mouthwash
   B.   Alka-Seltzer cold tablets
   C.   NYQUIL COLD MEDICATION
   D.   Arrid Extra Dry Deodorant

Rationale:

C. NyQuil is an over-the-counter cold product that contains 10% alcohol. This is equivalent to ingestion of 20-proof alcohol, which would denote a positive reading on the breath alcohol scale.

A. Many mouthwashes contain alcohol. Unless the mouthwash is ingested, it will dissipate from the mouth after a few minutes. In the procedure for a breath alcohol test, if a screening test is positive for alcohol, the patient is asked to wait 15 minutes to allow any "mouth" alcohol to dissipate.

B. Although Alka-Seltzer cold tablets may cause a change in mentation, they do not contain alcohol.

D. Unless Arrid Extra Dry Deodorant has been ingested, its use should not alter a breath alcohol test.

Content Category: Substance Abuse & Toxicological & Environmental

Reference: Department of Transportation, 2000.

136. A drug of choice for treatment of suspected organophosphate poisoning would be:
A. naloxone (Narcan).
B. physostigmine (Antilirium).
C. PRALIDOXIME (2-PAM).
D. flumazenil (Romazicon).

Rationale:

C. Pralidoxime (2-PAM) is utilized as an antidote for organophosphate poisoning because it releases binding of the insecticide. Atropine is given to ease symptoms.

A. Naloxone (Narcan) is a narcotic antidote.

B. Physostigmine (Antilirium) is an anticholinergic antidote.

D. Flumazenil (Romazicon) is a benzodiazepine antidote.

Content Category: Substance Abuse & Toxicological & Environmental

References: ENA, Core Curriculum, 2000; pp. 652–653; Skidmore-Roth, 2001.

137. A patient is discharged from the ED following an evaluation for dizziness. Upon evaluation, the patient is found to have mild hypertension. The provider has prescribed verapamil (Calan). In addition to returning to the family physician for follow-up and monitoring of blood pressure, what additional teaching point should be stressed with the patient and family?
A. Decrease fluid intake and discontinue any fiber.
B. Continue to drink 3–4 cups of regular coffee daily.
C. MONITOR AND RECORD HEART RATE PRIOR TO TAKING MEDICATION.
D. May take over-the-counter drugs except aspirin and acetaminophen (Tylenol).

Rationale:

C. Because of the potential for bradycardia posed by taking a calcium channel blocker, the heart rate should be closely monitored and recorded. The physician should be contacted and the medication withheld if the heart rate is less than 60 bpm.

A. Fluids and fiber should be increased to counteract constipation.

B. Caffeine consumption should be limited and no alcohol products should be consumed while the patient is taking calcium channel blockers.

D. All over-the-counter drugs should be avoided except as directed by the physician.

Content Category: Substance Abuse & Toxicological & Environmental

Reference: Skidmore-Roth, 2001.

138.   A patient in the hospital becomes confused and disoriented. S/he pulls leaves from a lily-of-the-valley plant and eats several of them. The floor nurse brings the patient to the ED for treatment. As the triage nurse, you would choose the following triage category:
A. EMERGENT
B. Urgent
C. Nonurgent
D. Refer back to medical floor

Rationale:

A. Because Lily-of-the-Valley ingestion may cause decreased cardiac excitability and hyperkalemia, this patient should receive emergent treatment. Extreme bradycardia may be noted.
B. As noted above, this patient should be triaged as emergent.
C. Same as above.
D. Same as above.

Content Category: Substance Abuse & Toxicological & Environmental
Reference: ENA, Core Curriculum, 2000; p. 658.

139.   A patient presents to the Urgent Care Center for treatment following an injury at work. The patient has a laceration to the left hand. The company protocol mandates that a urine drug screen be performed on all worker's compensation injuries. After you assess the wound and perform vital signs, you ask the patient to sign a permit for the urine drug screen. The patient refuses to sign the permit. You should:
A. collect a urine specimen as part of your assessment and send for drug screen.
B. note the refusal on the permit and continue to collect the specimen.
C. DISCONTINUE THE DRUG SCREEN PROCESS AND NOTIFY THE EMPLOYER.
D. omit the drug screen and continue treating the patient.

Rationale:

C. The drug screening procedure should be discontinued if the patient refuses to sign a permission form for it. Although the test has been requested by the employer, the employee must give permission before it can be done. The employer should be notified.
A. The patient must give permission for the drug screen to be done.
B. You should note the refusal in the nursing documentation, but the drug screen cannot be performed without the patient's permission.
D. Because the company has requested that a urine drug screen be done on the worker's compensation case, the company should be notified.

Content Category: Substance Abuse & Toxicological & Environmental
Reference: Herington & Morse, 1995.

140.   The drug of choice used for the reversal effects of opiates is:
A. N-acetylcysteine (Mucomyst).
B. flumazenil (Romazicon).
C. syrup of ipecac.
D. NALOXONE (NARCAN).

Rationale:

    D. Naloxone (Narcan) is an opioid receptor antagonist. It competes for binding sites at all opioid receptor types (mu, kappa, and delta). Naloxone reverses narcotic-induced respiratory depression, sedation, miosis, analgesia, euphoria, urinary and GI stasis, and bradycardia.

    A. N-acetylcysteine (Mucomyst) is an efficacious antidote for acetaminophen poisoning. It prevents toxicity by enhancing glutathione synthesis and neutralizes the toxicity of the intermediary metabolite N-acetyl-p-benzoquinone amine.

    B. Flumazenil (Romazicon) is the drug of choice for the reversal effects of benzodiazepines. It is a competitive antagonist at the benzodiazepine receptor site; it reverses the sedation effect of benzodiazepine.

    C. Syrup of ipecac is used for gastrointestinal decontamination by inducing vomiting.

Content Category: Substance Abuse & Toxicological & Environmental

Reference: Aghababian et al., 1998; pp. 1002–1005.

141. Upon assessing a victim of a head-on motor vehicle crash, you note that the patient has moderate respiratory difficulty. He is tachycardic and anxious and has jugular vein distention as well as decreased capillary refill. There is equal lung expansion, but on auscultation you note distant lung sounds in the left lower lobe and dullness to percussion. You would suspect what injury?

    A. Tension pneumothorax
    B. HEMOTHORAX
    C. Pneumothorax
    D. Pulmonary contusion

Rationale:

    B. A bleeding hemothorax can manifest in signs and symptoms of shock. Lung sounds are distant to the examiner listening through fluid. Percussion produces a dull sound.

    A. With a tension pneumothorax, you would have noted a deviated trachea toward the right, paradoxical movement of the chest, and distant heart sounds.

    C. A pneumothorax would present with tachypnea, and tachycardia. Hyperresonance would be produced on percussion.

    D. Hemoptysis and an ineffective cough are hallmarks of pulmonary contusion.

Content Category: Trauma & Shock

Reference: Sheehy & Lenehan, 1999; pp. 459–474.

142. How is the Glasgow Coma Scale (GCS) related to the Trauma Score?

    A. THE GLASGOW COMA SCALE IS PART OF THE TRAUMA SCORE.
    B. The Glasgow Coma Scale provides a survival percentage equivalency.
    C. A Glasgow Coma Scale score of less than 5 invalidates the Trauma Scale.
    D. The Trauma Score is part of the Glasgow Coma Scale.

Rationale:

    A. The Glasgow Coma Scale is one of the three factors examined in the Trauma Score.
    B. The Trauma Score provides a survival percentage to the GCS.
    C. The GCS is always incorporated into the Trauma Scale.
    D. The GCS is a portion of the Trauma Scale.

Content Category: Trauma & Shock

Reference: ENA, Trauma Nursing, 2000; pp. 63–66.

143.   An elderly patient who is a frequent visitor to your ED is being treated for injuries he sustained in a fall yesterday. His daughter has been providing all of the information and the patient appears reluctant to speak. You must screen for:
       A. lead contamination.
       B. ELDER ABUSE.
       C. alcohol poisoning.
       D. nutritional status.

Rationale:

       B. Abused elders often fear response of the caregiver. There was a delay in obtaining care. The patient has a history of being "accident prone."
       A. There are no indications of lead poisoning.
       C. Although alcoholism is a possibility, no data support the diagnosis.
       D. Concerns were not raised regarding the patient's nutrition status.

Content Category: Trauma & Shock

Reference: Sheehy & Lenehan, 1999; p. 658.

144.   After an indwelling urinary catheter and a nasogastric tube have been inserted, a peritoneal catheter is inserted. If no gross blood is obtained from the catheter, what action would the ED nurse expect?
       A. Instilling a liter of normal saline, then allowing gravity drainage and checking for return of gross blood
       B. Instilling 1 L of room temperature D5W, then sending a drainage specimen for electrolytes and cell count
       C. Further action is not indicated if gross blood is not seen after the tap.
       D. LAVAGING THE PERITONEUM WITH WARMED RINGER'S LACTATE AND SENDING THE SPECIMEN TO A LABORATORY TO BE TESTED FOR RED AND WHITE BLOOD CELLS.

Rationale:

       D. Warmed Ringer's lactate is the solution of choice for lavage. A positive DPL has a 98% accuracy rate in identifying intra-abdominal bleeding.
       A. Warmed Ringer's lactate is the solution of choice for lavage and instilling 1 L of fluid.
       B. This might worsen the injury. Warmed Ringer's lactate is the solution of choice. Laboratory electrolytes are not indicated.
       C. Although no overt blood has been found in the DPL, a small amount of bleeding may have been missed.

Content Category: Trauma & Shock

Reference: ENA, Trauma Nursing, 2000; pp. 63–66.

145.   In what way does a level I trauma center differ from centers at other levels?
       A. A level II trauma center is a regional trauma resource center.
       B. A LEVEL I CENTER HAS HIGHLY SOPHISTICATED TRAUMA EQUIPMENT.
       C. A level III trauma center is located in near proximity to other major trauma centers.
       D. A level II trauma center focuses on patient care and research.

Rationale:

B. Level I trauma centers invest in costly equipment and specialized trained personnel. They must handle a high volume of patients yearly in order to generate enough revenue to support the trauma program.

A. Level II trauma centers are known as area trauma centers.

C. Level II centers are typically located in remote outlying areas. These centers stabilize their patients and transfer them to distant, higher-level trauma centers.

D. Level I trauma centers have the resources to focus on research. Level II trauma centers focus on patient care and community education programs.

Content Category: Trauma & Shock

Reference: ENA, Core Curriculum, 2000.

146. Within the last decade, firearms have become the weapons of choice in penetrating trauma. What do the assailants and victims of penetrating injuries have in common?
    A. BOTH HAVE BECOME PROGRESSIVELY YOUNGER.
    B. More than 50% have handled a handgun.
    C. Both come from a household in which both parents work.
    D. None of the above.

Rationale:

A. According to trauma center and police department data, firearms have become the weapons of choice in penetrating trauma over the last decade. Both the assailants and victims of penetrating injuries have become progressively younger. The single largest group of assailants is 11–20 years old.

B. Of these groups, 28% had handled a gun without adult knowledge or supervision.

C. To an unprecedented degree, today's American adolescents are likely to come from a household lacking a male adult role model.

D. Incorrect.

Content Category: Trauma & Shock

Reference: Cornwell, 1998; pp. 115–121.

147. Trauma has become the third leading cause of death in the United States. Which of the following is also TRUE of this national crisis?
    A. The largest age range of trauma deaths is 16–25 years.
    B. Although males are victims more frequently, there has been no correlation with race.
    C. THE GREATER FREQUENCY OF MALE DEATHS HAS BEEN ATTRIBUTED TO INCREASED RISK TAKING.
    D. Homicides continue to outpace suicide as a leading cause of death.

Rationale:

C. Although increased risk is a factor, other factors, such as occupation and cultural norms, are considered as the cause of the greater number of male deaths.

A. The age group with the highest death rate from trauma is 25–34 years.

B. Death rates do vary by race. People of color die in much greater numbers than Caucasians.

D. Suicides rather than homicides result in a slightly greater number of trauma deaths.

Content Category: Trauma & Shock

Reference: ENA, Trauma Nursing, 2000.

148.   What type of force occurs when a body in motion comes to a sudden stop?
    A. External forces
    B. Velocity force
    C. Acceleration force
    D. DECELERATION FORCE

Rationale:

    D. As a body comes to a sudden stop, the energy load on tissue causes injury, mainly due to deceleration forces.
    A. External forces consist of mass and velocity.
    B. Velocity is the speed at which a body in motion travels.
    C. Acceleration forces occur when a body is in motion and sets the stage for the effect of deceleration force.

Content Category: Trauma & Shock

Reference: ENA, Trauma Nursing, 2000.

149.   What body system in an unrestrained passenger is most likely to be injured regardless of the direction from which a vehicle was struck?
    A. HEAD AND NECK
    B. Abdomen
    C. Extremities
    D. Face

Rationale:

    A. Head and neck injury is frequently seen in frontal, rear, and side-impact collisions.
    B. The abdomen is the area most likely to be injured when the occupant slides downward and under the dashboard.
    C. The extremities are injured in a lateral impact.
    D. Facial injuries are common in an up-and-over frontal collision.

Content Category: Trauma & Shock

Reference: ENA, Trauma Nursing, 2000.

150.   During your nursing assessment of the patient's airway, what would you address before proceeding to the next step?
    A. Any uncontrolled abdominal bleeding
    B. An angulated fractured femur
    C. Distended external jugular veins
    D. LOOSE TEETH OR FOREIGN OBJECTS IN THE MOUTH.

Rationale:

    D. Your assessment of the airway would include visualization of the mouth and any interventions necessary to relieve obstruction.
    A. Although such bleeding would be important to note, ensuring a patent airway takes precedence over the observation of bleeding.
    B. Disability and extremity evaluation should be performed after a patent airway and breathing have been assured.
    C. Distention of external jugular veins is an observation performed in the assessment of circulation.

Content Category: Trauma & Shock

Reference: ENA, Trauma Nursing, 2000.

Examination 3:
Self-Diagnostic Profile

Instructions

Step 1: Check your answers against the correct answers provided in Part 2 of this chapter. Then calculate your total score.

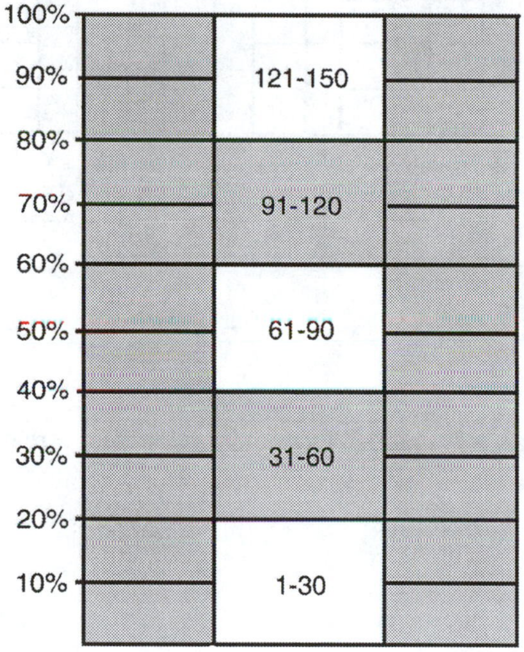

100%	
90%	121-150
80%	
70%	91-120
60%	
50%	61-90
40%	
30%	31-60
20%	
10%	1-30

Figure 1: Total Score

Step 2: For each category of the practice examination, determine the number of items that you answered correctly and plot that number in Figure 2. The result will assist you in diagnosing your areas of knowledge strength and in determing which areas benefit from review.

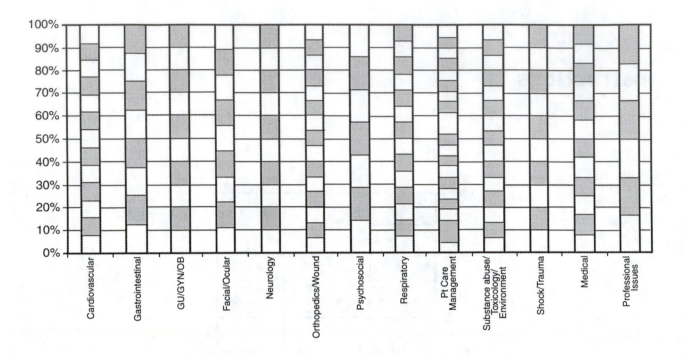

Figure 2: Practice Examination Content Areas

Practice Examination 4

Part I

1. A patient presents to the ED with a chief complaint of sore throat, stuffy nose, and a nonproductive cough that keeps him awake at night. A workup has been completed and his chest radiograph is negative. You suspect that this patient has:
   A. chronic obstructive pulmonary disease.
   B. asthma.
   C. acute bronchitis.
   D. pneumonia.

2. A 25-year-old male unrestrained driver was involved in a motor vehicle crash (MVC) in which the air bag was deployed. He is complaining of dyspnea. Your assessment reveals tachypnea, pale skin, and a Glasgow Coma Score of 15. Upon palpation of the left chest, the patient complains of chest pain, crepitus is noted, and left rib fractures are suspected. Auscultation reveals decreased breath sounds on the left. Based on these findings, which of the following concurrent injuries should be suspected?
   A. Cardiac contusion
   B. Pneumothorax
   C. Splenic injury
   D. Ruptured diaphragm

3. You are caring for an unrestrained passenger in a motor vehicle crash. EMS tells you that she was thrown forward and hit the dashboard. She is awake and alert. The radiograph shows two right-sided rib fractures. The priority nursing diagnosis for which this patient is at risk is which of the following?
   A. Fluid volume deficit
   B. Ineffective airway clearance
   C. Impaired gas exchange
   D. Pain

4. A patient is evaluated after receiving severe chest injuries in a motor vehicle crash (MVC) and presents with severe dyspnea, increasing subcutaneous emphysema of the neck, and decreased breath sounds on auscultation. What is the most appropriate position to relieve the patient's respiratory distress?
   A. Supine
   B. Modified Trendelenburg
   C. Semi-Fowler's position
   D. Lateral recumbent

5. An anxious, panic-stricken patient arrives in the ED with a chief complaint of dyspnea, rapid respirations, and periorbital numbness. All serious causes for this breathing pattern are eliminated. The ED nurse suspects that this patient has which of the following?
    A. Asthma
    B. Hyperventilation
    C. Pulmonary embolism
    D. Bronchitis

6. A patient with a history of chronic obstructive pulmonary disease (COPD) is admitted to the ED with moderate dyspnea. The patient has diminished breath sounds bilaterally and use of accessory muscles and appears anxious. Arterial blood gases on 2 L/min per nasal cannula are drawn and show a pH of 7.31, PaO_2 of 45, PCO_2 of 55, and HCO_3 of 26. The nurse anticipates that the physician will likely order the administration of which of the following?
    A. An intravenous aminophylline (Aminophyllin) infusion
    B. Albuterol/ipratropium (Combivent) nebulized treatment
    C. Epinephrine (Adrenalin) 0.03 subcutaneously
    D. Lorazepam (Ativan) 0.5 mg PO

7. A victim of an assault with a bat presents to the ED with blunt trauma to the head and neck The primary intervention for this patient should be to do which of the following?
    A. Start an IV, draw trauma bloods, infuse normal saline.
    B. Position airway, place on oxygen, prepare for possible intubation.
    C. Assess mental status, place on cardiac monitor, check vital signs.
    D. Place in cervical collar, administer pain meds and supplemental oxygen.

8. Respiratory syncytial virus (RSV) is most commonly associated with which childhood disease?
    A. Asthma
    B. Croup
    C. Pneumonia
    D. Bronchiolitis

9. To confirm your suspicion of a diaphragmatic tear, you would you expect to auscultate bowel sounds in which of the following areas?
    A. Right side of thorax
    B. Left side of thorax
    C. Upper abdomen
    D. Over gastric area, after nasogastric tube placement

10. If a patient is intubated and on a ventilator with positive end-expiratory pressure (PEEP), for what condition is the patient at risk?
    A. Airway obstruction
    B. Pneumothorax
    C. Fever
    D. Atelectasis

11. A 30-year-old nonsmoking patient in general good health is diagnosed with acute bronchitis. Patient education for this patient should include which of the following?
    A. Antibiotic therapy should be continued until sputum production ceases.
    B. Irritating substances such as smoke and pollen should be avoided.
    C. Physical activity should be reduced to help decrease induced bronchospasm.
    D. A repeat chest x-ray will be necessary to evaluate treatment effectiveness.

12.   A 40-year-old nonsmoking patient who is in general good health is diagnosed with acute bronchitis. In providing education regarding medications that can be used in treatment, which of the following should be included?
      A. Bronchodilator inhalers are of little benefit in this disorder.
      B. Cough suppressants should be avoided because of the potential for respiratory depression.
      C. Nonsteroidal anti-inflammatory agents are useful in treating associated symptoms.
      D. Antibiotic therapy should be continued until sputum production ceases.

13.   A 30-year-old nonsmoking patient who is in general good health is diagnosed with acute bronchitis and is now being discharged. Which of the following patient responses indicates a need for further patient education?
      A. "I need to drink about 8 to 10 glasses of water a day until I'm over this."
      B. "I should get a flu shot in about 6 weeks so i don't get this again."
      C. "I can take an over-the-counter cough suppressant to reduce my coughing at night."
      D. "I should come back to the hospital or see my own doctor if my sputum turns rusty colored."

14.   A 1-year-old child with bronchiolitis is being treated in the ED. The child is receiving blow-by oxygen and has been given several nebulized albuterol treatments over the past 1.5 hours. Which of the following findings would the ED nurse anticipate as an indication for admission of the child?
      A. Respiratory rate of 44/min with occasional wheezes on auscultation
      B. Pulse oximetry of 90% on room air
      C. Heart rate of 140/min at rest
      D. Rectal temperature of 101° F (38.4° C)

15.   An ED nursing colleague has been taking ginkgo biloba for several months to enhance thinking and sex drive. While on duty, the nurse experiences chest pain and is diagnosed with a myocardial infarction. Knowing the nurse has taken ginkgo, you as the primary nurse would be very hesitant to administer which of the following medication or treatment?
      A. Lidocaine (Xylocaine)
      B. Morphine sulfate
      C. Heparin
      D. Oxygen

16.   A patient is evaluated after an occupational exposure to cyanide. As the ED nurse, you would consider the primary nursing diagnosis to be which of the following?
      A. Impaired gas exchange
      B. Impaired physical mobility
      C. Fluid volume deficit
      D. Impaired tissue integrity

17.   While assisting with gardening at home, a 14-year-old collapses in the yard. When the patient arrives at the ED by EMS, a seizure is in progress. After approximately 1 minute, the seizure ends, but muscle fasciculations continue. The patient remains unresponsive. The pupils are constricted, skin is moist, and excessive salivation is noted. Vital signs are BP 80/40 mm Hg and HR 26/min. On the patient's admission to the ED, you suspect which of the following?
      A. Heat exhaustion
      B. Carbon monoxide toxicity
      C. Petroleum distillate ingestion
      D. Organophosphate poisoning

18. A depressed patient with a history of cardiac disease has taken an entire bottle of diltiazem (Cardizem). Approximately 50 pills had been in the bottle, which was labeled "Cardizem 120 mg." Toxicity to this medication would present with which of the following?
    A. Decreased cardiac output
    B. Increased heart rate
    C. Hypoglycemia with nausea
    D. Fatigue and hyperthermia

19. The purpose of administering amyl nitrite inhalants and sodium nitrite IV to a patient with cyanide toxicity is do which of the following?
    A. Increase oxygen concentration in the venous blood
    B. Induce methemoglobinemia
    C. Convert the cyanide to carbon dioxide
    D. Increase heart rate and decrease blood pressure

20. A middle-aged patient is brought to the ED by the person's significant other. There is a history of depression. A note was found on the table asking for forgiveness and a bottle of pills was found on the floor. The patient is breathing but unresponsive. Vital signs are BP 90/50 mm Hg, HR 136/min, respirations 8/min, and oxygen saturation 88% on room air. The pill bottle was labeled as phenobarbital (Luminal). What is your primary nursing diagnosis?
    A. Ineffective breathing pattern
    B. Impaired tissue integrity
    C. Ineffective individual coping
    D. Risk for poisoning

21. Which of the following drugs is NOT considered a sedative-hypnotic agent?
    A. Methaqualone (Quaalude)
    B. Tramadol (Ultram)
    C. Zolpidem (Ambien)
    D. Amitriptyline (Elavil)

22. You are working as an ED nurse in a ski resort. A patient is brought in after having been trapped in the snow for a considerable time. The patient is alert and oriented and states that the left foot and ankle was packed in snow for "a long time." Upon evaluation, you note a pale, slightly blue foot and ankle with moderate swelling. The skin is very cold to the touch and the patient does not feel your touch on the foot. As you are evaluating the wound, the patient demands to go outside and smoke a cigarette. Of course you say no. Your response should include which of the following statements?
    A. "You have not finished your assessment."
    B. "The nicotine will alter the effects of pain medication."
    C. "Your lungs need all their oxygen right now."
    D. "Smoking a cigarette would further damage your foot."

23. A wide QRS is noted on the ECG monitor of a patient who presented to the ED with cyclic antidepressant poisoning. The drug of choice for treatment would be which of the following?
    A. Sodium bicarbonate
    B. Physostigmine (Antilirium)
    C. Diazepam (Valium)
    D. Flumazenil (Romazicon)

24. The primary mode of decreasing systemic absorption of ingested toxins in the ED is which of the following?
    A. Gastric lavage
    B. Whole-bowel irrigation

C. Syrup of ipecac

D. Activated charcoal

25. A runner is brought to the ED after collapsing while participating in a road race. He is alert but perspiring profusely. Vital signs are BP 80/60 mm Hg, HR 132/min, respirations 34/min, and temperature 100.0° F (37.8° C). Treatment should include which of the following?

A. IV infusion of 5% dextrose in water (D5W) at a rapid rate

B. Two to 3 quarts of water orally

C. ECG observation of T waves

D. Wrapping the patient in a blanket to prevent rapid cooling

26. Which of the following drugs should be AVOIDED in the treatment of cocaine toxicity because it can interact with the cocaine, causing hyperthermia?

A. Diazepam (Valium)

B. Haloperidol (Haldol)

C. Sodium bicarbonate

D. Dopamine (Intropin)

27. A high school football player is starting practice in midsummer. He is instructed to run the track, along with other players, for 10 laps. On lap 6, he becomes dizzy and nauseated. As the trackside nurse, you note that he is pale, with moist skin, and is staggering to the sidelines. Vital signs are BP 90/50 mm Hg, HR 154/min, respirations 44/min, and temperature 99.0° F (37.2° C). You suspect which of the following?

A. Heat cramps

B. Heat exhaustion

C. Heat stroke

D. Heat intolerance

28. A food worker has been trapped in a meat cooler for 6 hours. Upon being discovered, he is very cold, unresponsive, and pale. Vital signs are BP 80/60 mm Hg, HR 36/min, respirations 8/min, and temperature 85° F (29.4° C). The priority nursing diagnosis for this patient is which of the following?

A. Ineffective airway clearance

B. Ineffective thermoregulation

C. Risk for infection

D. Hypothermia

29. A 28-year-old body builder was found unresponsive on the floor of the gym and brought to the ED by his friends. They state that he has recently been drinking "a health drink to build his muscles." Vital signs are BP 80/54 mm Hg, HR 48/min, respirations 4/ min, and temperature 97.0° F (36.1° C). The patient most likely has overdosed with which of the following?

A. Gamma hydroxybutyrate (GHB)

B. Lysergic acid diethylamide (LSD)

C. Methaqualone (Quaalude)

D. Ketalar (Ketamine)

30. You have performed an intraosseous cannulation for an 18-month-old pediatric patient. Which of the following would indicate that you performed the procedure correctly?

A. A blood flashback is seen in the catheter.

B. It is possible to thread an over-the-needle cannula.

C. A popping sound is heard during insertion, followed by lack of resistance to the needle.

D. The butterfly needle can stand upright without manual support.

31.   Your patient, a victim of a motor vehicle crash, has severe facial injury. Which of the following procedures is the correct way to test cranial nerve function?
A. Observe the patient for posturing patterns such as flexion or extension.
B. Observe for Battle's sign behind the ear.
C. Inspect the ears and nose for cerebral spinal fluid leakage.
D. Have the patient follow your moving finger with his eyes.

32.   You are preparing a motorcyclist crash victim for needle thoracentesis. Tension pneumothorax is suspected. After the necessary equipment has been assembled, in which of the following locations should a 14-gauge needle be inserted?
A. Unaffected side, fourth intercostal space, slightly anterior to the midaxillary line
B. Affected side, second intercostal space at the midclavicular line
C. Affected side, fifth intercostal space, slightly anterior to the midaxillary line
D. Unaffected side, third intercostal space at the midclavicular line.

33.   You are preparing to insert an indwelling urinary catheter for a trauma patient. What would you consider a contraindication for the procedure?
A. The patient tells you that she does not see a need for the catheter.
B. The patient felt discomfort during your abdominal palpation.
C. The patient tells you that s/he is allergic to latex.
D. There is blood at the urethral meatus.

34.   An example of an indirect or secondary injury is which of the following?
A. Hypoxia resulting from cerebral ischemia, cerebral edema, or bleeding
B. Hemorrhage from a massive head wound
C. Hemothorax from a penetrating stab wound
D. Paralysis from a cervical spine injury

35.   A 18-year-old male is transported to a small rural ED after a motorcycle crash. Once stabilized, he is transported to a Level I Trauma Center. Regarding this transfer, which of the following is TRUE?
A. Transfer must be accomplished expeditiously.
B. Once the decision to transfer has been made, it is necessary to access the full extent of all injuries.
C. Only a verbal report from the referring physician needs to be communicated to the receiving team.
D. Prehospital records do not have to accompany the patient. Only tests and procedures done in the sending hospital must accompany him.

36.   A complete history of a motor vehicle impact would include all of the following EXCEPT:
A. the amount of damage sustained to the passenger compartment.
B. the number of windows broken in the impact.
C. the speed of the vehicle and the point of impact.
D. the types of protective device used.

37.   Force is a physical factor that changes the motion of a body either at rest or already in motion. Which of the following is NOT considered one of these forces?
A. Acceleration
B. Deceleration
C. Shearing
D. Contusive force

38. A significant number of blunt injuries are associated with motor vehicle collisions (MVCs), motor-cycle collisions (MCCs), and falls. All of the following statements are true regarding blunt trauma EXCEPT which of the following?
    A. Injury is caused by forces that do not penetrate the body.
    B. Blunt trauma is usually less life threatening than penetration trauma.
    C. Explosion injuries may occur in air-filled organs such as the lungs and bowel.
    D. Solid organs sustain crush injuries, producing lacerations, fractures, or ruptures.

39. The driver of a motor vehicle commonly sustains the following injuries associated with side-impact collisions EXCEPT which of the following?
    A. Contralateral neck sprain
    B. Ruptured liver
    C. Fractured clavicle
    D. Pelvic and acetabular fractures

40. A 28-year-old female, 32 weeks pregnant, presents after a motor vehicle collision. She potentially has a ruptured uterus. The most appropriate intervention for this patient is probably:
    A. an emergency cesarean section.
    B. an abdominal ultrasound scan.
    C. peritoneal lavage.
    D. continuous fetal monitoring.

Questions 41 and 42

A 32-year-old female is pregnant and in her 34th week of gestation. She presents to the ED complaining of swelling in her lower extremities. She states that she has been having more headaches than usual. She denies visual disturbances. Vital signs are BP 192/110 mm Hg, HR 100/min, respirations 28, and temperature 99.2° F (37.4° C). You note that the patient has 3+ pitting edema to bilateral lower extremities and 3+ protein in her urine.

41. Based on the above assessment, you suspect that the patient has which of the following?
    A. Pregnancy-induced hypertension (PIH)
    B. Preeclampsia
    C. Eclampsia
    D. Normal findings of pregnancy

42. After the patient has been placed in a room for further evaluation, she begins to develop seizure activity. She is placed on her left side and on 100% nonrebreather mask. The seizures are eventually controlled after the administration of a loading dose of magnesium sulfate ($MgSO_4$). A maintenance infusion is started. Which of the following would suggest that the patient is developing magnesium sulfate toxicity?
    A. Respiratory rate 10/min
    B. Blood pressure 130/92 mm Hg
    C. Heart rate 98 beats/minute
    D. Temperature 97.4° F (36.3° C)

43. Which of the following anticonvulsants is the BEST choice for a woman with eclampsia?
    A. Phenytoin (Dilantin)
    B. Diazepam (Valium)
    C. Magnesium sulfate ($MGSO_4$)
    D. Lytic cocktail

Questions 44 and 45

A 26-year-old female presents to the ED complaining of severe left lower quadrant pain that began about 2 hours ago. Pain radiates to her left shoulder when she moves or takes a deep breath. She has vomited twice since the pain started. She states her last menstrual period was 10 weeks ago. She has had two positive home pregnancy tests. She has not received any prenatal care. Her prior reproductive history includes gravida 3, para 1, abortion 2, living children 1. She has had two episodes of pelvic inflammatory disease in the past 5 years. Vital signs are BP 94/56 mm Hg, HR 136/min, respirations 26/min, and temperature 97.8° F (36.5° C). Her skin is pale, cool, and diaphoretic. She admits to "spotty" vaginal bleeding. She denies any history of recent trauma to her abdomen.

44. The patient is most likely presenting with which of the following?
    A. Pelvic inflammatory disease (PID)
    B. Ruptured ectopic pregnancy
    C. Hyperemesis gravidarum
    D. Appendicitis

45. Your highest priority with this patient is do which of the following?
    A. Start 2 large-bore intravenous lines with Ringer's lactate
    B. Order a pelvic ultrasound scan
    C. Place the patient on her left side
    D. Infuse 2 units of O-positive blood as soon as it is available

Questions 46–49

A female patient who is 13 weeks pregnant by ultrasound presents to the ED with the complaint of vomiting for several days. She states that she vomits everything that she tries to eat or drink. She states that she feels very weak and dizzy. Vital signs are BP 88/52 mm Hg, HR 120/min, respirations 32/min, and temperature 99.8° F (37.7° C). Her urine has 3+ ketones and is negative for protein and negative for leukocytes.

46. The highest-priority nursing diagnosis for this patient is which of the following?
    A. Alteration in comfort related to weakness
    B. Fluid volume deficit related to persistent nausea and vomiting
    C. Anxiety related to diagnosis
    D. Alteration in safety related to dizziness

47. You suspect that the patient is experiencing which of the following?
    A. Viral gastroenteritis
    B. Hyperemesis gravidarum
    C. Pregnancy-induced hypotension
    D. Pelvic inflammatory disease (PID)

48. The most important intervention for the patient is which of the following?
    A. Initiate an intravenous line and rapidly administer a D5W solution.
    B. Initiate an intravenous line and rapidly administer 0.9% normal saline.
    C. Initiate an intravenous line and rapidly administer 2 units of O-negative blood.
    D. There is no indication that fluid resuscitation should be started at this time.

49. Which of the following antiemetics is considered the safest to administer to this patient?
    A. Promethazine (Phenergan)
    B. Prochlorperazine (Compazine)
    C. Ondansetron (Zofran)
    D. Droperidol (Inapsine)

50. A male patient presents to the ED with what he calls a panic attack. Objective findings include cool and clammy skin, tachycardia, and tachypnea. He is pacing. The priority medication for this patient is:
    A. thioridazine (Mellaril).
    B. lithium carbonate (Eskalith).
    C. lorazepam (Ativan).
    D. haloperidol (Haldol).

51. A 45-year-old teacher and father of two comes to the ED complaining of depression. He has a history of bipolar disease, is not taking any medication, and denies any plans to hurt himself. He was told by his therapist to come to the ED for a psychiatric admission. Which of the following statements by the ED nurse is most therapeutic?
    A. "You have so much to live for."
    B. "I know how you feel."
    C. "Everything will be OK."
    D. "This must be difficult for you."

52. A 48-year-old female presents to the ED with complaints of intermittent palpitations, chest tightness, and choking sensations. She reports having had these symptoms for about 6 weeks and states that the episodes are becoming more frequent. At triage she has an intact airway and her skin is cool and slightly diaphoretic to the touch. Vital signs are BP 168/72 mm Hg, HR 118/min, respirations 26/min, and temperature 99.2° F (37.3° C). The patient does not report any chest tightness, palpitations, or choking sensations at this time. Results of diagnostic tests are negative for cardiac disease. During discharge instruction, the patient reports that "something bad" is going to happen to her. At this point the ED nurse should do which of the following?
    A. Assure the patient that her cardiac monitor reading is perfectly normal
    B. Order another electrocardiogram to assure the absence of cardiac disease
    C. Leave the patient and locate the ED physician immediately
    D. Remain with the patient, perform a focused assessment to assure hemodynamic stability, and explore the patient's feelings of dread

53. A 35-year-old woman has just been treated in the ED after having been sexually assaulted. The patient is alert. Initial assessment reveals bruises and abrasions on her face, breasts, arms, and hands. She makes minimal eye contact with the nurse and responds only when asked a question. Discharge instructions for this patient must include which of the following?
    A. Partner notification, rape crisis counseling, STD treatment
    B. Rape crisis counseling, STD prophylaxis, HIV testing, prophylaxis if the exposure was assessed as high risk
    C. Importance of follow-up with law enforcement agencies
    D. Repeat STD testing in10 days, psychosocial counseling, chain of evidence

54.   A 25-year-old male is brought to the ED after a motor vehicle crash. He was a restrained driver whose vehicle ran out of control and struck a stone embankment. The front seat passenger, his girl-friend, was not restrained and was ejected through the windshield on impact. She was pronounced dead at the scene of the crash. As the ED nurse performs primary and secondary assessments on this patient, he insists that he must see his girlfriend and demands to know when the police are bringing her to visit him. Primary and secondary assessments reveal minor contusions and abrasions. The patient has completed his evaluation process and the physician states that he is ready to be dis-charged. As the ED nurse reviews the discharge instructions with this patient, he states, "Stop what you're doing and get this IV out of me! I need to find my girlfriend. The police and ambulance crew told me she didn't make it, but I know she's okay." The ED nurse recognizes that this patient's unre-solved crisis state, if left untreated, will result in which of the following?
    A. Psychosis
    B. Continued feelings of tension and heightened frustration
    C. Strengthened personality
    D. Enhanced ability to solve problems in the future

55.   A 13-year-old male is brought into the ED by EMS, police, and school officials after he drew a pic-ture of himself holding a gun to his class. He is withdrawn and does not freely interact with the triage nurse. School officials report that this is not the first time this student has received attention for his behavior and that his grandmother refuses to accept that he is having emotional problems. During psychiatric evaluation, the patient informs the psychiatric clinical nurse specialist that he is angry about the death of his mother and wants to join her. The child is becoming increasingly agitated dur-ing the assessment process. Which of the following interventions would be appropriate at this time?
    A. Isolate him in a seclusion room.
    B. Allow the grandmother, who has since calmed down, to remain with the patient during the interview.
    C. Obtain an order for IV conscious sedation.
    D. Restrain the patient to assure safety of all staff.

56.   A 16-year-old female arrives in the ED accompanied by her parents. She appears cachectic. Vital signs are BP 86/50 mm Hg, HR 50/min and irregular, respirations 20/min, and temperature 96° F (35.6° C). Her lips are dry and cracked. Skin turgor is tented. She has fine, downy hair growth on her face. She had her last menstrual period approximately 4 months ago. As an IV intravenous line is being started, she states, "There's no sugar in there, is there?" Your best response would be which of the following?
    A. "It is important to rehydrate you. We need to get you past this crisis."
    B. "I hear how frightened you are. Would you like to talk about it?"
    C. "Your doctor ordered it, yes."
    D. "Don't be afraid. It won't make you fat."

57.   Which of the following ophthalmic products produce constriction of the pupils?
    A. Cycloplegics
    B. Mydriatics
    C. Miotics
    D. Steroids

58.   Which of the following is true about otitis media?
    A. It occurs most frequently in the school-age child.
    B. Hearing is usually unaffected.
    C. It is often caused by a virus.
    D. Definitive treatment included placement of tubes.

59. A woman presents to the ED complaining of "shooting pains" in the left cheek region. The pain started when she was washing her face. Which of the following should be considered a likely diagnosis?
    A. Herpes zoster
    B. Trigeminal neuralgia
    C. Glossopharyngeal neuralgia
    D. Temporal arteritis

60. A swallowed meat bolus may be treated with a variety of methods, providing the patient can manage his or her own secretions. Which of the following treatment methods carries the greatest risk for perforation?
    A. Administration of glucagon intravenously
    B. Use of proteolytic enzymes such as meat tenderizer
    C. Use of sedation and waiting up to 12 hours before initiating treatment
    D. Endoscopy

61. When penetrating ocular injury is suspected, the ED nurse should do which of the following FIRST?
    A. Instill antibiotic eye drops
    B. Perform detailed range of motion of the extraocular muscles
    C. Apply a rigid shield over the eye
    D. Irrigate the eye with warmed saline

62. Labyrinthitis is characterized by acute onset of a severe vertiginous episode often accompanied by which of the following?
    A. Tinnitus
    B. Nausea and vomiting
    C. Hearing loss
    D. Otalgia

63. Anterior epistaxis accounts for 90% of nosebleeds. Most patients with anterior epistaxis can be managed by direct pressure and which of the following?
    A. Arterial ligation or embolization
    B. Nasal packing and cautery
    C. Nasal tampons and external carotid artery pressure
    D. Vasoconstrictive agents and use of epistaxis balloon

64. Discharge instructions for a patient with epistaxis should include humidification and which of the following?
    A. Use anti-inflammatory agents for 3–4 days.
    B. Hold any antihypertensive medications for 3–4 days.
    C. Apply petroleum jelly to affected naris with cotton swab daily.
    D. Apply antibiotic ointment to affected naris with finger daily.

65. A patient presents to triage complaining of sudden severe eye pain and a headache. The pupil is fixed and dilated. The ED nurse should suspect which of the following?
    A. Retinal detachment
    B. Keratitis
    C. Chalazion
    D. Acute glaucoma

66. Fluid volume deficit would be the priority nursing diagnosis in which of the following conditions?
    A. Diverticulitis
    B. Pancreatitis
    C. Cholecystitis
    D. Appendicitis

67. A 15-month-old child is being discharged from the ED with mild dehydration from gastroenteritis. The nurse is explaining the discharge instructions to the parents. What statement indicates the parents' understanding of the instructions?
    A. "If our child vomits again, we will attempt to give him/her oral replacement fluids right away, in sips."
    B. "Since our child wears diapers, s/he can return to day care if fever free."
    C. "Our child should take small, frequent sips of oral hydration fluids while home."
    D. "Our child is now stable and does not need follow-up with the family health care provider."

68. Which of the following inflammatory conditions requires surgical intervention?
    A. Crohn's disease
    B. Peritonitis
    C. Esophagitis
    D. Ulcerative colitis

69. Cirrhosis is a progressive, degenerative disease that results in INCREASED:
    A. flow of blood.
    B. function of the liver.
    C. pressure in the portal vein.
    D. clearing of metabolic wastes.

70. You are caring for a 25-year-old restrained male victim of a motor vehicle crash (MVC). He is complaining of abdominal pain in the right upper quadrant (RUQ) and has right shoulder pain. He is hypotensive. A seat belt abrasion is visible over the abdomen, which is firm, with hypoactive bowel sounds. You suspect this patient has an injury in which of the following areas?
    A. Stomach
    B. Spleen
    C. Bladder
    D. Liver

71. Discharge instructions for a patient diagnosed with diverticulitis should include instructions to do which of the following?
    A. Limit fluid intake.
    B. Avoid eating nuts and popcorn.
    C. Drink alcohol in moderation.
    D. Eat a high-fat diet.

72. The pharmacologic treatment of choice in patients with peptic ulcer disease caused by *Helicobacter pylori* (*H. pylori*) would be an antibiotic such as clarithromycin, bismuth subsalicylate (Pepto-Bismol), and which of the following?
    A. Prednisone
    B. Calcium carbonate (Os-Cal)
    C. Sodium bicarbonate
    D. Omeprazole (Prilosec)

73. Peritonitis can be life threatening. Which of the following statements about peritonitis is TRUE?
    A. The peritoneum is unable to produce an inflammatory reaction.
    B. Peristaltic activity increases with peritonitis.
    C. Respiratory difficulty is caused by increased abdominal pressure.
    D. Circulating volume increases with peritonitis.

74. A 35-year-old male jumped off a chair and landed on his right foot. On assessment, he is unable to flex his foot or stand on the ball of his foot and has a positive Thompson's sign. You suspect the patient has which of the following?
    A. Tibia fracture
    B. Achilles tendon rupture
    C. Jones fracture
    D. Ankle sprain

75. A female patient complains of worsening pain with numbness and tingling in both hands for 2 weeks. She has had no relief from acetaminophen (Tylenol). You are concerned that her symptoms represent which of the following?
    A. Carpal tunnel syndrome
    B. Tendinitis
    C. Bursitis
    D. Osteoarthritis

76. A child brought to the ED by his father is complaining of a painful index finger. The father tells you that the child tends to bite his nails. Exam reveals a tender, swollen, red fingertip with pus visible under the cuticle. The ED nurse should suspect that the child has which of the following?
    A. Felon
    B. Herpetic whitlow
    C. Paronychia
    D. Fungus infection

77. Supracondylar fractures in children are associated with neurovascular compromise of which of the following?
    A. Brachial plexus injury
    B. Brachial artery injury
    C. Ulnar nerve injury
    D. Ulnar artery injury

78. Acute compartment syndrome has been diagnosed in a patient with right tibia-fibula fractures. The patient will be scheduled in the operating room for closed reduction and:
    A. celiotomy.
    B. fasciotomy.
    C. escharotomy.
    D. casting.

79. Scaphoid (navicular) fractures classically have point tenderness in which area?
    A. Snuff box
    B. Ulnar styloid
    C. Radial head
    D. Olecranon

80. The motor function of the ulnar nerve includes:
    A. spreading and closing the fingers.
    B. elevating the wrist and extending the thumb.
    C. making a ring with thumb and small finger.
    D. crossing fingers.

81. A fracture with multiple splintered bone fragments is referred to as:
    A avulsion.
    B. oblique.
    C. comminuted.
    D. transverse.

82. An elderly male presents to the ED complaining of gradually increasing low back pain over a 3-month period. He denies any trauma and having done any lifting, pulling, or excessive bending. The ED nursing assessment should include:
    A. use of over-the-counter sleep aids.
    B. smoking history.
    C. recent travel to the tropics.
    D. family history of alcoholism.

83. A patient diagnosed with bursitis of the knee is ready for discharge. Which of the following statements by the patient indicates that discharge teaching has been successful?
    A "I will massage a mild hydrocortisone cream onto the knee twice a day."
    B. "I will see my doctor for a Lyme disease test."
    C "I will apply heat to the area six times a day."
    D "I will take an over-the-counter anti-inflammatory medication."

84. The minimum radiographic evaluation of the cervical spine includes:
    A. flexion and extension views.
    B. lateral, anteroposterior, and odontoid views.
    C. computed tomogram (CT) scans of the cervical spine.
    D. magnetic resonance imaging (MRI) films of the cervical spine.

85. The chin laceration of a 3-year-old child has been repaired and she is ready for discharge. The nurse advises the parents that the area should be protected from reinjury because full tensile strength will not return for:
    A. 7 days.
    B. 10 days.
    C. 2 months.
    D. 6 months.

Questions 86 and 87

A 10-year-old child is brought to the ED by her father. The child received a puncture wound to the foot on the previous day, when she stepped on a rusty nail. The father states the parental preference has been not to have their children immunized. His daughter has had no vaccines since birth.

86. In view of the girl's injury, her father wants her to receive tetanus immunization. The child should receive which of the following?
    A. Tetanus-diphtheria vaccine alone
    B. Tetanus immune globulin alone

C. Tetanus-diphtheria vaccine in the right deltoid and tetanus immune globulin in the right deltoid

D. Tetanus-diphtheria vaccine in the right deltoid and tetanus immune globulin in the right gluteus.

87. The patient received tetanus immunization in the ED. Discharge instructions for the father should include signs and symptoms of:
    A. wound infection.
    B. Stevens-Johnson syndrome.
    C. tetanus.
    D. Achilles tendinitis.

88. A 34-year-old female presents to triage complaining of right-sided chest and rib pain. She denies any unusual activities, but admits she was gardening for several hours the day before. She ranks the pain as 7 out of 10 on a 1-to-10 pain scale. The pain is sharp and worsens when she takes a deep breath. An ECG monitor is applied and demonstrates a normal, sinus rhythm. You suspect that the patient may be experiencing:
    A. a myocardial infarction.
    B. congestive heart failure.
    C. a pleural effusion.
    D. costochondritis.

89. A patient presents to the Urgent Care Center following an injury at work. Which of the following would require the company to make the visit a reportable incident according to the standards of the Occupational Safety and Health Administration (OSHA)?
    A. Puncture wound of the skin requiring a dressing application
    B. Prescription for over-the-counter ibuprofen (Advil) for 3-day use
    C. Administration of injectable antibiotic
    D. Recommendation of light duties for 3 days

90. An elderly patient falls from a stretcher in the ED. The patient was admitted with a history of confusion. The ED nurse did not raise the side rails and left the patient unattended. A suit is brought against the hospital and the ED nurse. Which of the following would be considered a cause for the suit?
    A. Breach of duty
    B. Proximate cause
    C. Duty to act
    D. Failure to act

91. An emergency nurse involved in a conflict with a peer should:
    A. focus on the behavior of the individual.
    B. establish a personal position at the beginning of the incident.
    C. use sentences that begin with "you."
    D. internalize personal feelings during the interaction.

92. The ED team decides that the current triage system is not working. Which of the following would indicate knowledge of evidenced-based practice?
    A. The team makes changes based on their past experiences of triage.
    B. The team conducts a literature review of current triage research and outcomes.
    C. The team decides to adopt the practice of other emergency departments in the same city.
    D. The team decides to write a new triage system based on emergency team experience.

93. During the absence of the ED manager, you are asked to interview a potential unit secretary. Which of the following questions should be AVOIDED?
    A. Work history
    B. Clinical and typing skills
    C. Marital status
    D. Educational preparation

94. The process by which data is collected, results are documented, and experiments and tests are validated in order to change a concept is considered to be which of the following?
    A. Research-focused theory
    B. Evidence-based practice
    C. Nursing process model
    D. Quantitative analysis approach

95. A 58-year-old male who recently had an aortic valve replacement is concerned that the valve is not working properly. Identify the landmark for auscultation of this valve.
    A. Second right intercostal space at right sternal border
    B. Second left intercostal space at left sternal border
    C. Fourth intercostal space at left sternal border
    D. Fifth intercostal space at the midclavicular line

96. A 72-year-old male is admitted to the ED with new onset of atrial fibrillation and a ventricular response of 160. He had no prior cardiovascular diagnosis but has been taking methylxanthine (Theo-Dur) for asthma. The following laboratory tests would be appropriate EXCEPT which of the following?
    A. Digitalis level
    B. Thyroid function studies
    C. Prothrombin time (PT)/partial thromboplastin time (PTT)
    D. Theophylline level

97. Ankle-brachial index (ABI) is a method used to assess arterial perfusion of the lower extremities. Which of the following is the correct formula for obtaining ABI?
    A. Ankle diastolic pressure divided by brachial diastolic pressure
    B. Ankle systolic pressure divided by brachial systolic pressure
    C. Brachial diastolic pressure divided by ankle diastolic pressure
    D. Brachial systolic pressure divided by ankle systolic pressure

98. A 70-year-old female presents with a chief complaint of "rest pain" in her foot. Which of the following data would correlate with the diagnosis of arterial occlusive disease?
    A. Pain aggravated by elevation of extremity
    B. Pain aggravated by dependent position of extremity
    C. Resting blood flow sufficient to meet metabolic requirements to extremity
    D. Pain occurs as isolated event during active/waking hours

99. An 88-year-old male with a history of chronic congestive heart failure (CHF) is admitted to the ED. He was seen 4 days ago in the ED because of respiratory distress and hypertension. Diuretics were administered and symptoms relieved. He was dismissed to the nursing home. At this time, bilateral midlobe crackles are auscultated. The patient is hypotensive, with distended neck veins. Weight gain of 20 lb is noted. The patient expresses discomfort of the upper right quadrant. These current findings indicate that he is in:
    A. biventricular failure.
    B. left ventricular failure.

C. right ventricular failure.

D. renal failure.

100. A specific diagnostic prognostic marker for congestive heart failure (CHF) is:

A. atrial natriuretic peptide (ANP).

B. angiotensin I.

C. aldosterone.

D. renin.

101. All of the following regarding possible interventions for torsade de pointes are true EXCEPT:

A. artificial pacing may be required.

B. isoproterenol (Isuprel) administration.

C. magnesium sulfate administration.

D. procainamide (Pronestyl) bolus and drip to lengthen refractory period.

102. Which of the following is TRUE regarding loss of atrial ventricular synchrony associated with atrial fibrillation?

A. Cardiac output is not affected.

B. Cardiac output is reduced by 10–15%.

C. Cardiac output is reduced by 25–30%.

D. Cardiac output is reduced by 50–60%.

103. The ED patient for whom you are caring requires close monitoring of mean arterial pressure (MAP). The function on the blood pressure cuff is not working and you must calculate this factor. The patient's BP is 110/70 mm Hg. What is the MAP for this patient?

A. 63

B. 73

C. 83

D. 93

104. Interpretation of the S-T segment in the following ECG strip indicates which of the following?

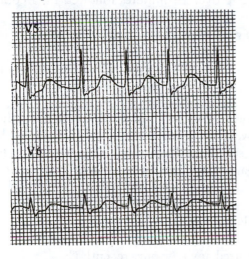

A. Acute infarct

B. Ischemia

C. ST segment is isoelectric

D. Nondiagnostic position

105.   Primary perfusion assessment includes all of the following EXCEPT:
       A. capillary refill.
       B. radial pulse.
       C. patient response.
       D. 12-lead ECG.

106.   A patient taking digoxin (Lanoxin) is most at risk for and would suffer the greatest adverse effects from which of the following?
       A. Increased serum potassium
       B. Decreased serum magnesium
       C. Increased serum calcium
       D. Decreased serum sodium

107.   An elderly patient comes to the ED with confusion and weakness. He has been taking digoxin (Lanoxin) for many years. While awaiting his laboratory results, you notice that his cardiac monitor shows a heart rate of 50/min with a PR interval of 0.28 sec and occasional PVCs. The most likely cause of this abnormality is which of the following?
       A. Hypercalcemia
       B. Hyponatremia
       C. Hypokalemia
       D. Hypomagnesemia

108.   A patient with neurologic deficits at the level of T10–11 is brought to your ED from an outlying hospital. S/he was involved in a motor vehicle collision approximately 5 hours before arrival. Initial evaluation at the outlying hospital reveals a T10–11 subluxation with neurologic deficits. CT scan of the head was negative for acute injury. CT scan of the abdomen revealed a grade II liver laceration with a small amount of free fluid in the peritoneal cavity. Hemoglobin is 10mg/dl. The ED physician orders high-dose steroids. The patient states s/he weighs 180 lb (81.8 kg). The correct dosing regimen for high-dose steroids for this patient is:
       A. methylprednisolone (Depo-Medrol) bolus of 2.5 g over 15 minutes followed by a continuous infusion of 443 mg/hr for 23 hours.
       B. methylprednisolone (Depo-Medrol) bolus of 2.5 g over 15 minutes followed by a continuous infusion of 443 mg/hour for 48 hours.
       C. methylprednisolone (Depo-Medrol) bolus of 2.5 g over 1 hour followed by a continuous infusion of 443 mg/hr for 48 hours.
       D. methylprednisolone (Depo-Medrol) bolus of 2.5 g over 15 minutes followed by a continuous infusion of 443 mg/hour for 23 hours and a second bolus of methylprednisolone.

109.   A 65-year-old female presents to the ED with a chief complaint of right-sided weakness. She states she noticed the weakness this morning when she awoke and tried to get out of bed. She is alert and oriented. She has right-sided facial droop and her speech is slurred but understandable. Her vital signs are stable. An important question to ask this patient during your assessment is which of the following?
       A. "Do you have a history of atrial fibrillation?"
       B. "Does anyone in your family have cerebrovascular disease?"
       C. "Are there signs of both expressive and receptive aphasia present?"
       D. "Have you stopped taking any medications or started any new ones recently?"

110.   A patient is admitted to the ED following an altercation and diagnosed as having a basilar skull fracture. The patient remains unconscious and has an ethanol level of 25 mg/dl. You prepare for:
   A.   insertion of a nasogastric tube.
   B.   nasal packing if there is a cerebrospinal fluid (CSF) leak.
   C.   administration of an anticoagulant to dissolve any potential blood clot.
   D.   protective observation due to possible combative behavior.

111.   A 60-year-old female is brought to the ED by her husband. He states she awoke this morning complaining of a headache and has gradually become more disoriented. She is now awake but confused and has difficulty standing. Upon further assessment, her left pupil is 6 mm in diameter and nonreactive to light; the right pupil is 4 mm in diameter and reacts briskly. Vital signs are BP 122/60 mm Hg, HR 60/min, and respirations 20/min. Based on these initial findings, you would anticipate interventions for possible:
   A.   calcium channel blocker toxicity.
   B.   meningitis.
   C.   subdural hematoma.
   D.   dehydration.

112.   A 2-year-old female is brought to the ED by her parents after a witnessed seizure lasting approximately 2 minutes. The child arouses to verbal stimuli. Skin is warm and dry to the touch, with brisk capillary refill. Vital signs are HR 140/min, respirations 36/min, and unlabored temperature 102° F (38.9° C) rectally. The parents begin asking you if their child will have to take anticonvulsants for the rest of her life. The most appropriate nursing diagnosis is which of the following?
   A.   Fluid volume deficit
   B.   Alterations in tissue perfusion
   C.   Ineffective breathing pattern
   D.   Knowledge deficit

113.   A teenager presents to the ED following a car crash. He is evaluated and determined to have a closed head injury with a possible cervical fracture. The ED nurse determines the following with a Glasgow Coma Scale (GCS) evaluation: no eye opening with stimulation, no verbal response prior to intubation, and no motor response with IV insertions. Which of the following GCS scores would be appropriate for this patient?
   A.   Eye: 0; Motor: 0; Verbal: 0
   B.   Eye: 1; Motor: 0; Verbal: 0
   C.   Eye: 1; Motor: 1; Verbal: 1
   D.   Eye: 0; Motor: 1; Verbal: 1

114.   An adult who is seizing should be placed in:
   A.   restraints.
   B.   a prone position.
   C.   a supine position.
   D.   left lateral decubitus position.

115.   In patients with severe closed head injury, fixed and dilated pupils result from increasing pressure on which cranial nerve(s)?
   A.   Cranial nerves IV and VI
   B.   Cranial nerve V
   C.   Cranial nerves II and III
   D.   Cranial nerve III

116.   A 45-year-old male is brought to the ED from a motor vehicle collision. He was unresponsive at the scene with agonal respirations. He is intubated and ventilations are assisted. On initial assessment, the patient's VS: BP 122/66 mm Hg, HR 100, Resp 16/min (assisted). He responds with decorticate posturing on the right side to painful stimuli. He remains immobilized with a rigid cervical collar and long spine board. IV fluids are being administered. As the patient is being prepared for CT scan, you notice his vital signs are now: BP 168/50 mm Hg, HR 58, Resp 16/min (assisted). This patient's signs and symptoms are most likely which of the following?
A. Cushing's response
B. Neurogenic shock
C. Horner's syndrome
D. Hypertensive crisis

117.   As an emergency nurse, you are asked to teach neurologic assessment in a First Responder class. You are teaching the class about orientation x 3. Your description of this assessment tool should be which of the following?
A. Oriented to name call three different times
B. Oriented to name, address, and phone number
C. Oriented to time, person, and place
D. Oriented to history, current medications, and allergies

118.   Which of the following laboratory studies is a classic finding in Reye's syndrome?
A. Metabolic alkalosis
B. Hypernatremia
C. Hyperglycemia
D. Hyperammonemia

119.   Patients who are immunocompromised and have an infection may present with which of the following signs and symptoms?
A. Swelling, localized redness, pus
B. Fever, pallor, malaise
C. Bradycardia; flushed, dry skin
D. Swollen glands, arthralgias

120.   An elderly woman presents to the ED at 5:00 AM. Chief complaint is fever and chills with sudden onset of pain and swelling in the first metatarsophalangeal joint. The pain awakened her from sleep. The most likely problem is:
A. septic arthritis.
B. rheumatoid arthritis.
C. cellulitis.
D. gout.

121.   Which of the following laboratory tests is indicative of hyperthyroidism?
A. Decreased T3
B. Decreased T4
C. Decreased TSH
D. Decreased free T4

122.   A 47-year-patient with type I diabetes is brought in by ambulance for the third time in 1 week for severe hypoglycemia. Before this past week, the patient never had any severe hypoglycemic episodes; she occasionally needed a glucose boost when feeling shaky or weak. The only change in her health has been the development of hypertension, which is now being treated with atenolol (Tenormin). What is the most likely cause of her frequent hypoglycemic episodes?

A. Not eating enough
B. Incorrect insulin dose
C. The new medication
D. Stress from hypertension diagnosis

123. Which category of medications is likely to cause significant increase in blood sugar levels in the diabetic patient?
A. Beta blockers
B. ACE inhibitors
C. Corticosteroids
D. Benzodiazepines

124. In the ED, a 4-year-old female who appears very ill is being triaged in a treatment room. She has a temperature of 104° F (40° C), severe headache, photophobia, and petechial rash. She cries when her head is bent forward. What should the ED nurse do next in caring for this child?
A. Don a mask
B. Give acetaminophen (Tylenol) per standing orders
C. Start an IV of lactated Ringer's
D. Administer oxygen by nasal cannula

125. The management of sickle cell crisis in children is most likely to include which of the following?
A. Active range of motion exercise
B. Transfusion of fresh frozen plasma
C. Hydration by oral and/or IV therapy
D. Administration of steroids

126. The emergency nurse knows that cancer is the second leading cause of death in children aged 1 to 14 years. The most frequent type of childhood cancer is which of the following?
A. Hodgkin's disease
B. Leukemia
C. Medulloblastoma
D. Osteogenic sarcoma

127. A 3-year-old is receiving immunosuppressive chemotherapy for acute leukemia at a tertiary children's hospital. The child presents to the ED of your community hospital with complaint of increased fever. You assess the temperature to be 101.4° F (38.7° C). The child received a weight-appropriate dose of acetaminophen (Tylenol) 1½ hours before arrival. What is a priority nursing intervention for this patient?
A. Place the child in protective isolation.
B. Administer another weight-appropriate does of acetaminophen.
C. Administer a weight-appropriate does of ibuprofen (Advil).
D. Place the child in a room with negative airflow.

128. Initial laboratory studies in a 45-year-old patient with insulin-dependent diabetes mellitus reveals a serum glucose level of 538 mg/dl. Which of the following factors might be contributing to his hyperglycemia?
A. Increased exercise
B. Decreased food intake
C. Recent infection
D. Excessive insulin dose

129.   A 19-year-old patient is brought to the ED with possible meningitis. The patient is most likely to be admitted if spinal fluid studies reveal a low:
A. white blood cell (WBC) count.
B. red blood cell (RBC) count.
C. protein level.
D. glucose level.

130.   An 18-month-old child with reactive airway disease is to be transported by ground ambulance. The best method of transporting the child is:
A. on the stretcher, with fastened seatbelt straps across the child.
B. in the mother's arms, with fastened seatbelt straps across the mother.
C. properly restrained in a child restraint seat that is the correct size for the child.
D. secured to a backboard, with a cervical collar, head blocks, and tape.

131.   A trauma patient is en route to your facility following a motor vehicle crash (MVC). Which of the following injuries should the nurse anticipate for the restrained driver with frontal impact?
A. Fractured sternum
B. Right clavicle fracture
C. Fractured pelvis
D. Aortic tear

Questions 132 and 133

A male patient sustained second- and third-degree burns 1 hour ago to anterior parts of his neck, chest, abdomen, and right leg (22% BSA total). He is coughing up carbonaceous sputum and complains of severe pain.

132.   Before he is transferred by air to a regional burn center, it is most appropriate to:
A. apply silver sulfadiazine (Silvadene Cream) to burns and fluid resuscitate.
B. insert a nasogastric tube and apply dry, sterile dressings to burns.
C. apply a condom catheter that is to gravity drainage and fluid resuscitate.
D. apply saline-moistened dressings to burns and insert an indwelling urinary catheter.

133.   To increase the potential for a positive outcome en route, it would be most appropriate for the sending facility to:
A. administer humidified oxygen by nasal cannula.
B. administer nonhumidified oxygen by nonrebreather mask.
C. administer humidified oxygen by nonrebreather mask.
D. perform rapid-sequence intubation and provide assisted ventilations.

134.   A sickle cell patient in crisis wishes to be transferred by air ambulance to a tertiary-care center near home. The transport will be approximately a 3-hour flight by jet. The patient is being hydrated, has received pain medication, is on oxygen, and is resting comfortably. This patient is a poor candidate for the noted transfer because:
A. the patient has not been adequately stabilized.
B. ED-to-ED transfers are illegal under the Consolidated Omnibus Reconciliation Act (COBRA) and the Emergency Medical Treatment and Active Labor Act (EMTALA).
C. the patient's insurance will not pay for the transfer.
D. the stressors of flight are likely to work in opposition to the patient's physiologic needs and prompt further exacerbation of disease.

135. A patient with significant alcohol intoxication is to be transported by ground ambulance from a small rural facility to a tertiary-care center. The ED physician has ordered oxygen by nonrebreather mask. What type of hypoxia is most likely in this patient?
   A. Hypoxic hypoxia
   B. Hyphemic hypoxia
   C. Stagnant hypoxia
   D. Histotoxic hypoxia

136. A 15.4-lb (7-kg) infant is brought to the ED in cardiac arrest. Because there is no intravenous access, epinephrine (Adrenalin) is administered via endotracheal tube. The appropriate dose is:
   A. 0.07 mg of 1:1,000 concentration.
   B. 0.7 mg of 1:1,000 concentration.
   C. 0.07 mg of 1:10,000 concentration.
   D. 0.7 mg of 1:10,000 concentration.

137. The most important factor to consider when permitting a family member to accompany a critically ill or injured child during transport from one ED to another is:
   A. the availability of emotional support for the family members.
   B. that the family member's presence calms the child.
   C. the travel distance between the two facilities.
   D. the transferring hospital's insurance coverage for the family member.

138. A 24-year-old male patient will be discharged from the ED following evaluation and treatment of a minor closed head injury and sprained ankle. Which of the following actions indicates that the patient understands his discharge instructions?
   A. He signs the instruction sheet and states that he understands what you have told him.
   B. He recalls 50% of the instructions listed on the discharge instructions sheet.
   C. He answers questions and restates information related to the teaching.
   D. He describes crutch walking and verbalizes how to ascend and descend stairs.

139. During emergent intubation, the physician requests that cricoid pressure be applied by the nurse. Which statement by the nurse indicates the need for further education regarding the principles of cricoid pressure?
   A. The thumb and forefinger are used to compress the cricoid cartilage downward toward C6.
   B. Cricoid pressure should be held until the cuff is inflated.
   C. The application of cricoid pressure reduces the risk of aspiration.
   D. Cricoid pressure is not used in the intubation of the traumatized uncooperative child.

140. A 56-year-old male presents with acute onset of right eye pain accompanied by blurred vision. A diagnosis of increased intraocular pressure is suspected. Which of the following is a CONTRA-INDICATION to tonometry?
   A. Patient is suspected to have acute angle-closure glaucoma.
   B. Patient has sustained blunt ocular injury.
   C. Patient has possible loss of integrity to the globe.
   D. Patient has iritis.

141.   A 32-year-old female with multiple injuries from a motor vehicle crash will be transferred to a trauma center by helicopter. The air-type splint device on her left lower leg will need to be replaced by another type of splinting device before air transport because:

A. air-filled devices do not provide appropriate immobilization.

B. changes in temperature and altitude that occur during flight may cause constriction of the extremity with the air-type splint.

C. air filled immobilization devices provide temporary immobilization.

D. air splints are not suitable for angulated fractures.

142.   A 26-year-old male who sustained a soft tissue injury to the lower leg returns to the ED complaining of pain and swelling. Assessment of the extremity reveals that it is swollen and cool to the touch, with decreased capillary refill and decreased sensation on palpation. Which of the steps below is CONTRAINDICATED in preparing the patient for measuring compartment pressure?

A   Remove any circumferential dressing or casts.

B. Keep the extremity at the level of the heart.

C. Do not give fluids or medications for hypotension.

D. Measure the systolic and diastolic blood pressure so that a differential pressure may be calculated.

143.   Which statement is FALSE regarding opportunities for teaching during the ED visit?

A. Teaching begins at triage.

B. Teaching opportunities generally end at the time of discharge.

C. Teaching is required before and after medications are administered.

D. Standardized discharge instructions must be used to provide consistency in patient discharge instructions.

144.   A 77-year-old patient reports to the triage area with many vague and varied complaints. Considering age-specific physiologic changes, which of the following would be an expected finding?

A. Upper abdominal pain

B. Ill appearance

C. Abnormal vital signs

D. Age-related deterioration of body system function

145.   Six patients report for treatment in 5 minutes. The triage nurse calls for additional help at triage because:

A. the primary assessment of a patient should occur within the first 2 to 5 minutes of arrival at the ED.

B. comprehensive triage takes approximately 10 to 15 minutes per patient.

C. all of the patient care areas in the triage area are full.

D. patient satisfaction may be diminished if patients wait too long at triage.

146.   A 6-year-old child arrives at the ED with several deep dog bite lacerations. The decision is made to use conscious sedation to facilitate closure of the wounds. "Dissociative sedation" can be defined as which of the following?

A. A state characterized by analgesia, sedation, amnesia, and catalepsy with relatively preserved ventilatory drive and airway protective reflexes

B. a state of reduced motor activity, reduced anxiety, and indifference to surroundings

C. A state of unconsciousness with partial or complete loss of protective reflexes, including the inability to maintain an airway independently

D. A state of controlled lessening of a patient's awareness and pain perception that leaves the patient able to respond to verbal or tactile stimulation and to continuously and independently maintain a patent airway and adequate ventilatory drive

147.   Failure to comply with discharge teaching may be the result of any of the following EXCEPT:
       A.   inability to recall the discharge instructions.
       B.   inability to comprehend the discharge instructions.
       C.   lack of resources to comply with the discharge instructions.
       D.   failure of the nurse to require a return demonstration.

148.   Inhaled nitrous oxide may be used to relieve pain associated with trauma, renal colic, or a minor surgical procedure. Which of the following conditions would be an indication for the use of inhaled nitrous oxide?
       A.   Pneumothorax
       B.   Recent middle-ear infection
       C.   Myocardial infarction
       D.   Bowel obstruction

149.   Eye donation is CONTRAINDICATED in which of the following circumstances?
       A.   Advanced age
       B.   Presence of eye condition
       C.   Non–heart beating donor
       D.   Intravenous (IV) drug use

150.   After brain death has been determined, the focus of care in supporting the viability of organs is on all of the following EXCEPT:
       A.   adequate hydration of the donor.
       B.   maintenance of normal blood pressure.
       C.   adequate oxygenation.
       D.   decreasing cardiac output.

Practice Examination 4

1. A patient presents to the ED with a chief complaint of sore throat, stuffy nose, and a nonproductive cough that keeps him awake at night. A workup has been completed and his chest radiograph is negative. You suspect that this patient has:
    A. chronic obstructive pulmonary disease.
    B. asthma.
    C. ACUTE BRONCHITIS.
    D. pneumonia.

Rationale:

C. This patient is exhibiting signs of acute bronchitis.
A. In a patient with chronic obstructive pulmonary disease, the chest radiograph would reveal hyperinflation and a flattened diaphragm.
B. A patient with asthma would have increased mucus secretion and reversible airway obstruction.
D. In a patient with pneumonia, the chest radiograph would show the presence of infiltrates.

Content Category: Respiratory

References: Kidd et al., 2000; pp. 566–592; Newberry, 1998; pp. 434–451.

2. A 25-year-old male unrestrained driver was involved in a motor vehicle crash (MVC) in which the air bag was deployed. He is complaining of dyspnea. Your assessment reveals tachypnea, pale skin, and a Glasgow Coma Score of 15. Upon palpation of the left chest, the patient complains of chest pain, crepitus is noted, and left rib fractures are suspected. Auscultation reveals decreased breath sounds on the left. Based on these findings, which of the following concurrent injuries should be suspected?
    A. Cardiac contusion
    B. PNEUMOTHORAX
    C. Splenic injury
    D. Ruptured diaphragm

Rationale:

B. Bony crepitus over rib fracture site, dyspnea, tachypnea, decreased or absent breath sounds, and pain at the site are very common signs and symptoms of rib fractures with a pneumothorax.
A. Angina chest pain, dyspnea, hypotension, and rhythm disturbances are likely symptoms of a cardiac contusion.
C. Peritoneal signs, Kerr's sign, shock not responsive to fluid replacement and a positive C.T. scan are all indicators of a splenic injury.
D. Dyspnea, Kerr's sign, and diminished breath sounds are all indicators of a ruptured diaphragm. Bowel sounds may be auscultated in the chest cavity.

Content Category: Respiratory

References: Kidd et al., 2000; pp. 689–697; Bayley & Turcke, 1998; p. 395.

3. You are caring for an unrestrained passenger in a motor vehicle crash. EMS tells you that she was thrown forward and hit the dashboard. She is awake and alert. The radiograph shows two right-sided rib fractures. The priority nursing diagnosis for which this patient is at risk is which of the following?
    A. Fluid volume deficit
    B. Ineffective airway clearance
    C. IMPAIRED GAS EXCHANGE
    D. Pain

Rationale:

C. Patients who have sustained rib fractures have impaired integrity to the thoracic cage, placing them at risk for impaired gas exchange.

A. There is no evidence to support a risk for circulatory impairment in this patient.

B. The patient is awake and alert and able to maintain her airway. There is no evidence that she is at risk for ineffective airway clearance.

D. Pain needs to be addressed with this patient, but it is not the priority at this time. Airway, breathing, and circulation should be assessed and maintained first.

Content Category: Respiratory

References: Newberry, 1998; pp. 295–296; ENA, Trauma Nursing, 2000; pp. 133–134.

4. A patient is evaluated after receiving severe chest injuries in a motor vehicle crash (MVC) and presents with severe dyspnea, increasing subcutaneous emphysema of the neck, and decreased breath sounds on auscultation. What is the most appropriate position to relieve the patient's respiratory distress?
    A. Supine
    B. Modified Trendelenburg
    C. SEMI-FOWLER'S POSITION
    D. Lateral recumbent

Rationale:

C. This patient is suspected to have a tracheobronchial injury. Semi-Fowler's position will permit better expansion of the chest wall, which will improve respiratory effort.

A. Lying supine or flat would potentially increase the patient's dyspnea.

B. Modified Trendelenburg position is used to treat hypotension. This position would increase the patient's dyspnea by placing increased pressure from the abdominal organs on the diaphragm.

D. The lateral recumbent position is useful for a patient who is vomiting but would not be helpful in supporting respiratory effort.

Content Category: Respiratory

References: ENA, Trauma Nursing, 2000; p. 122; Newberry, 1998; pp. 297–298; Blansfield et al., 1999; pp. 265–266; Tintinalli, 2000; p.1685.

5.   An anxious, panic-stricken patient arrives in the ED with a chief complaint of dyspnea, rapid respirations, and periorbital numbness. All serious causes for this breathing pattern are eliminated. The ED nurse suspects that this patient has which of the following?
      A. Asthma
      B. HYPERVENTILATION
      C. Pulmonary embolism
      D. Bronchitis

Rationale:

B. This patient's presentation is most consistent with hyperventilation. When a patient hyperventilates, carbon dioxide is blown off, causing the cerebral vasculature to constrict. This in turn causes anxiety, panic, shortness of breath, carpopedal spasms, and paresthesias of the fingers, toes, and periorbital area.

A. Asthma is the development of inflammation and hyperresponsiveness of the airway, causing the patient to cough, wheeze, and have a prolonged expiratory time and reduced peak expiratory flow. Periorbital numbness is usually not seen with asthma. Asthma is one of the conditions that would have been ruled out as a serious cause of this patient's condition.

C. A pulmonary embolism is a venous thrombus that has migrated to a pulmonary vessel. The most common cause is deep-vein thrombus, usually in a lower extremity. Dyspnea and chest pain are often present. This serious condition would also have been ruled out as a cause of this patient's distress.

D. Bronchitis is an acute inflammation of the bronchus. Bronchitis is usually viral and is associated with a recent upper respiratory infection such as a sore throat, stuffy nose, and cough. Dyspnea is not present unless there is underlying cardiopulmonary disease. There is no evidence that this patient has bronchitis.

Content Category: Respiratory

References: ENA, Core Curriculum, 2000; pp. 569–570; Newberry, 1998; pp. 436–437, 440–448, 451–452, 475–476.

6.   A patient with a history of chronic obstructive pulmonary disease (COPD) is admitted to the ED with moderate dyspnea. The patient has diminished breath sounds bilaterally and use of accessory muscles and appears anxious. Arterial blood gases on 2 L/min per nasal cannula are drawn and show a pH of 7.31, PaO_2 of 45, PCO_2 of 55, and HCO_3 of 26. The nurse anticipates that the physician will likely order the administration of which of the following?
      A. An intravenous aminophylline (Aminophyllin) infusion
      B. ALBUTEROL/IPRATROPIUM (COMBIVENT) NEBULIZED TREATMENT
      C. Epinephrine (Adrenalin) 0.03 subcutaneously
      D. Lorazepam (Ativan) 0.5 mg PO

Rationale:

B. Albuterol/ipratropium bronchodilators are the first-line treatment to improve air exchange.

A. IV aminophylline may or may not be given, depending on whether the patient is maintained on this drug. It is not the first-line treatment.

C. Epinephrine is not indicated for this patient. Its administration may increase cardiac side effects such as dysrhythmias.

D. COPD patients can have adverse effects of even low doses of sedatives. These drugs should not be given.

Content Category: Respiratory

References: Newberry, 1998; pp. 431–451; Kitt et al., 1995; pp.188–200; ENA, Core Curriculum, 2000; pp. 559–566.

7. A victim of an assault with a bat presents to the ED with blunt trauma to the head and neck The primary intervention for this patient should be to do which of the following?
    A. Start an IV, draw trauma bloods, infuse normal saline.
    B. POSITION AIRWAY, PLACE ON OXYGEN, PREPARE FOR POSSIBLE INTUBATION.
    C. Assess mental status, place on cardiac monitor, check vital signs.
    D. Place in cervical collar, administer pain meds and supplemental oxygen.

Rationale:

B. In treating trauma, remember the ABCs. In this case, airway needs are the priority, as there is high risk for obstruction or aspiration. Therefore, the patient should be positioned to assure a patent airway, placed on high-flow oxygen, and prepared for possible emergency intubation.

A. Starting an IV, drawing trauma bloods, and infusing normal saline should all be done to evaluate the patient's circulation, but the priority is to stabilize the airway, followed by an assessment of breathing status.

C. Assessing mental status, placing the patient on a cardiac monitor, and checking vital signs are important assessments and interventions, but the airway needs to be maintained first, followed by assessments of the patient's breathing and circulatory status.

D. Placing the patient in a cervical collar is a priority, as cervical spine immobilization is part of airway maintenance. Once the airway is maintained, the patient's breathing status is assessed and supplemental oxygen is administered. Administration of pain medication is not an initial priority but needs to be addressed after the patient's primary needs have been met and condition stabilized.

Content Category: Respiratory

References: ENA, Trauma Nursing, 2000; pp. 41–55, 92–108; ENA, Core Curriculum, 2000; pp. 165, 218.

8. Respiratory syncytial virus (RSV) is most commonly associated with which childhood disease?
    A. Asthma
    B. Croup
    C. Pneumonia
    D. BRONCHIOLITIS

Rationale:

D. Bronchiolitis is a viral illness of the lower respiratory tract that is commonly found in infants. RSV causes approximately 90% of these infections.

A. Bronchiolitis and RSV are risk factors for the later development of asthma.

B. Croup is a viral illness most commonly associated with parainfluenza virus.

C. While pneumonia may be caused by RSV, multiple bacteria and viruses are more common causes.

Content Category: Respiratory

References: ENA, Core Curriculum, 2000; p. 562; Newberry, 1998; p. 728.

9.   To confirm your suspicion of a diaphragmatic tear, you would you expect to auscultate bowel sounds in which of the following areas?
A. Right side of thorax
B. LEFT SIDE OF THORAX
C. Upper abdomen
D. Over gastric area, after nasogastric tube placement

Rationale:

B. A diaphragm tear allows abdominal organs such as the bowel to herniate into the thorax on the left side, since the right side is protected by the liver.
A. Herniation is more common on the left side because the liver protects the right side of the diaphragm.
C. It is possible to auscultate some bowel sounds in the abdomen; however, bowel sounds heard in the thorax will help verify the diagnosis.
D. No additional assessment data would be obtained by auscultation of the gastric area, even when decompressed with a nasogastric tube.

Content Category: Respiratory

References: Blansfield et al., 1999; p. 267; Goldy, 1998; p. 33; Newberry, 1998; pp. 302, 313; Tintinalli, 2000; p.1686.

10.   If a patient is intubated and on a ventilator with positive end-expiratory pressure (PEEP), for what condition is the patient at risk?
A. Airway obstruction
B. PNEUMOTHORAX
C. Fever
D. Atelectasis

Rationale:

B. Pneumothorax can be caused by the use of PEEP. Frequent assessment of lung sounds is crucial to monitor patient for this potential complication, which is more common in patients with COPD.
A. Airway obstruction is unlikely, as the patient's airway is being maintained with an endotracheal tube.
C. Fever is a symptom that is not caused by PEEP.
D. Atelectasis is already present because the alveolar-capillary membrane has been damaged. PEEP is used to expand the alveoli and to correct the ventilation-perfusion abnormality.

Content Category: Respiratory

References: Lombardi,1995; pp. 239–240; Newberry, 1998; pp. 452–455, 522; O'Hanlon-Nichols, 1995; p. 42.

11.   A 30-year-old nonsmoking patient in general good health is diagnosed with acute bronchitis. Patient education for this patient should include which of the following?
A. Antibiotic therapy should be continued until sputum production ceases.
B. IRRITATING SUBSTANCES SUCH AS SMOKE AND POLLEN SHOULD BE AVOIDED.
C. Physical activity should be reduced to help decrease induced bronchospasm.
D. A repeat chest x-ray will be necessary to evaluate treatment effectiveness.

Rationale:

B. Smoke and pollen frequently exacerbate and occasionally are the primary cause for episodes of acute bronchitis. They should be avoided.

A. Antibiotic therapy is not frequently used to treat bronchitis. If it is used, however the patient should complete the prescribed therapy and not base taking the medications on any symptoms.

C. Bronchospasm in acute bronchitis is caused by inflammation of the airway mucosa. Physical activity does not have a causal relationship to this inflammation and avoidance will not reduce its occurrence.

D. A repeat chest x-ray is not necessary unless the patient's condition worsens, and is not a marker of improvement. Decreased symptomatology; reduced fever, cough, sputum production; is used to determine effectiveness of treatments.

Content Category: Respiratory

References: Newberry, 1998; pp. 436–437; ENA, Core Curriculum, 2000; pp. 561–562.

12. A 40-year-old nonsmoking patient who is in general good health is diagnosed with acute bronchitis. In providing education regarding medications that can be used in treatment, which of the following should be included?
    A. Bronchodilator inhalers are of little benefit in this disorder.
    B. Cough suppressants should be avoided because of the potential for respiratory depression.
    C. NONSTEROIDAL ANTI-INFLAMMATORY AGENTS ARE USEFUL IN TREATING ASSOCIATED SYMPTOMS.
    D. Antibiotic therapy should be continued until sputum production ceases.

Rationale:

C. Nonsteroidals can be used to reduce inflammation in the bronchial passages and to manage associated fever. NSAIDs are one of the main medication treatments along with cough suppressants and bronchodilators.

A. Bronchodilators are frequently used to reduce bronchospasm caused by airway inflammation.

B. Cough suppressants are useful in treatment, particularly at night, in allowing patients to rest. They do not cause respiratory depression in prescribed dosages.

D. Antibiotic therapy is not frequently used to treat bronchitis. If it is used, however, the patient should complete the prescribed therapy regardless of symptoms.

Content Category: Respiratory

References: Newberry, 1998; pp. 436–437; ENA, Core Curriculum, 2000; pp. 561–562.

13. A 30-year-old nonsmoking patient who is in general good health is diagnosed with acute bronchitis and is now being discharged. Which of the following patient responses indicates a need for further patient education?
    A. "I need to drink about 8 to 10 glasses of water a day until I'm over this."
    B. "I SHOULD GET A FLU SHOT IN ABOUT 6 WEEKS SO I DON'T GET THIS AGAIN."
    C. "I can take an over-the-counter cough suppressant to reduce my coughing at night."
    D. "I should come back to the hospital or see my own doctor if my sputum turns rusty colored."

Rationale:

B. A flu shot is helpful for individuals who are at higher risk for respiratory complications. These include the elderly, people with chronic disease problems, and immunocompromised patients. The patient should understand that the timing of flu shot administration is related not to the current episode but to seasonal exposure to infectious agents and that it takes several weeks to achieve immunity.

A. Oral fluids should be increased to help liquefy secretions.

C. Cough suppressants are useful in reducing symptoms and allowing patients to rest.

D. Rust-colored sputum may indicate a bacterial infection and should be an indication for a reevaluation.

Content Category: Respiratory

References: Newberry, 1998; pp. 436–437; ENA, Core Curriculum, 2000; pp. 561–562.

14. A 1-year-old child with bronchiolitis is being treated in the ED. The child is receiving blow-by oxygen and has been given several nebulized albuterol treatments over the past 1.5 hours. Which of the following findings would the ED nurse anticipate as an indication for admission of the child?
A. Respiratory rate of 44/min with occasional wheezes on auscultation
B. PULSE OXIMETRY OF 90% ON ROOM AIR
C. Heart rate of 140/min at rest
D. Rectal temperature of 101° F (38.4° C)

Rationale:

B. Persistent pulse oximetry of < 90% despite treatment is an indication that the patient needs to be admitted.
A. A respiratory rate of > 60/min after treatment would be a criterion for admission. Wheezes on auscultation indicate bronchial narrowing and may not be completely resolved by treatment, but do not require admission.
C. An elevated heart rate is associated with temperature elevation and respiratory effort and is an expected finding.
D. Fever is also an associated finding with bronchiolitis. Fever requires management, but will not require admission unless it is accompanied by dehydration that cannot be managed by oral rehydration.

Content Category: Respiratory

References: Newberry, 1998; p. 728; ENA, Core Curriculum, 2000; pp. 562–564; Kitt et al., 1995; p. 417.

15. An ED nursing colleague has been taking ginkgo biloba for several months to enhance thinking and sex drive. While on duty, the nurse experiences chest pain and is diagnosed with a myocardial infarction. Knowing the nurse has taken ginkgo, you as the primary nurse would be very hesitant to administer which of the following medication or treatment?
A. Lidocaine (Xylocaine)
B. Morphine sulfate
C. HEPARIN
D. Oxygen

Rationale:

C. Ginkgo biloba may potentiate anticoagulants and antithrombotics because of its action of inhibiting platelet-activating factors. An increased bleeding tendency might occur if the anticoagulant heparin were administered.
A. There is no documented effect of ginkgo on lidocaine.
B. There is no documented effect of ginkgo on morphine sulfate.
D. There is no documented effect of ginkgo on oxygen therapy.

Content Category: Substance Abuse & Toxicological & Environmental

Reference: Newberry, 1998.

16. A patient is evaluated after an occupational exposure to cyanide. As the ED nurse, you would consider the primary nursing diagnosis to be which of the following?
A. IMPAIRED GAS EXCHANGE
B. Impaired physical mobility
C. Fluid volume deficit
D. Impaired tissue integrity

Rationale:

A. Cyanide is a lethal gas that can cause immediate death. It interferes with cellular respiration, causing a decreased utilization of oxygen by the tissue.
B. The main problem with cyanide toxicity is alterations in cellular respiration, not impaired physical mobility.
C. Fluid volumes are not affected by cyanide toxicity.
D. Tissue integrity is not a primary concern with cyanide toxicity.

Content Category: Substance Abuse & Toxicological & Environmental

Reference: ENA, Core Curriculum, 2000; pp. 651–652.

17. While assisting with gardening at home, a 14-year-old collapses in the yard. When the patient arrives at the ED by EMS, a seizure is in progress. After approximately 1 minute, the seizure ends, but muscle fasciculations continue. The patient remains unresponsive. The pupils are constricted, skin is moist, and excessive salivation is noted. Vital signs are BP 80/40 mm Hg and HR 26/min. On the patient's admission to the ED, you suspect which of the following?
A. Heat exhaustion
B. Carbon monoxide toxicity
C. Petroleum distillate ingestion
D. ORGANOPHOSPHATE POISONING

Rationale:

D. Toxicity from organophosphates causes a cholinergic crisis whereby the substance binds to acetylcholinesterase, resulting in an accumulation of acetylcholine at the receptor sites. Symptoms include excessive salivation, seizures, fasciculations, hypotension, and bradycardia.
A. Heat exhaustion would present with moist skin, but not the other symptoms described.
B. A patient with carbon monoxide toxicity would have respiratory compromise, but not the other symptoms listed.
C. A petroleum distillate ingestion would present with primary respiratory compromise.

Content Category: Substance Abuse & Toxicological & Environmental

Reference: ENA, Core Curriculum, 2000; pp. 652–653.

18. A depressed patient with a history of cardiac disease has taken an entire bottle of diltiazem (Cardizem). Approximately 50 pills had been in the bottle, which was labeled "Cardizem 120 mg." Toxicity to this medication would present with which of the following?
A. DECREASED CARDIAC OUTPUT
B. Increased heart rate
C. Hypoglycemia with nausea
D. Fatigue and hyperthermia

Rationale:

A. Calcium channel blockers such as diltiazem (Cardizem) inhibit the movement of calcium across the cell membrane. Toxicity results in severely decreased cardiac output and profound bradycardia.
B. A decreased heart rate, not an increased heart rate, would be present with a toxicity.
C. Hyperglycemia, not hypoglycemia, may be present secondary to the blockage of insulin release. Nausea with diarrhea is common in such cases.
D. Although fatigue may accompany depressed cardiac function, hyperthermia is not observed with a calcium channel blocker overdose.

Content Category: Substance Abuse & Toxicological & Environmental

Reference: ENA, Core Curriculum, 2000; pp. 654–655.

19.   The purpose of administering amyl nitrite inhalants and sodium nitrite IV to a patient with cyanide toxicity is do which of the following?
   A.   Increase oxygen concentration in the venous blood
   B.   INDUCE METHEMOGLOBINEMIA
   C.   Convert the cyanide to carbon dioxide
   D.   Increase heart rate and decrease blood pressure

Rationale:

   B.   The purpose of administering amyl nitrite, sodium nitrite, and sodium thiosulfate to a patient with cyanide toxicity is to induce methemoglobinemia to bind the cyanide, thus freeing cells to accept oxygen.
   A.   In cyanide toxicity, oxygen concentration is already increased in venous blood because cells are unable to utilize oxygen.
   C.   Cyanide is bound by methemoglobinemia and excreted, not as carbon dioxide.
   D.   Cyanide toxicity may cause tachycardia and hypotension.

Content Category: Substance Abuse & Toxicological & Environmental

Reference: ENA, Core Curriculum, 2000; pp. 650–651.

20.   A middle-aged patient is brought to the ED by the person's significant other. There is a history of depression. A note was found on the table asking for forgiveness and a bottle of pills was found on the floor. The patient is breathing but unresponsive. Vital signs are BP 90/50 mm Hg, HR 136/min, respirations 8/min, and oxygen saturation 88% on room air. The pill bottle was labeled as phenobarbital (Luminal). What is your primary nursing diagnosis?
   A.   INEFFECTIVE BREATHING PATTERN
   B.   Impaired tissue integrity
   C.   Ineffective individual coping
   D.   Risk for poisoning

Rationale:

   A.   Phenobarbital (Luminal) is a sedative-hypnotic, a central nervous system depressant with the chief effect of respiratory depression. This patient is in respiratory distress on admission with a respiratory rate of 8 and oxygen saturation of 88%. Immediate attention must be paid to the airway.
   B.   Tissue integrity would be of concern later in treatment.
   C.   Individual coping would be of major concern following the recovery phase of the ingestion.
   D.   The risk for poisoning is respiratory depression, which has already occurred. This patient's immediate problem, breathing compromise, must be addressed first.

Content Category: Substance Abuse & Toxicological & Environmental

Reference: ENA, Core Curriculum, 2000.

21.   Which of the following drugs is NOT considered a sedative-hypnotic agent?
   A.   Methaqualone (Quaalude)
   B.   Tramadol (Ultram)
   C.   Zolpidem (Ambien)
   D.   AMITRIPTYLINE (ELAVIL)

Rationale:

D. Amitriptyline (Elavil) is a tricyclic antidepressant, not a sedative-hypnotic agent.

A. Methaqualone (Quaalude) is a nonbenzodiazepine drug. Its predominant effect is CNS depression. Methaqualone also has sedative, hypnotic, anticonvulsant, and anxiolytic properties.

B. Tramadol (Ultram) is a nonbenzodiazepine drug. Its predominant effect is CNS depression. It also has sedative, hypnotic, anticonvulsant, and anxiolytic properties.

C. Zolpidem (Ambien) is a nonbenzodiazepine drug. Its predominant effect is CNS depression. It also has sedative, hypnotic, anticonvulsant, and anxiolytic properties.

Content Category: Substance Abuse & Toxicological & Environmental

Reference: Layton, 2000; pp. 626–627.

22. You are working as an ED nurse in a ski resort. A patient is brought in after having been trapped in the snow for a considerable time. The patient is alert and oriented and states that the left foot and ankle was packed in snow for "a long time." Upon evaluation, you note a pale, slightly blue foot and ankle with moderate swelling. The skin is very cold to the touch and the patient does not feel your touch on the foot. As you are evaluating the wound, the patient demands to go outside and smoke a cigarette. Of course you say no. Your response should include which of the following statements?

A. "You have not finished your assessment."
B. "The nicotine will alter the effects of pain medication."
C. "Your lungs need all their oxygen right now."
D. "SMOKING A CIGARETTE WOULD FURTHER DAMAGE YOUR FOOT."

Rationale:

D. The vasoconstrictive properties of nicotine could cause smoking a cigarette to restrict blood flow to the foot further. Alcohol, tobacco, and caffeine should be avoided during the treatment of frostbite.

A. Although this statement may be true, it would not persuade the patient to wait for that cigarette.

B. Nicotine does not affect pain medication.

C. While this statement is true, it is not related to the treatment of frostbite.

Content Category: Substance Abuse & Toxicological & Environmental

Reference: ENA, Core Curriculum, 2000.

23. A wide QRS is noted on the ECG monitor of a patient who presented to the ED with cyclic antidepressant poisoning. The drug of choice for treatment would be which of the following?

A. SODIUM BICARBONATE
B. Physostigmine (Antilirium)
C. Diazepam (Valium)
D. Flumazenil (Romazicon)

Rationale:

A. Sodium bicarbonate is the drug of choice in the treatment of wide QRS, which may occur in tricyclic antidepressant poisoning, because it enhances the protein binding of the drug.

B. The routine use of physostigmine (Antilirium) as an antidote is not recommended because of the serious toxic effects, such as bronchospasm, seizures, bradycardia, and asystole, that it can have.

C. Diazepam (Valium) is the drug of choice for controlling seizure activity.

D. Flumazenil (Romazicon) should be avoided in tricyclic antidepressant poisonings due the seizure potential of flumazenil as well as the seizure potential of the tricyclic antidepressants.

Content Category: Substance Abuse & Toxicological & Environmental

References: McDeed-Breault, 2000; pp. 641–643; Norton, 1998; pp.1045–1048; Shrestha, 1998; p. 1004.

24.   The primary mode of decreasing systemic absorption of ingested toxins in the ED is which of the following?
    A. Gastric lavage
    B. Whole-bowel irrigation
    C. Syrup of ipecac
    D. ACTIVATED CHARCOAL

Rationale:

    D. Activated charcoal is the primary mode of decreasing systemic absorption of ingested toxins. Activated charcoal has fewer side effects than other methods. It binds many compounds and is more effective than syrup of ipecac or gastric lavage.
    A. Data have demonstrated the effectiveness of activated charcoal alone in the absorption of many toxic compounds. Therefore, the use of gastric lavage has diminished.
    B. Whole-bowel irrigation is useful in the treatment of compounds that remain in the gut lumen for long periods of time, such as heavy metals and long-acting or slow-release compounds. This procedure is also useful for substances that are slowly absorbed from the gut lumen or not absorbed by charcoal.
    C. Syrup of ipecac is more effective if given immediately after ingestion of a toxin or an overdose.

Content Category: Substance Abuse & Toxicological & Environmental

Reference: Shrestha, 1998; pp. 998–999.

25.   A runner is brought to the ED after collapsing while participating in a road race. He is alert but perspiring profusely. Vital signs are BP 80/60 mm Hg, HR 132/min, respirations 34/min, and temperature 100.0° F (37.8° C). Treatment should include which of the following?
    A. IV infusion of 5% dextrose in water (D5W) at a rapid rate
    B. Two to 3 quarts of water orally
    C. ECG OBSERVATION OF T WAVES
    D. Wrapping the patient in a blanket to prevent rapid cooling

Rationale:

    C. T waves may be present on the electrocardiogram if there is significant electrolyte disturbance. Electrolytes should be replaced as cooling efforts are made.
    A. An IV infusion of normal saline or lactated Ringer's solution would be appropriate, but not dextrose. Dextrose could have a further dehydrating effect.
    B. Give 6 to 8 ounces of an electrolyte-containing solution. Two to 3 quarts of water would further dilute the remaining body electrolytes, worsening the condition.
    D. Rapid cooling should occur, not be prevented. The patient should be placed in a cool environment, not wrapped in blankets. Shivering should be prevented.

Content Category: Substance Abuse &Toxicological & Environmental

Reference: ENA, Core Curriculum, 2000.

26.   Which of the following drugs should be AVOIDED in the treatment of cocaine toxicity because it can interact with the cocaine, causing hyperthermia?
    A. Diazepam (Valium)
    B. HALOPERIDOL (HALDOL)
    C. Sodium bicarbonate
    D. Dopamine (Intropin)

Rationale:

    B. Haloperidol should be avoided in the treatment of cocaine toxicity. It could interact with the cocaine to cause hyperthermia.

    A. Diazepam is the benzodiazepine of choice for controlling agitation in cocaine toxicity. Diazepam is also the initial drug of choice to be used if seizures occur.

    C. Sodium bicarbonate is used to treat acidemia and used if QRS widening or dysrhythmia occurs.

    D. If hypotension occurs, treat initially with a bolus of isotonic fluid and place the patient in Trendelenburg position. If a vasopressor is needed, dopamine is preferred.

Content Category: Substance Abuse & Toxicological & Environmental

Reference: Cetaruk, 2000; pp. 330–331.

27. A high school football player is starting practice in midsummer. He is instructed to run the track, along with other players, for 10 laps. On lap 6, he becomes dizzy and nauseated. As the trackside nurse, you note that he is pale, with moist skin, and is staggering to the sidelines. Vital signs are BP 90/50 mm Hg, HR 154/min, respirations 44/min, and temperature 99.0° F (37.2° C). You suspect which of the following?

    A. Heat cramps

    B. HEAT EXHAUSTION

    C. Heat stroke

    D. Heat intolerance

Rationale:

    B. Heat exhaustion is precipitated by major exertion in hot weather. Peripheral vasodilation occurs to dissipate heat. Fluids and electrolytes are lost through profuse perspiration. Symptoms include pale color, diaphoresis, hypotension, tachycardia, tachypnea, and altered metal status along with dizziness and severe thirst.

    A. Heat cramps result from depletion of fluids and electrolytes in exerted muscles and do not present with such profound symptoms as heat exhaustion.

    C. Heat stroke is an acute medical emergency. The body has lost the ability to dissipate heat because of the failure of the thermoregulatory mechanisms. Core body temperature may rise to > 106° F (41.1° C).

    D. Heat intolerance is a term used casually to describe an inability to tolerate heat.

Content Category: Substance Abuse & Toxicological & Environmental

Reference: ENA, Core Curriculum, 2000.

28. A food worker has been trapped in a meat cooler for 6 hours. Upon being discovered, he is very cold, unresponsive, and pale. Vital signs are BP 80/60 mm Hg, HR 36/min, respirations 8/min, and temperature 85° F (29.4° C). The priority nursing diagnosis for this patient is which of the following?

    A. INEFFECTIVE AIRWAY CLEARANCE

    B. Ineffective thermoregulation

    C. Risk for infection

    D. Hypothermia

Rationale:

    A. The decrease in level of consciousness (patient is unconscious) and slow respirations require immediate gentle, careful attention to the airway.

    B. In the cold environment, the thermoregulation mechanisms were depleted and hypothermia developed. Primary attention must be given to the ABCs.

C. Risk for infection would be an important consideration, but not until lifesaving interventions and rewarming had been attended to.

D. Attention must be given to rewarming once the airway has been managed.

Content Category: Substance Abuse & Toxicological & Environmental

Reference: ENA, Core Curriculum, 2000.

29. A 28-year-old body builder was found unresponsive on the floor of the gym and brought to the ED by his friends. They state that he has recently been drinking "a health drink to build his muscles." Vital signs are BP 80/54 mm Hg, HR 48/min, respirations 4/ min, and temperature 97.0° F (36.1° C). The patient most likely has overdosed with which of the following?

A. GAMMA HYDROXYBUTYRATE (GHB)

B. Lysergic acid diethylamide (LSD)

C. Methaqualone (Quaalude)

D. Ketalar (Ketamine)

Rationale:

A. Gamma hydroxybutyrate (GHB) is used by weight lifters to build strength and muscles. Adverse effects include hypotension, bradycardia, and respiratory problems ranging from respiratory distress to respiratory arrest. Rapid airway management is essential.

B. Lysergic acid diethylamide (LSD) would present with a hallucinogenic effect.

C. Methaqualone (Quaalude) is a drug that was popularly used in the mid-1980s to give a boost and a "high."

D. Ketalar (Ketamine) is a hypnotic, used to alter mentation and release inhibitions.

Content Category: Substance Abuse & Toxicological & Environmental

References: Kokan & Heard, 2000; pp. 400–401; Layton, 2000; pp. 626–627; Millin, 2000; pp. 478–479.

30. You have performed an intraosseous cannulation for an 18-month-old pediatric patient. Which of the following would indicate that you performed the procedure correctly?

A. A blood flashback is seen in the catheter.

B. It is possible to thread an over-the-needle cannula.

C. A POPPING SOUND IS HEARD DURING INSERTION, FOLLOWED BY LACK OF RESISTANCE TO THE NEEDLE.

D. The butterfly needle can stand upright without manual support.

Rationale:

C. Hearing a popping sound while inserting the biopsy needle, followed by an absence of resistance and confirmation of bone marrow aspiration, would indicate correct tibial shaft placement.

A. In intraosseous insertion, blood does not flash back from the bone marrow space.

B. A large biopsy needle is used. It does not have an over-the-needle cannula.

D. A butterfly needle does not have the length, diameter, or strength for intraosseous cannulation.

Content Category: Trauma & Shock

Reference: Sheehy & Lenehan, 1999; pp.121–123.

31. Your patient, a victim of a motor vehicle crash, has severe facial injury. Which of the following procedures is the correct way to test cranial nerve function?

A. Observe the patient for posturing patterns such as flexion or extension.

B. Observe for Battle's sign behind the ear.

C. Inspect the ears and nose for cerebral spinal fluid leakage.

D. HAVE THE PATIENT FOLLOW YOUR MOVING FINGER WITH HIS EYES.

Rationale:

    D. Following your finger with the eyes will test extraocular movement and is a test of cranial nerves III, IV, and VI.

    A. Observing the patient for posturing pattern would determine whether he had a brainstem or high injury. Doing so would not, however, assess the cranial nerves.

    B. Battle's sign is usually an indication of a basal skull fracture and does not indicate cranial nerve injury.

    C. Cerebral spinal fluid leakage may be observed with a basal skull fracture but does not indicate cranial nerve function.

Content Category: Trauma & Shock

Reference: ENA, Trauma Nursing, 2000.

32.   You are preparing a motorcyclist crash victim for needle thoracentesis. Tension pneumothorax is suspected. After the necessary equipment has been assembled, in which of the following locations should a 14-gauge needle be inserted?
    A. Unaffected side, fourth intercostal space, slightly anterior to the midaxillary line
    B. AFFECTED SIDE, SECOND INTERCOSTAL SPACE AT THE MIDCLAVICULAR LINE
    C. Affected side, fifth intercostal space, slightly anterior to the midaxillary line
    D. Unaffected side, third intercostal space at the midclavicular line.

Rationale:

    B. The second intercostal space, midclavicular line on the affected side is the correct location.

    A. Although tension pneumothorax displaces the trachea and thoracic organs away from the affected side toward the unaffected side, inserting a thoracentesis needle in the unaffected side might compromise the patient.

    C. The fifth intercostal space slightly anterior to the midaxillary line would be the correct location for insertion of a chest tube if you suspected hemothorax. This location would permit drainage of accumulated blood.

    D. Although tension pneumothorax displaces the trachea and thoracic organs away from the affected side toward the unaffected side, inserting a thoracentesis needle in the unaffected side might compromise the patient.

Content Category: Trauma & Shock

Reference: Sheehy & Lenehan, 1999; p. 468.

33.   You are preparing to insert an indwelling urinary catheter for a trauma patient. What would you consider a contraindication for the procedure?
    A. The patient tells you that she does not see a need for the catheter.
    B. The patient felt discomfort during your abdominal palpation.
    C. The patient tells you that s/he is allergic to latex.
    D. THERE IS BLOOD AT THE URETHRAL MEATUS.

Rationale:

    D. You would not catheterize your patient if you found blood at the urethral meatus; this might indicate a urethral injury.

    A. Explain the reason for the need for the catheter to the patient. You have to obtain consent to insert the catheter.

    B. Inserting a urinary catheter will determine whether the bladder was ruptured. If so, that could be the cause of the abdominal pain.

    C. A latex allergy is pertinent. You would obtain a latex-free catheter and proceed.

Content Category: Trauma & Shock

Reference: ENA, Trauma Nursing, 2000.

34. An example of an indirect or secondary injury is which of the following?
    A. HYPOXIA RESULTING FROM CEREBRAL ISCHEMIA, CEREBRAL EDEMA, OR BLEEDING
    B. Hemorrhage from a massive head wound
    C. Hemothorax from a penetrating stab wound
    D. Paralysis from a cervical spine injury

Rationale:

    A. Hypoxia would eventually occur in a victim who had suffered a massive head injury. The cerebral edema, bleed, and eventual cerebral ischemia would lead to hypoxia if untreated.
    B. Hemorrhage from a massive head wound is a primary injury.
    C. A penetrating stab wound is a primary cause of hemothorax.
    D. A cervical spine injury is a primary cause of paralysis.

Content Category: Trauma & Shock

Reference: ENA, Core Curriculum, 2000; p. 375.

35. A 18-year-old male is transported to a small rural ED after a motorcycle crash. Once stabilized, he is transported to a Level I Trauma Center. Regarding this transfer, which of the following is TRUE?
    A. TRANSFER MUST BE ACCOMPLISHED EXPEDITIOUSLY.
    B. Once the decision to transfer has been made, it is necessary to access the full extent of all injuries.
    C. Only a verbal report from the referring physician needs to be communicated to the receiving team.
    D. Prehospital records do not have to accompany the patient. Only tests and procedures done in the sending hospital must accompany him.

Rationale:

    A. Once the need for transfer has been recognized, the patient should be stabilized and transferred as quickly as possible.
    B. It is not necessary to conduct a complete patient workup before transfer. The goal is for the patient to spend the least possible amount of time in the referral facility. Deferring all nonessential tests and interventions will expedite the transfer.
    C. A verbal report from the nurse and the referring physician need to be communicated to the receiving team.
    D. Prehospital records are an important aspect of the mechanism of injury and treatment. These records should accompany the patient.

Content Category: Trauma & Shock

Reference: Sheehy et al., 1999; pp. 50–59.

36. A complete history of a motor vehicle impact would include all of the following EXCEPT:
    A. the amount of damage sustained to the passenger compartment.
    B. THE NUMBER OF WINDOWS BROKEN IN THE IMPACT.
    C. the speed of the vehicle and the point of impact.
    D. the types of protective device used.

Rationale:

B. Depending on the type of crash, knowing these factors would not predict the severity of injury: rotational impact; vehicle rollover; front, side, or rear-end impact; broken or intact window.

A. The force of the impact is suggested by the vehicle deformity.

C. The speed at which the vehicles were traveling would help determine the significance of injury. Knowing whether the impact was frontal, rear, or side would be helpful in determining the types of injury suspected.

D. Correctly used restraints transfer energy from the impact to the restraint system instead of to the occupant. Injuries that occur when seat belts are used are usually non–life threatening.

Content Category: Trauma & Shock

Reference: Sheehy et al., 1999; pp. 29–30.

---

37. Force is a physical factor that changes the motion of a body either at rest or already in motion. Which of the following is NOT considered one of these forces?
    A. Acceleration
    B. Deceleration
    C. Shearing
    D. CONTUSIVE FORCE

Rationale:

D. A contusive force is a force that causes a bruise. Compression is the fourth type of force: the ability of an object or structure to resist squeezing forces or inward pressure.

A. Acceleration is the change in the rate of velocity or speed of a moving body. As velocity increases, so does tissue damage.

B. Deceleration is a decrease in the velocity of a moving object.

C. Shearing forces occur across a plane, with structures slipping relative to each other.

Content Category: Trauma Shock

Reference: ENA, Trauma Nursing, 2000.

---

38. A significant number of blunt injuries are associated with motor vehicle collisions (MVCs), motorcycle collisions (MCCs), and falls. All of the following statements are true regarding blunt trauma EXCEPT which of the following?
    A. Injury is caused by forces that do not penetrate the body.
    B. BLUNT TRAUMA IS USUALLY LESS LIFE THREATENING THAN PENETRATION TRAUMA.
    C. Explosion injuries may occur in air-filled organs such as the lungs and bowel.
    D. Solid organs sustain crush injuries, producing lacerations, fractures, or ruptures.

Rationale:

B. Blunt forces involve compression, deformation, or sudden change in atmospheric pressure. These result in more injuries and tend to be more difficult to manage due to the lack of external signs of occult injuries may delay diagnosis and patients experience more complications because the injury may be more life threatening than initially assessed to be.

A. Blunt injury is an injury that involves no opening in the skin or communication with the outside environment.

C. Air filled organs such as the lung and bowel are prone to compression injuries, which involve a squeezing inward when pressure is applied to tissue.

D. Solid organs undergo compression injuries when a squeezing inward pressure is applied.

Content Category: Trauma & Shock

Reference: Newberry, 1998; pp. 249–257.

39.   The driver of a motor vehicle commonly sustains the following injuries associated with side-impact collisions EXCEPT which of the following?
A. Contralateral neck sprain
B. RUPTURED LIVER
C. Fractured clavicle
D. Pelvic and acetabular fractures

Rationale:

B. A ruptured liver results when the impact occurs on the passenger's side of a motor vehicle. A ruptured spleen results when the impact is on the driver's side.
A. Strain on the lateral neck can cause spinal fractures or ligament tears.
C. Energy from the impact can pin the occupant's arm against the car, causing chest wall contusions and rib, clavicle, and sternal fractures.
D. Energy from the impact can force the femoral head through the pelvis, causing a pelvic or acetabular fracture.

Content Category: Trauma & Shock

Reference: Newberry, 1998; pp. 252–253.

40.   A 28-year-old female, 32 weeks pregnant, presents after a motor vehicle collision. She potentially has a ruptured uterus. The most appropriate intervention for this patient is probably:
A. AN EMERGENCY CESAREAN SECTION.
B. an abdominal ultrasound scan.
C. peritoneal lavage.
D. continuous fetal monitoring.

Rationale:

A. An emergency cesarean section is the treatment of choice for a ruptured uterus. In most cases an abdominal hysterectomy is performed.
B. An abdominal ultrasound is not indicated at this time.
C. Peritoneal lavage is not indicated in this situation.
D. Continuous fetal monitoring is not the priority intervention. It is an assessment performed pending the emergency cesarean section.

Content Category: Genitourinary & Obstetrics & Gynecology

Reference: Goodman, 1998; pp. 187–195.

Questions 41 and 42

A 32-year-old female is pregnant and in her 34th week of gestation. She presents to the ED complaining of swelling in her lower extremities. She states that she has been having more headaches than usual. She denies visual disturbances. Vital signs are BP 192/110 mm Hg, HR 100/min, respirations 28, and temperature 99.2° F (37.4° C). You note that the patient has 3+ pitting edema to bilateral lower extremities and 3+ protein in her urine.

41.   Based on the above assessment, you suspect that the patient has which of the following?
A. Pregnancy-induced hypertension (PIH)
B. PREECLAMPSIA

C. Eclampsia

D. Normal findings of pregnancy

Rationale:

B. Preeclampsia is a multisystem disorder that is found only during pregnancy. It is associated with an elevated blood pressure and proteinuria. Preeclampsia usually occurs after 20 weeks of gestation.

A. Pregnancy-induced hypertension is a rise in blood pressure without the presence of protein in the urine.

C. Eclampsia is the condition in which seizure activity occurs in the presence of preeclampsia.

D. These are not normal findings of pregnancy.

Content Category: Genitourinary & Obstetrics & Gynecology

Reference: Duley, 2000; pp. 804–813.

42. After the patient has been placed in a room for further evaluation, she begins to develop seizure activity. She is placed on her left side and on 100% nonrebreather mask. The seizures are eventually controlled after the administration of a loading dose of magnesium sulfate ($MgSO_4$). A maintenance infusion is started. Which of the following would suggest that the patient is developing magnesium sulfate toxicity?

A. RESPIRATORY RATE 10/MIN

B. Blood pressure 130/92 mm Hg

C. Heart rate 98 beats/minute

D. Temperature 97.4° F (36.3° C)

Rationale:

A. Patients who receive magnesium sulfate should be monitored closely for loss of deep tendon reflexes and respiratory depression.

B. Magnesium sulfate has no effect on blood pressure.

C. Magnesium sulfate has no effect on pulse rate.

D. Magnesium sulfate has no effect on temperature.

Content Category: Genitourinary & Obstetrics & Gynecology

Reference: Abbott, 1998.

43. Which of the following anticonvulsants is the BEST choice for a woman with eclampsia?

A. Phenytoin (Dilantin)

B. Diazepam (Valium)

C. MAGNESIUM SULFATE ($MgSO_4$)

D. Lytic cocktail

Rationale:

C. Magnesium sulfate has been found statistically to be the most appropriate drug of choice over phenytoin, diazepam, and a lytic cocktail to prevent further seizure activity.

A. Phenytoin is not so effective as magnesium sulfate for seizures related to eclampsia.

B. Diazepam not so effective as magnesium sulfate for seizures related to eclampsia.

D. Lytic cocktail is a mixture of pethidine (Demerol), chlorpromazine (Thorazine), and promethazine (Phenergan).

Content Category: Genitourinary & Obstetrics & Gynecology

References: Duley, 2000; pp. 804–813; Abbott, 1998.

Questions 44 and 45

A 26-year-old female presents to the ED complaining of severe left lower quadrant pain that began about 2 hours ago. Pain radiates to her left shoulder when she moves or takes a deep breath. She has vomited twice since the pain started. She states her last menstrual period was 10 weeks ago. She has had two positive home pregnancy tests. She has not received any prenatal care. Her prior reproductive history includes gravida 3, para 1, abortion 2, living children 1. She has had two episodes of pelvic inflammatory disease in the past 5 years. Vital signs are BP 94/56 mm Hg, HR 136/min, respirations 26/min, and temperature 97.8° F (36.5° C). Her skin is pale, cool, and diaphoretic. She admits to "spotty" vaginal bleeding. She denies any history of recent trauma to her abdomen.

44. The patient is most likely presenting with which of the following?
     A. Pelvic inflammatory disease (PID)
     B. RUPTURED ECTOPIC PREGNANCY
     C. Hyperemesis gravidarum
     D. Appendicitis

Rationale:

B. Presenting symptoms of ruptured ectopic pregnancy include increasing abdominal pain, abdominal distention, hypovolemia, and occasionally shoulder pain as a result of phrenic nerve irritation from intraperitoneal bleeding.

A. PID is an infection of the female's pelvic structure. Patients often present with a complaint of lower abdominal pain, fever and chills, nausea and vomiting, and vaginal discharge.

C. Hyperemesis gravidarum refers to intractable nausea and vomiting. The patient most often presents with weight loss, decreased skin turgor, and a dry, coated tongue.

D. Appendicitis is associated with inflammation of the vermiform appendix. Patients present with a complain of crampy abdominal pain. It may start in the epigastric or periumbilical area, eventually migrating to the right lower quadrant area.

Content Category: Genitourinary & Obstetrics & Gynecology

Reference: Abbott, 1998.

45. Your highest priority with this patient is do which of the following?
     A. START 2 LARGE-BORE INTRAVENOUS LINES WITH RINGER'S LACTATE
     B. Order a pelvic ultrasound scan
     C. Place the patient on her left side
     D. Infuse 2 units of O-positive blood as soon as it is available

Rationale:

A. Start 2 large-bore intravenous lines with Ringer's lactate. This patient is showing signs of hypovolemia; therefore, rapid volume resuscitation should be initiated. The patient should also have a baseline hematocrit and blood type and crossmatch should be obtained for surgery.

B. A pelvic ultrasound scan may be indicated, but this patient presents with symptoms of hypovolemia. Therefore, ultrasound would not be your highest priority.

C. Placing the patient on her left side may be helpful for comfort, but has no clinical significance in this situation.

D. If the patient were unstable and needed blood, you would infuse O-negative blood, not O-positive blood.

Content Category: Genitourinary & Obstetrics & Gynecology

Reference: Abbott, 1998.

Questions 46–49

A female patient who is 13 weeks pregnant by ultrasound presents to the ED with the complaint of vomiting for several days. She states that she vomits everything that she tries to eat or drink. She states that she feels very weak and dizzy. Vital signs are BP 88/52 mm Hg, HR 120/min, respirations 32/min, and temperature 99.8° F (37.7° C). Her urine has 3+ ketones and is negative for protein and negative for leukocytes.

46.   The highest-priority nursing diagnosis for this patient is which of the following?
A.   Alteration in comfort related to weakness
B.   FLUID VOLUME DEFICIT RELATED TO PERSISTENT NAUSEA AND VOMITING
C.   Anxiety related to diagnosis
D.   Alteration in safety related to dizziness

Reference: Rationale:

B.   The patient's presentation indicates dehydration secondary to nausea and vomiting; therefore, fluid volume deficit is of highest priority.
A.   Alteration in comfort, while important, is not the immediate priority.
C.   Anxiety, while important, is not the immediate priority.
D.   Alteration in safety is also an important diagnosis, but not the immediate priority.

Content Category: Genitourinary & Obstetrics & Gynecology

Reference: Abbott, 1998.

47.   You suspect that the patient is experiencing which of the following?
A.   Viral gastroenteritis
B.   HYPEREMESIS GRAVIDARUM
C.   Pregnancy-induced hypotension
D.   Pelvic inflammatory disease (PID)

Rationale:

B.   Hyperemesis gravidarum is a term used to describe intractable nausea and vomiting during pregnancy. The patient most often presents with weight loss, decreased skin turgor, and a dry, coated tongue.
A.   Although the patient could have viral gastroenteritis, her symptoms suggest the intractable vomiting during pregnancy that is associated with hyperemesis gravidarum.
C.   Pregnancy-induced hypotension is not a true syndrome or diagnosis.
D.   Pelvic inflammatory disease is not usually associated with nausea and vomiting.

Content Category: Genitourinary & Obstetrics & Gynecological

Reference: Nuwayhid et al., 1998; pp. 234–262.

48.   The most important intervention for the patient is which of the following?
      A. INITIATE AN INTRAVENOUS LINE AND RAPIDLY ADMINISTER A D5W SOLUTION.
      B. Initiate an intravenous line and rapidly administer 0.9% normal saline.
      C. Initiate an intravenous line and rapidly administer 2 units of O negative blood.
      D. There is no indication that fluid resuscitation should be started at this time.

Rationale:

      A. The patient is presenting with signs of hypovolemia and has unstable vital signs. Initially you would treat the hypovolemia with rapid infusion of an isotonic solution to correct the hypotensive state. You would then administer a solution of 5% glucose in saline or Ringer's lactate to correct the dehydration and ketonuria.
      B. Not appropriate replacement fluid.
      C. Not appropriate, as there is no indication of blood loss.
      D. The patient is severely dehydrated and has unstable vital signs; therefore interventions to correct this situation must be taken.

Content Category: Genitourinary & Obstetrics & Gynecological

Reference: Kuhn, 1998; pp. 694–702.

49.   Which of the following antiemetics is considered the safest to administer to this patient?
      A. Promethazine (Phenergan)
      B. Prochlorperazine (Compazine)
      C. ONDANSETRON (ZOFRAN)
      D. Droperidol (Inapsine)

Rationale:

      C. Ondansetron is a Category B drug. Drugs are classified for safety in pregnancy based on clinical trials. Class A drugs are considered safe based on human studies. Class B drugs are presumed safe based on animal studies. Class C drugs have uncertain reports concerning safety, although no human studies or animal studies have shown an adverse effect. Class D drugs are considered unsafe during pregnancy, yet the risk may be justifiable in certain clinical circumstances. Class X drugs are highly unsafe; the risk of use outweighs the possible benefit of the drug.
      A. Promethazine is a Class C drug.
      B. Prochlorperazine is a Class C drug.
      D. Droperidol is a Class C drug.

Content Category: Genitourinary & Obstetrics & Gynecological

Reference: Tarascon Publishing, 2001.

50.   A male patient presents to the ED with what he calls a panic attack. Objective findings include cool and clammy skin, tachycardia, and tachypnea. He is pacing. The priority medication for this patient is:
      A. thioridazine (Mellaril).
      B. lithium carbonate (Eskalith).
      C. LORAZEPAM (ATIVAN).
      D. haloperidol (Haldol).

Rationale:

      C. This patient is very anxious and requires an antianxiety medication such as lorazepam (Ativan).
      A. Thioridazine (Mellaril) is an antipsychotic mediation used in schizophrenic disorders.

B. Lithium carbonate (Eskalith) is an antimanic drug used in bipolar disorder.

D. Haloperidol (Haldol) is an antipsychotic mediation used in schizophrenic disorders. Although haloperidol may also be used for severe anxiety, lorazepam (Ativan) is more effective in reducing anxiety.

Content Category: Psychosocial

References: Copel, 1999; pp. 376–385; Varacolis, 1998; pp. 1014–1018.

51. A 45-year-old teacher and father of two comes to the ED complaining of depression. He has a history of bipolar disease, is not taking any medication, and denies any plans to hurt himself. He was told by his therapist to come to the ED for a psychiatric admission. Which of the following statements by the ED nurse is most therapeutic?

A. "You have so much to live for."

B. "I know how you feel."

C. "Everything will be OK."

D. "THIS MUST BE DIFFICULT FOR YOU."

Rationale:

D. Rapport with the patient needs to be developed. A therapeutic nurse-patient relationship requires caring and compassionate communication, while setting limits. This statement acknowledges the difficulty of most patients in being admitted for psychiatric reasons.

A. This response conveys little understanding and respect for the patient's feelings. It can block communication and create distance.

B. Therapeutic communication is patient centered, not nurse centered. This statement is untrue, as one person does not know how another person is feeling, even if s/he has experienced similar situations.

C. While it is important to offer hope to patients, this statement is likely to be premature if stated in the ED.

Content Category: Psychosocial

Reference: Stuart & Laraia, 1998; p. 365.

52. A 48-year-old female presents to the ED with complaints of intermittent palpitations, chest tightness, and choking sensations. She reports having had these symptoms for about 6 weeks and states that the episodes are becoming more frequent. At triage she has an intact airway and her skin is cool and slightly diaphoretic to the touch. Vital signs are BP 168/72 mm Hg, HR 118/min, respirations 26/min, and temperature 99.2° F (37.3° C). The patient does not report any chest tightness, palpitations, or choking sensations at this time. Results of diagnostic tests are negative for cardiac disease. During discharge instruction, the patient reports that "something bad" is going to happen to her. At this point the ED nurse should do which of the following?

A. Assure the patient that her cardiac monitor reading is perfectly normal

B. Order another electrocardiogram to assure the absence of cardiac disease

C. Leave the patient and locate the ED physician immediately

D. REMAIN WITH THE PATIENT, PERFORM A FOCUSED ASSESSMENT TO ASSURE HEMODYNAMIC STABILITY, AND EXPLORE THE PATIENT'S FEELINGS OF DREAD

Rationale:

D. Results of diagnostic testing do not support evidence of cardiac disease. Further assessment must be performed to determine the cause of this patient's problems. Patients with anxiety disorders often present to the ED with complaints that may be cardiac in origin. Exploration of feelings of dread reported by this patient will enhance acceptance and self-esteem by acknowledging the patient's anxiety and offering reassurance.

A. Verbal assurance that the cardiac monitor is not showing cardiac rhythm disturbances will not minimize the patient's perception of impending doom.

B. The original ECG does not support evidence of cardiac disease. It would be inappropriate for another ECG to be performed at this time.

C. Since the patient has expressed a sense of dread, it would be inappropriate for the emergency nurse to leave her alone at this time.

Content Category: Psychosocial

Reference: Kitt et al., 1995;) pp. 464–465.

53. A 35-year-old woman has just been treated in the ED after having been sexually assaulted. The patient is alert. Initial assessment reveals bruises and abrasions on her face, breasts, arms, and hands. She makes minimal eye contact with the nurse and responds only when asked a question. Discharge instructions for this patient must include which of the following?

A. Partner notification, rape crisis counseling, STD treatment

B. RAPE CRISIS COUNSELING, STD PROPHYLAXIS, HIV TESTING, PROPHYLAXIS IF THE EXPOSURE WAS ASSESSED AS HIGH RISK

C. Importance of follow-up with law enforcement agencies

D. Repeat STD testing in10 days, psychosocial counseling, chain of evidence

Rationale:

B. Rape crisis counseling, STD prophylaxis, and HIV testing and prophylaxis must be completed for sexual assault survivors. Counseling has decreased the incidence and negative impact of rape trauma syndrome.

A. Partner notification is inappropriate in sexual assault treatment unless the patient requests the nurse to do so.

C. Follow-up with law enforcement agencies is not within the domain of the ED staff.

D. STD testing should be repeated after 10 days of treatment. Counseling is needed. Supporting the chain of evidence is the responsibility of the ED staff, not the patient.

Content Category: Psychosocial

References: ENA, Core Curriculum, 2000; pp. 463–464; Kitt et al., 1995; pp. 265–268; Ledray, 1992; pp. 223–230.

54. A 25-year-old male is brought to the ED after a motor vehicle crash. He was a restrained driver whose vehicle ran out of control and struck a stone embankment. The front seat passenger, his girlfriend, was not restrained and was ejected through the windshield on impact. She was pronounced dead at the scene of the crash. As the ED nurse performs primary and secondary assessments on this patient, he insists that he must see his girlfriend and demands to know when the police are bringing her to visit him. Primary and secondary assessments reveal minor contusions and abrasions. The patient has completed his evaluation process and the physician states that he is ready to be discharged. As the ED nurse reviews the discharge instructions with this patient, he states, "Stop what you're doing and get this IV out of me! I need to find my girlfriend. The police and ambulance crew told me she didn't make it, but I know she's okay." The ED nurse recognizes that this patient's unresolved crisis state, if left untreated, will result in which of the following?

A. PSYCHOSIS

B. Continued feelings of tension and heightened frustration

C. Strengthened personality

D. Enhanced ability to solve problems in the future

Rationale:

A. A buildup of tension and frustration is the result of the person's ineffective attempt to problem solve.
B. Psychosis is generally not the result of crisis. It is an extreme response to stressors that affect a patient's affective, psychomotor, and physical behavior and is exhibited by hallucinations or delusions.
C. The development of newer coping mechanisms during crisis strengthens the personality.
D. Ineffective problem solving does not enhance future problem-solving ability.

Content Category: Psychosocial

Reference: Varcarolis, 1998; pp.371–375, 1034.

55.   A 13-year-old male is brought into the ED by EMS, police, and school officials after he drew a picture of himself holding a gun to his class. He is withdrawn and does not freely interact with the triage nurse. School officials report that this is not the first time this student has received attention for his behavior and that his grandmother refuses to accept that he is having emotional problems. During psychiatric evaluation, the patient informs the psychiatric clinical nurse specialist that he is angry about the death of his mother and wants to join her. The child is becoming increasingly agitated during the assessment process. Which of the following interventions would be appropriate at this time?
A. Isolate him in a seclusion room.
B. ALLOW THE GRANDMOTHER, WHO HAS SINCE CALMED DOWN, TO REMAIN WITH THE PATIENT DURING THE INTERVIEW.
C. Obtain an order for IV conscious sedation.
D. Restrain the patient to assure safety of all staff.

Rationale:

B. Since this child is 13 years old, it would be beneficial if his caregiver were to stay and support him during the evaluation process.
A. Placing the patient in seclusion would only worsen his feelings of isolation.
C. Manipulation of the environment to promote quiet and safety is the first step in reducing agitation.
D. Application of physical restraints is the last step. This intervention is performed only when the patient's behavior cannot be modified by other means. Restraint serves only to increase agitation.

Content Category: Psychosocial

Reference: Varcarolis, 1998.

56.   A 16-year-old female arrives in the ED accompanied by her parents. She appears cachectic. Vital signs are BP 86/50 mm Hg, HR 50/min and irregular, respirations 20/min, and temperature 96° F (35.6° C). Her lips are dry and cracked. Skin turgor is tented. She has fine, downy hair growth on her face. She had her last menstrual period approximately 4 months ago. As an IV intravenous line is being started, she states, "There's no sugar in there, is there?" Your best response would be which of the following?
A. "It is important to rehydrate you. We need to get you past this crisis."
B. "I HEAR HOW FRIGHTENED YOU ARE. WOULD YOU LIKE TO TALK ABOUT IT?"
C. "Your doctor ordered it, yes."
D. "Don't be afraid. It won't make you fat."

Rationale:

B. This answer validates the patient's fears and gives her an opportunity to verbalize them.

A. This response tells the patient that her fears are less important to you than they are to her. It may make her feel belittled and not in control.

C. This response also relays that her fears are not so important to you as to her. It may make her feel rejected because it does not give her an opportunity to express her thoughts and feelings.

D. This response makes the patient feel that her fears are not important. It underrates her feelings and belittles her concerns.

Content Category: Psychosocial

References: Varcarolis, 1998; pp. 188–196, 801–815, Copel, 1999; pp. 1–6, 235–245.

57. Which of the following ophthalmic products produce constriction of the pupils?
    A. Cycloplegics
    B. Mydriatics
    C. MIOTICS
    D. Steroids

Rationale:

C. Miotics constrict the pupils.

A. Cycloplegics paralyze ciliary muscles.

B. Mydriatics dilate the pupils.

D. Steroids decrease the inflammatory response.

Content Category: Maxillofacial & Ocular

Reference: Egging, 2000; pp. 689–706.

58. Which of the following is true about otitis media?
    A. It occurs most frequently in the school-age child.
    B. Hearing is usually unaffected.
    C. IT IS OFTEN CAUSED BY A VIRUS.
    D. Definitive treatment included placement of tubes.

Rationale:

C. Although otitis media can be bacterial, most otitis is viral.

A. The highest incidence of otitis media is in toddlers.

B. Otitis media produces fluid in the middle ear; the fluid alters hearing.

D. Chronic rather than acute otitis media is treated by placement of tubes.

Content Category: Maxillofacial & Ocular

Reference: Urdaneta & Lucchesi, 2000; pp. 1518–1526.

59. A woman presents to the ED complaining of "shooting pains" in the left cheek region. The pain started when she was washing her face. Which of the following should be considered a likely diagnosis?
    A. Herpes zoster
    B. TRIGEMINAL NEURALGIA
    C. Glossopharyngeal neuralgia
    D. Temporal arteritis

Rationale:

B. Trigeminal neuralgia produces electric shock-like stabbing pain, usually unilateral; patients may be pain free between attacks.

A. Herpes presents with a unilateral aching and burning jabs of pain.

C. Glossopharyngeal neuralgia presents with pain in the tonsillar fossa, pharynx, or base of the tongue.

D. Temporal arteritis presents with a temporal headache, fever, and localized pain.

Content Category: Maxillofacial & Ocular

References: Dains et al., 1998; pp. 371–400; Montgomery, 2000; pp. 577–600.

60. A swallowed meat bolus may be treated with a variety of methods, providing the patient can manage his or her own secretions. Which of the following treatment methods carries the greatest risk for perforation?

A. Administration of glucagon intravenously

B. USE OF PROTEOLYTIC ENZYMES SUCH AS MEAT TENDERIZER

C. Use of sedation and waiting up to 12 hours before initiating treatment

D. Endoscopy

Rationale:

B. Use of proteolytic enzymes, such as an aqueous solution of papain (e.g., Adolph's Meat Tenderizer), to dissolve a meat bolus is NOT recommended because of the number of reported complications. Several reports in the literature have described esophageal perforation secondary to the enzymatic action of the solution. Mucosal ischemia resulting from distention of the esophageal wall renders the esophagus more susceptible to enzymatic degradation. Hemorrhagic pulmonary edema also has been reported after aspiration of Adolph's Meat Tenderizer.

A. Administration of glucagon intravenously relaxes the esophageal smooth muscle to treat food impaction. A test dose should be given to ensure that hypersensitivity does not exist; then the recommended dose is 1 mg. If the food bolus is not passed in 20 minutes, an additional 2 mg is given intravenously.

C. Time and sedation often allow the meat to pass into the stomach, but the bolus should not be allowed to remain impacted for more than 12 hours.

D. Endoscopy is the preferred method of removal.

Content Category: Maxillofacial & Ocular

Reference: Gaasch & Barish, 2000; pp. 529–531.

61. When penetrating ocular injury is suspected, the ED nurse should do which of the following FIRST?

A. Instill antibiotic eye drops

B. Perform detailed range of motion of the extraocular muscles

C. APPLY A RIGID SHIELD OVER THE EYE

D. Irrigate the eye with warmed saline

Rationale:

C. A rigid shield should be applied to prevent pressure on the globe that could cause further damage or extrusion of intraocular contents.

A. Antibiotics are indicated, but should be administered intravenously.

B. All movement of the eye should be avoided to minimize additional injury.

D. Irrigation of the eye is contraindicated in the patient with possible penetrating ocular injury.

Content Category: Maxillofacial & Ocular

Reference: Egging, 1998; pp.689–706.

62. Labyrinthitis is characterized by acute onset of a severe vertiginous episode often accompanied by which of the following?
     A. Tinnitus
     B. NAUSEA AND VOMITING
     C. Hearing loss
     D. Otalgia

Rationale:

     B. Labyrinthitis is often accompanied by nausea and vomiting.
     A. Tinnitus does not usually accompany labyrinthitis.
     C. Hearing loss does not usually accompany labyrinthitis.
     D. Otalgia (ear pain) does not usually accompany labyrinthitis.

Content Category: Maxillofacial & Ocular

Reference: Urdaneta & Lucchesi, 2000; pp. 1518–1526.

63. Anterior epistaxis accounts for 90% of nosebleeds. Most patients with anterior epistaxis can be managed by direct pressure and which of the following?
     A. Arterial ligation or embolization
     B. NASAL PACKING AND CAUTERY
     C. Nasal tampons and external carotid artery pressure
     D. Vasoconstrictive agents and use of epistaxis balloon

Rationale:

     B. The majority of anterior nosebleeds can be managed by nasal packing and cautery.
     A. Arterial ligation and embolization are special techniques indicated for epistaxis that is refractive to first-line treatment.
     C. Nasal tampons can be used for anterior epistaxis, but external carotid artery pressure is not recommended.
     D. Vasoconstrictive agents are appropriate for anterior epistaxis, but balloons are indicated for posterior epistaxis.

Content Category: Maxillofacial & Ocular

Reference: Waters & Peacock, 2000; pp. 1532–1539.

64. Discharge instructions for a patient with epistaxis should include humidification and which of the following?
     A. Use anti-inflammatory agents for 3–4 days.
     B. Hold any antihypertensive medications for 3–4 days.
     C. APPLY PETROLEUM JELLY TO AFFECTED NARIS WITH COTTON SWAB DAILY.
     D. Apply antibiotic ointment to affected naris with finger daily.

Rationale:

     C. The application of petroleum jelly will help to keep the nasal mucosa from drying and becoming more susceptible for rebleeding. The cotton swab is a gentle method for application.
     A. Aspirin and nonsteroidal anti-inflammatory agents should be avoided for a minimum of 3–4 days to prevent further bleeding.

B. Hypertension is a common cause of epistaxis. Any antihypertensive medications should be taken as directed.

D. Although antibiotic ointment is indicated to keep the nasal mucosa from drying, the ointment should not be applied with a finger for fear of further trauma to the nasal mucosa. The ointment should be applied with a cotton swab to avoid rebleeding.

Content Category: Maxillofacial & Ocular

Reference: Waters & Peacock, 2000; pp. 1532–1539.

65. A patient presents to triage complaining of sudden severe eye pain and a headache. The pupil is fixed and dilated. The ED nurse should suspect which of the following?
A. Retinal detachment
B. Keratitis
C. Chalazion
D. ACUTE GLAUCOMA

Rationale:

D. Sudden, severe eye pain and headache are cardinal signs and symptoms for acute glaucoma. Additional symptoms include a hard globe, a foggy-appearing cornea, halos around lights, and decreased peripheral vision. Blindness can ensue quickly. Prompt identification and intervention are essential.

A. Retinal detachment is characterized by painless loss of vision.

B. Keratitis is an inflammation of the cornea characterized by light sensitivity and pain.

C. A patient with a chalazion presents with weeks of painless localized swelling. No pupil changes are present.

Content Category: Maxillofacial & Ocular

Reference: Egging, 1998; pp. 689–706.

66. Fluid volume deficit would be the priority nursing diagnosis in which of the following conditions?
A. Diverticulitis
B. PANCREATITIS
C. Cholecystitis
D. Appendicitis

Rationale:

B. Pancreatitis usually results in fluid volume deficit. The large fluid loss from volume shift into the abdominal cavity places the patient at high risk for hypotension and shock.

A. Diverticulitis, depending on severity, can present with pain management as well as knowledge deficit.

C. Cholecystitis does not usually present with fluid volume deficit as the primary nursing diagnosis. Pain management and preparation for surgical intervention are necessary.

D. Appendicitis does not initially present with fluid volume deficit. Pain management is important. A risk for fluid volume deficit exists.

Content Category: Gastrointestinal

References: Porth, 1998; pp. 769–771; Newberry, 1998; pp. 550–552.

67. A 15-month-old child is being discharged from the ED with mild dehydration from gastroenteritis. The nurse is explaining the discharge instructions to the parents. What statement indicates the parents' understanding of the instructions?
   A. "If our child vomits again, we will attempt to give him/her oral replacement fluids right away, in sips."
   B. "Since our child wears diapers, s/he can return to day care if fever free."
   C. "OUR CHILD SHOULD TAKE SMALL, FREQUENT SIPS OF ORAL HYDRATION FLUIDS WHILE HOME."
   D. "Our child is now stable and does not need follow-up with the family health care provider."

Rationale:

C. Children who are being discharged with acute gastroenteritis should be encouraged to take small, frequent sips of fluid replacement therapy after vomiting has subsided for 1 to 2 hours.

A. Resting the gastrointestinal gut after vomiting is encouraged. Fluids should be given 1 to 2 hours after vomiting.

B. Children with gastroenteritis are highly infectious through the oral-fecal route. Frequent hand washing and diaper changing should be done. Day care should be avoided until the acute stage of diarrhea and/or vomiting has subsided.

D. Children can deteriorate quickly from dehydration if a relapse occurs or if rehydration is unsuccessful in the home. Parents should follow up with their primary health care provider and observe the child for signs and symptoms of dehydration, especially if vomiting or diarrhea continues.

Content Category: Gastrointestinal

References: Soud & Rogers, 1998; pp. 333–362; Wyatt et al., 1999; pp. 516–533.

68. Which of the following inflammatory conditions requires surgical intervention?
   A. Crohn's disease
   B. PERITONITIS
   C. Esophagitis
   D. Ulcerative colitis

Rationale:

B. Peritonitis is the acute inflammation of the peritoneal membrane, indicating a contaminant in the peritoneal cavity. Antibiotics and surgery are appropriate interventions.

A. Crohn's disease is a chronic condition that causes inflammation of the intestine. The disease is treated with anticholinergics, antidiarrheals, and other supportive measures.

C. Esophagitis is a chronic condition that is treated with antibiotics, analgesics, and supportive care.

D. Ulcerative colitis is a nonspecific inflammatory response of the mucosa. This chronic condition is treated with antibiotics, steroids, and intravenous fluids as necessary.

Content Category: Gastrointestinal

References: Newberry, 1998; pp. 541–555; Black & Matassarin-Jacobs, 1997; pp. 1794–1801.

69. Cirrhosis is a progressive, degenerative disease that results in INCREASED:
   A. flow of blood.
   B. function of the liver.
   C. PRESSURE IN THE PORTAL VEIN.
   D. clearing of metabolic wastes.

Rationale:

C. The portal vein receives blood from the intestines and spleen. Increased pressure in the portal vein is the main complication of cirrhosis. It happens initially due to obstruction of flow caused by fibrous tissue and regenerative nodules. This elevated pressure results in the formation of fluid accumulation in the peritoneum (ascites). Obstruction of flow also leads to the formation of collateral blood flow, such as in veins in the esophagus. These collaterals, or varices, are a hallmark of cirrhosis.

A. Blood flow is not increased, but obstructed. The obstruction causes a reverse flow that in turn causes enlargement of the veins.

B. During cirrhosis, liver function decreases; it does not increase.

D. Clearing of metabolic wastes in cirrhosis is incomplete, not increased.

Content Category: Gastrointestinal

Reference: Black & Matassarin-Jacobs, 1997; pp. 1872–1884.

70. You are caring for a 25-year-old restrained male victim of a motor vehicle crash (MVC). He is complaining of abdominal pain in the right upper quadrant (RUQ) and has right shoulder pain. He is hypotensive. A seat belt abrasion is visible over the abdomen, which is firm, with hypoactive bowel sounds. You suspect this patient has an injury in which of the following areas?

A. Stomach

B. Spleen

C. Bladder

D. LIVER

Rationale:

D. Liver injuries must be suspected when the patient has received a direct blow to the RUQ. Clinical indicators include pain in the RUQ with possible bruising or abrasions and possibly a firm abdomen with hypoactive or diminished bowel sounds. Right shoulder pain can occur. The patient with a major liver injury almost always develops signs of shock.

A. Signs and symptoms of a stomach injury include left upper quadrant (LUQ) pain and tenderness, aspiration of blood via nasogastric tube, and the presence of free air on the abdominal x-ray.

B. Splenic injuries are suspected when the patient presents with pain to the LUQ. Kehr's sign may be present, with LUQ bruising and signs of shock.

C. Bladder injuries are suspected when a patient presents with a history of blunt lower abdominal trauma. Clinical signs include inability to void, suprapubic pain, and hematuria.

Content Category: Gastrointestinal

References: Newberry, 1998; pp. 311–323; ENA, Trauma Nursing, 2000; pp. 148–151.

71. Discharge instructions for a patient diagnosed with diverticulitis should include instructions to do which of the following?

A. Limit fluid intake.

B. AVOID EATING NUTS AND POPCORN.

C. Drink alcohol in moderation.

D. Eat a high-fat diet.

Rationale:

B. Patients diagnosed with diverticulitis are instructed to avoid nuts and popcorn, which may become trapped in the diverticula.

A. The patient should be encouraged to drink at least 8 glasses of water daily to facilitate bowel movements.

C. The patient should be instructed to avoid alcohol consumption.

D. The patient should be instructed to eat a low-fat diet.

Content Category: Gastrointestinal

Reference: ENA, Core Curriculum, 2000; p. 45.

72.   The pharmacologic treatment of choice in patients with peptic ulcer disease caused by *Helicobacter pylori* (*H. pylori*) would be an antibiotic such as clarithromycin, bismuth subsalicylate (Pepto-Bismol), and which of the following?
       A. Prednisone
       B. Calcium carbonate (Os-Cal)
       C. Sodium bicarbonate
       D. OMEPRAZOLE (PRILOSEC)

Rationale:

       D. Omeprazole (Prilosec) is a proton pump inhibitor that inhibits the final stage of hydrogen ion secretion. Prilosec in combination with bismuth and antibiotics such as clarithromycin (Biaxin) are used in combination to help eradicate *H. pylori*. This combination has been shown to have the greatest efficacy in fighting peptic ulcer disease by *H. pylori* when used as pharmacologic therapy.
       A. Prednisone is a steroid and should be avoided in patients who have peptic ulcer disease.
       B. Calcium carbonate causes constipation and may increase acid secretion.
       C. Sodium bicarbonate is not recommended, as it tends to cause metabolic alkalosis.

Content Category: Gastrointestinal

References: Porth, 1998; pp. 725–729, 769–771; Black & Matassarin-Jacobs, 1997; p. 1765.

73.   Peritonitis can be life threatening. Which of the following statements about peritonitis is TRUE?
       A. The peritoneum is unable to produce an inflammatory reaction.
       B. Peristaltic activity increases with peritonitis.
       C. RESPIRATORY DIFFICULTY IS CAUSED BY INCREASED ABDOMINAL PRESSURE.
       D. Circulating volume increases with peritonitis.

Rationale:

       C. The person with peritonitis has difficulty breathing because of increased abdominal pressure, which elevates the diaphragm and causing pain.
       A. The peritoneum is able to produce an inflammatory reaction and wall off a localized process to combat infection.
       B. Peristaltic activity decreases with peritonitis; it does not increase.
       D. Circulating volume decreases with peritonitis because of fluid shifts.

Content Category: Gastrointestinal

References: ENA, Core Curriculum, 2000; pp. 49–55; Black & Matassarin-Jacobs, 1997; pp. 1793–1794.

74.   A 35-year-old male jumped off a chair and landed on his right foot. On assessment, he is unable to flex his foot or stand on the ball of his foot and has a positive Thompson's sign. You suspect the patient has which of the following?
       A. Tibia fracture
       B. ACHILLES TENDON RUPTURE
       C. Jones fracture
       D. Ankle sprain

Rationale:

       B. Achilles tendon rupture results most often from a forceful dorsiflexion of the ankle. The patient complains of sharp pain from the heel into the back of the leg and is unable to use his foot. This patient has a positive Thompson's sign. This means that with the patient kneeling on a chair with legs extended over the edge, the clinician squeezes the calf muscle. In a positive result, the heel does not pull and no upward motion is seen.

A. A fractured tibia usually results from direct or indirect trauma or torsion. Patients are able to flex and extend the foot and have pain and a negative Thompson's sign.

C. A Jones fracture is a transverse fracture of the fifth metatarsal. Pain is usually present in the foot. The patient is able to flex and extend the foot and has a negative Thompson's sign.

D. A sprained ankle usually results from overstretching of a muscle where it is attached to the tendon. The patient is able to flex and extend the foot but has pain with movement and a negative Thompson's sign.

Content Category: Orthopedics & Wound Care

Reference: Sheehy, 1997; pp. 351–382.

75. A female patient complains of worsening pain with numbness and tingling in both hands for 2 weeks. She has had no relief from acetaminophen (Tylenol). You are concerned that her symptoms represent which of the following?
   A. CARPAL TUNNEL SYNDROME
   B. Tendinitis
   C. Bursitis
   D. Osteoarthritis

Rationale:

A. Carpal tunnel syndrome results from compression of the median nerve in the carpal canal, causing pain, tingling, and numbness in the hands and fingers.

B. Tendinitis is caused by an inflammation of the tendon. It usually results in an aching pain with motion and swelling.

C. Bursitis is an inflammation of the sac (bursa) that covers a bony prominence between bones, muscles, and tendons. Bursitis usually involves the elbow, shoulder, knee, heel, or hip.

D. Osteoarthritis is a chronic disease involving the joints that causes articular cartilage deterioration and bony overgrowth of the joint surface. The patient has pain with movement and activity that is relieved with rest.

Content Category: Orthopedics & Wound Care

References: Buttaravoli & Stair, 2000; pp. 267–270; Strauss, 1999; pp. 487–536.

76. A child brought to the ED by his father is complaining of a painful index finger. The father tells you that the child tends to bite his nails. Exam reveals a tender, swollen, red fingertip with pus visible under the cuticle. The ED nurse should suspect that the child has which of the following?
   A. Felon
   B. Herpetic whitlow
   C. PARONYCHIA
   D. Fungus infection

Rationale:

C. Paronychia is an infection of the distal phalanx along the edge of the nail.

A. Felon is an infection of the closed space of the pulp of the distal phalanx.

B. Herpetic whitlow is a viral infection of the fingertip with intracutaneous vesicles.

D. A fungus infection usually presents with a nail that is discolored and pitted.

Content Category: Orthopedics& Wound Care

References: Buttaravoli & Stair, 2000; pp. 398–402; Allison & Gough, 1996; pp.1118–1121; Simon & Slobodkin, 1996; pp. 1338–1322.

77. Supracondylar fractures in children are associated with neurovascular compromise of which of the following?
    A. Brachial plexus injury
    B. BRACHIAL ARTERY INJURY
    C. Ulnar nerve injury
    D. Ulnar artery injury

Rationale:

B. Brachial artery injury is a risk with this fracture. The incidence of neurovascular compromise is 6–16%. Once the problem has been identified, immediate surgical intervention is needed to avoid Volkmann's ischemic contracture.
A. The brachial plexus is above the supracondylar area and is therefore not at risk in this situation.
C. Ulnar nerve injury is a potential complication with pin insertion, but not likely upon presentation.
D. Injury to the ulnar artery is unlikely because it is positioned distally in the arm.

Content Category: Orthopedics & Wound Care

References: Bailey, 1998; pp. 415–447; Hammond et al., 1998; pp. 186–199.

78. Acute compartment syndrome has been diagnosed in a patient with right tibia-fibula fractures. The patient will be scheduled in the operating room for closed reduction and:
    A. celiotomy.
    B. FASCIOTOMY.
    C. escharotomy.
    D. casting.

Rationale:

B. Fasciotomy is performed to release pressure. Lateral and medial incisions are made into the four compartments.
A. Celiotomy is an abdominal operation.
C. Escharotomy is performed to release pressure under burned skin.
D. Casting would increase pressure. Generally bivalving is done to relieve the pressure.

Content Category: Orthopedics & Wound Care

References: Bailey, 1998; pp.415–447; Tumbarella, 2000; pp. 30–35.

79. Scaphoid (navicular) fractures classically have point tenderness in which area?
    A. SNUFF BOX
    B. Ulnar styloid
    C. Radial head
    D. Olecranon

Rationale:

A. The snuff box is an anatomic location between the radial styloid and the first metacarpal. It directly overlies the navicular bone.
B. The ulnar styloid is on the opposite side of the wrist.
C. The radial head is located in the elbow.
D. The olecranon is at the point of the elbow.

Content Category: Orthopedics & Wound Care

Reference: Bailey, 1998; pp.415–447.

80. The motor function of the ulnar nerve includes:
    A. SPREADING AND CLOSING THE FINGERS.
    B. elevating the wrist and extending the thumb.
    C. making a ring with thumb and small finger.
    D. crossing fingers.

Rationale:

    A. This is the motor function of the ulnar nerve.
    B. This is the motor function of the radial nerve.
    C. This is the motor function of the median nerve.
    D. This is not a specific motor function.

Content Category: Orthopedic & Wound Care

Reference: Bailey, 1998; pp.415–447.

81. A fracture with multiple splintered bone fragments is referred to as:
    A. avulsion.
    B. oblique.
    C. COMMINUTED.
    D. transverse.

Rationale:

    C. A comminuted fracture is a fracture with multiple splintered bone fragments.
    A. An avulsion fracture is a fracture consisting of a fragment and ligamentous attachment that is avulsed from the bone.
    B. An oblique fracture is an angulated fracture through the bone with no fragments.
    D. A transverse fracture is a horizontal linear fracture through the bone with no fragments.

Content Category: Orthopedics & Wound Care

Reference: Walker, 2000; pp. 501–535.

82. An elderly male presents to the ED complaining of gradually increasing low back pain over a 3-month period. He denies any trauma and having done any lifting, pulling, or excessive bending. The ED nursing assessment should include:
    A. use of over-the-counter sleep aids.
    B. SMOKING HISTORY.
    C. recent travel to the tropics.
    D. family history of alcoholism.

Rationale:

    B. Metastatic bone disease may be the initial presentation in a patient with undiagnosed cancer. Lung tumors have a propensity to metastasize to bones, especially the spine.
    A. Over-the-counter sleep aids have no role in back pain.
    C. Travel to the tropics would not produce isolated back pain.
    D. A family history of alcoholism has no relationship to back pain.

Content Category: Orthopedics & Wound Care

Reference: Rosen et al., 1999.

83. A patient diagnosed with bursitis of the knee is ready for discharge. Which of the following statements by the patient indicates that discharge teaching has been successful?
    A. "I will massage a mild hydrocortisone cream onto the knee twice a day."
    B. "I will see my doctor for a Lyme disease test."
    C. "I will apply heat to the area six times a day."
    D. "I WILL TAKE AN OVER-THE-COUNTER ANTI-INFLAMMATORY MEDICATION."

Rationale:

    D. Anti-inflammatory medication will help to decrease the inflammation of the bursa.
    A. Topical steroid cream will have no effect on the bursa.
    B. A Lyme disease test is indicated if the knee joint appears arthritic. In bursitis, the bursa, not the joint, is involved.
    C. Ice, not heat, should be applied to the area of bursitis.

Content Category: Orthopedics & Wound Care

Reference: Walker, 2000; pp. 501–535.

84. The minimum radiographic evaluation of the cervical spine includes:
    A. flexion and extension views.
    B. LATERAL, ANTEROPOSTERIOR, AND ODONTOID VIEWS.
    C. computed tomogram (CT) scans of the cervical spine.
    D. magnetic resonance imaging (MRI) films of the cervical spine.

Rationale:

    B. These three views represent the minimum views needed to assess all seven cervical vertebrae.
    A. Flexion and extension views would not be performed unless the minimum films were normal.
    C. CT is performed if fracture is seen on the plain films.
    D. MRI is performed to evaluate ligament or soft tissue injury.

Content Category: Orthopedics & Wound Care

Reference: Barkin et al., 1999.

85. The chin laceration of a 3-year-old child has been repaired and she is ready for discharge. The nurse advises the parents that the area should be protected from reinjury because full tensile strength will not return for:
    A. 7 days.
    B. 10 days.
    C. 2 months.
    D. 6 MONTHS.

Rationale:

    D. Scar remodeling takes several months. Full tensile strength is achieve at around 6 months post injury.
    A. There is an increase in tensile strength at 7 days, but it is transient.
    B. There is a decrease in tensile strength at 10 days.
    C. There is only a 50% achievement of full tensile strength at 2 months.

Content Category: Orthopedics & Wound Care

Reference: Trott, 1997; pp.20–37.

Questions 86 and 87

A 10-year-old child is brought to the ED by her father. The child received a puncture wound to the foot on the previous day, when she stepped on a rusty nail. The father states the parental preference has been not to have their children immunized. His daughter has had no vaccines since birth.

86.   In view of the girl's injury, her father wants her to receive tetanus immunization. The child should receive which of the following?
   A. Tetanus-diphtheria vaccine alone
   B. Tetanus immune globulin alone
   C. Tetanus-diphtheria vaccine in the right deltoid and tetanus immune globulin in the right deltoid
   D. TETANUS-DIPHTHERIA VACCINE IN THE RIGHT DELTOID AND TETANUS IMMUNE GLOBULIN IN THE RIGHT GLUTEUS.

Rationale:

   D. Because primary immunization was never completed, this child needs passive immunization with globulin as well as the start of active immunization with vaccine. When both injections are administered at the same time, each should be deposited in a muscle distant from the other site.
   A. Vaccine is not sufficient in this instance; there must also be passive immunization.
   B. While the globulin will provide passive immunization, vaccine must also be administered to stimulate the production of antibodies.
   C. Depositing the globulin too close to the vaccine might blunt the body's response and therefore antibody production.

Content Category: Orthopedics & Wound Care

Reference: Gilbert et al., 2001.

87.   The patient received tetanus immunization in the ED. Discharge instructions for the father should include signs and symptoms of:
   A. WOUND INFECTION.
   B. Stevens-Johnson syndrome.
   C. tetanus.
   D. Achilles tendinitis.

Rationale:

   A. Puncture wounds carry an increased risk of infection because bacteria may be deposited deep in the tissues.
   B. Stevens-Johnson syndrome occurs after the administration of certain drugs, most notably the sulfas.
   C. Tetanus should have been prevented once active and passive immunization were completed.
   D. The Achilles tendon is rarely involved when the plantar surface of the foot is punctured.

Content Category: Orthopedics & Wound Care

Reference: Trott, 1997; pp. 285–301.

88. A 34-year-old female presents to triage complaining of right-sided chest and rib pain. She denies any unusual activities, but admits she was gardening for several hours the day before. She ranks the pain as 7 out of 10 on a 1-to-10 pain scale. The pain is sharp and worsens when she takes a deep breath. An ECG monitor is applied and demonstrates a normal, sinus rhythm. You suspect that the patient may be experiencing:
   A. a myocardial infarction.
   B. congestive heart failure.
   C. a pleural effusion.
   D. COSTOCHONDRITIS.

Rationale:

   D. Costochondritis is an inflammation in the rib, sternal junction, or both, caused by physical exertion or repetitive movements. Patient will present with chest pain that is sharp in nature and usually worsens with deep inspiration.
   A. MI is a result of prolonged ischemia resulting in necrosis of the myocardium. The patient generally complains of shortness of breath, nausea, vomiting, and diaphoresis. The pain is generally dull, but may vary accordingly. Electrocardiography changes may or may not be present.
   B. Congestive heart failure is the inability of the heart to maintain adequate output to meet the demands of the body. Patients will complain of shortness of breath because of pulmonary congestion. Patients will also complain of chest pain, fatigue, and possibly coughing up pinkish sputum.
   C. A pleural effusion is the buildup of fluids in the pleural space. Patients will complain of coughing, shortness of breath, and chest pain.

Content Category: Orthopedics & Wound Care

References: Walker, 2000; pp. 501–535; Howard-Gradman & Kitt, 1995; pp. 138–187.

89. A patient presents to the Urgent Care Center following an injury at work. Which of the following would require the company to make the visit a reportable incident according to the standards of the Occupational Safety and Health Administration (OSHA)?
   A. Puncture wound of the skin requiring a dressing application
   B. Prescription for over-the-counter ibuprofen (Advil) for 3-day use
   C. Administration of injectable antibiotic
   D. RECOMMENDATION OF LIGHT DUTIES FOR 3 DAYS

Rationale:

   D. Recordable or reportable injuries under OSHA regulations involve loss of consciousness, prescription medication, sutures, restriction of work or motion, and treatment beyond that described as first aid.
   A. A puncture wound treated with a dressing application would be considered first aid and not defined as an OSHA recordable or reportable incident.
   B. Over-the-counter medication use is not considered an OSHA recordable or reportable incident.
   C. A single dose of medication administered in the office would not be considered an OSHA recordable or reportable incident.

Content Category: Professional Issues

Reference: Herington & Morse, 1995; p. 3.

90. An elderly patient falls from a stretcher in the ED. The patient was admitted with a history of confusion. The ED nurse did not raise the side rails and left the patient unattended. A suit is brought against the hospital and the ED nurse. Which of the following would be considered a cause for the suit?
   A. Breach of duty
   B. PROXIMATE CAUSE

C. Duty to act

D. Failure to act

Rationale:

B. Proximate cause is defined as being determined by foreseeability. The ED nurse should have fore-seen that injury would occur in this particular situation or form of conduct. A confused, elderly patient should never have been left alone with the side rails down.

A. Breach of duty occurs when commission or omission falls below established standards of care. While the current situation may also be considered breach of duty, it more closely resembles proximate cause.

C. Duty to act is a lay term and not defined by the legal system in medical negligence issues.

D. Failure to act is a lay terms and not defined by the legal system in medical negligence issues.

Content Category: Professional Issues

Reference: Newberry, 1998.

91. An emergency nurse involved in a conflict with a peer should:

A. FOCUS ON THE BEHAVIOR OF THE INDIVIDUAL.

B. establish a personal position at the beginning of the incident.

C. use sentences that begin with "you."

D. internalize personal feelings during the interaction.

Rationale:

A. By focusing on the behavior of the individual, the emergency nurse avoids personal criticism and creates an effective environment for discussion of concerns.

B. Establishing a personal position at the beginning of the incident would create the impression that you believe you are right and might cause further conflict.

C. Sentences that begin with "you" are considered aggressive and often viewed as attacking or labeling. Such comments may lead to further conflict.

D. Internalizing personal feelings would not resolve the conflict.

Content Category: Professional Issues

Reference: Salluzzo et al., 1997.

92. The ED team decides that the current triage system is not working. Which of the following would indicate knowledge of evidenced-based practice?

A. The team makes changes based on their past experiences of triage.

B. THE TEAM CONDUCTS A LITERATURE REVIEW OF CURRENT TRIAGE RESEARCH AND OUTCOMES.

C. The team decides to adopt the practice of other emergency departments in the same city.

D. The team decides to write a new triage system based on emergency team experience.

Rationale:

B. Application of nursing research to practice includes identifying a patient care problem and iden-tifying and assessing research-based knowledge before adapting and adopting nursing innova-tion. A current literature review would provide data to support triage design decisions.

A. Although past experiences in triage may be a part of the discussion, current literature and data should be reviewed.

C. Other triage systems in the area may experience the same dilemmas. An appropriate benchmark study should be conducted.

D. Research data should be included in the decision process to design an evidence-based system.

Content Category: Professional Issues

Reference: Newberry, 1998; p. 101

93.   During the absence of the ED manager, you are asked to interview a potential unit secretary. Which of the following questions should be AVOIDED?
A. Work history
B. Clinical and typing skills
C. MARITAL STATUS
D. Educational preparation

Rationale:

C. During an interview process, questions cannot be asked about marital status, dependent children, health history, or areas covered under the Americans with Disabilities Act.
A. A complete review of work history should be included in an interview.
B. An employee applying for a position as unit secretary should be asked about secretarial skills.
D. Educational preparation should be included in an interview process.

Content Category: Professional Issues

Reference: Salluzzo et al., 1997.

94.   The process by which data is collected, results are documented, and experiments and tests are validated in order to change a concept is considered to be which of the following?
A. Research-focused theory
B. EVIDENCE-BASED PRACTICE
C. Nursing process model
D. Quantitative analysis approach

Rationale:

B. Evidence-based practice is the model for validating a need for a practice guideline or verifying a process to create one. Emergency nursing practice should be evidence based and based on current research validating change concepts.
A. The described plan is that of an evidence-based practice concept.
C. The nursing process model looks at assessment, planning/analysis, intervention, and evaluation.
D. Quantitative analysis is data collection and review, part of evidence-based practice.

Content Category: Professional Issues

Reference: ENA, Core Curriculum, 2000.

95.   A 58-year-old male who recently had an aortic valve replacement is concerned that the valve is not working properly. Identify the landmark for auscultation of this valve.
A. SECOND RIGHT INTERCOSTAL SPACE AT RIGHT STERNAL BORDER
B. Second left intercostal space at left sternal border
C. Fourth intercostal space at left sternal border
D. Fifth intercostal space at the midclavicular line

Rationale:

A. The aortic valve is auscultated best at this landmark.
B. The pulmonic valve is auscultated best at this landmark.
C. The tricuspid valve is auscultated best at this landmark.
D. The mitral valve is auscultated best at this landmark.

Content Category: Cardiovascular

Reference: Kasper et al., 1998.

96. A 72-year-old male is admitted to the ED with new onset of atrial fibrillation and a ventricular response of 160. He had no prior cardiovascular diagnosis but has been taking methylxanthine (Theo-Dur) for asthma. The following laboratory tests would be appropriate EXCEPT which of the following?
    A. DIGITALIS LEVEL
    B. Thyroid function studies
    C. Prothrombin time (PT)/partial thromboplastin time (PTT)
    D. Theophylline level

Rationale:

A. The patient has not been on digitalis.
B. Thyroid function studies are recommended for all new-onset atrial fibrillation.
C. PT/PTT would be needed for baseline levels, as the patient has the potential to be anticoagulated.
D. Because the patient is taking Theo-Dur, a theophylline level is indicated to determine whether the level is therapeutic or toxic.

Content Category: Cardiovascular

Reference: Kasper et al., 1998.

97. Ankle-brachial index (ABI) is a method used to assess arterial perfusion of the lower extremities. Which of the following is the correct formula for obtaining ABI?
    A. Ankle diastolic pressure divided by brachial diastolic pressure
    B. ANKLE SYSTOLIC PRESSURE DIVIDED BY BRACHIAL SYSTOLIC PRESSURE
    C. Brachial diastolic pressure divided by ankle diastolic pressure
    D. Brachial systolic pressure divided by ankle systolic pressure

Rationale:

B. Ankle systolic pressure divided by brachial systolic pressure gives the significant value of perfusion to extremity.
A. Diastolic pressure is not used to determine perfusion.
C. Diastolic pressure is not used to determine perfusion.
D. You need perfusion pressure, which equals ankle systolic pressure (usually equal to or a little higher than brachial pressure) divided by brachial systolic pressure.

Content Category: Cardiovascular

Reference: Fahey, 1999; p. 67.

98. A 70-year-old female presents with a chief complaint of "rest pain" in her foot. Which of the following data would correlate with the diagnosis of arterial occlusive disease?
    A. PAIN AGGRAVATED BY ELEVATION OF EXTREMITY
    B. Pain aggravated by dependent position of extremity
    C. Resting blood flow sufficient to meet metabolic requirements to extremity
    D. Pain occurs as isolated event during active/waking hours

Rationale:

A. Pain is increased with elevation because of decreased blood supply to the foot, resulting in decreased perfusion and pain.
B. In a dependent position, there is increased blood supply to the foot; pain is decreased.

C. During the resting state, there is a decrease in cardiac output. Metabolic needs are not met.

D. The experience of "resting pain" is a nocturnal event.

Content Category: Cardiovascular

Reference: Fahey & McCarthy, 1999; p. 235.

99.   An 88-year-old male with a history of chronic congestive heart failure (CHF) is admitted to the ED. He was seen 4 days ago in the ED because of respiratory distress and hypertension. Diuretics were administered and symptoms relieved. He was dismissed to the nursing home. At this time, bilateral midlobe crackles are auscultated. The patient is hypotensive, with distended neck veins. Weight gain of 20 lb is noted. The patient expresses discomfort of the upper right quadrant. These current findings indicate that he is in:

A. BIVENTRICULAR FAILURE.

B. left ventricular failure.

C. right ventricular failure.

D. renal failure.

Rationale:

A. The patient presents with symptoms of both left and right ventricular failure. The most common cause of right heart failure is the progression of left heart failure.

B. Symptoms of left ventricular failure include edema, neck vein distension, and hepatic engorgement (signs of right heart failure).

C. Pulmonary symptoms (crackles) indicate left heart failure as well as right heart failure.

D. The clinical presentation is not specific for renal failure. No information on acid-base status or creatinine levels has been provided.

Content Category: Cardiovascular

Reference: Goran & Johantgen, 1998; p. 436.

100.   A specific diagnostic prognostic marker for congestive heart failure (CHF) is:

A. ATRIAL NATRIURETIC PEPTIDE (ANP).

B. angiotensin I.

C. aldosterone.

D. renin.

Rationale:

A. Atrial natriuretic peptide (ANP) is a compensatory response to stretching of the atria by increased filling.

B. Angiotension increases with decreased volume in the renal artery.

C. Aldosterone increases with decreased circulating volume (shock states and decreased renal artery perfusion).

D. Renin increases with decreased circulating volume (shock states and decreased renal artery perfusion).

Content Category: Cardiovascular

Reference: Goran & Johantgen, 1998; p. 434.

101. All of the following regarding possible interventions for torsade de pointes are true EXCEPT:
    A. artificial pacing may be required.
    B. isoproterenol (Isuprel) administration.
    C. magnesium sulfate administration.
    D. PROCAINAMIDE (PRONESTYL) BOLUS AND DRIP TO LENGTHEN REFRACTORY PERIOD.

Rationale:

    D. Pronestyl bolus and drip may lengthen the refractory period and further worsen torsade.
    A. Artificial pacing may be done to shorten the refractory period.
    B. Isoproterenol administration may assist in shortening the refractory period.
    C. Magnesium is effective in the management of torsade.

Content Category: Cardiovascular

Reference: Eagan, 1998; p. 481.

102. Which of the following is TRUE regarding loss of atrial ventricular synchrony associated with atrial fibrillation?
    A. Cardiac output is not affected.
    B. Cardiac output is reduced by 10–15%.
    C. CARDIAC OUTPUT IS REDUCED BY 25–30%.
    D. Cardiac output is reduced by 50–60%.

Rationale:

    C. Cardiac output is reduced by 25–30%.
    A. Incorrect.
    B. Incorrect. The reduction percentage is too small.
    D. Incorrect. The reduction percentage is too large.

Content Category: Cardiovascular

Reference: Eagan, 1998; p. 485.

103. The ED patient for whom you are caring requires close monitoring of mean arterial pressure (MAP). The function on the blood pressure cuff is not working and you must calculate this factor. The patient's BP is 110/70 mm Hg. What is the MAP for this patient?
    A. 63
    B. 73
    C. 83
    D. 93

Rationale:

    C. Systolic BP + (diastolic BP × 2) divided by 3 = 83 mm Hg.
    A. Incorrect.
    B. Incorrect.
    D. Incorrect.

Content Category: Cardiovascular

Reference: Hogsten, 1996; p. 247.

104.   Interpretation of the S-T segment in the following ECG strip indicates which of the following?

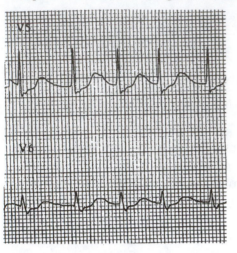

    A. Acute infarct
    B. ISCHEMIA
    C. ST segment is isoelectric
    D. Nondiagnostic position

Rationale:

    B. Ischemic depression of the S-T segment indicates ischemia.
    A. Acute infarct S-T segment is not elevated.
    C. Isoelectric S-T segment is depressed, not a straight line (not at 0 point).
    D. It is diagnostic; it indicates ischemia.

Content Category: Cardiovascular

Reference: Newberry, 1998.

105.   Primary perfusion assessment includes all of the following EXCEPT:
    A. capillary refill.
    B. radial pulse.
    C. patient response.
    D. 12-LEAD ECG.

Rationale:

    D. A 12-lead ECG will provide information about electrical conduction and depolarization of the heart, but not about perfusion.
    A. Capillary refill shows distal vascular filling.
    B. Radial pulse gives information about heart rate, stroke volume, and systolic BP (if palpable SBP is at or about 80).
    C. Patient response and level of consciousness are important factors in assessing the perfusion state.

Content Category: Cardiovascular

Reference: Kidd, 1996; p. 295.

106. A patient taking digoxin (Lanoxin) is most at risk for and would suffer the greatest adverse effects from which of the following?
A. INCREASED SERUM POTASSIUM
B. Decreased serum magnesium
C. Increased serum calcium
D. Decreased serum sodium

Rationale:

A. The increased digoxin affects the sodium-potassium pump and displaces the potassium from the cells, thus causing an increase in serum potassium. This situation may potentate lethal cardiac dysrhythmias.
B. Incorrect.
C. Calcium is the other major electrolyte affected by digoxin toxicity. The calcium will also increase. Patients who are digoxin toxic should not receive calcium. Potassium is more likely than calcium to induce a potentially lethal response in the patient.
D. Incorrect.

Content Category: Cardiovascular

References: ENA, Core Curriculum, 2000; Kee & Hayes, 2000.

107. An elderly patient comes to the ED with confusion and weakness. He has been taking digoxin (Lanoxin) for many years. While awaiting his laboratory results, you notice that his cardiac monitor shows a heart rate of 50/min with a PR interval of 0.28 sec and occasional PVCs. The most likely cause of this abnormality is which of the following?
A. Hypercalcemia
B. Hyponatremia
C. HYPOKALEMIA
D. Hypomagnesemia

Rationale:

C. Hypokalemia is a common electrolyte imbalance, particularly in patients taking digitalis preparations. Additionally, the elderly are at risk because of decreased dietary intake of potassium due to poor nutrition (from poor dentition, limited income, poor appetite, social isolation, and other factors). Heart blocks and ventricular irritability are common findings in severe hypokalemia.
A. While hypercalcemia may cause similar ECG findings, nothing in this patient's history indicates calcium imbalance.
B. Hyponatremia does not cause these ECG abnormalities; confusion and weakness are symptoms of hyponatremia, but the use of digoxin makes hypokalemia the most likely cause.
D. Magnesium deficiency may be seen in conjunction with low potassium levels, but it does not cause these ECG changes.

Content Category: Cardiovascular

References: Newberry, 2000; pp. 275–317; Ross, 1998; pp. 575–591; Wilson & Barton, 1996; pp. 118–140.

108.   A patient with neurologic deficits at the level of T10–11 is brought to your ED from an outlying hospital. S/he was involved in a motor vehicle collision approximately 5 hours before arrival. Initial evaluation at the outlying hospital reveals a T10–11 subluxation with neurologic deficits. CT scan of the head was negative for acute injury. CT scan of the abdomen revealed a grade II liver laceration with a small amount of free fluid in the peritoneal cavity. Hemoglobin is 10mg/dl. The ED physician orders high-dose steroids. The patient states s/he weighs 180 lb (81.8 kg). The correct dosing regimen for high-dose steroids for this patient is:

    A.   methylprednisolone (Depo-Medrol) bolus of 2.5 g over 15 minutes followed by a continuous infusion of 443 mg/hr for 23 hours.

    B.   METHYLPREDNISOLONE (DEPO-MEDROL) BOLUS OF 2.5 G OVER 15 MINUTES FOLLOWED BY A CONTINUOUS INFUSION OF 443 MG/HOUR FOR 48 HOURS.

    C.   methylprednisolone (Depo-Medrol) bolus of 2.5 g over 1 hour followed by a continuous infusion of 443 mg/hr for 48 hours.

    D.   methylprednisolone (Depo-Medrol) bolus of 2.5 g over 15 minutes followed by a continuous infusion of 443 mg/hour for 23 hours and a second bolus of methylprednisolone.

Rationale:

    B.   Methylprednisolone bolus of 2.5 g over 15 minutes followed by a continuous infusion of 443 mg/hour for 48 hours is recommended when started 3–8 hours after injury.

    A.   Methylprednisolone bolus of 2.5 g over 15 minutes followed by a continuous infusion of 443 mg/hour for 23 hours is recommended when started within 3 hours of injury.

    C.   The bolus dose should be infused over 15 minutes, followed by a 45-minute pause.

    D.   There should be no repeat bolus dose when the infusion is to run for 48 hours.

Content Category: Neurological

Reference: Bracken et al., 1997; pp. 1597–1604.

109.   A 65-year-old female presents to the ED with a chief complaint of right-sided weakness. She states she noticed the weakness this morning when she awoke and tried to get out of bed. She is alert and oriented. She has right-sided facial droop and her speech is slurred but understandable. Her vital signs are stable. An important question to ask this patient during your assessment is which of the following?

    A.   "DO YOU HAVE A HISTORY OF ATRIAL FIBRILLATION?"

    B.   "Does anyone in your family have cerebrovascular disease?"

    C.   "Are there signs of both expressive and receptive aphasia present?"

    D.   "Have you stopped taking any medications or started any new ones recently?"

Rationale:

    A.   Atrial fibrillation is a major risk factor for ischemic stroke. Approximately 20% of ischemic strokes are caused by cardiogenic embolisms.

    B.   Family history gives information about other risk factors the patient may have.

    C.   Assessing for both expressive and receptive aphasia may help determine the location of the stroke.

    D.   Medication regimen is a routine part of the history.

Content Category: Neurological

References: Boss, 1998; pp. 510–571; ENA, Core Curriculum, 2000.

110.   A patient is admitted to the ED following an altercation and diagnosed as having a basilar skull fracture. The patient remains unconscious and has an ethanol level of 25 mg/dl. You prepare for:
   A. insertion of a nasogastric tube.
   B. nasal packing if there is a cerebrospinal fluid (CSF) leak.
   C. administration of an anticoagulant to dissolve any potential blood clot.
   D. PROTECTIVE OBSERVATION DUE TO POSSIBLE COMBATIVE BEHAVIOR.

Rationale:

   D. A basilar skull fracture develops when enough force is exerted on the base of the skull to cause deformity. Neurologic changes that occur with a basilar skull fracture range from mild changes in mentation to combativeness. Combative behavior is often considered a hallmark of a basilar skull fracture. The small amount of alcohol observed with this patient would not be a cause for altered behavior.
   A. A nasogastric or nasotracheal tube should be avoided in patients with a potential basilar skull fracture. The tube might penetrate the cranium.
   C. There should be no attempt to stop a cerebrospinal fluid leak.
   D. There are no indications to administer anticoagulant therapy to this patient, since the possibilities for intracerebral bleeding, epidural hematoma, and subgaleal hematoma exist.

Content Category: Neurological

References: Newberry, 1998; p. 271; Sheehy & Lenehan, 1998; p. 395.

111.   A 60-year-old female is brought to the ED by her husband. He states she awoke this morning complaining of a headache and has gradually become more disoriented. She is now awake but confused and has difficulty standing. Upon further assessment, her left pupil is 6 mm in diameter and nonreactive to light; the right pupil is 4 mm in diameter and reacts briskly. Vital signs are BP 122/60 mm Hg, HR 60/min, and respirations 20/min. Based on these initial findings, you would anticipate interventions for possible:
   A. calcium channel blocker toxicity.
   B. meningitis.
   C. SUBDURAL HEMATOMA.
   D. dehydration.

Rationale:

   C. A patient with acute subdural hematoma presents with headache, confusion, and a steady decline in level of consciousness. History should be evaluated for a fall or injury to the head. Ipsilateral, unilateral pupil dilation and contralateral hemiparesis are associated with acute and chronic subdural hematomas.
   A. Calcium channel blocker toxicity usually presents with hypotension, shortness of breath, dizziness, and irregular heart rate. Unequal pupils are not associated with toxicity.
   B. Meningitis is not usually associated with unequal sluggish pupils and extremity weakness.
   D. Severe dehydration may be associated with disorientation, hypotension, and tachycardia. Unequal pupils are not found with dehydration.

Content Category: Neurological

References: ENA, Core Curriculum, 2000; Boss, 1998; pp. 510–571.

112.   A 2-year-old female is brought to the ED by her parents after a witnessed seizure lasting approximately 2 minutes. The child arouses to verbal stimuli. Skin is warm and dry to the touch, with brisk capillary refill. Vital signs are HR 140/min, respirations 36/min, and unlabored temperature 102° F (38.9° C) rectally. The parents begin asking you if their child will have to take anticonvulsants for the rest of her life. The most appropriate nursing diagnosis is which of the following?
   A. Fluid volume deficit
   B. Alterations in tissue perfusion
   C. Ineffective breathing pattern
   D. KNOWLEDGE DEFICIT

Rationale:

   D. This child has most likely experienced a febrile seizure. Febrile seizures are most common in children between the ages of 6 months and 3 years. They do not normally require management with anticonvulsant therapy.
   A. Fluid volume deficit is a potential problem from prolonged hyperthermia, vomiting, or diarrhea from infection. The heart and respiratory rates are mildly elevated, probably from the increased metabolic rate of the seizure activity.
   B. Alterations in tissue perfusion may occur if the heart and respiratory rates are not restored to within normal limits.
   C. Ineffective breathing pattern is a potential problem during seizure activity. A respiratory rate of 36 is within normal limits for a toddler.

Content Category: Neurological

References: Farley & Mooney, 1998; pp. 591–693; ENA, Core Curriculum, 2000.

113.   A teenager presents to the ED following a car crash. He is evaluated and determined to have a closed head injury with a possible cervical fracture. The ED nurse determines the following with a Glasgow Coma Scale (GCS) evaluation: no eye opening with stimulation, no verbal response prior to intubation, and no motor response with IV insertions. Which of the following GCS scores would be appropriate for this patient?
   A. Eye: 0; Motor: 0; Verbal: 0
   B. Eye: 1; Motor: 0; Verbal: 0
   C. EYE: 1; MOTOR: 1; VERBAL: 1
   D. Eye: 0; Motor: 1; Verbal: 1

Rationale:

   C. On the Glasgow Coma Scale, the lowest possible score is 3—a score of 1 in each of the 3 categories evaluated (eye, verbal, and motor response). This patient's score totaled 3.
   A. A score of 0 is not possible on the GCS.
   B. A score of 1 is not possible on the GCS. The lowest score in each category is 1.
   D. A score of 2 is not possible on the GCS. The lowest score in each category is 1. Notations should be made if the patient is paralyzed due to medication effect, injury, or intubation.

Content Category: Neurological

Reference: Dolan & Holt, 2000.

114.   An adult who is seizing should be placed in:
   A. restraints.
   B. a prone position.
   C. a supine position.
   D. LEFT LATERAL DECUBITUS POSITION.

Rationale:

    D. The left lateral decubitus position is the best position in which to place a patient who is having seizures. This position minimizes the likelihood of aspiration of vomitus and other secretions. The left position is preferred over the right because of the anatomic superiority of the right mainstem bronchus.

    A. Restraints are not indicated for a patient who is having a seizure.

    B. A prone position would be face down, not recommended for a person who is having a seizure.

    C. A supine position, lying on the back, would not permit adequate secretion removal and might increase the likelihood of aspiration.

Content Category: Neurological

Reference: Newberry, 1998.

115.   In patients with severe closed head injury, fixed and dilated pupils result from increasing pressure on which cranial nerve(s)?

    A. Cranial nerves IV and VI

    B. Cranial nerve V

    C. Cranial nerves II and III

    D. CRANIAL NERVE III

Rationale:

    D. Cranial nerve III (oculomotor) controls pupil constriction and dilation. As intracranial pressure rises, pupils become fixed and dilated.

    A. Cranial nerve IV (trochlear) controls downward and inward movement of the eye. Cranial nerve VI (abducens) controls lateral eye movement.

    B. Cranial nerve V (trigeminal) has three divisions. The ophthalmic division controls the blink reflex.

    C. Cranial nerve I is the olfactory nerve, which controls the sense of smell. Cranial nerve II is the optic nerve and is not affected by increasing intracranial pressure.

Content Category: Neurological

References: Allerton, 1998; pp. 343–366; Hickey, 1997; pp. 385–417.

116.   A 45-year-old male is brought to the ED from a motor vehicle collision. He was unresponsive at the scene with agonal respirations. He is intubated and ventilations are assisted. On initial assessment, the patient's VS: BP 122/66 mm Hg, HR 100, Resp 16/min (assisted). He responds with decorticate posturing on the right side to painful stimuli. He remains immobilized with a rigid cervical collar and long spine board. IV fluids are being administered. As the patient is being prepared for CT scan, you notice his vital signs are now: BP 168/50 mm Hg, HR 58, Resp 16/min (assisted). This patient's signs and symptoms are most likely which of the following?

    A. CUSHING'S RESPONSE

    B. Neurogenic shock

    C. Horner's syndrome

    D. Hypertensive crisis

Rationale:

    A. Cushing's response is an attempt by the body to maintain cerebral blood flow in the presence of rising intracranial pressure. As intracranial pressure rises, the systolic blood pressure increases, resulting in a widened pulse pressure and a reflex bradycardia.

B. Neurogenic shock may be seen in spinal cord injuries in which there is loss of sympathetic innervation and unopposed parasympathetic innervation that results in hypotension, bradycardia,
and loss of the ability to sweat below the level of the lesion.

C. Horner's syndrome may be seen in partial spinal cord transection and is associated with miosis,
ptosis, and loss of sweating on the ipsilateral side.

D. Herniation syndromes occur when a portion of the brain is displaced due to increased intracranial pressure. The most common is uncal herniation, in which the medial aspect of the temporal
lobe is displaced over the tentorium into the posterior fossa. Symptoms include pupil dilation
and abnormal motor posturing.

Content Category: Neurological

References: ENA, Core Curriculum, 2000; Hickey, 1997; pp. 385–417.

117.   As an emergency nurse, you are asked to teach neurologic assessment in a First Responder class. You
are teaching the class about orientation × 3. Your description of this assessment tool should be which
of the following?
A. Oriented to name call three different times
B. Oriented to name, address, and phone number
C. ORIENTED TO TIME, PERSON, AND PLACE
D. Oriented to history, current medications, and allergies

Rationale:

C. Level of awareness in a neurologic assessment can be determined by an assessment of orientation. The classic three parameters are time, person, and place.

A. Orientation to name call times three is not defined as "oriented × 3."

B. Orientation to name, address and phone number is not the classic definition of "oriented × 3."

D. History, current medications, and allergies are vital information to be determined during an
assessment.

Content Category: Neurological

Reference: ENA, Core Curriculum, 2000.

118.   Which of the following laboratory studies is a classic finding in Reye's syndrome?
A. Metabolic alkalosis
B. Hypernatremia
C. Hyperglycemia
D. HYPERAMMONEMIA

Rationale:

D. The liver enzyme system that converts ammonia to urea for excretion is not functional. Liver
enzymes and ammonia levels increase in patients with Reye's syndrome.

A. Metabolic acidosis and respiratory alkalosis both occur because of hyperventilation and the
body's inability to remove acids.

B. Hypernatremia is more likely to be accompanied by diarrhea, not the persistent vomiting seen in
Stage I Reye's syndrome.

C. In a child under age 4 years, it is not uncommon to find hypoglycemia due to a dysfunction of
the glyconeogenesis enzyme pathways.

Content Category: General Medical

References: ENA, Core Curriculum, 2000; pp. 278–280, 289–292; Beers & Berkow, 1999; pp. 2357–
2359.

119. Patients who are immunocompromised and have an infection may present with which of the following signs and symptoms?
      A. Swelling, localized redness, pus
      B. FEVER, PALLOR, MALAISE
      C. Bradycardia; flushed, dry skin
      D. Swollen glands, arthralgias

Rationale:

   B. With the immune system severely compromised, normal signs and symptoms are absent. The key finding is fever. The effect of neutrophils and the body's phagocytic response are not able to give further clues toward localizing the infection.
   A. These signs occur with an intact white blood cell system, since neutrophils must be present for phagocytosis, the body's protective system to ingest invading organisms, to take place.
   C. Fever does increase the metabolic rate, thus increasing the pulse rate.
   D. Macrophages circulate attacking infection in the tissues as well as in the lymphatic system. An adequate number must be present to perform this task, which leads to swollen glands and arthralgias.

Content Category: General Medical

References: ENA, Core Curriculum, 2000; pp. 315–316; Guyton & Hall, 1996; pp. 435–449.

120. An elderly woman presents to the ED at 5:00 AM. Chief complaint is fever and chills with sudden onset of pain and swelling in the first metatarsophalangeal joint. The pain awakened her from sleep. The most likely problem is:
      A. septic arthritis.
      B. rheumatoid arthritis.
      C. cellulitis.
      D. GOUT.

Rationale:

   D. Severe, sudden onset of pain in the middle of the night, most often affecting the joint under consideration in this case, is a classic presentation of gout. Fever and chills are common, with many precipitating factors. Although gout occurs more commonly among men, elderly women are also affected.
   A. Septic arthritis often strikes a large weight-bearing joint due to *Staphylococcus aureus* infection with a progressively swollen, painful, warm joint.
   B. Rheumatoid arthritis is progressive, with 3 or more joints involved, often in the hands or feet, usually symmetrical and diffuse.
   C. Cellulitis appears over 2 to 4 days, presenting with erythema, warmth, swelling, and tenderness. Fever and chills may be present. .

Content Category: General Medical

Reference: Humes, 2000; pp. 1370–1375, 1963, 1350, 1889–1890.

121.   Which of the following laboratory tests is indicative of hyperthyroidism?
   A. Decreased T3
   B. Decreased T4
   C. DECREASED TSH
   D. Decreased free T4

Rationale:

   C. Thyroid-stimulating hormone (TSH) is suppressed in hyperthyroidism by
   increased levels of T3 and T4.
   A. An accurate indicator of thyroid function, T3 is increased in primary hyperthyroidism, despite
       the lack of TSH.
   B. T4, which constitutes 90% of the thyroid hormone, is increased in hyperthyroidism.
   D. Free T4, total T4, T3 uptake, and free thyroxine index are elevated in
   hyperthyroidism. The free T4 measurement reflects the metabolically active portion of the hor-
       mone.

Content Category: General Medical

Reference: Pagana & Pagana, 1998; pp. 410–441.

122.   A 47-year-patient with type I diabetes is brought in by ambulance for the third time in 1 week for
        severe hypoglycemia. Before this past week, the patient never had any severe hypoglycemic episodes;
        she occasionally needed a glucose boost when feeling shaky or weak. The only change in her health
        has been the development of hypertension, which is now being treated with atenolol (Tenormin).
        What is the most likely cause of her frequent hypoglycemic episodes?
   A. Not eating enough
   B. Incorrect insulin dose
   C. THE NEW MEDICATION
   D. Stress from hypertension diagnosis

Rationale:

   C. Beta blocker medications such as atenolol (Tenormin) must be used with caution in diabetics
       because these medications tend to mask the symptoms of hypoglycemia. Many of the symptoms
       of hypoglycemia are induced by the release of epinephrine when blood sugar levels start to drop.
       Since beta-adrenergic receptors are blocked, the patient is unaware that her blood sugar is drop-
       ping until it is so low that level of consciousness changes and she is no longer able to care for
       herself.
   A. It can be inferred from the fact that this patient has type I diabetes that she has had the disease
       since childhood and has managed well until now. There is nothing in the history to indicate a
       change in diet, but even if so, she should recognize and treat hypoglycemia early.
   B. A medication error is always possible; however, one would not expect a longtime well-controlled
       diabetic to make a significant error three times in 1 week. Additionally, there is no mention of a
       physician-ordered change in insulin dose.
   D. Any diabetic who develops hypertension is at greater risk for cardiovascular disease. This diag-
       nosis might be stressful. This patient, however, should still recognize the symptoms of hypoglyce-
       mia in herself and respond appropriately.

Content Category: General Medical

References: Peabody, 2000; pp. 227–274; Wood, 1998; pp. 593–610.

123. Which category of medications is likely to cause significant increase in blood sugar levels in the diabetic patient?
    A. Beta blockers
    B. ACE inhibitors
    C. CORTICOSTEROIDS
    D. Benzodiazepines

Rationale:

    C. One of the adverse affects of all corticosteroids is increase in blood glucose levels in any patient. In the diabetic patient, this can be a serious problem and, if undetected, can lead to hyperglycemic hyperosmolar coma. Steroids are commonly used in the treatment of cancer, in which attention of focused on life-threatening issues. It is crucial for people with diabetes to monitor their own glucose levels closely and to report any unusual elevations to the doctor immediately. Elderly type II diabetics are particularly at risk.
    A. Beta blockers commonly cause hypotension and bradycardia, but not hyperglycemia.
    B. ACE inhibitors have many potential adverse reactions, including hypotension, syncope, headache, and dizziness. They do not cause hyperglycemia.
    D. Benzodiazepines cause respiratory depression, sedation, and dependence. They do not directly affect blood sugar. If, however, the patient is overly sedated, s/he may be unable to care for her/his diabetes properly.

Content Category: General Medical

Reference: Turkoski et al., 2000.

124. In the ED, a 4-year-old female who appears very ill is being triaged in a treatment room. She has a temperature of 104° F (40° C), severe headache, photophobia, and petechial rash. She cries when her head is bent forward. What should the ED nurse do next in caring for this child?
    A. DON A MASK
    B. Give acetaminophen (Tylenol) per standing orders
    C. Start an IV of lactated Ringer's
    D. Administer oxygen by nasal cannula

Rationale:

    A. Whenever a patient presents with fever and rash, there is a possibility that the illness is infectious. The important clue here is that the rash is petechial. When this is coupled with the other findings, the nurse must suspect meningococcal meningitis and septicemia. This highly infectious disease is spread by droplet infection. It is crucial to add a mask to normal standard precautions as soon as this type of meningitis is suspected. Other bacteria can cause petechial rash, but this one is easily spread and often fatal. It takes only seconds to put on a mask.
    B. This child needs fever control, but protection of the staff takes priority.
    C. An IV is indicated and lactated Ringer's is a safe choice, but prevention of infection spread comes first.
    D. Oxygen therapy is indicated, but infection precautions come first.

Content Category: General Medical

References: Anderson & Kozak, 1996; pp. 1049–1055; Cosby, 1998; pp. 721–741; Mellis, 1996; pp. 618–621.

125.   The management of sickle cell crisis in children is most likely to include which of the following?
       A. Active range of motion exercise
       B. Transfusion of fresh frozen plasma
       C. HYDRATION BY ORAL AND/OR IV THERAPY
       D. Administration of steroids

Rationale:

       C. The main objectives in treating sickle cell crisis include bed rest, hydration, electrolyte replacement, analgesics, blood replacement, and antibiotics.
       A. Bed rest is encouraged to minimize energy expenditure and oxygen utilization.
       B. Transfusions of packed red blood cells may be indicated.
       D. Incorrect.

Content Category: General Medical

Reference: ENA, Core Curriculum, 2000; p. 1670.

126.   The emergency nurse knows that cancer is the second leading cause of death in children aged 1 to 14 years. The most frequent type of childhood cancer is which of the following?
       A. Hodgkin's disease
       B. LEUKEMIA
       C. Medulloblastoma
       D. Osteogenic sarcoma

Rationale:

       B. Leukemia is the most common form of childhood cancer.
       A. Incorrect.
       C. Incorrect.
       D. Incorrect.

Content Category: General Medical

Reference: Wong, 1999; p.1727.

127.   A 3-year-old is receiving immunosuppressive chemotherapy for acute leukemia at a tertiary children's hospital. The child presents to the ED of your community hospital with complaint of increased fever. You assess the temperature to be 101.4° F (38.7° C). The child received a weight-appropriate dose of acetaminophen (Tylenol) 1½ hours before arrival. What is a priority nursing intervention for this patient?
       A. PLACE THE CHILD IN PROTECTIVE ISOLATION.
       B. Administer another weight-appropriate does of acetaminophen.
       C. Administer a weight-appropriate does of ibuprofen (Advil).
       D. Place the child in a room with negative airflow.

Rationale:

       A. Place the child in protective isolation.
       B. Another dose of acetaminophen is not indicated.
       C. Ibuprofen may be contraindicated for use in children who are receiving immunosuppressive chemotherapy.
       D. Negative airflow may expose the patient to other potentially harmful agents in the ambient air.

Content Category: General Medical

Reference: ENA, Core Curriculum, 2000; pp. 315–317.

128.   Initial laboratory studies in a 45-year-old patient with insulin-dependent diabetes mellitus reveals a serum glucose level of 538 mg/dl. Which of the following factors might be contributing to his hyper-glycemia?
   A.   Increased exercise
   B.   Decreased food intake
   C.   RECENT INFECTION
   D.   Excessive insulin dose

Rationale:

   C.   Infection and stressful events are the usual precipitating factors for patients presenting with dia-betic ketoacidosis.
   A.   Increased exercise would cause a decrease in glucose levels.
   B.   Decreased food intake would cause a decrease in glucose levels.
   D.   Excessive insulin dose would cause a decrease in glucose levels.

Content Category: General Medical

Reference: ENA, Core Curriculum, 2000; pp.263–265.

129.   A 19-year-old patient is brought to the ED with possible meningitis. The patient is most likely to be admitted if spinal fluid studies reveal a low:
   A.   white blood cell (WBC) count.
   B.   red blood cell (RBC) count.
   C.   protein level.
   D.   GLUCOSE LEVEL.

Rationale:

   D.   Glucose levels are decreased in the spinal fluid of a patient with bacterial meningitis. The fluid is cloudy. Bacteria will be present on the Gram's stain.
   A.   WBC would be elevated in patients with bacterial meningitis.
   B.   RBC would be elevated in patients with bacterial meningitis.
   C.   Protein level would be elevated in patients with bacterial meningitis.

Content Category: General Medical

Reference: ENA; Core Curriculum, 2000; pp. 245–247.

130.   An 18-month-old child with reactive airway disease is to be transported by ground ambulance. The best method of transporting the child is:
   A.   on the stretcher, with fastened seatbelt straps across the child.
   B.   in the mother's arms, with fastened seatbelt straps across the mother.
   C.   PROPERLY RESTRAINED IN A CHILD RESTRAINT SEAT THAT IS THE CORRECT SIZE FOR THE CHILD.
   D.   secured to a backboard, with a cervical collar, head blocks, and tape.

Rationale:

   C.   Children that are transported by ambulance warrant size-appropriate child restraint devices in that vehicle, with proper restraining techniques.
   A.   An 18-month-old is too small for the stretcher with fastened seat belts.
   B.   Children in ambulances must be properly restrained. Restraining a mother to the stretcher and expecting her to hold the child safely is unrealistic.
   D.   Full immobilization with a backboard, cervical collar, and head blocks is primarily for trauma patients.

Content Category: Patient Care

Reference: American Academy of Pediatrics, 2000; pp. 11, 148–149.

131. A trauma patient is en route to your facility following a motor vehicle crash (MVC). Which of the following injuries should the nurse anticipate for the restrained driver with frontal impact?
    A. Fractured sternum
    B. Right clavicle fracture
    C. FRACTURED PELVIS
    D. Aortic tear

Rationale:

C. A pelvic fracture is a predicted injury for a restrained driver. This is especially true if the person was wearing a lap belt without a shoulder harness.
A. A fractured sternum is a predicted injury for an unrestrained driver.
B. A right clavicle fracture is a predicted injury for an unrestrained driver.
D. n aortic tear is a predicted injury for an unrestrained driver.

Content Category: Patient Care

Reference: Holleran, 1996; p. 101.

Questions 132 and 133

A male patient sustained second- and third-degree burns 1 hour ago to anterior parts of his neck, chest, abdomen, and right leg (22% BSA total). He is coughing up carbonaceous sputum and complains of severe pain.

132. Before he is transferred by air to a regional burn center, it is most appropriate to:
    A. apply silver sulfadiazine (Silvadene Cream) to burns and fluid resuscitate.
    B. INSERT A NASOGASTRIC TUBE AND APPLY DRY, STERILE DRESSINGS TO BURNS.
    C. apply a condom catheter that is to gravity drainage and fluid resuscitate.
    D. apply saline-moistened dressings to burns and insert an indwelling urinary catheter.

Rationale:

B. Patients burned in excess of 20% of body surface may develop an ileus. Patients transported by air are in even greater need of gastric decompression because of the added factor of gas expansion as altitude increases. Burns should be dressed with dry, sterile dressings or linen.
A. Fluid resuscitation is necessary for burn patients. Burns should be dressed with dry, sterile dressings or linen. Moist dressings can prompt heat loss. Burn centers generally prefer receive wounds treated in ways that do not require removal of ointments or creams for examination.
C. A condom catheter may be helpful in the rehabilitation process, but frequent urine output monitoring is critical in the acute phase of treatment for patients with significant burns. An indwelling urinary catheter should be inserted in these patients.
D. Moist dressings can prompt heat loss. Burn centers generally prefer to receive wounds treated in ways that do not require removal of ointments or creams for examination. Frequent urine output monitoring is critical in the acute phase of treatment for patients with significant burns; thus an indwelling urinary catheter is warranted.

Content Category: Patient Care

Reference: Holleran, 1996; pp. 298–300.

133. To increase the potential for a positive outcome en route, it would be most appropriate for the sending facility to:
    A. administer humidified oxygen by nasal cannula.
    B. administer nonhumidified oxygen by nonrebreather mask.
    C. administer humidified oxygen by nonrebreather mask.
    D. PERFORM RAPID-SEQUENCE INTUBATION AND PROVIDE ASSISTED VENTILATIONS.

Rationale:

    D. A patient with carbonaceous sputum is assumed to have airway burns until proven otherwise. With that considered, this patient warrants intubation early in the resuscitation process, since airway swelling may quickly make the procedure impossible. Rapid-sequence intubation is one of the best methods of accomplishing the task.
    A. A nasal cannula is not an appropriate device for this patient.
    B. A nonrebreather mask might suffice up to the point at which intubation equipment is ready, but is not appropriate beyond that point.
    C. A nonrebreather mask might suffice up to the point at which intubation equipment is ready, but is not appropriate beyond that point.

Content Category: Patient Care

Reference: Holleran, 1996; pp. 298–300, 345.

134. A sickle cell patient in crisis wishes to be transferred by air ambulance to a tertiary-care center near home. The transport will be approximately a 3-hour flight by jet. The patient is being hydrated, has received pain medication, is on oxygen, and is resting comfortably. This patient is a poor candidate for the noted transfer because:
    A. the patient has not been adequately stabilized.
    B. ED-to-ED transfers are illegal under the Consolidated Omnibus Reconciliation Act (COBRA) and the Emergency Medical Treatment and Active Labor Act (EMTALA).
    C. the patient's insurance will not pay for the transfer.
    D. THE STRESSORS OF FLIGHT ARE LIKELY TO WORK IN OPPOSITION TO THE PATIENT'S PHYSIOLOGIC NEEDS AND PROMPT FURTHER EXACERBATION OF DISEASE.

Rationale:

    D. Infection, hypoxia, dehydration, cold, and a number of other stressors can trigger sickle cell crisis. Noise, cold, vibration, dehydration, hypoxia, and fatigue are stressors of flight. Any stressor can potentially exacerbate or worsen sickle cell crisis.
    A. Hydration, analgesia, oxygen augmentation, and decreased stimuli are appropriate treatments for a patient with sickle cell crisis. The information provided gives no indication that the patient has not been stabilized.
    B. COBRA and EMTALA do not limit the areas of a facility to which or from which a patient can be transferred.
    C. The patient's insurance coverage is irrelevant. If the transfer were not covered by insurance, the patient could choose to pay from personal finances.

Content Category: Patient Care

References: Holleran, 1996; pp. 14–15, 22–25; Newberry, 1998; pp. 644, 734.

135. A patient with significant alcohol intoxication is to be transported by ground ambulance from a small rural facility to a tertiary-care center. The ED physician has ordered oxygen by nonrebreather mask. What type of hypoxia is most likely in this patient?
    A. Hypoxic hypoxia
    B. Hyphemic hypoxia
    C. Stagnant hypoxia
    D. HISTOTOXIC HYPOXIA

Rationale:

D. Cellular poisoning (histotoxic hypoxia) occurs when poisoned cells or metabolic disorders inhibit the use of oxygen by the cell. Alcohol, carbon monoxide, and cyanide are among the possible causes.

A. Hypoxic hypoxia is a deficiency in alveolar oxygen exchange. This is also known as altitude hypoxia.

B. A reduction in the oxygen-carrying capacity of the blood is hyphemic hypoxia. An example of this phenomenon is anemia.

C. Stagnant hypoxia occurs in the presence of pooling or decreased flow of blood. Heart failure, pulmonary embolism, and shock are possible causes.

Content Category: Patient Care

Reference: Holleran, 1996; pp. 14–15.

136. A 15.4-lb (7-kg) infant is brought to the ED in cardiac arrest. Because there is no intravenous access, epinephrine (Adrenalin) is administered via endotracheal tube. The appropriate dose is:
    A. 0.07 mg of 1:1,000 concentration.
    B. 0.7 MG OF 1:1,000 CONCENTRATION.
    C. 0.07 mg of 1:10,000 concentration.
    D. 0.7 mg of 1:10,000 concentration.

Rationale:

B. The recommended dose for endotracheal epinephrine is 0.1 mg/kg of 1:1,000 concentration.

A. This dose is too low for endotracheal administration.

C. This is the correct dose for intravenous or intraosseous administration.

D. This is not the appropriate endotracheal dose.

Content Category: Patient Care

Reference: American Heart Association, 1995; p. 6.

137. The most important factor to consider when permitting a family member to accompany a critically ill or injured child during transport from one ED to another is:
    A. the availability of emotional support for the family members.
    B. THAT THE FAMILY MEMBER'S PRESENCE CALMS THE CHILD.
    C. the travel distance between the two facilities.
    D. the transferring hospital's insurance coverage for the family member.

Rationale:

B. The presence of a family member who is able to calm the child is an important consideration when transferring a child to another facility. When the critically ill or injured child is calm, physiologic stability is enhanced.

A. The availability of emotional support from other family members has no bearing on the ability of the family members in attendance to accompany the child.

C. Travel distance should not be a consideration in permitting or discouraging family presence. Children need their families regardless of the transport time.
D. The transferring hospital's insurance coverage is not an issue.

Content Category: Patient Care

Reference: Holleran, 1996; spp. 14–15, 22–25.

138. A 24-year-old male patient will be discharged from the ED following evaluation and treatment of a minor closed head injury and sprained ankle. Which of the following actions indicates that the patient understands his discharge instructions?
A. He signs the instruction sheet and states that he understands what you have told him.
B. He recalls 50% of the instructions listed on the discharge instructions sheet.
C. HE ANSWERS QUESTIONS AND RESTATES INFORMATION RELATED TO THE TEACHING.
D. He describes crutch walking and verbalizes how to ascend and descend stairs.

Rationale:

C. Asking the patient a question about what he has been taught is an appropriate method to evaluate effectiveness of patient and family education.
A. Signing the discharge instruction sheet does not assure understanding.
B. Partial recall of instructions does not demonstrate adequate knowledge acquisition of essential information.
D. The ability to demonstrate partial instructions does not show adequate knowledge acquisition of essential information.

Content Category: Patient Care

Reference: ENA, Core Curriculum, 2000; pp. 757–761.

139. During emergent intubation, the physician requests that cricoid pressure be applied by the nurse. Which statement by the nurse indicates the need for further education regarding the principles of cricoid pressure?
A. The thumb and forefinger are used to compress the cricoid cartilage downward toward C6.
B. Cricoid pressure should be held until the cuff is inflated.
C. The application of cricoid pressure reduces the risk of aspiration.
D. CRICOID PRESSURE IS NOT USED IN THE INTUBATION OF THE TRAUMATIZED UNCOOPERATIVE CHILD.

Rationale:

D. Incorrect statement. Cricoid pressure is indicated in the intubation of the traumatized uncooperative child using rapid-sequence intubation. Cricoid pressure occludes the esophagus, reducing the risk of aspiration.
A. Cricoid pressure is correctly applied by using the thumb and forefinger to compress the cricoid cartilage downward toward C6.
B. True statement.
C. True statement.

Content Category: Patient Care

Reference: Holleran, 1996; pp. 14–15, 22–25.

140.   A 56-year-old male presents with acute onset of right eye pain accompanied by blurred vision. A diagnosis of increased intraocular pressure is suspected. Which of the following is a CONTRAINDI-CATION to tonometry?

A. Patient is suspected to have acute angle-closure glaucoma.
B. Patient has sustained blunt ocular injury.
C. PATIENT HAS POSSIBLE LOSS OF INTEGRITY TO THE GLOBE.
D. Patient has iritis.

Rationale:

C. Application of pressure to the eye during tonometry may cause extrusion of the contents of a nonintact globe.
A. Tonometry is indicated in patients suspected to have acute angle-closing glaucoma.
B. Tonometry is indicated in blunt ocular injury.
D. Tonometry is indicated in iritis, which may be a precursor to both open-angle and closed-angle glaucoma.

Content Category: Patient Care

Reference: Proehl, 1999; p. 516.

141.   A 32-year-old female with multiple injuries from a motor vehicle crash will be transferred to a trauma center by helicopter. The air-type splint device on her left lower leg will need to be replaced by another type of splinting device before air transport because:

A. air-filled devices do not provide appropriate immobilization.
B. CHANGES IN TEMPERATURE AND ALTITUDE THAT OCCUR DURING FLIGHT MAY CAUSE CONSTRICTION OF THE EXTREMITY WITH THE AIR-TYPE SPLINT.
C. air filled immobilization devices provide temporary immobilization.
D. air splints are not suitable for angulated fractures.

Rationale:

B. Air pressure with a pneumatic splint device is subject to fluctuations with temperature and altitude variation, which may cause overinflation or underinflation of the splint device.
A. Air splints can provide immobilization; however, they must be replaced before air transport.
C. Although this is a true statement, it is not a reason an air-type splint should be replaced before transport.
D. Although this is a true statement, it is not a reason an air-type splint should be replaced before transport.

Content Category: Patient Care

Reference: Schaffler, 1999; pp. 389–390.

142.   A 26-year-old male who sustained a soft tissue injury to the lower leg returns to the ED complaining of pain and swelling. Assessment of the extremity reveals that it is swollen and cool to the touch, with decreased capillary refill and decreased sensation on palpation. Which of the steps below is CONTRAINDICATED in preparing the patient for measuring compartment pressure?

A   Remove any circumferential dressing or casts.
B. Keep the extremity at the level of the heart.
C. DO NOT GIVE FLUIDS OR MEDICATIONS FOR HYPOTENSION.
D. Measure the systolic and diastolic blood pressure so that a differential pressure may be calculated.

Rationale:

C. Treat systemic hypotension with fluids, medications, or both. Metabolically, the differential pressure between diastolic blood pressure and compartment pressure may be more important then absolute compartment pressure. Hypotension may actually reduce blood flow and perfusion to the injured extremity.

A. Removing any circumferential dressing or casts prevents further constriction due to swelling.

B. Keeping the extremity at heart level optimizes blood flow to the tissues until compartmental syndrome has been ruled out.

D. Knowing the diastolic blood pressure is necessary in order to calculate the differential pressure.

Content Category: Patient Care

Reference: Proehl, 1999; pp. 428–433.

143. Which statement is FALSE regarding opportunities for teaching during the ED visit?
    A. Teaching begins at triage.
    B. Teaching opportunities generally end at the time of discharge.
    C. Teaching is required before and after medications are administered.
    D. STANDARDIZED DISCHARGE INSTRUCTIONS MUST BE USED TO PROVIDE CONSISTENCY IN PATIENT DISCHARGE INSTRUCTIONS.

Rationale:

D. A standardized teaching tool must be used to provide consistency in patient discharge instructions. Patient discharge instructions must be customized to the patient's age and developmental level.

A. Teaching does begin at triage.

B. Teaching opportunities do generally end at discharge. Teaching may be a "one-moment, one-visit" opportunity.

C. All opportunities for teaching during the ED visit should be used. Teaching is required before and after medication is administered.

Content Category: Patient Care

Reference: ENA, Core Curriculum, 2000; pp.757–758.

144. A 77-year-old patient reports to the triage area with many vague and varied complaints. Considering age-specific physiologic changes, which of the following would be an expected finding?
    A. Upper abdominal pain
    B. Ill appearance
    C. Abnormal vital signs
    D. AGE-RELATED DETERIORATION OF BODY SYSTEM FUNCTION

Rationale:

D. Age-related deterioration of body system function is an expected finding in the geriatric population.

A. Upper abdominal pain is a triage red flag.

B. Ill appearance is a triage red flag.

C. Presentation with abnormal vital signs is a triage red flag.

Content Category: Patient Care

Reference: ENA, Core Curriculum, 2000.

145.   Six patients report for treatment in 5 minutes. The triage nurse calls for additional help at triage because:
   A.   THE PRIMARY ASSESSMENT OF A PATIENT SHOULD OCCUR WITHIN THE FIRST 2 TO 5 MINUTES OF ARRIVAL AT THE ED.
   B.   comprehensive triage takes approximately 10 to 15 minutes per patient.
   C.   all of the patient care areas in the triage area are full.
   D.   patient satisfaction may be diminished if patients wait too long at triage.

Rationale:

   A.   The primary assessment of a patient should occur within the first 2 to 5 minutes of his or her arrival at the ED to determine whether the condition is life threatening.
   B.   While this statement is true, primary assessment takes precedence.
   C.   Not a triage priority.
   D.   While this statement is true, patient satisfaction is not a triage priority.

Content Category: Patient Care

Reference: ENA, Core Curriculum, 2000.

146.   A 6-year-old child arrives at the ED with several deep dog bite lacerations. The decision is made to use conscious sedation to facilitate closure of the wounds. "Dissociative sedation" can be defined as which of the following?
   A.   A STATE CHARACTERIZED BY ANALGESIA, SEDATION, AMNESIA, AND CATALEPSY WITH RELATIVELY PRESERVED VENTILATORY DRIVE AND AIRWAY PROTECTIVE REFLEXES
   B.   A state of reduced motor activity, reduced anxiety, and indifference to surroundings
   C.   A state of unconsciousness with partial or complete loss of protective reflexes, including the inability to maintain an airway independently
   D.   A state of controlled lessening of a patient's awareness and pain perception that leaves the patient able to respond to verbal or tactile stimulation and to continuously and independently maintain a patent airway and adequate ventilatory drive

Rationale:

   A.   This is a definition of dissociative sedation, which occurs with the administration of anesthetic medications such as ketamine (Ketalar).
   B.   This is a definition of neurolepsis.
   C.   This is a definition of general anesthesia.
   D.   This is a definition of light sedation.

Content Category: Patient Care

Reference: ENA, Core Curriculum, 2000.

147.   Failure to comply with discharge teaching may be the result of any of the following EXCEPT:
   A.   inability to recall the discharge instructions.
   B.   inability to comprehend the discharge instructions.
   C.   lack of resources to comply with the discharge instructions.
   D.   FAILURE OF THE NURSE TO REQUIRE A RETURN DEMONSTRATION.

Rationale:

  D. Failure to comply with teaching instruction is not an inevitable result of the patient's inability to perform a return demonstration.
  A. Compliance with teaching requires recall ability.
  B. Compliance with teaching requires comprehension.
  C. Compliance with teaching requires availability of resources.

Content Category: Patient Care

Reference: ENA, Core Curriculum, 2000; pp. 760–761.

148.   Inhaled nitrous oxide may be used to relieve pain associated with trauma, renal colic, or a minor surgical procedure. Which of the following conditions would be an indication for the use of inhaled nitrous oxide?
  A. Pneumothorax
  B. Recent middle-ear infection
  C. MYOCARDIAL INFARCTION
  D. Bowel obstruction

Rationale:

  C. Pain associated with MI is an indication for use of inhaled nitrous oxide.
  A. Use of inhaled nitrous oxide is contraindicated for use in patients with a pneumothorax because the gas collects in dead-air spaces and can expand preexisting pockets of air associated with pneumothorax.
  B. Use of inhaled nitrous oxide is contraindicated for use in patients with recent middle-ear infections because the gas collects in dead-air spaces and can expand preexisting pockets of air associated with otitis media.
  D. Use of inhaled nitrous oxide is contraindicated for use in patients with a bowel obstruction because the gas collects in dead-air spaces and can expand preexisting pockets of air associated with bowel obstruction.

Content Category: Patient Care

Reference: Proehl, 1999; pp. 560–562.

149.   Eye donation is CONTRAINDICATED in which of the following circumstances?
  A. Advanced age
  B. Presence of eye condition
  C. Non–heart beating donor
  D. INTRAVENOUS (IV) DRUG USE

Rationale:

  D. IV drug use is a contraindication to eye donation.
  A. Acceptable eye donors may be of any age.
  B. The presence of an eye condition is not a contraindication to eye donation.
  C. Eye donation may be accepted from non–heart beating donors.

Content Category: Patient Care

Reference: ENA, Core Curriculum, 2000; p. 489.

150.   After brain death has been determined, the focus of care in supporting the viability of organs is on all of the following EXCEPT:
A. adequate hydration of the donor.
B. maintenance of normal blood pressure.
C. adequate oxygenation.
D. DECREASING CARDIAC OUTPUT.

Rationale:

D. Adequate cardiac output is needed to perfuse donor organs.
A. The focus of care is in supporting the viability of the organ through adequate hydration.
B. The focus of care is in supporting the viability of the organ through maintenance of normal blood pressure.
C. The focus of care is in supporting the viability of the organ through adequate oxygenation.

Content Category: Patient Care

Reference: ENA, Core Curriculum, 2000; p. 492.

Examination 4:
Self-Diagnostic Profile

Instructions

Step 1: Check your answers against the correct answers provided in Part 2 of this chapter. Then calculate your total score.

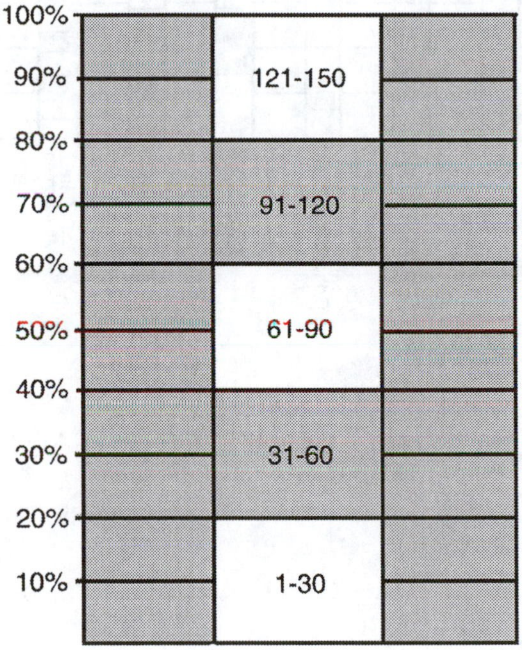

Figure 1: Total Score

Step 2: For each category of the practice examination, determine the number of items that you answered correctly and plot that number in Figure 2. The result will assist you in diagnosing your areas of knowledge strength and in determing which areas benefit from review.

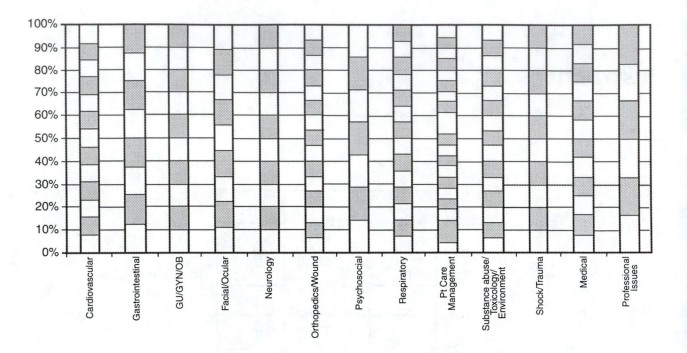

Figure 2: Practice Examination Content Areas

Practice Examination 5

Questions 1–4

A 19-year-old female presents to the ED with a complaint of pelvic pain and fever. In reviewing her reproductive history, you determine that she has had 3 sex partners in the past 2 months. She does not use contraceptive devices and denies a pregnancy history. Her last menstrual period was 10 days ago. She states that she has a thick vaginal discharge with vaginal itching and dysuria. Pelvic pain is aggravated by sexual intercourse and walking. Vital signs are BP 110/60 mm Hg, HR 110/min, respirations 20/min, and temperature 102.6° F (39.2° C).

1. The above signs and symptoms suggest that the patient has:
   A. ectopic pregnancy
   B. pelvic inflammatory disease (PID).
   C. Mittelschmerz.
   D. ovarian cyst.

2. The most probable cause of this patient's vaginal discharge is which of the following?
   A. Bacterial vaginosis
   B. Neisseria gonorrhoeae
   C. Candidal vulvovaginitis
   D. Normal vaginal discharge

3. A pelvic exam is performed. The most likely finding would be which of the following?
   A. An adnexal mass
   B. An open cervical os
   C. Cervical motion tenderness
   D. None of the above

4. You would expect the medical provider to order which of the following?
   A. Benzathine penicillin G (Permapen)
   B. Ceftriaxone (Tazidime)
   C. Metronidazole (Flagyl)
   D. None of the above

Questions 5 and 6

A 29-year-old female presents to the ED complaining of severe pain and swelling in her vaginal area. Upon evaluation you note swelling and erythema to her left vulvar area.

5. These symptoms are most consistent with which of the following?
   A. Herpes simplex virus
   B. A volvulus
   C. A chancroid
   D. Bartholin's abscess

6. Definitive treatment for this patient should include which of the following?
   A. An oral antiviral agent
   B. Surgical consult
   C. A fluoroquinolone antibiotic
   D. Incision and drainage

7. A 5-day-old female is brought to the ED by her parents for a blood-tinged vaginal discharge. Her parents deny trauma and state that no one else has cared for the infant except them. Examination of the patient does not reveal evidence of gross trauma. Your intervention for this child should be:
   A. Contact Child Protective Services to evaluate for child abuse.
   B. Separate the parents and question each separately to determine whether their stories differ.
   C. Obtain cultures and wet mount of the vaginal discharge.
   D. Reassure the parents that this is a normal finding in the newborn.

8. A 16-year-old female presents to the ED with a complaint of abnormal vaginal bleeding for 2 weeks. A possible cause of the bleeding is which of the following?
   A. Hypothyroidism
   B. Idiopathic thrombocytopenia
   C. Neoplasia
   D. All of the above

9. A 50-year-old construction worker presents to the ED with complaints of severe flank pain, nausea, vomiting, and diaphoresis and is unable to stand still or converse. The patient is most likely exhibiting signs of:
   A. acute heat exhaustion.
   B. renal calculi.
   C. acute food poisoning.
   D. dissecting aneurysm.

10. A female patient presents to the ED triage nurse with complaints of dysuria, urinary frequency, and lower abdominal pain. One of the first procedures the ED nurse should initiate is which of the following?
    A. Prepare for a pelvic examination.
    B. Administer analgesia.
    C. Obtain clean-catch urine.
    D. Check the patient's rectal temperature.

11. A 40-year-old nonsmoking patient who is in general good health is diagnosed with acute bronchitis. Which of the following pieces of information about the disease process should be included in patient education?
    A. The risk of subsequent development of pneumonia is high with this disorder.
    B. Acute bronchitis is often a precursor to development of chronic obstructive pulmonary disease.

C. The causative agent of acute bronchitis is frequently viral rather than bacterial.

D. Acute bronchitis is a lifelong disease that requires continued medical management.

12.   Discharge instructions have been given to the caregiver of a 1-year-old child with bronchiolitis. Which of the following statements by the caregiver indicates a need for further clarification?

A. "I will use Tylenol for fever control and comfort as needed."

B. "I will make sure she drinks extra fluids over the next few days."

C. "I can take her to day care tomorrow as long as she is on the medications."

D. "My 5-year-old may get this, too, but he should have milder cold symptoms."

13.   You are caring for a patient diagnosed with rib fractures and a pneumothorax. He is tachypneic and dyspneic. Decreased breath sounds are auscultated on the right side. A patent airway has been assured. C-spine precautions are in effect. The next priority intervention would be to insert:

A. a nasogastric tube.

B. a chest tube.

C. two large-bore IVs.

D. a urinary catheter.

14.   The priority treatment for a patient diagnosed with rib fractures includes:

A. chest tube placement.

B. aggressive pulmonary toilet.

C. IV crystalloid bolus infusion.

D. nasogastric tube placement.

15.   As you assess a patient with increasing respiratory distress, you suspect a tracheobronchial injury. For which of the following life-threatening conditions would this patient be at a high risk?

A. Distributive shock

B. Tension pneumothorax

C. Pulmonary contusion

D. Pericardial tamponade

16.   What other medical condition can imitate similar signs and symptoms as you assess a patient who is hyperventilating?

A. Asthma attack

B. Diabetic ketoacidosis

C. Myocardial infarct

D. Pertussis

17.   A patient sustains chest trauma resulting in a pulmonary contusion. Which of the following medical history findings places this patient at high risk for developing complications from this injury?

A. Emphysema

B. Environmentally triggered asthma

C. Gastroesophageal reflux

D. Pulmonary tuberculosis

18.   A 2-year-old girl is brought to the ED by her mother, who states the child was playing with beads and pushed one up her nose. The mother cannot get the bead out. After ensuring that the child's oxygenation is adequate, the ED nurse should prepare for which of the following interventions?

A. Oxymetazoline (Afrin) and a tracheostomy setup

B. Diazepam (Valium) and a rigid esophagoscopy

C. Phenylephrine (Neo-Synephrine) and balloon-tipped catheter

D. Meperidine (Demerol) and flexible endoscopy

19.   A 58-year-old male presents to the ED with increasing shortness of breath, pleuritic pain, and fever of 101.2° F (38.5° C). Breath sounds are decreased over the lower half of the left lung. Chest x-ray shows a large pleural effusion. The ED nurse should anticipate and prepare for which of the following interventions?
A.   Thoracentesis
B.   Rapid diuresis
C.   Emergent intubation
D.   Arterial line placement

20.   When the nurse is caring for a patient with a diaphragmatic tear, early recognition and treatment is important to prevent which of the following?
A.   Displaced bowel
B.   Infection
C.   Hypoxia
D.   Respiratory distress

21.   What nursing diagnosis would be a priority in a patient with respiratory distress syndrome?
A.   Anxiety related to dyspnea
B.   Fluid volume excess related to overhydration during resuscitation
C.   Pain
D.   Impaired gas exchange related to noncompliant lungs

22.   When teaching an asthma patient about the disease, it is important to remember that:
A.   asthma is caused primarily by airway inflammation and hyperresponsiveness to stimuli.
B.   physiologic changes seen in asthma exacerbation are often irreversible.
C.   asthma exacerbations are most frequently a result of a respiratory infection.
D.   most asthma attacks occur suddenly and without warning in the early morning.

23.   When teaching an asthma patient about medication usage, it is important to discuss that:
A.   inhaled steroids are addictive and their use should be limited to acute exacerbations.
B.   patients often develop a tolerance to daily asthma medications and require increased doses.
C.   inhaled bronchodilators should not be used with inhaled corticosteroids.
D.   oral corticosteroids are often used for short-term treatment of exacerbations.

24.   When teaching an asthma patient how to avoid potential triggers of the disease, it is important to discuss that:
A.   avoidance of spicy foods can help to reduce asthma attacks.
B.   exacerbations of asthma can be reduced by decreasing physical activity.
C.   a chronic postnasal drip can contribute to recurrent asthma attacks.
D.   most triggers of asthma cannot be avoided.

25.   Which of the following classes of drugs is a contributing factor in the development of gout?
A.   Thiazide diuretics
B.   Corticosteroids
C.   Oral anticoagulants
D.   Estrogen replacement

26.   A 4-month-old infant is brought to the ED by his parents. He has been crying for 6 hours and will not take his bottle. He has a fever of 101°F (38.3°C), is listless, and appears very ill. When the mother tries to comfort him by rocking, the baby screams and becomes dusky. The nurse notices that when the baby was placed on the bed to have vital signs taken, he became quiet and appeared to be sleeping. What should the ED nurse suspect the underlying problem with this infant to be?

A. Child abuse
B. Pneumonia
C. Dehydration
D. Meningitis

27. A young woman is treated in the ED after reporting that she was raped by an unknown male. She is healthy and the only medication she takes is an oral contraceptive. In addition to the trauma of rape, she is very concerned about having possibly contracted HIV. What patient education should she receive?
A. Oral contraceptives protect against HIV infection.
B. As long as there was no vaginal bleeding, she won't get HIV from one contact.
C. If today's HIV test is negative, she does not have to worry.
D. She will need to wait 6 weeks to 6 months to know whether she was infected.

28. Anna is a 13-year-old girl with a 2-year history of diabetes. She is poorly controlled and has been treated in your ED four times this year. She presents today lethargic and with an Accu-Chek of 620. You understand that the reason for the problem may be which of the following?
A. Puberty is the most likely cause of Anna's poor control of her disease.
B. Adolescents are "magical thinkers" who cannot accept responsibility for their own care.
C. Poor control of diabetes is the result of failure to follow the plan of care.
D. Most children can control their diabetes with periodic adjustments of insulin, diet, and activity.

29. The ED nurse advises parents to avoid using aspirin for fever control for children with influenza or varicella because of its potential association with which of the following?
A. Fifth disease
B. Kawasaki disease
C. Schönlein-Henoch purpura
D. Reye's syndrome

30. Which of the following vaccines provides protection against epiglottitis?
A. DTP
B. MMR
C. HIB
D. HBV

31. A 65-year-old female is found unresponsive on the floor. The patient has no significant medical history, but prior to this event she complained of headache and neck stiffness. Vital signs are BP 130/84 mm Hg, HR 100/min, respirations 10/min and shallow and snorting. Glasgow Coma Score is 7. The initial intervention to be performed by the ED nurse is:
A. administer oxygen by nasal cannula.
B. prepare for endotracheal intubation.
C. prepare for a lumbar puncture.
D. initiate antibiotic therapy.

32. An elderly woman visiting from Russia is brought to the ED by her family. She became ill with fever, night sweats, cough, and weight loss about 2 weeks ago. Her chest x-ray has findings consistent with active tuberculosis (TB). She refuses hospital admission and the family agrees to care for her at home. What information should the ED nurse give the family regarding transmission of TB?
A. Clean house thoroughly; launder patient's clothing in hot water and dryer.
B. Boil dishes, glasses, and silverware used by the patient.
C. Keep the house well ventilated, exhausting old air to the outside.
D. All family members should wear surgical masks when caring for the patient.

33. An elderly woman with profound lethargy is brought to the ED by EMS. Caregivers report a gradual decline in activity and mentation over a 6-month period. History is significant for hypothyroidism and a recent urinary tract infection treated with antibiotics. On exam, the woman is lethargic but responsive, with slow speech. The skin is pale and dry and the tongue is swollen. Vital signs are BP 82/40 mm Hg, HR 50/min, respirations 16/min, and rectal temperature 94° F (34.4° C). Intravenous access has been secured and lab specimens have been drawn. Careful fluid resuscitation is under way. Which of the following should be AVOIDED?
   A. Intravenous levothyroxine (Levoxyl)
   B. Vasopressors
   C. Hydrocortisone (Solu-Cortef)
   D. Normal saline

34. A 40-year-old woman with a known history of hyperthyroidism is brought to the ED with agitation and confusion. Family members report thyroid surgery had been performed 2 weeks prior. The patient is noted to be restless, diaphoretic, and oriented to person and place. Vital signs are BP 174/100 mm Hg, HR 160/min, respirations 32/min, and temperature 103.6° F (39.8° C). Thyroid storm is suspected. Following initial stabilization, the ED nurse should reduce fever by:
   A. rapid infusion of 1,000 ml of normal saline.
   B. administration of acetaminophen (Tylenol) 650 mg orally.
   C. infusion of 50 ml of D50W.
   D. administration of acetylsalicylic acid (Aspirin) 600 mg orally.

35. Which of the following statements by the patient who has herpes zoster indicates an understanding of discharge instructions?
   A. "A similar rash will break out on my right chest in about 2 weeks."
   B. "I should stay away from pregnant women."
   C. "I can return to work in 3 days."
   D. "I cannot use calamine lotion on this rash."

36. Which of the following ECG changes may be associated with hypokalemia?
   A. Elevated ST segment
   B. Peaked, tented T waves
   C. Q waves
   D. Ventricular irritability

37. A patient is escorted to the ED by the local police after being found in a department store preaching to the customers and stating he is an apostle of Jesus. He is dressed in a bright fluorescent green blazer and top hat and is talking nonstop in a loud, bellowing tone, changing topics frequently. The priority nursing diagnosis for this patient is which of the following?
   A. Risk for injury
   B. Ineffective individual or family coping
   C. Knowledge deficit
   D. Impaired social interaction

38. Antipsychotic drugs may cause:
   A. reduction in sleep patterns.
   B. a decrease in activity.
   C. reduction in disruptive behavior.
   D. an increase in paranoid reactions.

39. A male patient presents to the ED with a self-defined panic attack. Objective findings include cool and clammy skin, tachycardia, and tachypnea. He is pacing. The priority for this patient is to:
   A. place him in a quiet area on constant observation.
   B. give a complete detailed explanation of what to expect.
   C. tell the patient to sit in the chair.
   D. get the physician.

40. An elderly male is brought to the ED with his home health attendant for evaluation of increased weakness. The attendant states that the patient has dementia. Accurate assessment includes:
   A. asking the patient about recent activities of daily living.
   B. obtaining a health history from the patient.
   C. asking questions loudly to ensure that the patient understands.
   D. assess regimen of both prescription and over-the-counter drugs with the family and/or home health assistant.

41. A 28-year-old woman with a history of bipolar disease is brought to the ED at 11 A.M. by her family, who state that she has been out for the last 3 days and nights and has just come home with a new car filled with purchases she made for the family, including a new TV and clothes. She is wearing a short skirt, a tight top, and a lot of makeup. She has difficulty sitting in the chair at triage and is talking rapidly about many different things. Which of the following is the ED nurse's first priority?
   A. Set limits, especially concerning necessary tasks.
   B. Start the lithium (Lithobid) that the physician has ordered.
   C. Keep the patient awake during daytime hours.
   D. Encourage the patient to focus on the things around her.

42. A 48-year-old female is referred to the ED from a community ambulatory care center for evaluation of intermittent palpitations, chest tightness, and choking sensations. The patient reports having had these symptoms for about 6 weeks and states that the episodes are becoming more frequent. Triage assessment reveals an intact airway. Skin is cool and slightly diaphoretic to the touch. Vital signs are BP 168/72 mm Hg, HR 118/min, respirations 26/min, and temperature 99.2° F (37.3° C). The patient does not report any chest tightness, palpitations, or choking sensations at this time. Priority interventions for this patient include:
   A. draw blood specimens for cardiac enzymes and markers.
   B. initiate oxygen therapy via nasal cannula at 5 L/min.
   C. obtain an arterial blood sample for blood gas analysis.
   D. obtain a chest x-ray.

43. A 17-year-old high school student is brought to the ED by her parents, who state that she has been crying incessantly and has been withdrawn and unable to sleep since breaking up with her boyfriend 3 weeks ago. Parents express concern to the triage nurse by stating that they feel their daughter will harm herself if she is not admitted to the hospital for observation. Triage assessment reveals a tearful young female who is wringing her hands constantly. There is no evidence of physical injury and the patient denies ingestion of any medication or harmful substance. Vital signs are BP 90/60 mm Hg, HR 126/min, and respirations 22/min. During her stay in the ED, this patient becomes agitated and hostile toward her parents and the staff. Which of the following would be the most appropriate action for the ED nurse to take?
   A. Call security and have the patient restrained immediately.
   B. Notify the consulting psychiatrist to obtain an order for a sedative.
   C. Assure the safety of the patient by minimizing environmental stimuli and politely request that the parents wait outside in a nearby location.
   D. Speak quietly to the patient in a calm, compassionate manner for the purpose of defining the source of her agitation.

44. When caring for a patient with an acute gouty arthritis attack, the ED nurse should anticipate an order to administer:
    A. oxycodone/acetaminophen (Percocet).
    B. prednisone (Delta-Cortef).
    C. indomethacin (Indocin).
    D. acetylsalicylic acid (aspirin).

45. A patient presents to the ED with possible contamination by a hazardous material. The patient is rinsed with another reactive agent that is known to alter the chemical structure of the hazardous material, thus producing a less harmful substance. This process is known as which of the following?
    A. Dilution
    B. Absorption
    C. Degradation
    D. Chelation

46. A passenger train has derailed. First responders indicate that at least 56 people have been injured. An ED nurse has gone in an ambulance to assist with care at the scene. Which of the following patients is the LOWEST PRIORITY for treatment and transport ("black" category)?
    A. A 75-year-old with femur, tibia, and fibula fractures and pelvis tenderness and mobility on palpation; skin is pale and moist
    B. A 45-year-old with a metal rod impaled in the right forearm, which is neurovascularly intact; patient is ambulatory
    C. A 63-year-old with second- and third-degree burns over 95% of body surface areas; patient is unconscious and has a thready pulse
    D. A 25-year-old with pain to the left lateral lower chest and a 5-inch laceration to the left forearm; wound squirts blood when uncovered; patient is controlling bleeding by applying pressure with a bandanna; skin is pink and dry

47. An off-duty ED nurse stops at a motor vehicle crash (MVC). The nurse's first priority in rendering aid is:
    A. stabilization of the patient's cervical spine with simultaneous airway control.
    B. breathing assessment and assistance.
    C. circulatory assessment and assistance.
    D. his/her own safety.

48. Which of the following patients should be transferred to a tertiary-care center?
    A. Adult with grand mal seizures
    B. Adolescent with single long-bone injury
    C. Adult with chest injury and widened mediastinum
    D. Adult with second-degree burns over less than 15% of body surface area

49. An elderly patient with right ventricular failure secondary to right ventricular infarction is admitted to the ICU. Because no bed is available, the patient must stay in the ED. The ED nurse should anticipate administration of large quantities of:
    A. morphine.
    B. intravenous fluids.
    C. diuretics.
    D. nitrates.

50. Which of the following situations increases ED nursing responsibility for patient teaching?
    A. Patient education level has decreased.
    B. Hospital admissions have been restricted.

C. Lawsuits against health care providers have decreased.

D. The public has lost interest in preventive health care.

51. A 4-year-old girl treated for accidental drug ingestion will be discharged home with her parents. Which of the following statements by the parents suggests that the parents understand home safety?

A. "We will store all medications in child safety containers in locked cabinets."

B. "We will be more careful watching her and won't let her out of our sight."

C. "We plan to keep all the medications in our highest cupboards in the kitchen."

D. "We think this trip to the hospital has convinced her never to take these pills again."

52. The most effective intervention to overcome obstacles to teaching in the ED setting is to:

A. use videotaped teaching materials for all patients.

B. allocate a minimum of 15 minutes to provide patient education for each patient.

C. provide group teaching in the waiting area to promote group support among the patients.

D. establish rapport between the nurse and patient.

53. A 16-year-old female presents with limb-threatening injuries following a motor vehicle crash. Although the patient is a minor, health care providers begin treatment while attempting to reach her parents. In this case, consent for treatment is which of the following?

A. Informed express consent

B. Involuntary

C. Implied

D. Assumed, since the patient is obviously emancipated.

54. A mother brings her 6-year-old son to triage, stating, "My child was scratched by a raccoon and needs rabies shots." The triage nurse informs the mother that rabies vaccine is not administered in the ED and refers her to the health department. This is an example of an EMTALA violation because:

A. A triage screening exam is not a replacement for a medical screening exam.

B. Rabies vaccine should be available at all emergency departments.

C. The triage nurse failed to contact the health department.

D. The triage nurse failed to clean the wound.

55. A 50-year-old patient who received a heart transplant 6 months ago reports to the ED complaining of a low-grade fever, fatigue, and shortness of breath. The triage nurse assesses the patient's vital signs as normal. The triage nurse correctly classifies this patient as:

A. Emergent: immediate threat to life or limb.

B. Urgent: No immediate threat to life or limb but needs reassessment every 15 minutes.

C. Nonurgent: No immediate threat to life or limb, reassessment in 1–2 hours.

D. Stable: No immediate threat to life or limb, reassessment in 30–60 minutes.

56. Elements of an organized emergency disaster preparedness plan include all of the following EXCEPT:

A. security.

B. communications.

C. coordination of patient care.

D. hospital-based transportation services.

57. A patient who opens his eyes spontaneously, obeys motor commands, and is oriented to person and place has a Glasgow Coma Scale score of:

A. 8

B. 10

C. 12

D. 15

58. Your ED has received 3 patients from a motor vehicle crash. Which patient needs to be stabilized and transferred to a Level 1 facility first?
    A. A 16-year-old female; driver, no seat belt. Injuries to right arm and leg, with abdominal trauma. Vital signs stable.
    B. An 18-year-old male; front seat passenger. Multiple facial lacerations and fractures, positive loss of consciousness. Decreasing oxygen saturation and positive chest trauma.
    C. A 17-year-old female; rear seat passenger, no seat belt. She is 22 weeks pregnant, with abdominal trauma, low BP, tachycardia, and respiratory distress.
    D. A 15-year-old female; rear seat passenger with seat belt. Injuries to right leg and chest. Vital signs stable.

59. Before a patient is transferred, documentation must include all of the following EXCEPT:
    A. care given during the patient's stay.
    B. planned length of stay at the receiving facility.
    C. all laboratory tests and x-rays performed at the sending facility.
    D. signed consent for transfer.

60. Which of the following equipment should be avoided on a rotary wing aircraft?
    A. Heimlich valve
    B. IV solution in a pressure bag
    C. MAST trousers
    D. Traction splint

61. Which of the following accurately describes the sequence for disaster preparation?
    A. Education, planning, practice, evaluation
    B. Planning, practice, evaluation, education
    C. Planning, education, evaluation, practice
    D. Planning, education, practice, evaluation

62. When discharging a patient home, the most important component of the process is which of the following?
    A. The removal of all medical apparatus prior to discharge.
    B. A verbal review of the discharge instructions.
    C. Providing the patient with written discharge instructions.
    D. Making transportation arrangements for the patient's follow-up appointment.

63. Documentation at triage must include which of the following?
    A. Whom to notify in case of emergency
    B. The name and address of the patient's doctor
    C. The chief complaint and a set of vital signs
    D. A list of medications and a set of vital signs

64. When a patient is being discharged with a cast, which of the following is the MOST ESSENTIAL discharge information?
    A. The name of the physician who will provide follow-up care
    B. The name of the physician who cared for the patient in the ED
    C. Documentation of the care provided in the ED
    D. Review of cast care and discussion of reasons to call or return to the Emergency Department

65. Rabies postexposure prophylaxis includes human rabies immune globulin (Hyperab, Imogam) and:
    A. human diploid cell vaccine (Imovax, HDCV).
    B. diphtheria/tetanus (DT).

    C. hepatitis B vaccine (Engerix-B).

    D. Lyme vaccine (LYMErix).

66. A subungual hematoma is caused by a:
    A. laceration to the palmar aspect of a finger.
    B. contusion to the tongue.
    C. fracture of the wrist.
    D. crush injury to the finger or nailbed.

67. Your neurovascular assessment of an anterior shoulder dislocation includes the upper extremity nerves and vascular tests for sensory and motor functioning. The area of concern is most likely which of the following?
    A. Axillary nerve, sensory branch
    B. Radial nerve, motor branch
    C. Ulnar artery
    D. Median nerve, motor branch

68. An open tibial fracture, Grade III, is prepared for debridement procedures and irrigation. The ideal time frame for these procedures is within:
    A. 26–36 hours.
    B. 16–24 hours.
    C. 9–12 hours.
    D. 6–8 hours.

69. Acute compartment syndrome most commonly occurs in the:
    A. abdominal cavity.
    B. forearm.
    C. thigh.
    D. lower leg.

70. A patient is en route to the operating room for repair of a midshaft femur fracture. A possible lethal complication of a femur fracture is:
    A. deep-vein thrombosis.
    B. nonunion of the fracture.
    C. rhabdomyolysis.
    D. fat emboli.

71. Radial head fractures classically involve pain and point tenderness, particularly with:
    A. wrist flexion.
    B. wrist extension.
    C. finger extension.
    D. supination.

Questions 72–74

An 18-month-old female is brought into the ED. The mother states that the child was sitting in her high chair and pulled a cup of hot coffee off the counter. You note that the child has superficial and partial thickness burns to her mouth, chin, and anterior chest. Intact blisters are noted on her chest.

72. What type of burn has the child sustained?
    A. Chemical burn
    B. Electrical burn
    C. Inhalation burn
    D. Thermal burn

73. Which of the following is most appropriate for care of the toddler who burned herself with coffee?
    A. Undress the child and leave her uncovered in ambient air.
    B. Apply ice to cool the burned areas.
    C. Undress the patient and keep warm with sterile sheets and/or heating lamp.
    D. Apply hydrocortisone ointment to decrease inflammation.

74. Upon further examination of the child, the nurse notes multiple bruises of various ages over the back and lower extremities. There also appear to be well-healed circumferential scars above both ankles. The child is crying and inconsolable. The ED nurse should suspect:
    A. abuse/neglect.
    B. careless child care/parenting.
    C. the child is acting normally.
    D. the child is spoiled and out of control.

75. An elderly woman slips and falls onto her left forearm. The arm just below the shoulder has extensive swelling and bruising and is tender to palpation. A fractured humerus is suspected. As part of the assessment, the ED nurse should evaluate the patient's ability to:
    A. extend the hand at the wrist against pressure.
    B. make a clenched fist.
    C. spread the fingers apart.
    D. flex the hand at the wrist.

76. A patient presents to the ED after catching his great toe nail in the track of his shower stall. The proximal aspect of the nail has lifted away from the nailbed. There is no bleeding from the bed or surrounding tissues. This injury would best be described as:
    A. avulsion injury of the toe.
    B. nail root avulsion.
    C. contusion of the toe.
    D. nailbed laceration.

Questions 77 and 78

An adolescent male is being evaluated after he jammed his finger playing basketball. On exam, capillary refill is brisk and sensation is intact. The finger is held in flexion at the proximal interphalangeal joint and he is unable to extend it.

77. The ED nurse should suspect that this patient has:
    A. fractured the distal phalangis.
    B. lacerated the digital artery.
    C. ruptured the extensor tendon.
    D. contused the digital nerve.

78. Prior to discharge, the ED nurse should immobilize the finger by:
    A. taping it to an adjacent finger.
    B. splinting it in extension.
    C. splinting it in the position of comfort.
    D. splinting it in flexion.

79. When the emergency nurse is evaluating foreign bodies in soft tissues, which of the following is considered a reactive object?
    A. Sewing needle
    B. Glass fragment
    C. Wood splinter
    D. Graphite from a pencil

80. Your trauma patient has been diagnosed with neurogenic shock. You note no movement of any extremity, hypotension, and bradycardia. His respirations are 40/minute and shallow. After you have assessed and maintained the patient's airway, what is your next intervention?
    A. Administer 100% oxygen via nonrebreather mask.
    B. Administer 100% oxygen via bag-valve-mask device.
    C. Intubate the patient with rapid-sequence inline intubation.
    D. Intubate via nasotracheal intubation.

81. The most important stabilization treatment of an unconscious victim with a closed head injury from motor vehicle collision is which of the following?
    A. Maintain spinal immobilization
    B. Control of the airway
    C. Establish intravenous access
    D. Determine history of bleeding dyscrasias

82. The test that is done to determine the degree of a LeFort fracture is:
    A. computed tomography (CT) of orbits.
    B. magnetic resonance imaging (MRI) of maxillofacial bones.
    C. Waters' view of skull.
    D. temporal mandibular x-rays.

83. A 12-year-old child presents to the ED after being struck in the head with a baseball bat. The patient complaints of headache and pain in his deltoid region. The triage nurse should perform which of the following first?
    A. Determine if there was loss of consciousness
    B. Apply ice to area of injury
    C. Obtain pulse oximetry and vital signs
    D. Apply cervical spine immobilization

84. A patient who is brought to the ED was the known driver in a high-speed motor vehicle crash. The patient was not belted, was ejected from the vehicle, and is now complaining of severe substernal chest pain, dyspnea, stridor, and hoarseness on exam. The patient has swelling of the neck and cyanosis of the lower extremities. This patient may be exhibiting signs of:
    A. cervical spine subluxation.
    B. fractures of the first ribs.
    C. aortic tear.
    D. fractured sternum.

85. After you have performed an intraosseous cannulation for your 18-month-old pediatric patient, what would indicate that you had performed the procedure correctly?
    A. A blood flashback is seen in the catheter.
    B. It is possible to thread the over-the-needle cannula.
    C. A popping sound is heard during insertion, followed by lack of resistance to the needle.
    D. The butterfly needle can stand upright without manual support.

86.   Your patient is a victim of a motor vehicle crash. He has severe facial injury. You select the following manner to test cranial nerve function:
    A. Observe the patient for posturing patterns such as flexion or extension.
    B. Observe for Battle's sign behind the ear.
    C. Inspect the ears and nose for cerebrospinal fluid leakage.
    D. Have the patient follow your moving finger with his eyes.

87.   You are preparing a motorcycle crash victim for a needle thoracentesis. A tension pneumothorax is suspected. After assembling the needed equipment, you would know that insertion of a 14-gauge needle would be placed in which location?
    A. Unaffected side, fourth intercostal space slightly anterior to the midaxillary line
    B. Affected side, second intercostal space at the midclavicular line
    C. Affected side, fifth intercostal space slightly anterior to the midaxillary line
    D. Unaffected side, third intercostal space at the midclavicular line.

88.   You are preparing to insert an indwelling urinary catheter. What would you consider a contraindication for the procedure?
    A. The patient tells you that she does not see a need for the catheter.
    B. There had been discomfort during your abdominal palpation.
    C. The patient tells you that she allergic to latex.
    D. There is blood at the urethral meatus.

89.   The proper positioning of the multitrauma patient with suspected flat chest injury is which of the following?
    A. High Fowler's position to prevent aspiration of hemoptysis
    B. Flail side downward to stabilize flail segment and improve ventilation
    C. Flail side splinted with sandbags keeping patient dorsorecumbent
    D. Flail side upward to avoid hemopneumothorax from penetrating fractured ribs

90.   A 30-year-old male presents to the ED with new onset of profound lower extremity weakness and numbness and tingling in the abdomen, chest, and upper extremities. S/he has absent superficial and deep tendon reflexes. The patient reports burning and aching in both legs that have increased over the last week. Based on the patient's history and presenting symptoms, the nurse would assess for:
    A. respiratory rate; depth and work of breathing.
    B. presence of rectal tone.
    C. changes in level of consciousness.
    D. recent history of upper respiratory illness.

91.   A 33-year-old female patient involved in a motor vehicle collision is brought to the ED via EMS. Prehospital providers report she was responsive only to painful stimuli at the scene. The patient is intubated and has 2 large-bore IVs with normal saline infusing. Pupils are equal and reactive at 4 mm. The patient withdraws to painful stimuli. The ED nurse should anticipate which of the following interventions?
    A. Hyperventilating to maintain $pCO_2 < 30$ mm Hg
    B. Mannitol (Osmitrol) 100 g IV
    C. Dexamethasone (Decadron) 10 mg IV
    D. Fluid administration to maintain mean arterial pressure (MAP) > 90 mm Hg

92.   A 26-year-old patient is brought to the ED after falling out a second-story window. He responds only to deep pain and has blood oozing from the right ear and right naris. The right pupil is 7 mm in diameter and nonreactive to light. The left pupil is 4 mm in diameter and sluggish. The Glasgow Coma Scale is determined to be 4. Prehospital providers have immobilized the patient with a rigid

cervical collar and long spine board. The patient has an 18-gauge IV with lactated Ringer's infusing. The initial priority for the ED nurse is do which of the following?

A. Initiate a second large-bore IV with warmed crystalloid
B. Prepare to administer mannitol (Osmitrol)
C. Assist with rapid-sequence induction and intubation
D. Hyperventilate to maintain $pCO_2 < 30$ mm Hg

93. A patient is admitted to the ED with a diagnosis of Alzheimer's disease. The patient appears very disoriented and confused. Which of the following nursing diagnoses would be MOST appropriate for this patient?

A. Injury, high risk, related to altered thought processes
B. Tissue perfusion, altered cerebral, related to interruption in blood flow
C. Anxiety, fear, related to onset of symptoms
D. Knowledge deficit, risk factors and prevention

94. A 24-year-old male presents to the ED after falling 10 feet from a roof. He is lethargic but easily aroused to verbal stimuli. He is confused and perseverating. Witnesses report the patient was unconscious for at least 5 minutes. On initial exam he is found to have multiple abrasions on the left side of his face, blood oozing from the left ear, ecchymosis around both eyes, and a laceration on his left arm. As part of the assessment, the ED nurse should do which of the following?

A. Assess for hemotympanum and pack the external canal
B. Assess for cerebrospinal fluid (CSF) in the ear drainage
C. Prepare to administer prophylactic antibiotics
D. Prepare the patient for computed tomography (CT) scan of the head

95. A 45-year-old male presents to the ED with complaints of severe pain and burning around the left eye, pain in the left side of the head, increased tearing, and nausea. You note ptosis of the left eye, which is red. The patient states that these symptoms started approximately 30 minutes prior to arrival. This patient's symptoms are most commonly associated with:

A. cluster headache.
B. tension headache.
C. intracerebral neoplasm.
D. optic neuritis.

96. A 60-year-old female is brought to the ED by her husband. He states that she awoke this morning complaining of a headache and has gradually become more disoriented. She is now awake but confused and has difficulty standing. Upon further assessment, her left pupil is 6 mm in diameter and nonreactive to light. The right pupil is 4 mm in diameter and reacts briskly. Vital signs are BP 122/60 mm Hg, HR 60/min, and respirations 20/min. Based on these initial findings, you would anticipate interventions for possible:

A. calcium channel blocker toxicity.
B. meningitis.
C. subdural hematoma.
D. dehydration.

97. The priority nursing diagnosis for a patient in the ED awaiting admission for an acoustic neuroma would be:

A. dysreflexia.
B. risk for aspiration.
C. risk for injury.
D. impaired verbal communication.

98. A 40-year-old male involved in a house fire presents to the ED with dyspnea, sooty sputum, and a brassy cough. He is conscious; 100% oxygen via nonrebreather reservoir mask is being administered. The priority nursing diagnosis for this patient would be:
    A. fluid volume deficit.
    B. impaired gas exchange.
    C. airway clearance, ineffective.
    D. pain.

99. 45-year-old man falls 8 feet onto his shoulder, sustaining a scapular fracture. Concomitant injuries associated with a scapular fracture are which of the following?
    A. Pneumothorax and pulmonary contusion
    B. Head injury and abdominal injury
    C. Elbow and wrist fractures
    D. Scaphoid and capitate fractures

100. Patient comfort and cooperation during eye irrigation can be facilitated by the administration of:
    A. pilocarpine (Pilocar).
    B. tetracycline (Achromycin).
    C. tetracaine (Pontocaine).
    D. lidocaine (Xylocaine).

101. A complication found in patients with a LeFort II fracture is:
    A. cerebrospinal fluid leak.
    B. Ludwig's angina.
    C. otitis externa.
    D. spinal shock.

102. A 54-year-old patient presents to triage clutching bloody tissues and complaining of a nosebleed. Vital signs are BP 154/100 mm Hg, HR 88/min, respirations 16/min, and temperature 98.5°F (36.9°C). An appropriate intervention for this patient would be to:
    A. place patient in Trendelenburg position.
    B. apply pinch pressure to nose.
    C. administer a rapid infusion of 250 ml of normal saline.
    D. tilt head backwards until bleeding subsides.

103. Which of the following patients represents the highest triage acuity level?
    A. A 12-year-old reporting a "stye" in the left eye
    B. A 34-year-old with "pepper spray to both eyes"
    C. A 22-year-old who is "unable to remove my contact lens"
    D. A 4-year-old with "itchy, sticky eyes"

104. Pediatric patients presenting with nasal obstruction and purulent, unilateral, foul-smelling rhinorrhea most likely have which of the following conditions?
    A. Epistaxis
    B. Sinusitis
    C. Foreign body of the nose
    D. Acute or chronic pharyngitis

105. The patient with a hyphema should be placed in which of the following positions?
    A. Trendelenburg
    B. Supine
    C. Elevated head of bed
    D. Prone

106.   Signs and symptoms of globe rupture of the eye include:
        A. teardrop-shaped pupil and decreased intraocular pressure.
        B. shallow anterior chamber and increased intraocular pressure.
        C. hyphema and increased intraocular pressure.
        D. corneal ulcer and decreased intraocular pressure.

107.   Which cranial nerves (CN) are measured in assessing extraocular muscle function?
        A. CN III, V, VIII
        B. CN III, IV, VI
        C. CN II, VII, X
        D. CN III, VI, VIII

108.   Which of the following is true about temporomandibular joint (TMJ) dislocation?
        A. The cause is usually a blow to the chin.
        B. The patient presents with the mandible tightly clenched against the maxilla.
        C. Unilateral dislocations are common.
        D. It is often seen in toddlers who fall on the chin when learning to walk.

109.   The endpoint for the administration of procainamide (Pronestyl) includes all of the following
        EXCEPT:
        A. The arrhythmia is suppressed.
        B. A total of 17mg/kg of the drug is given.
        C. The QRS complex is narrowed by 50% from its original duration.
        D. Hypotension ensues.

110.   The first medication indicated for any pulseless patient is which of the following?
        A. Epinephrine (Adrenalin)
        B. Atropine
        C. Lidocaine (Xylocaine)
        D. Sodium bicarbonate

111.   When defibrillating with the initial three shocks, the ED nurse should:
        A. wait until after intubation has occurred to begin the shocks.
        B. assess the cardiac rhythm between stacked shocks.
        C. continue CPR between stacked shocks.
        D. check the pulse after each shock.

112.   The most common lethal arrhythmia in the first hour of an acute myocardial infarction (AMI) is
        which of the following?
        A. Atrial fibrillation
        B. Asystole
        C. Third-degree heart block
        D. Ventricular fibrillation

113.   All of the following statements about atropine sulfate are true EXCEPT:
        A. Atropine can result in paradoxical bradycardia if given in high doses.
        B. Atropine can be administered endotracheally.
        C. Atropine can cause bradycardia if given by slow IV push.
        D. Atropine is an antidote for anticholinesterase insecticide poisoning.

114.   A patient is brought to the ED after a motor vehicle crash. He is pulseless and apneic. The monitor shows a sinus tachycardia at a rate of 120. The nurse anticipates which of the following?
   A. Administration of epinephrine (Adrenalin)
   B. Administration of epinephrine (Adrenalin) and atropine
   C. Attempt immediate defibrillation
   D. Administration of adenosine (Adenocard)

115.   Which of the following medications should NOT be administered endotracheally?
   A. Lidocaine (Xylocaine)
   B. Adenosine (Adenocard)
   C. Atropine
   D. Epinephrine (Adrenalin)

116.   When administering intravenous Adenosine (Adenocard), the nurse realizes that all of the following are true EXCEPT that:
   A. adenosine (Adenocard) must be administered slowly to prevent hypotension.
   B. adenosine (Adenocard) should be followed by a 20-ml saline bolus.
   C. adenosine (Adenocard) may cause a brief period of asystole after rapid administration.
   D. adenosine (Adenocard) may cause flushing.

117.   Sodium bicarbonate may be effective treatment in all of the following cases EXCEPT which of the following?
   A. Preexisting metabolic acidosis
   B. Hyperkalemia
   C. Tricyclic or phenobarbital overdose
   D. Hypoxic lactic acidosis

118.   When you are establishing IV access during cardiopulmonary resuscitation (CPR), your first choice should be:
   A. the back of the hand.
   B. antecubital.
   C. femoral.
   D. a central line.

119.   To assist medications into the central circulation after peripheral IV administration during cardiopulmonary resuscitation (CPR), the ED nurse should:
   A. defibrillate after each medication.
   B. give a 20-ml fluid bolus and elevate the patient's arm.
   C. bag vigorously.
   D. turn the patient on his left side.

120.   Which statement regarding ventricular tachycardia is TRUE?
   A. The rhythm is always irregular.
   B. Patients with sustained ventricular tachycardia are usually asymptomatic.
   C. Frequent PVCs and short runs of ventricular tachycardia commonly precede ventricular tachycardia.
   D. The QRS duration is < 0.12.

121. A patient presents to the ED with a sinus bradycardia and frequent PVCs. Vital signs are 80/60 mm/Hg and HR 38/min. Which of the following interventions is MOST appropriate?
    A. Administer a lidocaine (Xylocaine) bolus.
    B. Insert a transvenous pacemaker.
    C. Administer an atropine bolus.
    D. Initiate a dopamine (Intropin) drip.

122. The emergency nurse manager wishes to evaluate staffing as part of a continuous improvement plan. The manager would benchmark information such as:
    A. staff senses that patients are staying longer while awaiting in house beds.
    B. actual staffing, wait times, and length of stay by patient triage classification.
    C. Chief Financial Officer statement that ED is overstaffed by full-time equivalents for unit of service.
    D. patient compliant letter stating ED is understaffed.

123. During an interview, which of the following questions would be reasonable to ask a potential nurse who is applying for a position in the ED?
    A. "What are your expectations of the ED management team?"
    B. "Do you have transportation to and from work?"
    C. "What hobbies do you engage in after work hours?"
    D. "Do you speak Spanish or French?"

124. A hospital can be charged with the unfair labor practice known as interference if the hospital:
    A. refuses to meet with union representatives.
    B. gives union leaders a special meeting room.
    C. threatens to close if a union is elected.
    D. does not stop the distribution of union material.

125. Following the death of a child in the ED, a stress debriefing session is arranged. Personnel invited to this session should include:
    A. all ED personnel with small children.
    B. ED nursing staff from all shifts.
    C. nursing management responsible for staff in the ED.
    D. ED personnel involved with the situation.

126. The process by which data are collected, results are documented, and experiments and tests are validated in order to change a concept is which of the following?
    A. Research-focused theory
    B. Evidence-based practice
    C. Nursing process model
    D. Quantitative analysis approach

127. The job description of an employee in the ED reads as follows: "To focus on education, system analysis, research, and research utilization and the provision of direct and indirect nursing care. Job requirement: minimum of master's degree in nursing; area of specialization, Emergency Care." This description is for a/an:
    A. nurse practitioner.
    B. clinical nurse specialist.
    C. ED educator.
    D. case manager.

128.   You are caring for a 30-year-old female victim of domestic violence. She experienced an assault to the chest and upper abdomen. She has a pneumothorax, which has been treated with a chest tube. The patient is hypotensive. You note particulate matter in the chest tube. She also has crepitus over the mediastinal area. You suspect:
A. ruptured diaphragm.
B. ruptured esophagus.
C. stomach injury.
D. mesenteric injury.

129.   A 38-year-old male patient presents to the ED in severe distress from upper gastrointestinal bleeding. He has been vomiting bright-red blood at home for 2 hours and is now experiencing rectal bleeding. The ED nurse who must prioritize his care immediately performs which of the following?
A. Ensures that the patient is on 100% nonrebreather oxygen mask
B. Initiates intravenous therapy for fluid rehydration
C. Inserts nasogastric tube
D. Sends for a type and crossmatch of packed red blood cells

130.   When a patient with peptic ulcer disease presents to the ED, the ED nurse must first consider which of the following?
A. Insertion of a nasogastric tube
B. Administration of antiemetics
C. Administration of pain medication/analgesics
D. Obtaining a serum electrolyte profile

131.   A 24-year-old female presents to the ED complaining, "It's my Crohn's disease acting up again. I overdid it this weekend." She admits to some abdominal pain and diarrhea. "Just give me some prednisone and I will be fine," she states. The priority nursing diagnosis for this patient is which of the following?
A. Altered nutrition related to less than body requirements.
B. Altered nutrition related to more than body requirements.
C. Knowledge deficit related to diet and medications.
D. Altered health maintenance.

132.   A patient presents to the ED with a chief complaint of sudden onset of colicky abdominal pain and nausea after eating a meal of fried chicken and French fries. Vital signs are BP 140/80 mm Hg, HR 116/min, respirations 18/min, and temperature 100.4° F (38.0° C). The ED nurse suspects:
A. diverticulitis.
B. appendicitis.
C. cholecystitis.
D. esophagitis.

133.   A 39-year-old female patient presents to the ED with abdominal distention, severe epigastric pain, and hypoactive bowel sounds following a heavy meal. She has a history of alcohol abuse. The ED nurse should be concerned with what potential complications besides fluid volume deficit?
A. Intestinal obstruction
B. Ruptured appendix
C. Sepsis
D. Acute respiratory distress syndrome

134. The patient presents with periumbilical pain and fever. Appendicitis is suspected. The diagnosis of appendicitis will largely be derived from:
    A. ultrasonography of the abdomen.
    B. physical examination.
    C. white blood cell count (WBC).
    D. computed tomography (CT) of the abdomen.

135. Nursing care for the patient who has suspected appendicitis will most likely include:
    A. repeated physical examinations.
    B. medicating the patient with a narcotic.
    C. discharge instructions to follow up with a surgeon.
    D. insertion of a nasogastric tube.

136. A snake handler is bitten on the left arm by a rattlesnake. He presents to the ED for treatment, but tells you that he is OK. He states this has happened many times and all he needs is a shot, after which he will be ready to go back to work. Which of the following symptoms would lead you to believe that he has had a systemic reaction to the venom and will require more extensive treatment than he describes?
    A. Two puncture wounds located on the left forearm, approximately 8 mm apart
    B. A burning sensation at the site of the puncture wounds
    C. He asks for a glass of water to cleanse the metallic taste in his mouth.
    D. He is very dry mouthed and has unequal pupils.

137. A patient is being discharged from the ED following a cat bite and scratch by a neighbor's cat the patient was emptying the garbage. Instructions should include which of the following?
    A. "Return if you note swelling of your arm, even several weeks later."
    B. "Cat bites and scratches are fairly clean, but local antibiotics will be helpful."
    C. "Rates of infection are fairly low, but observe for a fever for the next 3 days."
    D. "Although the scratch is near your elbow, any bacteria would be limited to the skin."

138. You are a camp nurse providing emergency care to a group on an outing. Which of the following campers would you suspect to have the highest likelihood of experiencing frostbite?
    A. An 18-year-old female who jogs frequently
    B. A 25-year-old black male who smokes less than 1 pack per day
    C. A 45-year-old female with a history of recent cataract surgery
    D. A 60-year-old male with asthma and a cold

139. Which of the following bites has the highest rate of infection?
    A. Cat
    B. Dog
    C. Snake
    D. Human

140. Immediate treatment for a skier presenting to the ED with suspected frostbite to the foot would include:
    A. Removing the boot and rubbing the foot and ankle
    B. Opening the blisters and applying antibiotic cream to the entire area
    C. Application of warm soaks to the extremity
    D. Placing the foot in immobilization lower than the heart

141. In evaluating the chart of a patient brought to the ED with hypothermia, you note a treatment that is not appropriate for this patient. The following chart entry was part of your evaluation: "Patient admitted to the ED after being found under bridge early this A.M. Vital signs are BP 140/90 mm Hg, HR 120/min, respirations 24/min, and temperature 90° F (32.2° C). The wet cloths were removed and warm blankets were applied. The patient was given a cola to drink and warmed IV lactated Ringer's was started at 125 ml/hour. Warmed humidified oxygen was started via mask at 6 L. An NG tube was inserted with warm lavage, completed after about 30 minutes. Lab analysis and an ECG were completed. After 30 minutes, repeated vital signs were BP 140/80 mm Hg, HR 100/min, respirations 20/min, and temperature 91° F (32.8° C)." You would have a concern about which entry?
      A. Warmed gastric lavage
      B. Administration of oral cola
      C. Warmed IV lactated Ringer's
      D. Performance of an electrocardiogram

142. What proportion of people die when infected with West Nile virus?
      A. Case fatality rates range from 3–15% and are highest in the elderly.
      B. The case fatality rate is 100%.
      C. Case fatality rates range from 25% to 50% and are highest in children under 5 years of age.
      D. The case fatality rate is 80% and is highest in the adult population.

143. Which of the following statements concerning snakebites is TRUE?
      A. Of the approximately 50,000 snakebites recorded annually, approximately 30% patients die.
      B. Most poisonous snakebites in the United States are made by pit vipers, usually rattlesnakes.
      C. Pit viper venom is neurotoxic and is delivered from the fangs of the snake.
      D. The U.S. has only one family of poisonous snakes: the *Crotalidae*.

144. A teenager who is visiting a roadside animal show places a hand in the Gila monster (Heloderma) cage. The teen is bitten on the arm and the lizard has to be physically removed from the arm. On the patient's arrival in the ED, you would anticipate:
      A. mild irritation, since lizard bites are benign
      B. an order for immediate administration of antivenin.
      C. nausea, vomiting, hypotension, syncope, and shock.
      D. only local symptoms, with irritation, swelling, bruising, and petechiae.

145. An unconscious patient is being treated for the ingestion of an unknown quantity of hydrocodone tablets. The patient is given naloxone (Narcan). The ED nurse would suspect which of the following actions from the naloxone?
      A. Increase the duration of the amphetamine
      B. Decrease the intracranial pressure
      C. Alter the peripheral vascular resistance
      D. Reverse the narcotic effect

146. As ED Nurse Educator, you are invited to speak at an industry concerning various first aid procedures. During your presentation, an employee asks you to discuss emergency treatment for chemicals on the skin, especially hydrofluoric acid. Which of the following statements would demonstrate an understanding of the immediate treatment for hydrofluoric acid contact?
      A. The skin should be coated with a calcium gluconate gel.
      B. Copious water irrigation should be performed.
      C. Neutralization should begin with baking soda and water.
      D. Evaluation by a physician should occur within 2–4 hours.

147.   Following admission for a new onset of atrial fibrillation, a patient's discharge medications included warfarin (Coumadin). Upon arriving home, the patient became confused and took the entire bottle. Once the patient's adult daughter learned what had happened, she immediately returned the patient to the ED. You would prepare which of the following for the patient?
   A. Protamine sulfate
   B. Phytonadione (Aqua-Mephyton) (vitamin K)
   C. Thiamine (vitamin B_1)
   D. Nicotinic acid (Nicobid) (vitamin B_3)

•148.   Mild radiation exposure occurs with radiation levels of less than 125 units of absorbed radiation (rads). Symptoms of mild radiation exposure include:
   A. gastrointestinal bleeding.
   B. nausea and vomiting.
   C. tremors and muscle weakness.
   D. tachycardia and hypertension.

149.   A 25-year-old male is returning home after a weekend scuba expedition. He suddenly develops throbbing pain over the shoulders and upper torso. He is brought to the ED with those complaints in addition to that of a burning sensation with intense itching. As the ED nurse, you would suspect:
   A. barotrauma.
   B. decompression sickness.
   C. nitrogen narcosis.
   D. air embolism.

150.   A patient has been treated in the ED for decompression sickness. Upon discharge, which of the following statements would indicate the need for additional discharge teaching?
   A. "Next time, I will shorten the length of my dive."
   B. "From now on, I will carry a scuba identification card."
   C. "I need to watch how fast I reach the bottom."
   D. "I will never try a long scuba dive alone."

Practice Examination 5
Part 2

Questions 1–4

A 19-year-old female presents to the ED with a complaint of pelvic pain and fever. In reviewing her reproductive history, you determine that she has had 3 sex partners in the past 2 months. She does not use contraceptive devices and denies a pregnancy history. Her last menstrual period was 10 days ago. She states that she has a thick vaginal discharge with vaginal itching and dysuria. Pelvic pain is aggravated by sexual intercourse and walking. Vital signs are BP 110/60 mm Hg, HR 110/min, respirations 20/min, and temperature 102.6° F (39.2° C).

1. The above signs and symptoms suggest that the patient has:
    A. ectopic pregnancy
    B. PELVIC INFLAMMATORY DISEASE (PID).
    C. Mittelschmerz.
    D. ovarian cyst.

Rationale:

B. PID is an infection of the female pelvic structure. The patient most often presents with complaint of lower abdominal pain, fever and chills, nausea and vomiting, and vaginal discharge. Dysuria may also be a presenting complaint in the face of a negative urinary analysis. Cervical motion tenderness is a hallmark finding on pelvic exam.

A. An ectopic pregnancy usually presents with a classic triad of symptoms: abdominal pain with spotting and vaginal bleeding in a woman who has had amenorrhea.

C. Mittelschmerz is associated with ovulation. It is the rupture of an ovarian follicle. The pain is usually described as mild to moderate and located in the lower abdomen or pelvic area during midcycle.

D. There are two classic types of ovarian cysts. The first is a follicular cyst. It develops when the ovarian follicle fails to rupture during follicular development and ovulation. A follicular cyst is usually asymptomatic. It seldom grows to more than 8 cm in diameter. It usually regressed during the menstrual cycle. The second is a lutein cyst. It develops if the corpus luteum becomes cystic or hemorrhagic. A lutein cyst is more likely to cause pain and signs of peritoneal irritation. It is generally larger and more firm and has a solid consistency when compared to a follicle cyst. Fever and vaginal discharge are not associated with ovarian cysts.

Content Category: Genitourinary & Obstetrics & Gynecological

Reference: Hacker & Moore, 1998.

2. The most probable cause of this patient's vaginal discharge is which of the following?
    A. Bacterial vaginosis
    B. NEISSERIA GONORRHOEAE
    C. Candidal vulvovaginitis
    D. Normal vaginal discharge

Rationale:

B. *Neisseria gonorrhoeae* and *Chlamydia trachomatis* are the two most common causes of PID. Both can be traced to a recent sexual exposure to an infected partner. Gonorrhea exposure most likely occurred within 2 weeks of the onset of symptoms, whereas exposure may have occurred up to 2 months before onset of symptoms in a chlamydial infection.

A. Bacterial vaginosis (*Gardnerella vaginalis*) is characterized by a moderate to profuse vaginal discharge. The discharge is usually ivory to gray in color. It usually has a fishy odor that can be enhanced by adding 10% KOH to the discharge. Vaginal itching and burning are usually present.

C. Candidal vulvovaginitis is often referred called yeast infection. The discharge is often a thick and white, with the consistency of cottage cheese. Vaginal itching and burning are not uncommon.

D. The patient's symptoms do not represent normal vaginal discharge.

Content Category: Genitourinary & Obstetrics & Gynecological

Reference: Hacker & Moore, 1998.

3. A pelvic exam is performed. The most likely finding would be which of the following?
A. An adnexal mass
B. An open cervical os
C. CERVICAL MOTION TENDERNESS
D. None of the above

Rationale:

C. Cervical motion tenderness is a hallmark sign of PID.
A. Adnexal mass is not associated with PID.
B. An open cervical os is not associated with PID.
D. Incorrect.

Content Category: Genitourinary & Obstetrics & Gynecology

Reference: Hacker & Moore, 1998.

4. You would expect the medical provider to order which of the following?
A. Benzathine penicillin G (Permapen)
B. CEFTRIAXONE (TAZIDIME)
C. Metronidazole (Flagyl)
D. None of the above

Rationale:

B. Ceftriaxone 125–250 mg IM is the drug of choice to treat *Neisseria gonorrhoeae*.
A. Benzathine penicillin G is used to treat syphilis.
C. Metronidazole is used to treat *Trichomonas vaginalis*.
D. Incorrect.

Content Category: Genitourinary & Obstetrics & Gynecological

Reference: Hacker & Moore, 1998.

Questions 5 and 6

A 29-year-old female presents to the ED complaining of severe pain and swelling in her vaginal area. Upon evaluation you note swelling and erythema to her left vulvar area.

5.   These symptoms are most consistent with which of the following?
A. Herpes simplex virus
B. A volvulus
C. A chancroid
D. BARTHOLIN'S ABSCESS

Rationale:

D. Bartholin's cyst is very common. The cyst is usually a unilateral swelling, measuring about 2–8 cm in diameter, located posterolaterally in the Bartholin's gland. It contains sterile mucus and is usually asymptomatic. When the cyst becomes infected, it becomes inflamed, swollen, and painful. At that point it is called a Bartholin's abscess.
A. Herpes simplex virus (genital herpes) often presents with painful vesicles and shallow ulcers on the vulva. The herpes infection will generally appear 3 to 7 days after the initial exposure.
B. A volvulus is a malrotation of the intestine that results in an obstruction and strangulation. This can often lead to vascular compromise and intestinal loss. This is often found in very young children.
C. A chancroid is caused by the bacillus *Haemophilus ducreyi*. It is a highly contagious sexually transmitted disease that occurs most frequently in tropical and subtropical climates. Therefore, it is only seen in a few areas of the United States. Chancroid presents with vulvar pain and tenderness. A small papule will occur within 3 to 5 days of exposure. The papule rapidly turns into a grayish-based ulceration with a foul odor. It is extremely painful to the touch.

Content Category: Genitourinary & Obstetrics & Gynecological

Reference: Hacker & Moore, 1998.

6.   Definitive treatment for this patient should include which of the following?
A. An oral antiviral agent
B. Surgical consult
C. A fluoroquinolone antibiotic
D. INCISION AND DRAINAGE

Rationale:

D. Incision and drainage of the abscess are the most common treatment of choice.
A. Oral antiviral agents are used to treat the herpes simplex virus.
B. A surgical consult is needed to treat a volvulus.
C. A fluoroquinolone antibiotic is used to treat gonorrhea.

Content Category: Genitourinary & Obstetrics & Gynecological

Reference: Hacker & Moore, 1998.

7.   A 5-day-old female is brought to the ED by her parents for a blood-tinged vaginal discharge. Her parents deny trauma and state that no one else has cared for the infant except them. Examination of the patient does not reveal evidence of gross trauma. Your intervention for this child should be:
A. Contact Child Protective Services to evaluate for child abuse.
B. Separate the parents and question each separately to determine whether their stories differ.
C. Obtain cultures and wet mount of the vaginal discharge.
D. REASSURE THE PARENTS THAT THIS IS A NORMAL FINDING IN THE NEWBORN.

Rationale:

    D. A decrease in circulating maternal estrogen, which was diffused across the placenta, occurs during the neonatal period. This results in a physiologic vaginal discharge, which may range from blood-tinged to frank blood. The discharge usually disappears within 10 days of birth.

    A. Appropriate only if child abuse is suspected.

    B. Appropriate only if child abuse is suspected.

    C. Appropriate only if child abuse is suspected.

Content Category: Genitourinary & Obstetrics & Gynecological

Reference: Hacker & Moore, 1998.

8. A 16-year-old female presents to the ED with a complaint of abnormal vaginal bleeding for 2 weeks. A possible cause of the bleeding is which of the following?

    A. Hypothyroidism

    B. Idiopathic thrombocytopenia

    C. Neoplasia

    D. ALL OF THE ABOVE

Rationale:

    D. There are many causes of abnormal vaginal bleeding. If the bleeding is persistent, the patient should be referred to a gynecologist for further evaluation.

    A. One possible reason for abnormal vaginal bleeding.

    B. One possible reason for abnormal vaginal bleeding.

    C. One possible reason for abnormal vaginal bleeding.

Content Category: Genitourinary & Obstetrics & Gynecological

Reference: Hacker & Moore, 1998.

9. A 50-year-old construction worker presents to the ED with complaints of severe flank pain, nausea, vomiting, and diaphoresis and is unable to stand still or converse. The patient is most likely exhibiting signs of:

    A. acute heat exhaustion.

    B. RENAL CALCULI.

    C. acute food poisoning.

    D. dissecting aneurysm.

Rationale:

    B. Patients with renal calculi are unable to sit or speak because of severe flank pain. Occupations such as construction may predispose patients to dehydration, which can cause renal calculi.

    A. Acute heat exhaustion is manifested by an increase in temperature as high as 104° F. These patients have severe weakness and altered mental status.

    C. Patients with acute food poisoning complain of severe abdominal discomfort and have symptoms of vomiting and severe diarrhea.

    D. Patients with dissecting aneurysm present with severe pain and hypertension. They usually do not present with vomiting when symptoms start acutely.

Content Category: Genitourinary & Obstetrics & Gynecological

Reference: ENA, Core Curriculum, 2000.

10. A female patient presents to the ED triage nurse with complaints of dysuria, urinary frequency, and lower abdominal pain. One of the first procedures the ED nurse should initiate is which of the following?
A. Prepare for a pelvic examination.
B. Administer analgesia.
C. OBTAIN CLEAN-CATCH URINE.
D. Check the patient's rectal temperature.

Rationale:

C. Obtaining a clean-catch urine specimen is of the utmost importance to determine which organism is responsible for the infection and thereby ensuring that the correct antibiotic will be chosen.
A. The patient may require a pelvic exam, but she should empty her bladder first and provide a urine specimen.
B. Analgesia may be offered after a brief exam and history to specify the origin of pain.
D. Since the patient is an adult, an oral temperature should be sufficient for first evaluation.

Content Category: Genitourinary & Obstetrics & Gynecological
Reference: ENA, Core Curriculum, 2000.

11. A 40-year-old nonsmoking patient who is in general good health is diagnosed with acute bronchitis. Which of the following pieces of information about the disease process should be included in patient education?
A. The risk of subsequent development of pneumonia is high with this disorder.
B. Acute bronchitis is often a precursor to development of chronic obstructive pulmonary disease.
C. THE CAUSATIVE AGENT OF ACUTE BRONCHITIS IS FREQUENTLY VIRAL RATHER THAN BACTERIAL.
D. Acute bronchitis is a lifelong disease that requires continued medical management.

Rationale:

C. Patient education should include the fact that the most common causes are viral and that antibiotic therapy is less often being used to treat the disorder. Antibiotics may be prescribed when a superimposed bacterial infection is suspected.
A. Bronchitis develops into pneumonia in less than 5% of cases in normally healthy individuals without other risk factors such as underlying lung disease, diabetes, or smoking history.
B. Acute bronchitis is an episodic disorder commonly associated with incidences of the common cold and flu. It rarely precedes the development of chronic bronchitis or emphysema in a normal healthy individual without other risk factors.
D. A repeat chest x-ray is not necessary unless the patient's condition worsens and is not a marker of improvement. Decreased symptomatology and reduced fever, cough, and sputum production are used to determine the effectiveness of treatments.

Content Category: Respiratory
References: Newberry, 1998; pp. 436–437; ENA, Core Curriculum, 2000; pp. 561–562.

12. Discharge instructions have been given to the caregiver of a 1-year-old child with bronchiolitis. Which of the following statements by the caregiver indicates a need for further clarification?
A. "I will use Tylenol for fever control and comfort as needed."
B. "I will make sure she drinks extra fluids over the next few days."
C. "I CAN TAKE HER TO DAY CARE TOMORROW AS LONG AS SHE IS ON THE MEDICATIONS."
D. "My 5-year-old may get this, too, but he should have milder cold symptoms."

Rationale:

C. Because the common viral diseases are highly contagious, the ill child should not be taken to day care until symptoms have cleared. The course of the disease is 7–10 days.

A. Acetaminophen is acceptable to use for fever and analgesia.

B. Increased fluid intake will help prevent dehydration associated with fever and increased respiratory effort.

D. Older children with bronchiolitis have upper respiratory symptoms, including cough, low-grade fever, and minor rhinorrhea, but usually do not progress beyond this stage.

Content Category: Respiratory

References: Newberry, 1998; p. 728; ENA, Core Curriculum, 2000; pp. 562–564; Kitt et al., 1995; p. 417.

13. You are caring for a patient diagnosed with rib fractures and a pneumothorax. He is tachypneic and dyspneic. Decreased breath sounds are auscultated on the right side. A patent airway has been assured. C-spine precautions are in effect. The next priority intervention would be to insert:
    A. a nasogastric tube.
    B. A CHEST TUBE.
    C. two large-bore IVs.
    D. a urinary catheter.

Rationale:

B. Placement of a chest tube is the priority to restore intrapulmonary pressure and prevent further compromise to this patient's breathing. This is accomplished during the primary survey.

A. Placement of a nasogastric tube is appropriate in trauma, but this is done as part of the secondary survey after airway, breathing, and circulation have been addressed.

C. Placement of two large-bore IVs is appropriate, but the patient's breathing must be protected first. When breathing is compromised, it is necessary to intervene before proceeding to circulation assessments and interventions.

D. Placement of a urinary catheter is appropriate in trauma, but this is done as part of the secondary survey after airway, breathing, and circulation have been addressed.

Content Category: Respiratory

References: Kidd et al., 2000; pp. 689–697; ENA, Trauma Nursing, 2000; pp. 43–44, 134–137.

14. The priority treatment for a patient diagnosed with rib fractures includes:
    A. chest tube placement.
    B. AGGRESSIVE PULMONARY TOILET.
    C. IV crystalloid bolus infusion.
    D. nasogastric tube placement.

Rationale:

B. Treatment for most rib fractures includes analgesia and good pulmonary toilet. This is particularly important in the elderly because they have decreased chest wall compliance and diminished vital capacity.

A. Chest tube placement is appropriate for a pneumothorax, when there is a loss of intrapleural pressure.

C. A fluid bolus of crystalloid may be appropriate after airway and breathing have been preserved. Care must be taken about the amount of volume infused because of the potential of an underlying pulmonary contusion.

D. Insertion of a nasogastric tube is a necessary intervention during the management of most trauma victims; however, airway and breathing must be assessed and managed first.

Content Category: Respiratory

References: Bayley & Turcke, 1998; pp. 379–380, 562–563; ENA, Core Curriculum, 2000; pp. 8–11, 385; Newberry, 1998; pp. 291–306.

15.   As you assess a patient with increasing respiratory distress, you suspect a tracheobronchial injury. For which of the following life-threatening conditions would this patient be at a high risk?
   A. Distributive shock
   B. TENSION PNEUMOTHORAX
   C. Pulmonary contusion
   D. Pericardial tamponade

Rationale:

   B. Tension pneumothorax can occur as increased mediastinal emphysema occurs.
   A. Distributive shock is associated with vasodilation of blood vessels relating to events of sepsis, spinal cord injuries, and anaphylaxis.
   C. Pulmonary contusion results from blunt trauma and is often associated with rib fractures or a flail chest.
   D. Pericardial tamponade is most commonly caused by penetrating trauma that causes blood to be released into the pericardial sac, thus compromising ventricular filling

Content Category: Respiratory

References: Newberry, 1998; pp. 297–298; Blansfield et al., 1999; pp. 265–266.

16.   What other medical condition can imitate similar signs and symptoms as you assess a patient who is hyperventilating?
   A. Asthma attack
   B. DIABETIC KETOACIDOSIS
   C. Myocardial infarct
   D. Pertussis

Rationale:

   B. Signs and symptoms of diabetic ketoacidosis include hyperglycemia, Kussmaul's respirations, dehydration, and acid-base imbalance, which can mimic hyperventilation relating to anxiety. It is crucial to obtain a past medical history.
   A. Asthma is a disease that involves bronchial constriction and inflammation and usually presents with cough and/or wheezing. The patient is not hyperventilating.
   C. Myocardial infarction presentation varies, but patients usually complain of some type of chest discomfort. They may have gastrointestinal symptoms and can be pale and diaphoretic. They are usually able to converse as well as to control their respiratory rate.
   D. Pertussis is a communicable disease that presents with a paroxysmal cough, low-grade fever, and nasal congestion.

Content Category: Respiratory

References: ENA, Trauma Nursing, 2000; pp. 569–570, 263–265, 559–561, 250–252; Kidd et al., 2000; pp. 276, 328–330, 572–573.

17.   A patient sustains chest trauma resulting in a pulmonary contusion. Which of the following medical history findings places this patient at high risk for developing complications from this injury?
   A. EMPHYSEMA
   B. Environmentally triggered asthma
   C. Gastroesophageal reflux
   D. Pulmonary tuberculosis

Rationale:

A. The structural changes of emphysema—breakdown of alveoli, loss of elasticity, and increased diameter of the chest wall—contribute to a decrease in the vital capacity of the respiratory system. A pulmonary contusion may develop into atelectasis and/or pneumonia.

B. Environmentally triggered asthma should not be triggered by the events described and the patient should have no complications from it.

C. Gastroesophageal reflux is a major contributing factor to asthma and is not related to this condition.

D. A history of tuberculosis does not necessarily suggest that the patient has active disease and does not pose an increased risk for other respiratory complications due to a contusion, although it could pose a risk to the caregiver.

Content Category: Respiratory

References: Newberry, 1998; pp. 431–451; Kitt et al., 1995; pp. 188–200; ENA, Core Curriculum, 2000; pp. 559–566.

18. A 2-year-old girl is brought to the ED by her mother, who states the child was playing with beads and pushed one up her nose. The mother cannot get the bead out. After ensuring that the child's oxygenation is adequate, the ED nurse should prepare for which of the following interventions?
   A. Oxymetazoline (Afrin) and a tracheostomy setup
   B. Diazepam (Valium) and a rigid esophagoscopy
   C. PHENYLEPHRINE (NEO-SYNEPHRINE) AND BALLOON-TIPPED CATHETER
   D. Meperidine (Demerol) and flexible endoscopy

Rationale:

C. Phenylephrine (Neo-Synephrine) is used to reduce swelling in the nasal passage. The balloon-tipped catheter can be used to remove the bead.

A. While oxymetazoline (Afrin) would reduce nasal swelling, the child has an adequate airway and does not need a tracheostomy at this time.

B. Diazepam (Valium) and rigid esophagoscopy are not necessary. The foreign body is not in the esophagus, but in the nasal cavity.

D. Meperidine (Demerol) and flexible endoscopy are not needed. The bead is in the nasal passage, not in the gastrointestinal tract.

Content Category: Respiratory

Reference: ENA, Core Curriculum, 2000; p. 162.

19. A 58-year-old male presents to the ED with increasing shortness of breath, pleuritic pain, and fever of 101.2° F (38.5° C). Breath sounds are decreased over the lower half of the left lung. Chest x-ray shows a large pleural effusion. The ED nurse should anticipate and prepare for which of the following interventions?
   A. THORACENTESIS
   B. Rapid diuresis
   C. Emergent intubation
   D. Arterial line placement

Rationale:

A. A thoracentesis is a procedure to remove the effusion and help to determine whether the fluid is purulent. Breathing should improve substantially once the fluid has been removed.

B. Rapid diuresis would be helpful in treating diffuse congestion associated with congestive heart failure. It would not help to remove the pleural fluid consolidation, however; in fact, overly aggressive diuresis might result in dehydration.

C. Emergent intubation is a possibility; however, if the fluid collection is removed, the need for intubation may resolve.

D. Arterial line placement would not reduce or resolve the pleural effusion.

Content Category: Respiratory

Reference: ENA, Core Curriculum, 2000; p. 571.

20. When the nurse is caring for a patient with a diaphragmatic tear, early recognition and treatment is important to prevent which of the following?
A. Displaced bowel
B. Infection
C. HYPOXIA
D. Respiratory distress

Rationale:

C. When abdominal contents herniate into the chest, the lungs and mediastinum are compressed, decreasing both venous return and cardiac output. The mediastinal shift applies pressure to the contralateral lung, eventually causing hypoxia.

A. Displaced bowel occurs as a consequence of injury to the diaphragm.

B. Infection is ultimately a potential risk if the bowel becomes strangulated or perforates in the chest; however, assessment and correction of hypoxia take priority.

D. Respiratory distress is a symptom associated with a diaphragmatic tear. Abdominal herniated contents apply pressure against the lungs.

Content Category: Respiratory

References: Blansfield et al., 1999; p. 267; Goldy, 1998; p. 33; Newberry, 1998; pp. 302, 313.

21. What nursing diagnosis would be a priority in a patient with respiratory distress syndrome?
A. Anxiety related to dyspnea
B. Fluid volume excess related to overhydration during resuscitation
C. Pain
D. IMPAIRED GAS EXCHANGE RELATED TO NONCOMPLIANT LUNGS

Rationale:

D. Impaired gas exchange is a priority for this patient due to the damage of the alveolar- capillary membranes. If left untreated, this damage will cause an increase in hypoxia.

A. Anxiety can be present and may increase due to the already present dyspnea, but is not a priority at this time.

B. Fluid volume is a concern and potentially may increase any present pulmonary edema, but ventilation and gas exchange take priority.

C. Pain may be present due to injuries and may increase dyspnea, but is not a priority at this time.

Content Category: Respiratory

References: Lombardi & Sheehy, 1995; pp. 239–240; Newberry, 1998; pp. 452–455, 522; O'Hanlon-Nichols, 1995; p. 42.

22.   When teaching an asthma patient about the disease, it is important to remember that:
A. ASTHMA IS CAUSED PRIMARILY BY AIRWAY INFLAMMATION AND HYPER-RESPONSIVENESS TO STIMULI.
B. physiologic changes seen in asthma exacerbation are often irreversible.
C. asthma exacerbations are most frequently a result of a respiratory infection.
D. most asthma attacks occur suddenly and without warning in the early morning.

Rationale:

A. The patient needs to understand that inflammation and response to stimuli are key factors in the treatment and prevention of asthma.
B. Asthma changes are episodic and reversible with treatment and medication.
C. While infection can trigger an asthma exacerbation, most patients have specific triggers that can be identified and avoided.
D. Asthma attacks are not without warning and can be predicted by identifying triggers and using peak flow rate measurements.

Content Category: Respiratory

References: Newberry, 1998; pp. 440–451; Kitt et al., 1995; pp. 194–197; ENA, Core Curriculum, 2000; pp. 559–561.

23.   When teaching an asthma patient about medication usage, it is important to discuss that:
A. inhaled steroids are addictive and their use should be limited to acute exacerbations.
B. patients often develop a tolerance to daily asthma medications and require increased doses.
C. inhaled bronchodilators should not be used with inhaled corticosteroids.
D. ORAL CORTICOSTEROIDS ARE OFTEN USED FOR SHORT-TERM TREATMENT OF EXACERBATIONS.

Rationale:

D. Oral corticosteroids are frequently given for acute exacerbation to gain control of the inflammatory process.
A. Inhaled steroids are not the same as anabolic steroids and are not addictive.
B. Patients are frequently maintained on the same dosages for many years and do not experience increasing tolerance to medication with continued usage.
C. Inhaled bronchodilators and inhaled corticosteroids are common treatments for asthma and can safely be administered together.

Content Category: Respiratory

References: Newberry, 1998; pp. 440–451; Kitt et al., 1995; pp. 194–197; ENA, Core Curriculum, 2000; pp. 559–561.

24.   When teaching an asthma patient how to avoid potential triggers of the disease, it is important to discuss that:
A. avoidance of spicy foods can help to reduce asthma attacks.
B. exacerbations of asthma can be reduced by decreasing physical activity.
C. A CHRONIC POSTNASAL DRIP CAN CONTRIBUTE TO RECURRENT ASTHMA ATTACKS.
D. most triggers of asthma cannot be avoided.

Rationale:

C. Sinusitis and allergic rhinitis with postnasal drip are common asthma triggers in adult patients.
A. Food allergens are not common triggers. Spicy foods in particular have not been found to induce asthma attacks.

B. Developing a sedentary lifestyle does not improve the asthma condition. Exercise and physical activity should be included in the plan of care.

D. A great majority of asthma triggers can be identified and lifestyle modifications made to reduce their impact on the patient's disease.

Content Category: Respiratory

References: Newberry, 1998; pp. 440–451; Kitt et al., 1995; pp. 194–197; ENA, Core Curriculum, 2000; pp. 559–561.

25.   Which of the following classes of drugs is a contributing factor in the development of gout?
    A. THIAZIDE DIURETICS
    B. Corticosteroids
    C. Oral anticoagulants
    D. Estrogen replacement

Rationale:

A. Hyperuricemia may develop with thiazide diuretic use due to decreased secretion of uric acid by the tubular cells, increased renal reabsorption of uric acid, and dehydration. If the patient has a hereditary predisposition to gout or has chronic renal failure, increased uric acid levels may cause symptoms.

B. Corticosteroids decrease the levels of uric acid.

C. Warfarin binds to protein sites in the plasma and interferes with vitamin K production in the gut. Interference with protein metabolism decreases uric acid levels.

D. Estrogen decreases levels of uric acid.

Content Category: General Medical

References: ENA, Core Curriculum, 2000; pp. 281–282; Humes, 2000; pp. 1370–1375; Pagana & Pagana, 1998; pp. 410–441; Kuhn, 1998; pp. 522–523.

26.   A 4-month-old infant is brought to the ED by his parents. He has been crying for 6 hours and will not take his bottle. He has a fever of 101°F (38.3°C), is listless, and appears very ill. When the mother tries to comfort him by rocking, the baby screams and becomes dusky. The nurse notices that when the baby was placed on the bed to have vital signs taken, he became quiet and appeared to be sleeping. What should the ED nurse suspect the underlying problem with this infant to be?
    A. Child abuse
    B. Pneumonia
    C. Dehydration
    D. MENINGITIS

Rationale:

D. The clue that this baby has meningitis is that he cries when rocked and is quiet when left alone. Meningitis causes irritation of the meninges, which, when stretched, result in pain. In older children and adults, flexing the head and neck results in severe pain and hip flexion; this is known as Brudzinski's sign. A positive Kernig's sign, also a sign of meningeal irritation, is noted when the hip and knee are flexed to about 90 degrees. When the hip is kept immobile and the knee is extended, there will be pain in the hamstring muscles. Infants do not exhibit these signs, nor do they have nuchal rigidity. Health care professionals must look for the sometimes subtle sign of "paradoxical irritability," a disinclination to be held and comforted because the movement results in pain. It is also important to remember that infants with meningitis may NOT have high fever.

A. One might mistake the disinclination to be held that occurs in meningitis with fear of injury. However, this child is very young and would be unlikely to be afraid of its mother even if the mother were inflicting injury.

B. Pneumonia in infants might present with fever, listlessness, and crying, but such babies are usually comforted when held by a parent.

C. Any infant who is seriously ill is at risk for dehydration from fever and decreased intake, but one would expect the baby to feel better when cradled by a parent.

Content Category: General Medical

References: Cosby, 1998; pp. 721–741.

27. A young woman is treated in the ED after reporting that she was raped by an unknown male. She is healthy and the only medication she takes is an oral contraceptive. In addition to the trauma of rape, she is very concerned about having possibly contracted HIV. What patient education should she receive?

A. Oral contraceptives protect against HIV infection.

B. As long as there was no vaginal bleeding, she won't get HIV from one contact.

C. If today's HIV test is negative, she does not have to worry.

D. SHE WILL NEED TO WAIT 6 WEEKS TO 6 MONTHS TO KNOW WHETHER SHE WAS INFECTED.

Rationale:

D. Most people infected with HIV seroconvert within 45 days. However, it may take up to 6 months for HIV testing to be positive or for the patient to be declared uninfected. This wait can be extremely stressful for victims of sexual assault.

A. Oral contraceptives offer no protection against HIV infection. Women taking protease inhibitors (ritonavir, nelfinavir) to treat HIV infection should understand that these drugs interfere with the action of oral contraceptives. Another form of contraception should be used in addition to the oral agents.

B. The HIV virus can penetrate intact vaginal tissue. If the viral load of the male is high, this patient could be infected from a single exposure.

C. One test is not adequate to rule out HIV infection because of the delayed seroconversion nature of this virus. Each health care facility should have a protocol in place to ensure repeat testing at a minimum of 6 weeks, 3 months, and 6 months. The purpose of the HIV test at the time of reported sexual assault is to document that the patient is not already infected, whether knowingly or unknowingly.

Content Category: General Medical

References: Marco, 1996; pp. 701–707; Peabody, 2000; pp. 227–274.

28. Anna is a 13-year-old girl with a 2-year history of diabetes. She is poorly controlled and has been treated in your ED four times this year. She presents today lethargic and with an Accu-Chek of 620. You understand that the reason for the problem may be which of the following?

A. Puberty is the most likely cause of Anna's poor control of her disease.

B. Adolescents are "magical thinkers" who cannot accept responsibility for their own care.

C. Poor control of diabetes is the result of failure to follow the plan of care.

D. MOST CHILDREN CAN CONTROL THEIR DIABETES WITH PERIODIC ADJUSTMENTS OF INSULIN, DIET, AND ACTIVITY.

Rationale:

D. Given a supportive home environment and adequate medical supervision, periodic adjustments of insulin, diet, and activity will enable children to control their disease.

A. Puberty may certainly be contributing to Anna's poor control, but other factors must be considered equally likely to be doing so.

B. With adequate and ongoing education and supervision, most adolescents can accept responsibility for the management of their disease.

C. Poor control of diabetes may be caused by any number of factors and needs careful evaluation to determine the cause or causes.

Content Category: General Medical

Reference: Wong, 1999; pp.1872–1884.

29. The ED nurse advises parents to avoid using aspirin for fever control for children with influenza or varicella because of its potential association with which of the following?
A. Fifth disease
B. Kawasaki disease
C. Schönlein-Henoch purpura
D. REYE'S SYNDROME

Rationale:

D. The potential association between aspirin therapy for the treatment of fever in children with varicella or influenza and the development of Reye's syndrome (RS) precludes its use in these patients. RS is manifested clinically by encephalopathy and coma and is usually preceded by a viral illness.

A. There is no known association between the use of aspirin in the treatment of fifth disease (erythema infectiosum) and the subsequent development of Reye's syndrome. Fifth disease is caused by the human parvovirus B19 and is characterized by a rash that begins on the face and spreads distally.

B. There is no known association between the use of aspirin in the treatment of Kawasaki disease and the subsequent development of Reye's syndrome. Kawasaki disease is an acute systemic vasculitis of unknown etiology.

C. There is no known association between the use of aspirin in the treatment of Schönlein-Henoch purpura and the subsequent development of Reye's syndrome. Schönlein-Henoch purpura (allergic vasculitis) is a relatively common acquired disease in children. It is characterized by a non-thrombocytopenic purpura, arthritis, nephritis, and abdominal pain.

Content Category: General Medical

Reference: Wong, 1999; p. 1806.

30.   Which of the following vaccines provides protection against epiglottitis?
A. DTP
B. MMR
C. **HIB**
D. HBV

Rationale:

C. HIB conjugate vaccines provide protection against a number of serious infections caused by *Haemophilus influenzae* type B, especially bacterial meningitis, epiglottitis, bacterial pneumonia, and sepsis.

A. DTP is the diphtheria, tetanus, and pertussis vaccine.

B. MMR is the measles, mumps, and rubella vaccine.

D. HBV is the hepatitis B vaccine.

Content Category: General Medical

Reference: Wong, 1999; p. 600.

31. A 65-year-old female is found unresponsive on the floor. The patient has no significant medical history, but prior to this event she complained of headache and neck stiffness. Vital signs are BP 130/84 mm Hg, HR 100/min, respirations 10/min and shallow and snoring. Glasgow Coma Score is 7. The initial intervention to be performed by the ED nurse is:
    A. administer oxygen by nasal cannula.
    B. PREPARE FOR ENDOTRACHEAL INTUBATION.
    C. prepare for a lumbar puncture.
    D. initiate antibiotic therapy.

Rationale:

   B. Patient is unable to maintain her airway adequately; therefore, intubation is necessary to maintain airway and breathing.
   A. Endotracheal intubation would not assist with airway maintenance.
   C. A lumbar puncture is not the treatment of choice for cardiovascular accidents.
   D. Antibiotic therapy is not the treatment of choice for cardiovascular accidents.

Content Category: General Medical

Reference: ENA, Core Curriculum, 2000; pp. 409–411.

32. An elderly woman visiting from Russia is brought to the ED by her family. She became ill with fever, night sweats, cough, and weight loss about 2 weeks ago. Her chest x-ray has findings consistent with active tuberculosis (TB). She refuses hospital admission and the family agrees to care for her at home. What information should the ED nurse give the family regarding transmission of TB?
    A. Clean house thoroughly; launder patient's clothing in hot water and dryer.
    B. Boil dishes, glasses, and silverware used by the patient.
    C. KEEP THE HOUSE WELL VENTILATED, EXHAUSTING OLD AIR TO THE OUTSIDE.
    D. All family members should wear surgical masks when caring for the patient.

Rationale:

   C. TB is transmitted through exhaled air and by small droplets inhaled directly into the bronchioles and alveoli. Droplets can remain suspended in still air for several days. A well-ventilated home with at least 20 air exchanges a day greatly reduces the possibility of transmission. The patient should be isolated in a room with a door or window opening to the outside to provide adequate air exchange.
   A. Special cleaning of the home and clothing is unnecessary unless the patient is expectorating onto her clothing or furniture. She should be taught to cough and expectorate into tissues and immediately place them in a plastic receptacle lined with a plastic or paper bag for disposal.
   B. No special washing of eating and drinking utensils is needed. TB is not transmitted by the hand-mouth route; the bacteria must be inhaled.
   D. It is useful for the patient to wear a surgical mask to control droplet spread, but masks provide no protection for close contact or health care workers. Special filtration masks and adequate room air exchange provide the best protection.

Content Category: General Medical

References: Almeida, 1998; pp. 611–618; Peabody, 2000; pp. 227–274; Welch, 1996; pp. 422–425.

33.   An elderly woman with profound lethargy is brought to the ED by EMS. Caregivers report a gradual decline in activity and mentation over a 6-month period. History is significant for hypothyroidism and a recent urinary tract infection treated with antibiotics. On exam, the woman is lethargic but responsive, with slow speech. The skin is pale and dry and the tongue is swollen. Vital signs are BP 82/40 mm Hg, HR 50/min, respirations 16/min, and rectal temperature 94° F (34.4° C). Intravenous access has been secured and lab specimens have been drawn. Careful fluid resuscitation is under way. Which of the following should be AVOIDED?
    A. Intravenous levothyroxine (Levoxyl)
    B. VASOPRESSORS
    C. Hydrocortisone (Solu-Cortef)
    D. Normal saline

Rationale:

B. Vasopressors should be avoided because they may produce dysrhythmias in the setting of hypothyroidism.
A. Intravenous thyroid replacement should be started as soon as possible.
C. Profound hypothyroidism is accompanied by hypoadrenalism, which also needs correction.
D. Normal saline is an appropriate fluid for resuscitation.

Content Category: General Medical

Reference: Peabody, 2000; pp. 227–274.

34.   A 40-year-old woman with a known history of hyperthyroidism is brought to the ED with agitation and confusion. Family members report thyroid surgery had been performed 2 weeks prior. The patient is noted to be restless, diaphoretic, and oriented to person and place. Vital signs are BP 174/100 mm Hg, HR 160/min, respirations 32/min, and temperature 103.6° F (39.8° C). Thyroid storm is suspected. Following initial stabilization, the ED nurse should reduce fever by:
    A. rapid infusion of 1,000 ml of normal saline.
    B. ADMINISTRATION OF ACETAMINOPHEN (TYLENOL) 650 MG ORALLY.
    C. infusion of 50 ml of D50W.
    D. administration of acetylsalicylic acid (Aspirin) 600 mg orally.

Rationale:

B. Acetaminophen is the drug of choice to reduce fever of thyroid storm. Aspirin should be avoided because it would increase levels of free T3 and T4.
A. Although thyroid storm causes fluid loss, the patient is not hemodynamically unstable and does not require rapid saline infusion.
C. A patient with thyroid storm may require glucose to treat hypoglycemia; however, D50W does not reduce fever.
D. Aspirin should be administered to patients with thyroid storm.

Content Category: General Medical

Reference: Peabody, 2000; pp. 227–274.

35.   Which of the following statements by the patient who has herpes zoster indicates an understanding of discharge instructions?
    A. "A similar rash will break out on my right chest in about 2 weeks."
    B. "I SHOULD STAY AWAY FROM PREGNANT WOMEN."
    C. "I can return to work in 3 days."
    D. "I cannot use calamine lotion on this rash."

Rationale:

    B. Herpesvirus poses a threat to the fetus; therefore, contact with pregnant women should be avoided.

    A. Herpes zoster is unilateral and does not cross the midline.

    C. Patients should not return to work until all lesions are crusted. Typically, lesions continue to erupt for about a week.

    D. Calamine lotion can be used on the lesions.

Content Category: General Medical

Reference: Peabody, 2000; pp. 227–274.

36.   Which of the following ECG changes may be associated with hypokalemia?
    A. Elevated ST segment
    B. Peaked, tented T waves
    C. Q waves
    D. VENTRICULAR IRRITABILITY

Rationale:

    D. Hypokalemia refers to serum potassium below 3.5 mEq/L. Dysrhythmias (heart blocks) are expected ECG findings in these patients due to ventricular irritability.

    A. Elevated ST segment is seen in patients with acute MI.

    B. Peaked, tented T waves are seen in patients with hyperkalemia.

    C. Q waves are seen in MI patients.

Content Category: General Medical

Reference: ENA, Core Curriculum, 2000; pp. 292–293.

37.   A patient is escorted to the ED by the local police after being found in a department store preaching to the customers and stating he is an apostle of Jesus. He is dressed in a bright fluorescent green blazer and top hat and is talking nonstop in a loud, bellowing tone, changing topics frequently. The priority nursing diagnosis for this patient is which of the following?
    A. RISK FOR INJURY
    B. Ineffective individual or family coping
    C. Knowledge deficit
    D. Impaired social interaction

Rationale:

    A. This patient is exhibiting a manic phase of bipolar disease and is at risk for injury due to his extreme hyperactivity, agitation, and poor impulse control. Safety is the priority. This patient requires a quiet environment, frequent rest periods, high-calorie fluids, and potential seclusion to minimize physical harm. He may also need to be protected from his "generosity" caused by irrational, grandiose thinking.

    B. This patient does have a problem of ineffective individual or family coping that must be addressed on a long-term basis.

    C. There is no evidence in this scenario that this patient has a knowledge deficit about his disease.

    D. This patient does have impaired social interaction related to his altered thought processes and his intrusive, aggressive behavior. However, his risk for injury must be addressed first, as it will take a while for the mania to subside well enough for him to be involved in activities that provide a focus and social contact.

Content Category: Psychosocial

References: Newberry, 1998; pp. 780–782; Varacolis, 1998; pp. 595–623.

38.   Antipsychotic drugs may cause:
       A. reduction in sleep patterns.
       B. a decrease in activity.
       C. REDUCTION IN DISRUPTIVE BEHAVIOR.
       D. an increase in paranoid reactions.

Rationale:

       C. Antipsychotic drugs target the symptoms of schizophrenia and reduce disruptive behavior.
       A. Sleep patterns are improved with antipsychotics.
       B. Antipsychotics cause an increase in activity, speech, and sociability.
       D. Antipsychotics cause a decrease in the intensity of paranoid reactions.

Content Category: Psychosocial

Reference: Varacolis, 1998; pp. 644–645.

39.   A male patient presents to the ED with a self-defined panic attack. Objective findings include cool
       and clammy skin, tachycardia, and tachypnea. He is pacing. The priority for this patient is to:
       A. PLACE HIM IN A QUIET AREA ON CONSTANT OBSERVATION.
       B. give a complete detailed explanation of what to expect.
       C. tell the patient to sit in the chair.
       D. get the physician.

Rationale:

       A. This patient is exhibiting anxiety and should be placed in a quiet room to decrease excessive
           stimuli and provide the ability to concentrate. This patient should be placed on constant obser-
           vation to minimize self-injury and loss of control.
       B. This patient is anxious and unable to interpret details. A brief discussion limits indecision and
           conveys the nurse's belief that the patient can respond in a healthy manner.
       C. This patient is unable to sit in a chair as he has a substantial amount of anxiety-generated
           energy. It would be more appropriate to walk with the patient to give him support.
       D. Before summoning the physician, it is important to place the patient in a quiet area, complete
           your assessment, and establish a trusting relationship. This patient also requires constant obser-
           vation to assure safety and minimize loss of control.

Content Category: Psychosocial

References: Varacolis, 1998; pp. 458–459; ENA, Core Curriculum, 2000; pp. 347–351.

40.   An elderly male is brought to the ED with his home health attendant for evaluation of increased
       weakness. The attendant states that the patient has dementia. Accurate assessment includes:
       A. asking the patient about recent activities of daily living.
       B. obtaining a health history from the patient.
       C. asking questions loudly to ensure that the patient understands.
       D. ASSESS REGIMEN OF BOTH PRESCRIPTION AND OVER-THE-COUNTER DRUGS
           WITH THE FAMILY AND/OR HOME HEALTH ASSISTANT.

Rationale:

       D. Polypharmacy and nonadherence to medication can cause many adverse symptoms in the geriat-
           ric population. Family members and caregivers are the best sources of information for a patient
           with dementia.
       A. Impairment of short-term memory is a problem with dementia. Simple closed questions can
           facilitate a more appropriate response from the patient.

B. The demented patient has diminished communication skills, which can be exacerbated by the busy ED environment. Family members and caregivers are the best sources of history.

C. The patient has dementia but may not be hard of hearing and could be offended by loud talking.

Content Category: Psychosocial

References: ENA, Core Curriculum, 2000; pp. 24, 411–412; Hayes, 2000; pp. 430–435; Royner, 1998; pp. 331–332; Wallis, 2000; pp. 58–61.

41. A 28-year-old woman with a history of bipolar disease is brought to the ED at 11 A.M. by her family, who state that she has been out for the last 3 days and nights and has just come home with a new car filled with purchases she made for the family, including a new TV and clothes. She is wearing a short skirt, a tight top, and a lot of makeup. She has difficulty sitting in the chair at triage and is talking rapidly about many different things. Which of the following is the ED nurse's first priority?

A. SET LIMITS, ESPECIALLY CONCERNING NECESSARY TASKS.

B. Start the lithium (Lithobid) that the physician has ordered.

C. Keep the patient awake during daytime hours.

D. Encourage the patient to focus on the things around her.

Rationale:

A. Manic patients need limit setting, which should be well coordinated and consistent. Otherwise, the manic patient can become very disruptive.

B. While lithium can limit manic behavior, it does not become effective for 1 to 2 weeks. Treating symptoms fully may take up to 1 month.

C. The manic patient usually exhibits a decreased need for sleep and often needs to be encouraged to rest at appropriate times, including periods during the day.

D. The manic patient is focused on a variety of different things and has difficulty maintaining a single focus; thus, s/he needs a structured direction and routine.

Content Category: Psychosocial

Reference: Stuart & Laraia, 1998; pp. 366–370.

42. A 48-year-old female is referred to the ED from a community ambulatory care center for evaluation of intermittent palpitations, chest tightness, and choking sensations. The patient reports having had these symptoms for about 6 weeks and states that the episodes are becoming more frequent. Triage assessment reveals an intact airway. Skin is cool and slightly diaphoretic to the touch. Vital signs are BP 168/72 mm Hg, HR 118/min, respirations 26/min, and temperature 99.2° F (37.3° C). The patient does not report any chest tightness, palpitations, or choking sensations at this time. Priority interventions for this patient include:

A. draw blood specimens for cardiac enzymes and markers.

B. INITIATE OXYGEN THERAPY VIA NASAL CANNULA AT 5 L/MIN.

C. obtain an arterial blood sample for blood gas analysis.

D. obtain a chest x-ray.

Rationale:

B. Standards of care for patients presenting to the ED with complaints that may be cardiac in origin should be treated as if infarction is present. Therefore, oxygen therapy should be initiated, followed by placing the patient on a cardiac monitor.

A. Although diagnostic evaluation for cardiac problems involves serum enzyme and marker analysis, obtaining specimens is not a priority over oxygen therapy and cardiac monitoring for dysrhythmias.

C. Arterial blood sampling is not appropriate in initial evaluation of chest pain, since thrombolytic therapy may be used if the diagnosis of myocardial infarction is made.

D. A chest x-ray would not assist in determining the origin of this patient's presenting problems.

Content Category: Psychosocial

References: ENA, Core Curriculum, 2000; p. 12; Handysides, 1996; pp. 162–166.

43.   A 17-year-old high school student is brought to the ED by her parents, who state that she has been crying incessantly and has been withdrawn and unable to sleep since breaking up with her boyfriend 3 weeks ago. Parents express concern to the triage nurse by stating that they feel their daughter will harm herself if she is not admitted to the hospital for observation. Triage assessment reveals a tearful young female who is wringing her hands constantly. There is no evidence of physical injury and the patient denies ingestion of any medication or harmful substance. Vital signs are BP 90/60 mm Hg, HR 126/min, and respirations 22/min. During her stay in the ED, this patient becomes agitated and hostile toward her parents and the staff. Which of the following would be the most appropriate action for the ED nurse to take?

A. Call security and have the patient restrained immediately.

B. Notify the consulting psychiatrist to obtain an order for a sedative.

C. Assure the safety of the patient by minimizing environmental stimuli and politely request that the parents wait outside in a nearby location.

D. SPEAK QUIETLY TO THE PATIENT IN A CALM, COMPASSIONATE MANNER FOR THE PURPOSE OF DEFINING THE SOURCE OF HER AGITATION.

Rationale:

D. If triggers for increased agitation are identified, the emergency nurse should be able to manipulate the patient's environment of care to minimize their incidence.

A. Interventions that are less likely to limit the patient's freedom should be tried prior to any restrictive devices.

B. Although this patient will probably be referred for a mental health consultation, obtaining an order for chemical sedation is inappropriate at this time.

C. Assurance of patient and family safety is paramount to all care interactions. However, this patient is calling attention to her need for human interaction and assistance.

Content Category: Psychosocial

Reference: Kitt et al., 1995; pp. 470–472.

44.   When caring for a patient with an acute gouty arthritis attack, the ED nurse should anticipate an order to administer:

A. oxycodone/acetaminophen (Percocet).

B. prednisone (Delta-Cortef).

C. INDOMETHACIN (INDOCIN).

D. acetylsalicylic acid (aspirin).

Rationale

C. Indocin is the NSAID of choice for gouty arthritis.

A. Oxycodone/acetaminophen is a general pain reliever but has minimal anti-inflammatory effects.

B. Prednisone is a steroidal anti-inflammatory; NSAIDS are preferred for gouty arthritis.

D. Although aspirin is an NSAID, indomethacin is the NSAID of choice for gouty arthritis.

Content Category: Patient Care

Reference: Snider, 1997; pp. 1–69.

45. A patient presents to the ED with possible contamination by a hazardous material. The patient is rinsed with another reactive agent that is known to alter the chemical structure of the hazardous material, thus producing a less harmful substance. This process is known as which of the following?
A. DILUTION
B. Absorption
C. Degradation
D. Chelation

Rationale:

A. Dilution is a process to reduce the chemical concentration of a hazardous substance until it is no longer harmful.
B. Absorption is the process of picking up the hazardous material with an absorptive material.
C. Degradation is the process of mixing a hazardous material with another reactive agent to alter the chemical structure and produce a less harmful substance.
D. Chelation is a process of forming a complex with a metal to change its function, render it harmless, or promote excretion of the metal. For example, an iron-poisoning patient may be given deferoxamine as a chelating agent to change the structure of the molecule to ferrioxamine complex, which is excreted in the urine.

Content Category: Patient Care

References: Holleran, 1994; pp. 94–95; Jaimovich & Vidyasagar, 1996; pp. 387–388.

46. A passenger train has derailed. First responders indicate that at least 56 people have been injured. An ED nurse has gone in an ambulance to assist with care at the scene. Which of the following patients is the LOWEST PRIORITY for treatment and transport ("black" category)?
A. A 75-year-old with femur, tibia, and fibula fractures and pelvis tenderness and mobility on palpation; skin is pale and moist
B. A 45-year-old with a metal rod impaled in the right forearm, which is neurovascularly intact; patient is ambulatory
C. A 63-YEAR-OLD WITH SECOND- AND THIRD-DEGREE BURNS OVER 95% OF BODY SURFACE AREAS; PATIENT IS UNCONSCIOUS AND HAS A THREADY PULSE
D. A 25-year-old with pain to the left lateral lower chest and a 5-inch laceration to the left forearm; wound squirts blood when uncovered; patient is controlling bleeding by applying pressure with a bandanna; skin is pink and dry

Rationale:

C. An unconscious patient with burns to 80% to 90% of the body and a thready pulse is considered terminal ("black" category). This patient is the lowest priority.
A. An unstable pelvic fracture with signs of shock warrants immediate intervention to decrease the potential of death. This patient is first priority.
B. A stable patient with an arm injury and neurovascular intactness is not first priority. This patient is currently minor ("green" category), but should be monitored for deterioration to delayed ("yellow") or critical ("red") categories.
D. A stable patient with a controlled arterial bleed and left lateral lower chest pain is currently delayed ("yellow" category). Part of the concern is the potential for injuries in the left lower chest and left upper abdomen.

Content Category: Patient Care

Reference: Holleran, 1994; p. 82.

47.   An off-duty ED nurse stops at a motor vehicle crash (MVC). The nurse's first priority in rendering aid is:
A. stabilization of the patient's cervical spine with simultaneous airway control.
B. breathing assessment and assistance.
C. circulatory assessment and assistance.
D. HIS/HER OWN SAFETY.

Rationale:

D. Securing the scene is the first priority in all prehospital situations. *After* the caregiver has determined that the scene is safe, patient care may begin.
A. Cervical spine stabilization and airway control are important, but occur after the scene has been secured.
B. Breathing follows scene security, cervical spine stabilization, and airway control.
C. Circulation follows scene security, cervical spine stabilization, airway control, and breathing assessment and intervention.

Content Category: Patient Care

Reference: Holleran, 1994; pp. 72, 117–118.

48.   Which of the following patients should be transferred to a tertiary-care center?
A. Adult with grand mal seizures
B. Adolescent with single long-bone injury
C. ADULT WITH CHEST INJURY AND WIDENED MEDIASTINUM
D. Adult with second-degree burns over less than 15% of body surface area

Rationale:

C. A widened mediastinum in a patient with chest trauma suggests the possibility of cardiac tamponade or mediastinum disruption. This patient should be transferred to a trauma center for further evaluation and treatment.
A. A patient who has a grand mal seizure does not require treatment at a tertiary-care center.
B. A patient with a single long-bone injury that does not have neurovascular compromise can be adequately treated in most hospitals.
D. Adults with second-degree burns over less than 15% of body surface area do not require treatment in burn care facilities.

Content Category: Patient Care

Reference: Newberry, 1998.

49.   An elderly patient with right ventricular failure secondary to right ventricular infarction is admitted to the ICU. Because no bed is available, the patient must stay in the ED. The ED nurse should anticipate administration of large quantities of:
A. morphine.
B. INTRAVENOUS FLUIDS.
C. diuretics.
D. nitrates.

Rationale:

B. The patient with right ventricular infarction requires large volumes of intravenous fluids to maintain adequate perfusion. The fluid increases ventricular stretch, which in turn increases cardiac output. Giving up to 6 L of fluid during the first 24 hours may be necessary to maintain adequate tissue perfusion.

A. Morphine reduces preload and should be used with caution in the patient with right ventricular infarction.

C. Diuretics remove fluid and reduce cardiac output from the damaged right ventricle.

D. Nitrates dilate the venous vasculature, thereby reducing venous return. Nitrates should be used with caution in the patient with right ventricular infarction.

Content Category: Patient Care

Reference: American Heart Association, 2000; I-1–I-384.

50. Which of the following situations increases ED nursing responsibility for patient teaching?
    A. Patient education level has decreased.
    B. HOSPITAL ADMISSIONS HAVE BEEN RESTRICTED.
    C. Lawsuits against health care providers have decreased.
    D. The public has lost interest in preventive health care.

Rationale:

B. Changes in health care regulations have led to significant restriction of hospital admissions. Patients who might previously have been admitted overnight for observation are now discharged home from the ED with more complex instructions for follow-up and self-care.

A. The educational level of patients has increased in recent years.

C. Lawsuits filed for alleged malpractice are increasing.

D. The public is very conscious of health prevention and health improvement.

Content Category: Patient Care

Reference: ENA, Core Curriculum, 2000; pp. 757–761.

51. A 4-year-old girl treated for accidental drug ingestion will be discharged home with her parents. Which of the following statements by the parents suggests that the parents understand home safety?
    A. "WE WILL STORE ALL MEDICATIONS IN CHILD SAFETY CONTAINERS IN LOCKED CABINETS."
    B. "We will be more careful watching her and won't let her out of our sight."
    C. "We plan to keep all the medications in our highest cupboards in the kitchen."
    D. "We think this trip to the hospital has convinced her never to take these pills again."

Rationale:

A. This statement indicates a clear understanding of child safety measures.

B. This statement expresses great concern for the child's safety but does not indicate a comprehensive action plan for child safety.

C. This statement presents a partial action plan. It would be more complete if childproof containers and locked cabinets had been mentioned.

D. This statement does not suggest an action plan for child safety in the home.

Content Category: Patient Care

Reference: ENA, Core Curriculum, 2000; pp.757–761.

52.   The most effective intervention to overcome obstacles to teaching in the ED setting is to:
      A. use videotaped teaching materials for all patients.
      B. allocate a minimum of 15 minutes to provide patient education for each patient.
      C. provide group teaching in the waiting area to promote group support among the patients.
      D. ESTABLISH RAPPORT BETWEEN THE NURSE AND PATIENT.

Rationale:

D. Establishing rapport between nurse and patient is essential to ensure that the patient views the nurse as credible. Without this rapport, the patient may not see value in the information provided by the nurse.

A. Videotaped materials may be useful in some situations; however, using a videotape to explain extensive, in-depth material is usually not appropriate in the ED.

B. Allocating 15 minutes for teaching may be unrealistic. Teaching should be specific and individualized for the patient, not based on a predetermined time frame.

C. On rare occasions, group teaching in the ED may be appropriate. However, issues such as space availability and material suitable for an entire group should be evaluated first.

Content Category: Patient Care

Reference: ENA, Core Curriculum, 2000; pp.757–761.

53.   A 16-year-old female presents with limb-threatening injuries following a motor vehicle crash. Although the patient is a minor, health care providers begin treatment while attempting to reach her parents. In this case, consent for treatment is which of the following?
      A. Informed express consent
      B. Involuntary
      C. IMPLIED
      D. Assumed, since the patient is obviously emancipated.

Rationale:

C. Because of the threat to the patient's limb, emergency treatment may be initiated while attempting to obtain informed express consent from the parents.

A. Informed express consent consists of either oral or written consent by an adult—in this case, a parent, since the patient is a minor.

B. Involuntary consent is obtained when the patient is either physically or mentally unable to give consent.

D. There is no indication that the patient is emancipated. Therefore, she cannot legally consent to treatment for this condition herself.

Content Category: Patient Care

Reference: ENA, Core Curriculum, 2000; p. 37.

54.   A mother brings her 6-year-old son to triage, stating, "My child was scratched by a raccoon and needs rabies shots." The triage nurse informs the mother that rabies vaccine is not administered in the ED and refers her to the health department. This is an example of an EMTALA violation because:
      A. A TRIAGE SCREENING EXAM IS NOT A REPLACEMENT FOR A MEDICAL SCREENING EXAM.
      B. Rabies vaccine should be available at all emergency departments.
      C. The triage nurse failed to contact the health department.
      D. The triage nurse failed to clean the wound.

Rationale:

    A. A common EMTALA violation is failure to distinguish triage from appropriate medical screening.

    B. Rabies vaccine is not available at all emergency departments.

    C. Failure to contact the health department is not an EMTALA violation, but may violate local and state statutes.

    D. Failure to clean the wound does not constitute an EMTALA violation.

Content Category: Patient Care

Reference: Frank, 2001; pp. 65–67.

55. A 50-year-old patient who received a heart transplant 6 months ago reports to the ED complaining of a low-grade fever, fatigue, and shortness of breath. The triage nurse assesses the patient's vital signs as normal. The triage nurse correctly classifies this patient as:
   A. EMERGENT: IMMEDIATE THREAT TO LIFE OR LIMB.
   B. Urgent: No immediate threat to life or limb but needs reassessment every 15 minutes.
   C. Nonurgent: No immediate threat to life or limb, reassessment in 1–2 hours.
   D. Stable: No immediate threat to life or limb, reassessment in 30–60 minutes.

Rationale:

    A. Although vital signs are normal, a low-grade fever, fatigue, and shortness of breath may indicate early signs of organ rejection.

    B. Signs and symptoms of threat to the organ are present.

    C. Signs and symptoms of threat to the organ are present.

    D. Signs and symptoms of threat to the organ are present.

Content Category: Patient Care

Reference: Zavotsky et al., 2001; pp.33–39.

56. Elements of an organized emergency disaster preparedness plan include all of the following EXCEPT:
   A. security.
   B. communications.
   C. coordination of patient care.
   D. HOSPITAL-BASED TRANSPORTATION SERVICES.

Rationale:

    D. Hospital-based transportation services are not essential to disaster preparedness plans.

    A. Security is an essential component of disaster preparedness plans.

    B. Communications is an essential component of disaster preparedness plans.

    C. Coordination of patient care is an essential component of disaster preparedness plans.

Content Category: Patient Care

Reference: ENA, Core Curriculum, 2000; pp. 697–699.

57.   A patient who opens his eyes spontaneously, obeys motor commands, and is oriented to person and place has a Glasgow Coma Scale score of:
    A. 8
    B. 10
    C. 12
    D. **15**

Rationale:

    D. This patient has a Glasgow Coma Scale score of 15, the highest score obtainable, because he can respond appropriately to eye opening and has verbal and motor responses.
    A. A score of less than 15 would represent a deficit in one or more of the three categories.
    B. A score of less than 15 would represent a deficit in one or more of the three categories.
    C. A score of less than 15 would represent a deficit in one or more of the three categories.

Content Category: Patient Care

Reference: ENA, Core Curriculum, 2000; p. 787.

58.   Your ED has received 3 patients from a motor vehicle crash. Which patient needs to be stabilized and transferred to a Level 1 facility first?
    A. A 16-year-old female; driver, no seat belt. Injuries to right arm and leg, with abdominal trauma. Vital signs stable.
    B. An 18-year-old male; front seat passenger. Multiple facial lacerations and fractures, positive loss of consciousness. Decreasing oxygen saturation and positive chest trauma.
    C. A 17-YEAR-OLD FEMALE; REAR SEAT PASSENGER, NO SEAT BELT. SHE IS 22 WEEKS PREGNANT, WITH ABDOMINAL TRAUMA, LOW BP, TACHYCARDIA, AND RESPIRATORY DISTRESS.
    D. A 15-year-old female; rear seat passenger with seat belt. Injuries to right leg and chest. Vital signs stable.

Rationale:

    C. The 17-year-old female who is pregnant is at high risk for a uterine rupture, which would endanger not only her life but that of the fetus as well.
    A. This patient will need close monitoring and further evaluation.
    B. This patient will need intubation and probable transfer to a Level 1 facility.
    D. This patient can be evaluated, monitored, and treated at the local ED

Content Category: Patient Care

Reference: ENA, Trauma Nursing, 2000.

59.   Before a patient is transferred, documentation must include all of the following EXCEPT:
    A. care given during the patient's stay.
    B. PLANNED LENGTH OF STAY AT THE RECEIVING FACILITY.
    C. all laboratory tests and x-rays performed at the sending facility.
    D. signed consent for transfer.

Rationale:

    B. At the time of the transfer, it would be impossible to determine the length of time that the patient would have to stay in the receiving facility.
    A. This is a required component of documentation prior to patient transfer.
    C. This is a required component of documentation prior to patient transfer.
    D. This is a required component of documentation prior to patient transfer.

Content Category: Patient Care

Reference: ENA, Core Curriculum, 2000; p. 728.

60. Which of the following equipment should be avoided on a rotary wing aircraft?
    A. Heimlich valve
    B. IV solution in a pressure bag
    C. MAST TROUSERS
    D. Traction splint

Rationale:

C. Medical Anti-Shock Trousers (MAST Trousers) cannot be used in unpressurized aircraft. Because they are a pressure device, their pressure fluctuates during flight.

A. A Heimlich valve is a medical device that is typically found on unpressurized aircraft.

B. IV solution in a pressure bag is a medical device that is typically found on unpressurized aircraft.

D. A traction splint is a medical device that is typically found on unpressurized aircraft.

Content Category: Patient Care

Reference: Newberry, 1998; pp.129–145.

61. Which of the following accurately describes the sequence for disaster preparation?
    A. Education, planning, practice, evaluation
    B. Planning, practice, evaluation, education
    C. Planning, education, evaluation, practice
    D. PLANNING, EDUCATION, PRACTICE, EVALUATION

Rationale:

D. The process of planning for a disaster is continuous. To begin the process, you must plan, educate, practice, and then evaluate your disaster plan.

A. Incorrect.

B. Incorrect.

C. Incorrect.

Content Category: Patient Care

Reference: Newberry, 1998; pp. 199–206.

62. When discharging a patient home, the most important component of the process is which of the following?
    A. The removal of all medical apparatus prior to discharge.
    B. A verbal review of the discharge instructions.
    C. PROVIDING THE PATIENT WITH WRITTEN DISCHARGE INSTRUCTIONS.
    D. Making transportation arrangements for the patient's follow-up appointment.

Rationale:

C. Although answers A, B, and D are important components of the discharge process, providing the patient with written instructions in a language that s/he can understand will allow the patient to review and remember the information after arriving at home.

A. Incorrect.

B. Incorrect.

D. Incorrect.

Content Category: Patient Care

Reference: ENA, Core Curriculum, 2000; p. 731.

63.   Documentation at triage must include which of the following?
    A. Whom to notify in case of emergency
    B. The name and address of the patient's doctor
    C. THE CHIEF COMPLAINT AND A SET OF VITAL SIGNS
    D. A list of medications and a set of vital signs

Rationale:

    C. Even a brief triage note must include a chief complaint and at least a limited set of vital signs.
    A. Whom to notify in case of emergency is important information that can be completed after the patient has been assigned to a nurse in the ED.
    B. The name and address of the patient's doctor is important information that can be completed after the patient has been assigned to a nurse in the ED.
    D. A list of the medications that the patient is taking and a set of vital signs provide important information that can be completed after the patient has been assigned to a nurse in the ED.

Content Category: Patient Care

Reference: ENA, Triage, 2000.

64.   When a patient is being discharged with a cast, which of the following is the MOST ESSENTIAL discharge information?
    A. The name of the physician who will provide follow-up care
    B. The name of the physician who cared for the patient in the ED
    C. Documentation of the care provided in the ED
    D. REVIEW OF CAST CARE AND DISCUSSION OF REASONS TO CALL OR RETURN TO THE EMERGENCY DEPARTMENT

Rationale:

    D. The most essential information to give the patient is cast care and a review of situations that would warrant a return to the ED.
    A. Important information; however, giving cast care instructions is essential.
    B. Important information; however, giving cast care instructions is essential.
    C. Important information; however, giving cast care instructions is essential.

Content Category: Patient Care

Reference: ENA, Core Curriculum, 2000; p. 731.

65.   Rabies postexposure prophylaxis includes human rabies immune globulin (Hyperab, Imogam) and:
    A. HUMAN DIPLOID CELL VACCINE (IMOVAX, HDCV).
    B. diphtheria/tetanus (DT).
    C. hepatitis B vaccine (Engerix-B).
    D. Lyme vaccine (LYMErix).

Rationale:

    A. Human diploid cell vaccine (Imovax, HDCV) is given on the same day as the human rabies immune globulin (Imogam) and then on days 3, 7, 14, and 28.
    B. Diphtheria and tetanus (DT) is indicated for all tetanus-prone wounds but is not part of rabies prophylaxis.
    C. Hepatitis B vaccine (Engerix-B) is indicated for immunization against hepatitis B, which is transmitted through contact with blood and body fluids.
    D. Lyme vaccine (LYMErix) is indicated for prevention of Lyme disease but is not part of rabies pro- phylaxis.

Content Category: Orthopedics & Wound Care

References: Newberry, 1998; pp. 251–261; Garcia, 1999; pp. 91–107.

66.   A subungual hematoma is caused by a:
    A.   laceration to the palmar aspect of a finger.
    B.   contusion to the tongue.
    C.   fracture of the wrist.
    D.   CRUSH INJURY TO THE FINGER OR NAILBED.

Rationale:

    D.   A crush injury to the finger or nailbed can cause bleeding underneath the nail. This can be accompanied by a distal phalanx fracture. The patient feels throbbing pain in the distal finger tip.
    A.   A laceration to the palmar aspect of a finger is unlikely to cause a subungual hematoma unless the laceration was caused by a crush injury.
    B.   A contusion of the tongue is not a subungual hematoma.
    C.   A fracture to the wrist would not cause a subungual hematoma.

Content Category: Orthopedics & Wound Care

References: Newberry, 1998; pp. 351–382; Sheehy & Lenehan, 1999; pp. 487–536.

67.   Your neurovascular assessment of an anterior shoulder dislocation includes the upper extremity nerves and vascular tests for sensory and motor functioning. The area of concern is most likely which of the following?
    A.   AXILLARY NERVE, SENSORY BRANCH
    B.   Radial nerve, motor branch
    C.   Ulnar artery
    D.   Median nerve, motor branch

Rationale:

    A.   This occurs as the humeral head dislocates and stretches or tears the nerve. The occurrence rate has been reported as high as 33–50%. Documenting the finding before any reduction attempts are made is important.
    B.   Injury to the motor branch of the radial nerve is uncommon to an anterior shoulder dislocation. The nerve does not travel through that area.
    C.   Vascular compromise is uncommon in an anterior shoulder dislocation. The ulnar artery arises more distally in the extremity.
    D.   This is uncommon with this injury.

Content Category: Orthopedics & Wound Care

References: Urquhart & Kearney, 2001; pp. 33–35; Bayley & Turcke, 1998; pp. 415–447.

68.   An open tibial fracture, Grade III, is prepared for debridement procedures and irrigation. The ideal time frame for these procedures is within:
    A.   26–36 hours.
    B.   16–24 hours.
    C.   9–12 hours.
    D.   6–8 HOURS.

Rationale:

    D.   Removing gross contaminants, debriding devitalized issue, irrigating the wound, and obtaining cultures are best done early.
    A.   This would be a more appropriate time frame for a second look and irrigation.

B. This is probably too long.

C. This is probably too long.

Content Category: Orthopedics & Wound Care

References: Bayley & Turcke, 1998; pp. 415–447; Brown et al., 1998; pp. 875–895.

69. Acute compartment syndrome most commonly occurs in the:
    A. abdominal cavity.
    B. forearm.
    C. thigh.
    D. LOWER LEG.

Rationale:

D. The lower leg is the most common site. There are four compartments in this area.

A. The abdominal cavity is possible, but less common.

B. The forearm is the second most common site.

C. It is rare in the thigh.

Content Category: Orthopedics & Wound Care

References: Bayley & Turcke, 1998; pp. 415–447; Tumbarella, 2000; pp. 30–35.

70. A patient is en route to the operating room for repair of a midshaft femur fracture. A possible lethal complication of a femur fracture is:
    A. deep-vein thrombosis.
    B. nonunion of the fracture.
    C. rhabdomyolysis.
    D. FAT EMBOLI.

Rationale:

D. Fat emboli occur in a low percentage of long-bone fractures, but are potentially fatal. Usually such emboli occur after the first 72 hours.

A. Deep-vein thrombosis is not lethal, but embolization may be.

B. Nonunion signifies that a fracture is not healing. This is not lethal.

C. Rhabdomyolysis occurs when myoglobin is released from injured muscle. Rhabdomyolysis is not lethal, but the sequela of acute renal failure is.

Content Category: Orthopedics & Wound Care

Reference: D'Heere et al., 1999; pp. 73–76.

71. Radial head fractures classically involve pain and point tenderness, particularly with:
    A. wrist flexion.
    B. wrist extension.
    C. finger extension.
    D. SUPINATION.

Rationale:

D. Supination and pronation cause pain and point tenderness in the elbow.

A. Wrist flexion may cause discomfort, but not point tenderness, in the elbow, where the radial head is located.

B. Wrist extension should not exacerbate pain in the elbow with this injury.

C. Finger extension should have no painful effect on the elbow.

Content Category: Orthopedics & Wound Care

Reference: Bayley & Turcke, 1998; pp. 415–447.

Questions 72–74

An 18-month-old female is brought into the ED. The mother states that the child was sitting in her high chair and pulled a cup of hot coffee off the counter. You note that the child has superficial and partial thickness burns to her mouth, chin, and anterior chest. Intact blisters are noted on her chest.

72. What type of burn has the child sustained?
    A. Chemical burn
    B. Electrical burn
    C. Inhalation burn
    D. THERMAL BURN

Rationale:

D. The child sustained a thermal burn as a result of contact with hot liquid.
A. A chemical burn results from contact with three types of chemicals: acids, alkali and organic compounds.
B. An electrical burn results from contact with heat generated from electrical current passing through human tissue.
C. An inhalation burn results from the inhalation of toxic substances and heat.

Content Category: Orthopedics & Wound Care

References: Jordan, 2000; pp.171–205; Kitt et al., 1995; pp. 578–600.

73. Which of the following is most appropriate for care of the toddler who burned herself with coffee?
    A. Undress the child and leave her uncovered in ambient air.
    B. Apply ice to cool the burned areas.
    C. UNDRESS THE PATIENT AND KEEP WARM WITH STERILE SHEETS AND/OR HEATING LAMP.
    D. Apply hydrocortisone ointment to decrease inflammation.

Rationale:

C. The patient should be kept warm with clean or sterile sheets. An overhead heating lamp may be carefully used to keep the patient normothermic.
A. The child should be undressed. Toddlers may become hypothermic from cooling measures unless precautions are take to conserve body heat.
B. Direct application of ice increases cellular damage.
D. Hydrocortisone products should not be applied to traumatized body surfaces.

Content Category: Orthopedics & Wound Care

Reference: Jordan, 2000; pp. 171–205.

74. Upon further examination of the child, the nurse notes multiple bruises of various ages over the back and lower extremities. There also appear to be well-healed circumferential scars above both ankles. The child is crying and inconsolable. The ED nurse should suspect:
   A. ABUSE/NEGLECT.
   B. careless child care/parenting.
   C. the child is acting normally.
   D. the child is spoiled and out of control.

Rationale:

   A. The nurse should have a fairly high suspicion of child abuse/ neglect. Child abuse is a nonaccidental act committed by a caregiver that results in physical, emotional, or sexual injury. Physical examination will note detachment, withdrawal, inappropriate behavior, ecchymosis in various planes or stages of healing, or injuries inconsistent with age.
   B. Although there may be careless parenting in regard to the burns, the presence of bruising and scars suggests a more serious problem.
   C. A toddler with superficial partial-thickness burns should be consolable by the mother.
   D. The child is acting appropriate for age.

Content Category: Orthopedics & Wound Care
Reference: Jordan, 2000; pp. 343–370.

75. An elderly woman slips and falls onto her left forearm. The arm just below the shoulder has extensive swelling and bruising and is tender to palpation. A fractured humerus is suspected. As part of the assessment, the ED nurse should evaluate the patient's ability to:
   A. EXTEND THE HAND AT THE WRIST AGAINST PRESSURE.
   B. make a clenched fist.
   C. spread the fingers apart.
   D. flex the hand at the wrist.

Rationale:

   A. The radial nerve lies in close proximity to the humeral shaft, particularly in the upper humerus. Therefore, fractures in this area can injure the radial nerve. Extension at the wrist, particularly against pressure, is a test of radial nerve function.
   B. Clenching the fist does not evaluate radial nerve function.
   C. Spreading the fingers is a test of ulnar nerve function.
   D. Flexion of the wrist does not evaluate radial nerve function.

Content Category: Orthopedics & Wound Care
Reference: Jordan, 2000; pp. 501–535.

76. A patient presents to the ED after catching his great toe nail in the track of his shower stall. The proximal aspect of the nail has lifted away from the nailbed. There is no bleeding from the bed or surrounding tissues. This injury would best be described as:
   A. avulsion injury of the toe.
   B. NAIL ROOT AVULSION.
   C. contusion of the toe.
   D. nailbed laceration.

Rationale:

B. The nail has been avulsed, or lifted off the nailbed, by the force of catching on the track. The proximal aspect is the nail root; therefore, this is a nail root avulsion.

A. An avulsion injury of the toe involves loss of soft tissue and skin from the toe.

C. Contusion of the toe occurs when blood is extravasated into the soft tissues after a direct blow.

D. While nailbed lacerations frequently occur with nail avulsions, the lack of bleeding suggests that there is no laceration in this situation.

Content Category: Orthopedics & Wound Care

Reference: Trott, 1997; pp. 208–247.

Questions 77 and 78

An adolescent male is being evaluated after he jammed his finger playing basketball. On exam, capillary refill is brisk and sensation is intact. The finger is held in flexion at the proximal interphalangeal joint and he is unable to extend it.

77.   The ED nurse should suspect that this patient has:
A. fractured the distal phalangis.
B. lacerated the digital artery.
C. RUPTURED THE EXTENSOR TENDON.
D. contused the digital nerve.

Rationale:

C. The unopposed and intact flexor tendon holds the joint in flexion. Rupture of the extensor tendon prevents the patient from extending the joint.

A. The injury involves the proximal and middle phalanges; the distal phalangis is not involved.

B. Brisk capillary refill indicates that the digital artery is intact.

D. Normal sensation suggests that the digital nerve is uninjured.

Content Category: Orthopedics & Wound Care

Reference: Snider, 1999; pp. 162–262.

78.   Prior to discharge, the ED nurse should immobilize the finger by:
A. taping it to an adjacent finger.
B. SPLINTING IT IN EXTENSION.
C. splinting it in the position of comfort.
D. splinting it in flexion.

Rationale:

B. The joint must be splinted in extension or the finger may heal with a permanent boutonnière deformity.

A. Taping it to an adjacent finger will permit movement of the finger and will not maintain it in full extension.

C. The position of comfort will not be full extension.

D. Splinting in flexion would increase the distance between the ruptured fragments of the extensor, making it less likely to achieve functional healing.

Content Category: Orthopedics & Wound Care

Reference: Snider, 1997; pp. 162–262.

79. When the emergency nurse is evaluating foreign bodies in soft tissues, which of the following is considered a reactive object?
    A. Sewing needle
    B. Glass fragment
    C. WOOD SPLINTER
    D. Graphite from a pencil

Rationale:

    C. Wood is considered organic and therefore reactive. Failure to remove it would cause infection and chronic inflammation.
    A. Metal is considered inert and nonreactive. The decision to remove it is based on accessibility, potential damage to surrounding structures, and patient discomfort.
    B. Glass is considered inert and nonreactive; however, it is generally removed because it will normally cause discomfort.
    D. Graphite is considered inert and nonreactive; however, it is generally removed to prevent tattooing.

Content Category: Orthopedics & Wound Care

Reference: Trott, 1997; pp. 285–301.

80. Your trauma patient has been diagnosed with neurogenic shock. You note no movement of any extremity, hypotension, and bradycardia. His respirations are 40/minute and shallow. After you have assessed and maintained the patient's airway, what is your next intervention?
    A. Administer 100% oxygen via nonrebreather mask.
    B. ADMINISTER 100% OXYGEN VIA BAG–VALVE–MASK DEVICE.
    C. Intubate the patient with rapid-sequence inline intubation.
    D. Intubate via nasotracheal intubation.

Rationale:

    B. Use of the bag-valve-mask device is the next intervention BEFORE intubation to help build oxygen reserves in preparation for the procedure.
    A. The patient's respiratory rate and depth are inadequate for necessary gas exchange. The patient's respirations need to be assisted.
    C. This patient is unable to sustain his own respirations. Intubation should not be performed until the patient has been preoxygenated.
    D. This patient is unable to sustain his own respirations. Intubation should not be performed until the patient has been preoxygenated.

Content Category: Trauma & Shock

Reference: ENA, Core Curriculum, 2000.

81. The most important stabilization treatment of an unconscious victim with a closed head injury from motor vehicle collision is which of the following?
    A. Maintain spinal immobilization
    B. CONTROL OF THE AIRWAY
    C. Establish intravenous access
    D. Determine history of bleeding dyscrasias

Rationale:

    B. Keeping the airway open is always the first and most important stabilizing factor.

    A. Although maintaining spinal immobilization is important to prevent spinal cord injury, always do the ABCs first: airway, breathing, circulation.

    C. Intravenous access should be established after the airway has been secured.

    D. Bleeding dyscrasia history is important, as is the history of the patient's taking any blood-thinning medications, such as coumadin. These factors can increase the potential for hemorrhage.

Content Category: Trauma and Shock

Reference: ENA, Trauma Nursing, 2000.

82.   The test that is done to determine the degree of a LeFort fracture is:
    A. computed tomography (CT) of orbits.
    B. magnetic resonance imaging (MRI) of maxillofacial bones.
    C. WATERS' VIEW OF SKULL.
    D. temporomandibular x-rays.

Rationale:

    C. Waters' view will reveal a bony fracture or asymmetry and subcutaneous emphysema. The test can be done relatively quickly.

    A. CT of orbits might show occult orbital fractures.

    B. MRI is not usually used for facial bones.

    D. Temporomandibular x-rays would not necessarily show all facial involvement.

Content Category: Trauma & Shock

Reference: ENA, Trauma Nursing, 2000.

83.   A 12-year-old child presents to the ED after being struck in the head with a baseball bat. The patient complaints of headache and pain in his deltoid region. The triage nurse should perform which of the following first?
    A. Determine if there was loss of consciousness
    B. Apply ice to area of injury
    C. Obtain pulse oximetry and vital signs
    D. APPLY CERVICAL SPINE IMMOBILIZATION

Rationale:

    D. The mechanism of injury suggests possible cervical spine involvement as well as pain referred to the deltoid area.

    A. Loss of consciousness is important in determining the possibility of intracranial bleed and when taking the history.

    B. Ice will help swelling and pain, but is not the most important step.

    C. Vital signs should be taken in every patient.

Content Category: Trauma & Shock

Reference: ENA, Trauma Nursing, 2000.

84.   A patient who is brought to the ED was the known driver in a high-speed motor vehicle crash. The patient was not belted, was ejected from the vehicle, and is now complaining of severe substernal chest pain, dyspnea, stridor, and hoarseness on exam. The patient has swelling of the neck and cyanosis of the lower extremities. This patient may be exhibiting signs of:
   A. cervical spine subluxation.
   B. fractures of the first ribs.
   C. AORTIC TEAR.
   D. fractured sternum.

Rationale:

   C. An aortic tear would produce pain, stridor, and hoarseness of the neck in response to an expanding hematoma and cyanosis of the extremities due to lack of blood flow.
   A. Cervical spine subluxation may cause extremity paraplegia and numbness.
   B. Fractures of the first ribs are serious but would not have led to the severe symptoms listed here. Cyanosis from lack of blood flow has not been accounted for.
   D. Fractured sternum may be painful and cause cardiac arrhythmias.

Content Category: Trauma & Shock

Reference: ENA, Trauma Nursing, 2000.

85.   After you have performed an intraosseous cannulation for your 18-month-old pediatric patient, what would indicate that you had performed the procedure correctly?
   A. A blood flashback is seen in the catheter.
   B. It is possible to thread the over-the-needle cannula.
   C. A POPPING SOUND IS HEARD DURING INSERTION, FOLLOWED BY LACK OF RESISTANCE TO THE NEEDLE.
   D. The butterfly needle can stand upright without manual support.

Rationale:

   C. Popping is indictive of piercing the bone and, when followed by the ability of the needle to progress, indicates sucessful intraosseous cannulation.
   A. You would not see flashback as you are not using a plastic needle.
   B. You would not be using an over-the-needle cannula for intraosseous cannulation.
   D. The butterfly needle would not be used for intraosseous cannulation.

Content Category: Trauma & Shock

Reference: Sheehy & Lenehan, 1999; pp. 121–123.

86.   Your patient is a victim of a motor vehicle crash. He has severe facial injury. You select the following manner to test cranial nerve function:
   A. Observe the patient for posturing patterns such as flexion or extension.
   B. Observe for Battle's sign behind the ear.
   C. Inspect the ears and nose for cerebrospinal fluid leakage.
   D. HAVE THE PATIENT FOLLOW YOUR MOVING FINGER WITH HIS EYES.

Rationale:

   D. Having the patient follow your finger with his eyes will test extraocular movement, which is a test of cranial nerves III, IV, and VI.
   A. Observing the patient for posturing pattern would determine whether he had a brainstem or high injury. It would not assess the cranial nerves.

B. Battle's sign is usually an indication of a basal skull fracture and does not indicate cranial nerve injury.

C. Cerebrospinal fluid leakage may be observed with a basal skull fracture but does not indicate cranial nerve function.

Content Category: Trauma & Shock

Reference: ENA, Trauma Nursing, 2000.

87. You are preparing a motorcycle crash victim for a needle thoracentesis. A tension pneumothorax is suspected. After assembling the needed equipment, you would know that insertion of a 14-gauge needle would be placed in which location?

A. Unaffected side, fourth intercostal space slightly anterior to the midaxillary line

B. AFFECTED SIDE, SECOND INTERCOSTAL SPACE AT THE MIDCLAVICULAR LINE

C. Affected side, fifth intercostal space slightly anterior to the midaxillary line

D. Unaffected side, third intercostal space at the midclavicular line.

Rationale:

B. The second intercostal space at the midclavicular line is the correct location.

A. Although a tension pneumothorax displaces the trachea and thoracic organs away from the affected side toward the unaffected side, inserting a thoracentesis needle in the unaffected side may compromise the patient.

C. The fifth intercostal space slightly anterior to the midaxillary line would be the correct location for insertion of a chest tube if you suspected a hemothorax. This location would allow for drainage of accumulated blood.

D. Although a tension pneumothorax displaces the trachea and thoracic organs away from the affected side toward the unaffected side, inserting a thoracentesis needle in the unaffected side might compromise the patient.

Content Category: Trauma & Shock

Reference: Sheehy & Lenehan, 1999; p. 468.

88. You are preparing to insert an indwelling urinary catheter. What would you consider a contraindication for the procedure?

A. The patient tells you that she does not see a need for the catheter.

B. There had been discomfort during your abdominal palpation.

C. The patient tells you that she allergic to latex.

D. THERE IS BLOOD AT THE URETHRAL MEATUS.

Rationale:

D. You would not catheterize your patient if you found blood at the urethral meatus. It might indicate a urethral injury.

A. Explain to the patient the reason for the need for the catheter. You would need consent to insert it.

B. Inserting a urinary catheter will determine if the bladder was ruptured, a possible cause of the abdominal pain.

C. A latex allergy is pertinent. You would obtain a latex-free catheter and proceed.

Content Category: Trauma & Shock

Reference: ENA, Trauma Nursing, 2000.

89.   The proper positioning of the multitrauma patient with suspected flat chest injury is which of the following?
    A.   High Fowler's position to prevent aspiration of hemoptysis
    B.   FLAIL SIDE DOWNWARD TO STABILIZE FLAIL SEGMENT AND IMPROVE VENTILATION
    C.   Flail side splinted with sandbags keeping patient dorsorecumbent
    D.   Flail side upward to avoid hemopneumothorax from penetrating fractured ribs

Rationale:

    B.   Placing the patient with flail downward will stabilize the chest and improve ventilation in the noninjured hemothorax.
    A.   While airway maintenance is important, the patient may be hypotensive and too uncomfortable to sit in high Fowler's position.
    C.   Sandbags will not help flail. Position may not be comfortable to patient.
    D.   Flail side upward will not facilitate ventilation from uninjured hemothorax and would put the patient at risk of hypoxia.

Content Category: Trauma & Shock

Reference: ENA, Trauma Nursing, 2000.

90.   A 30-year-old male presents to the ED with new onset of profound lower extremity weakness and numbness and tingling in the abdomen, chest, and upper extremities. S/he has absent superficial and deep tendon reflexes. The patient reports burning and aching in both legs that have increased over the last week. Based on the patient's history and presenting symptoms, the nurse would assess for:
    A.   RESPIRATORY RATE; DEPTH AND WORK OF BREATHING.
    B.   presence of rectal tone.
    C.   changes in level of consciousness.
    D.   recent history of upper respiratory illness.

Rationale:

    A.   Respiratory rate and depth and work of breathing are a priority assessment and part of an ongoing evaluation in a patient with Guillain-Barré syndrome. The ascending weakness may cause respiratory muscle fatigue, decreased ventilatory capacity, and respiratory failure.
    B.   Presence of rectal tone is not a priority in the assessment of a patient with Guillain-Barré syndrome.
    C.   Changes in level of consciousness do not normally occur with Guillain-Barré syndrome.
    D.   Recent history of upper respiratory illness will help establish a diagnosis of Guillain-Barré syndrome but is not a priority.

Content Category: Neurological

References: McCance & Huether, 1998; pp. 510–571; Hickey, 1997; pp. 665–703.

91.   A 33-year-old female patient involved in a motor vehicle collision is brought to the ED via EMS. Prehospital providers report she was responsive only to painful stimuli at the scene. The patient is intubated and has 2 large-bore IVs with normal saline infusing. Pupils are equal and reactive at 4 mm. The patient withdraws to painful stimuli. The ED nurse should anticipate which of the following interventions?
    A.   Hyperventilating to maintain $pCO_2 < 30$ mm Hg
    B.   Mannitol (Osmitrol) 100 g IV
    C.   Dexamethasone (Decadron) 10 mg IV
    D.   FLUID ADMINISTRATION TO MAINTAIN MEAN ARTERIAL PRESSURE (MAP) > 90 MM HG

Rationale:

    D. Fluid administration to maintain mean arterial pressure (MAP) > 90 mm Hg is the best solution. Hypotension is a major cause of secondary injury. Inadequate systemic blood pressure in a patient with traumatic brain injury may result in inadequate cerebral perfusion pressure.

    A. Hyperventilating to maintain pCO_2 < 30 mm Hg is no longer indicated in severe head injury.

    B. Mannitol (Osmitrol) 100 g IV is indicated when there is evidence of neurologic deterioration, herniation, or increased intracranial pressure refractory to other interventions.

    C. Dexamethasone (Decadron) 10 mg IV is contraindicated in severe head injury

Content Category: Neurological

Reference: ENA, Trauma Nursing, 2000.

92.   A 26-year-old patient is brought to the ED after falling out a second-story window. He responds only to deep pain and has blood oozing from the right ear and right naris. The right pupil is 7 mm in diameter and nonreactive to light. The left pupil is 4 mm in diameter and sluggish. The Glasgow Coma Scale is determined to be 4. Prehospital providers have immobilized the patient with a rigid cervical collar and long spine board. The patient has an 18-gauge IV with lactated Ringer's infusing. The initial priority for the ED nurse is do which of the following?

    A. Initiate a second large-bore IV with warmed crystalloid

    B. Prepare to administer mannitol (Osmitrol)

    C. ASSIST WITH RAPID-SEQUENCE INDUCTION AND INTUBATION

    D. Hyperventilate to maintain pCO_2 < 30 mm Hg

Rationale:

    C. Assisting with rapid-sequence induction and intubation is the priority in patients with a Glasgow Coma Scale (GCS) score less than 8 and traumatic brain injury.

    A. Initiating a second large-bore IV with warmed crystalloid is necessary for fluid resuscitation, but only after an adequate airway has been secured.

    B. Mannitol should be considered in patients with traumatic brain injury who have signs and symptoms of herniation or neurologic deterioration.

    D. Although mannitol may be indicated for this patient, the priority is to secure the airway. Mild hyperventilation in the presence of neurologic deterioration may be indicated after securing the airway. Decreasing the pCO_2 to less than 30 mm Hg would not be indicated. Empiric hyperventilation is not recommended.

Content Category: Neurological

Reference: ENA, Core Curriculum, 2000.

93.   A patient is admitted to the ED with a diagnosis of Alzheimer's disease. The patient appears very disoriented and confused. Which of the following nursing diagnoses would be MOST appropriate for this patient?

    A. INJURY, HIGH RISK, RELATED TO ALTERED THOUGHT PROCESSES

    B. Tissue perfusion, altered cerebral, related to interruption in blood flow

    C. Anxiety, fear, related to onset of symptoms

    D. Knowledge deficit, risk factors and prevention

Rationale:

    A. Patients with Alzheimer's disease may become progressively confused and disoriented. The risk for injury increases as the patient loses the sense of awareness and has increasing difficulty in performing the activities of daily living.

B. There are many causes of dementia. The exact agent for Alzheimer's disease is still undetermined. There is no proof that altered tissue perfusion is the causative factor.
C. Although patients with dementia may be anxious, their sense of awareness is diminished.
D. The loss of awareness and inability to perform activities of daily living are not a result of knowledge deficit.

Content Category: Neurological

Reference: ENA, Core Curriculum, 2000.

94. A 24-year-old male presents to the ED after falling 10 feet from a roof. He is lethargic but easily aroused to verbal stimuli. He is confused and perseverating. Witnesses report the patient was unconscious for at least 5 minutes. On initial exam he is found to have multiple abrasions on the left side of his face, blood oozing from the left ear, ecchymosis around both eyes, and a laceration on his left arm. As part of the assessment, the ED nurse should do which of the following?
A. Assess for hemotympanum and pack the external canal
B. ASSESS FOR CEREBROSPINAL FLUID (CSF) IN THE EAR DRAINAGE
C. Prepare to administer prophylactic antibiotics
D. Prepare the patient for computed tomography (CT) scan of the head

Rationale:

B. Periorbital ecchymosis and CSF leaks are signs and symptoms of a basilar skull fracture.
A. Hemotympanum may be present with basilar skull fractures and should be assessed. A dressing should be placed over the ear, but the canal should not be packed if a CSF leak is suspected.
C. Antibiotics should be administered when a CSF leak is present. This patient should be evaluated for a CSF leak.
D. CT imaging is a diagnostic procedure that will identify intracranial lesions.

Content Category: Neurological

References: ENA, Core Curriculum, 2000.

95. A 45-year-old male presents to the ED with complaints of severe pain and burning around the left eye, pain in the left side of the head, increased tearing, and nausea. You note ptosis of the left eye, which is red. The patient states that these symptoms started approximately 30 minutes prior to arrival. This patient's symptoms are most commonly associated with:
A. CLUSTER HEADACHE.
B. tension headache.
C. intracerebral neoplasm.
D. optic neuritis.

Rationale:

A. Cluster headaches occur primarily in men 20 to 50 years of age. They are called cluster headaches because several attacks can occur during the day for a period of days followed by a long period of remission. They are characterized by severe unilateral tearing, burning, periorbital, or temporal pain lasting 30 minutes to 2 hours. Associated symptoms include lacrimation, reddening of the eye, nasal stuffiness, eyelid ptosis, and nausea. Pain may be referred to the midface and teeth.
B. Tension headaches are mild to moderate bilateral headaches with a sensation of a tight band or pressure around the head. They occur in both men and women and are the most common type of headache.
C. Clinical manifestations of intracerebral tumor are a result of invasion and destruction of local tissue as well as increased intracranial pressure. Focal deficits depend on the site of the tumor. Clinical manifestations of increased intracranial pressure include headache, vomiting, papilledema, unsteady gait, and diminishing cognitive function.

D. Optic neuritis is a presenting complaint in approximately 25% of persons with multiple sclerosis. The condition is a result of optic nerve demyelination. It evolves rapidly. Subjective symptoms are blurring, foggy or hazy vision, and impaired color perception. There is decreased central visual acuity, color vision deficit, and visual field deficits.

Content Category: Neurological

Reference: McCance & Huether, 1998; pp. 510–571.

96. A 60-year-old female is brought to the ED by her husband. He states that she awoke this morning complaining of a headache and has gradually become more disoriented. She is now awake but confused and has difficulty standing. Upon further assessment, her left pupil is 6 mm in diameter and nonreactive to light. The right pupil is 4 mm in diameter and reacts briskly. Vital signs are BP 122/60 mm Hg, HR 60/min, and respirations 20/min. Based on these initial findings, you would anticipate interventions for possible:
    A. calcium channel blocker toxicity.
    B. meningitis.
    C. SUBDURAL HEMATOMA.
    D. dehydration.

Rationale:

C. A patient with a subdural hematoma (acute) presents with headache, confusion, and a steady decline in level of consciousness. History should be evaluated for a fall or injury to head. Ipsilateral pupil dilation and contralateral hemiparesis are associated with acute and chronic subdural hematomas.

A. Calcium channel blocker toxicity usually presents with hypotension, shortness of breath, dizziness, and irregular heart rate. Unequal pupils are not associated with toxicity.

B. Meningitis is not usually associated with unequal sluggish pupils and extremity weakness.

D. Severe dehydration may be associated with disorientation, hypotension, and tachycardia. Unequal pupils are not found with dehydration.

Content Category: Neurological

References: ENA, Core Curriculum, 2000; McCance & Huether, 1998; pp. 510–571.

97. The priority nursing diagnosis for a patient in the ED awaiting admission for an acoustic neuroma would be:
    A. dysreflexia.
    B. risk for aspiration.
    C. RISK FOR INJURY.
    D. impaired verbal communication.

Rationale:

C. Acoustic neuroma is a tumor of cranial nerve VIII. It affects vestibular function, balance, and hearing. Dizziness and poor balance place the patient at risk for injury.

A. Dysreflexia is not associated with an acoustic neuroma.

B. Aspiration is not a complication of acoustic neuroma, since cranial nerve VIII does not affect swallowing or respirations.

D. Speech is not affected by impairment of cranial nerve VIII.

Content Category: Neurological

Reference: ENA, Core Curriculum, 2000.

98.   A 40-year-old male involved in a house fire presents to the ED with dyspnea, sooty sputum, and a brassy cough. He is conscious; 100% oxygen via nonrebreather reservoir mask is being administered. The priority nursing diagnosis for this patient would be:
      A. fluid volume deficit.
      B. impaired gas exchange.
      C. AIRWAY CLEARANCE, INEFFECTIVE.
      D. pain.

Rationale:

C. Ineffective airway clearance is the priority nursing diagnosis because of the potential for edema and obstruction of the airway. If the airway is not patent you will be unable to ventilate and oxygenate the patient.

A. Fluid volume deficit could be a potential diagnosis depending of the extent of the burn, total body surface area involved and time of the burn but ineffective airway clearance remains the highest priority.

B. Impaired gas exchange will certainly be another nursing diagnosis for this patient due to the inhalation of carbon monoxide and possible other toxins. However the priority diagnosis remains ineffective airway clearance.

D. Pain and pain management are important to consider, but the highest priority remains ineffective airway clearance.

Content Category: Trauma & Shock

Reference: Kitt et al., 1995; pp. 590, 593.

99.   45-year-old man falls 8 feet onto his shoulder, sustaining a scapular fracture. Concomitant injuries associated with a scapular fracture are which of the following?
      A. PNEUMOTHORAX AND PULMONARY CONTUSION
      B. Head injury and abdominal injury
      C. Elbow and wrist fractures
      D. Scaphoid and capitate fractures

Rationale:

A. A scapular fracture is a harbinger of serious underlying conditions. Pneumothorax and pulmonary contusion may necessitate chest tubes and a mechanical ventilator.

B. These are possible associated injuries, but not so directly related.

C. Elbow and wrist fractures are possible, but not probable.

D. Scaphoid and capitate fractures are not likely.

Content Category: Trauma & Shock

Reference: Bayley & Turcke, 1998; pp. 415–447.

100. Patient comfort and cooperation during eye irrigation can be facilitated by the administration of:
      A. pilocarpine (Pilocar).
      B. tetracycline (Achromycin).
      C. TETRACAINE (PONTOCAINE).
      D. lidocaine (Xylocaine).

Rationale:

C. Tetracaine is a safe, fast-acting topical local anesthetic for ophthalmologic use.

A. Pilocarpine is a miotic, used primarily to treat glaucoma.

B. Tetracycline is an antibiotic with no anesthetic properties.

D. Lidocaine is a local anesthetic for wound closure, not ophthalmologic use.

Content Category: Maxillofacial & Ocular

Reference: Newberry, 1998; pp. 689–706.

101.   A complication found in patients with a LeFort II fracture is:
A. CEREBROSPINAL FLUID LEAK.
B. Ludwig's angina.
C. otitis externa.
D. spinal shock.

Rationale:

A. Due to the high energy and force needed to sustain a LeFort II fracture, skull fracture may also be present. Clear drainage from the ears or nasal passage testing positive for glucose is suggestive of cerebrospinal fluid leak.
B. Ludwig's angina is a dental condition characterized by pain, tenderness, drooling, and fever as a result of infected dental caries.
C. Otitis externa is an ear infection and unrelated to LeFort fractures. Ear problems such as avulsion, laceration, and hematoma are seen in patients with maxillofacial trauma.
D. Spinal shock is a shock state that occurs in patients with spinal cord injury. Although patients with maxillofacial injury can also have spinal injury, especially c-spine trauma, spinal shock is a complication of spinal cord trauma, not maxillofacial trauma.

Content Category: Maxillofacial & Ocular

Reference: Newberry, 1998; pp. 373–387.

102.   A 54-year-old patient presents to triage clutching bloody tissues and complaining of a nosebleed. Vital signs are BP 154/100 mm Hg, HR 88/min, respirations 16/min, and temperature 98.5° F (36.9° C). An appropriate intervention for this patient would be to:
A. place patient in Trendelenburg position.
B. APPLY PINCH PRESSURE TO NOSE.
C. administer a rapid infusion of 250 ml of normal saline.
D. tilt head backwards until bleeding subsides.

Rationale:

B. Pinch pressure to the nares is an effective initial method to control bleeding in epistaxis.
A. The patient should sit upright with head slightly forward. Trendelenburg position is contraindicated unless there is profound shock.
C. Intravenous fluids are not indicated at this time since vital signs are stable.
D. The head should be tilted forward.

Content Category: Maxillofacial & Ocular

Reference: Newberry, 1998; pp. 673–688.

103.   Which of the following patients represents the highest triage acuity level?
A. A 12-year-old reporting a "stye" in the left eye
B. A 34-YEAR-OLD WITH "PEPPER SPRAY TO BOTH EYES"
C. A 22-year-old who is "unable to remove my contact lens"
D. A 4-year-old with "itchy, sticky eyes"

Rationale:

B. Pepper spray is a chemical burn. Chemical burns are the most urgent of all ocular emergencies. This patient requires eye irrigation without delay.

A. A stye is a nonurgent problem.

C. Contact lens removal would not take priority over a patient with a chemical burn.

D. Itchy, sticky eyes consistent with conjunctivitis are a nonurgent problem.

Content Category: Maxillofacial & Ocular

Reference: Handysides & Hanscom, 1996; pp. 117–153.

104. Pediatric patients presenting with nasal obstruction and purulent, unilateral, foul-smelling rhinorrhea most likely have which of the following conditions?

A. Epistaxis

B. Sinusitis

C. FOREIGN BODY OF THE NOSE

D. Acute or chronic pharyngitis

Rationale:

C. Foreign body of the nose should be suspected in a child who presents with a sensation of unilateral nasal obstruction; persistent, foul-smelling rhinorrhea despite proper antibiotic treatment; and persistent unilateral epistaxis.

A. A patient with epistaxis would have a bloody, not purulent, nasal discharge. There is generally no odor associated with this condition.

B. This patient has an infection of the sinuses with nasal discharge, which is usually bilateral. The odor associated with this condition is limited to the nasal and oropharyngeal areas.

D. This patient often has bad breath, but no bad body odor. There is also no purulent nasal discharge.

Content Category: Maxillofacial & Ocular

References: Buttaravoli & Stair, 2000; Tintinalli et al., 2000; pp. 1532–1539.

105. The patient with a hyphema should be placed in which of the following positions?

A. Trendelenburg

B. Supine

C. ELEVATED HEAD OF BED

D. Prone

Rationale:

C. The patient's head should be elevated to promote settling of suspended red blood cells inferiorly in the anterior chamber. This position will prevent clogging of the entire 360 degrees of the trabecular meshwork, which would cause further increased intraocular pressure.

A. The Trendelenburg position would further increase intraocular pressure and potentially cause further bleeding.

B. The supine position would increase intraocular pressure and could worsen the patient's condition.

D. The prone position would increase intraocular pressure and could worsen the patient's condition.

Content Category: Maxillofacial & Ocular

Reference: Tintinalli et al., 2000; pp. 1501–1518.

106.   Signs and symptoms of globe rupture of the eye include:
   A.   TEARDROP-SHAPED PUPIL AND DECREASED INTRAOCULAR PRESSURE.
   B.   shallow anterior chamber and increased intraocular pressure.
   C.   hyphema and increased intraocular pressure.
   D.   corneal ulcer and decreased intraocular pressure.

Rationale:

   A.   The pupil of the patient with a globe rupture assumes a teardrop shape with the point toward the rupture site. In addition, intraocular pressure is decreased by the leak from the rupture site.
   B.   Signs of globe rupture include a shallow anterior chamber, but with decreased intraocular pressure from the rupture site.
   C.   Signs of globe rupture do include hyphema, but with decreased intraocular pressure from the rupture site.
   D.   Corneal ulcer occurs in the unconscious patient or in the patient who leaves contact lenses in place for an inordinate period of time. Corneal ulcer is not associated with globe rupture. Intraocular pressure is decreased in globe rupture.

Content Category: Maxillofacial & Ocular

Reference: Newberry, 1998; pp. 689–706.

107.   Which cranial nerves (CN) are measured in assessing extraocular muscle function?
   A.   CN III, V, VIII
   B.   CN III, IV, VI
   C.   CN II, VII, X
   D.   CN III, VI, VIII

Rationale:

   B.   CN III, oculomotor (medial, superior, and inferior rectus muscles of the eye), CN IV, trochlear (superior oblique muscle of the eye), and CN VI. abducens (lateral rectus muscle of the eye).
   A.   CN VIII is the acoustic nerve. CN V is the trigeminal nerve.
   C.   CN II is the optic nerve. CN X is the vagus nerve.
   D.   CN VIII is the acoustic nerve.

Content Category: Maxillofacial & Ocular

Reference: Newberry, 1998.

108.   Which of the following is true about temporomandibular joint (TMJ) dislocation?
   A.   THE CAUSE IS USUALLY A BLOW TO THE CHIN.
   B.   The patient presents with the mandible tightly clenched against the maxilla.
   C.   Unilateral dislocations are common.
   D.   It is often seen in toddlers who fall on the chin when learning to walk.

Rationale:

   A.   The usual cause of a dislocation is the result of a direct blow to the chin while the mouth is open. If the patient is predisposed to dislocation, a vigorous yawn can cause this condition.
   B.   The patient with TMJ dislocation presents with the mouth open and is unable to close the mouth.
   C.   Unilateral dislocations are rare.
   D.   TMJ dislocation rarely occurs in toddlers.

Content Category: Maxillofacial & Ocular

Reference: Knoop et al., 1997; pp.141–175.

109.   The endpoint for the administration of procainamide (Pronestyl) includes all of the following EXCEPT:
    A. The arrhythmia is suppressed.
    B. A total of 17mg/kg of the drug is given.
    C. THE QRS COMPLEX IS NARROWED BY 50% FROM ITS ORIGINAL DURATION.
    D. Hypotension ensues.

Rationale:

    C. The endpoint for the administration of procainamide is indicated when the QRS is *prolonged* by 50% from its original duration.
    A. The endpoint for the administration of procainamide is indicated when the arrhythmia is suppressed.
    B. The endpoint for the administration of procainamide is indicated when a total of 17mg/kg of the drug is given.
    D. The endpoint for the administration of procainamide is indicated when hypotension ensues

Content Category: Cardiovascular

Reference: American Heart Association, 2000; pp. 102–124.

110.   The first medication indicated for any pulseless patient is which of the following?
    A. EPINEPHRINE (ADRENALIN)
    B. Atropine
    C. Lidocaine (Xylocaine)
    D. Sodium bicarbonate

Rationale:

    A. Epinephrine is indicated in the treatment of asystole, pulseless electrical activity, ventricular fibrillation, and pulseless ventricular tachycardia.
    B. Atropine is indicated in the treatment of symptomatic bradycardia.
    C. Lidocaine is administered in the treatment of ventricular tachycardia and ventricular fibrillation after administration of epinephrine.
    D. Sodium bicarbonate is considered as a buffering agent in the treatment of preexisting metabolic acidosis, hyperkalemia, or tricyclic or phenobarbital overdose.

Content Category: Cardiovascular

Reference: American Heart Association, 2000; pp. 102–134.

111.   When defibrillating with the initial three shocks, the ED nurse should:
    A. wait until after intubation has occurred to begin the shocks.
    B. ASSESS THE CARDIAC RHYTHM BETWEEN STACKED SHOCKS.
    C. continue CPR between stacked shocks.
    D. check the pulse after each shock.

Rationale:

    B. The three shocks are delivered one after the other as soon as the defibrillator can be charged and the rhythm checked on the monitor.
    A. Defibrillation should not be delayed in order to intubate the patient.
    C. Personnel should not resume CPR between shocks unless an unavoidable delay is required.
    D. A pulse is checked only at the end of the third shock unless the rhythm is restored.

Content Category: Cardiovascular

Reference: American Heart Association, 2000; pp. 102–147.

112. The most common lethal arrhythmia in the first hour of an acute myocardial infarction (AMI) is which of the following?
    A. Atrial fibrillation
    B. Asystole
    C. Third-degree heart block
    D. VENTRICULAR FIBRILLATION

Rationale:

    D. Half of the patients who die of AMI do so early, before reaching a hospital. In most of these deaths, ventricular fibrillation is the presenting rhythm.
    A. Atrial fibrillation is not considered a lethal rhythm.
    B. Asystole is a lethal rhythm, but not the most common initial rhythm associated with AMI.
    C. Third-degree heart block may be associated with an MI, but it is not the most common initial rhythm.

Content Category: Cardiovascular

Reference: American Heart Association, 2000; pp. 102–172.

113. All of the following statements about atropine sulfate are true EXCEPT:
    A. ATROPINE CAN RESULT IN PARADOXICAL BRADYCARDIA IF GIVEN IN HIGH DOSES.
    B. Atropine can be administered endotracheally.
    C. Atropine can cause bradycardia if given by slow IV push.
    D. Atropine is an antidote for anticholinesterase insecticide poisoning.

Rationale:

    A. Atropine can result in paradoxical bradycardia if given in low doses.
    B. Atropine can be administered endotracheally.
    C. Atropine should be administered rapidly to avoid inducing bradycardia.
    D. Atropine is an antidote for anticholinesterase insecticide poisoning.

Content Category: Cardiovascular

Reference: Hodgson & Kizor, 2000.

114. A patient is brought to the ED after a motor vehicle crash. He is pulseless and apneic. The monitor shows a sinus tachycardia at a rate of 120. The nurse anticipates which of the following?
    A. ADMINISTRATION OF EPINEPHRINE (ADRENALIN)
    B. Administration of epinephrine (Adrenalin) and atropine
    C. Attempt immediate defibrillation
    D. Administration of adenosine (Adenocard)

Rationale:

    A. Epinephrine 1 mg IV is recommended in the treatment of pulseless electrical activity.
    B. Atropine is recommended in the treatment of pulseless electrical activity only when the heart rate is less than 60 beats per minute or a relative bradycardia.
    C. Defibrillation is not indicated in the treatment of pulseless electrical activity.
    D. Adenosine is not indicated in the treatment of pulseless electrical activity.

Content Category: Cardiovascular

Reference: American Heart Association, 2000; pp.102–150.

115. Which of the following medications should NOT be administered endotracheally?
    A. Lidocaine (Xylocaine)
    B. ADENOSINE (ADENOCARD)
    C. Atropine
    D. Epinephrine (Adrenalin)

Rationale:

    B. Adenosine is not recommended for endotracheal administration.
    A. Lidocaine is recommended for endotracheal administration when an intravenous or intraosseous line is unavailable.
    C. Atropine is recommended for endotracheal administration when an intravenous or intraosseous line is unavailable.
    D. Epinephrine is recommended for endotracheal administration when an intravenous or intraosseous line is unavailable.

Content Category: Cardiovascular

Reference: American Heart Association, 2000; pp. 102–113.

116. When administering intravenous Adenosine (Adenocard), the nurse realizes that all of the following are true EXCEPT that:
    A. ADENOSINE (ADENOCARD) MUST BE ADMINISTERED SLOWLY TO PREVENT HYPOTENSION.
    B. adenosine (Adenocard) should be followed by a 20-ml saline bolus.
    C. adenosine (Adenocard) may cause a brief period of asystole after rapid administration.
    D. adenosine (Adenocard) may cause flushing.

Rationale:

    A. The recommended initial dosage of adenosine is a 6-mg rapid bolus over 1 to 3 seconds.
    B. The initial dose should be quickly followed by a 20-ml saline flush.
    C. A brief period of asystole (up to 15 seconds) is common after rapid administration.
    D. Flushing, dyspnea, and chest pain are the most frequently observed side effects.

Content Category: Cardiovascular

Reference: American Heart Association, 2000; pp.102–114.

117. Sodium bicarbonate may be effective treatment in all of the following cases EXCEPT which of the following?
    A. Preexisting metabolic acidosis
    B. Hyperkalemia
    C. Tricyclic or phenobarbital overdose
    D. HYPOXIC LACTIC ACIDOSIS

Rationale:

    D. Ventilation is indicated for the treatment of hypoxic lactic acidosis.
    A. Sodium bicarbonate is indicated in the treatment of preexisting metabolic acidosis.
    B. Sodium bicarbonate is indicated in the treatment of hyperkalemia.
    C. Sodium bicarbonate is indicated in the treatment of tricyclic or phenobarbital overdose.

Content Category: Cardiovascular

Reference: American Heart Association, 2000; pp. 102–133.

118. When you are establishing IV access during cardiopulmonary resuscitation (CPR), your first choice should be:
    A. the back of the hand.
    B. ANTECUBITAL.
    C. femoral.
    D. a central line.

Rationale:

    B. Ideally, only the antecubital veins should be used for drug administration during CPR.
    A. This site is located distal to the antecubital site and would prolong entrance of the drug into the central circulation.
    C. Blind cannulation of the femoral vein during CPR poses special problems because of limited space around the patient.
    D. The primary disadvantage of central venous cannulation is an increased complication rate.

Content Category: Cardiovascular

Reference: American Heart Association, 2000; pp. 102–113.

119. To assist medications into the central circulation after peripheral IV administration during cardiopulmonary resuscitation (CPR), the ED nurse should:
    A. defibrillate after each medication.
    B. GIVE A 20-ML FLUID BOLUS AND ELEVATE THE PATIENT'S ARM.
    C. bag vigorously.
    D. turn the patient on his left side.

Rationale:

    B. To assist medication into the central circulation during CPR, administer a 20-ml fluid bolus and elevate the extremity.
    A. Immediate defibrillation is a priority for ventricular defibrillation.
    C. Vigorous bagging will assist the placement of endotracheal drugs into the lungs, speeding the entry of the drug into circulation.
    D. Turning the patient on the left side is not appropriate during CPR.

Content Category: Cardiovascular

Reference: American Heart Association, 2000; pp. 102–113.

120. Which statement regarding ventricular tachycardia is TRUE?
    A. The rhythm is always irregular.
    B. Patients with sustained ventricular tachycardia are usually asymptomatic.
    C. FREQUENT PVCS AND SHORT RUNS OF VENTRICULAR TACHYCARDIA COMMONLY PRECEDE VENTRICULAR TACHYCARDIA.
    D. The QRS duration is < 0.12.

Rationale:

    C. Frequent PVCs and short runs of ventricular tachycardia commonly precede ventricular tachycardia.
    A. Ventricular tachycardia is often regular.
    B. Patients with sustained ventricular tachycardia are usually symptomatic.
    D. The QRS duration is > 0.12.

Content Category: Cardiovascular

Reference: American Heart Association, 2000; pp. 102–124.

121.   A patient presents to the ED with a sinus bradycardia and frequent PVCs. Vital signs are 80/60 mm/Hg and HR 38/min. Which of the following interventions is MOST appropriate?
        A. Administer a lidocaine (Xylocaine) bolus.
        B. Insert a transvenous pacemaker.
        C. ADMINISTER AN ATROPINE BOLUS.
        D. Initiate a dopamine (Intropin) drip.

Rationale:

        D. An atropine bolus is indicated in the treatment of symptomatic bradycardia.
        A. PVCs may be compensatory and should not be suppressed.
        B. A transvenous pacemaker may be indicated if the patient does not respond to the atropine.
        C. Dopamine may be administered to increase blood pressure but is not the first-line intervention.

Content Category: Cardiovascular

Reference: American Heart Association, 2000; pp. 102–124.

122.   The emergency nurse manager wishes to evaluate staffing as part of a continuous improvement plan. The manager would benchmark information such as:
        A. staff senses that patients are staying longer while awaiting in house beds.
        B. ACTUAL STAFFING, WAIT TIMES, AND LENGTH OF STAY BY PATIENT TRIAGE CLASSIFICATION.
        C. Chief Financial Officer statement that ED is overstaffed by full-time equivalents for unit of service.
        D. patient compliant letter stating ED is understaffed.

Rationale:

        B. Benchmarking includes current databases and comparisons with emergency departments of similar size. Actual data rather than comments or opinions are used to benchmark.
        A. Although staff awareness issues should be addressed, data collection should be instituted and evaluated.
        C. A Chief Financial Officer's statement should be supported by documentation of data analysis that supports the rationale.
        D. The complaint letter should be evaluated and actual data analysis should be conducted, using benchmark data from hospitals of similar size and volume.

Content Category: Professional Issues

Reference: ENA, 1999; pp. 1–3.

123.   During an interview, which of the following questions would be reasonable to ask a potential nurse who is applying for a position in the ED?
        A. "WHAT ARE YOUR EXPECTATIONS OF THE ED MANAGEMENT TEAM?"
        B. "Do you have transportation to and from work?"
        C. "What hobbies do you engage in after work hours?"
        D. "Do you speak Spanish or French?"

Rationale:

A. Reasonable questions in an interview process focus on the work experience and not personal issues. Other questions may include the employee's greatest assets, how the person would create a positive environment, and challenges the person perceives in the position.
B. Questions concerning personal issues such as transportation, child care, and marital status are illegal to ask in an interview process.
C. Simple conversation concerning hobbies is illegal during an interview process.
D. Foreign language fluency may be asked if it is a job requirement.

Content Category: Professional Issues

Reference: Salluzzo et al., 1997.

124. A hospital can be charged with the unfair labor practice known as interference if the hospital:
A. refuses to meet with union representatives.
B. gives union leaders a special meeting room.
C. THREATENS TO CLOSE IF A UNION IS ELECTED.
D. does not stop the distribution of union material.

Rationale:

C. Threatening to close a hospital if a union is elected is considered interference, since it may unduly influence employees to vote against a union.
A. Hospital officials' refusing to meet with union representatives is an example of refusal to bargain.
B. Hospitals that give union representatives special treatment or pay union dues are displaying dominance.
D. Hospitals may not stop the distribution of union materials.

Content Category: Professional Issues

Reference: Salluzzo et al., 1997.

125. Following the death of a child in the ED, a stress debriefing session is arranged. Personnel invited to this session should include:
A. all ED personnel with small children.
B. ED nursing staff from all shifts.
C. nursing management responsible for staff in the ED.
D. ED PERSONNEL INVOLVED WITH THE SITUATION.

Rationale:

D. Anyone who cared for this child may experience a stress reaction. Each should be offered Critical Incidence Stress Debriefing.
A. Although many ED personnel may feel the impact of a child's death, only those directly involved in the situation should participate in the group debriefing.
B. Programs should be available concerning the Critical Incidence Stress Debriefing program, but only those employees directly involved in the situation should participate in the debriefing.
C. Management should be supportive of personnel that attend the sessions and offer assistance as needed.

Content Category: Professional Issues

Reference: Salluzzo et al., 1997.

126.   The process by which data are collected, results are documented, and experiments and tests are vali-
       dated in order to change a concept is which of the following?
       A. Research-focused theory
       B. EVIDENCE-BASED PRACTICE
       C. Nursing process model
       D. Quantitative analysis approach

Rationale:

       B. Evidence-based practice is the model for validating a need for a practice guideline or verifying a
           process to create one. Emergency nursing practice should be evidence based. Current research
           should validate any planned change.
       A. The described plan is that of an evidence-based practice concept.
       C. The nursing process model looks at assessment, planning and analysis, intervention, and evalua-
           tion.
       D. Quantitative analysis is data collection and review. These are part of evidence-based practice.

Content Category: Professional Issues

Reference: ENA, Core Curriculum, 2000.

127.   The job description of an employee in the ED reads as follows: "To focus on education, system analy-
       sis, research, and research utilization and the provision of direct and indirect nursing care. Job
       requirement: minimum of master's degree in nursing; area of specialization, Emergency Care." This
       description is for a/an:
       A. nurse practitioner.
       B. CLINICAL NURSE SPECIALIST.
       C. ED educator.
       D. case manager.

Rationale:

       B. A clinical nurse specialist is a master's-prepared nurse, at minimum, who focuses on education,
           system analysis, research, and research utilization. This nurse also serves as a preceptor and men-
           tor to staff, providing consulting both in direct and nondirect patient care roles.
       A. A nurse practitioner focuses on the diagnosis and treatment of patients in the department.
       C. An ED educator typically focuses on educational training components.
       D. The case manager typically focuses on system analysis and improvement of care delivery by man-
           aging various types of patients or care paths in the department.

Content Category: Professional Issues

Reference: ENA, Core Curriculum, 2000.

128.   You are caring for a 30-year-old female victim of domestic violence. She experienced an assault to
       the chest and upper abdomen. She has a pneumothorax, which has been treated with a chest tube.
       The patient is hypotensive. You note particulate matter in the chest tube. She also has crepitus over
       the mediastinal area. You suspect:
       A. ruptured diaphragm.
       B. RUPTURED ESOPHAGUS.
       C. stomach injury.
       D. mesenteric injury.

Rationale:

B. Blunt trauma may cause a ruptured esophagus. Clinical signs that present with a ruptured esophagus are particulate matter draining from the chest tube, subcutaneous and/or mediastinal air noted on palpation, and chest x-ray and shock out of proportion to the injury.

A. A ruptured diaphragm may clinically present with a spectrum of clinical signs. This patient may present with a range of symptoms from none to profound shock. The patient also presents with dyspnea, decreased breath sounds on the affected side, and bowel sounds on the affected side in the lower lung fields.

C. Signs and symptoms of a stomach injury include left upper quadrant pain and tenderness, aspiration of blood via nasogastric tube, and the presence of free air on abdominal x-ray.

D. Patients with mesenteric and small-intestine injuries may show no symptoms. Small-bowel pH is neutral and therefore causes less peritoneal irritation.

Content Category: Gastrointestinal

References: Bayley & Turcke, 1998; pp. 376–399.

129. A 38-year-old male patient presents to the ED in severe distress from upper gastrointestinal bleeding. He has been vomiting bright-red blood at home for 2 hours and is now experiencing rectal bleeding. The ED nurse who must prioritize his care immediately performs which of the following?
    A. ENSURES THAT THE PATIENT IS ON 100% NONREBREATHER OXYGEN MASK
    B. Initiates intravenous therapy for fluid rehydration
    C. Inserts nasogastric tube
    D. Sends for a type and crossmatch of packed red blood cells

Rationale:

A. In the patient with any massive intestinal bleeding, airway, breathing, and circulation (ABCs) are priority care. Therefore, ensuring that the patient has oxygen in place for airway and breathing is the nurse's first priority. All the other options are important and must be considered afterward.

B. Initiation of intravenous therapy should be established immediately after the ABCs have been established.

C. Insertion of a nasogastric tube may be necessary but is not the priority nursing intervention.

D. Because the patient will need blood replacement, type and crossmatch are necessary, but not until the ABCs of care have been initiated.

Content Category: Gastrointestinal

References: ENA, Core Curriculum, 1994; pp.29–45; Kidd et al., 2000; pp. 93–116; Newberry, 1998; pp. 537–555.

130. When a patient with peptic ulcer disease presents to the ED, the ED nurse must first consider which of the following?
    A. Insertion of a nasogastric tube
    B. Administration of antiemetics
    C. ADMINISTRATION OF PAIN MEDICATION/ANALGESICS
    D. Obtaining a serum electrolyte profile

Rationale:

C. Pain management related to epigastric burning is a priority in the patient with peptic ulcer disease without perforation.

A. Although insertion of a nasogastric tube may be indicated during patient assessment, it is not the initial action of the ED nurse. If a patient might require surgery, nasogastric tube insertion would be indicated.

B. Administration of antiemetics would not be indicated initially, as most such patients are in severe pain but not vomiting.

D. A serum electrolyte profile, along with other laboratory work, is indicated for diagnostic and evaluation purposes. However, this would not be the nurse's first consideration in this particular patient population.

Content Category: Gastrointestinal

References: ENA, Core Curriculum, 2000; pp. 29–34; Porth, 1998; pp.725–729, 769–771.

131. A 24-year-old female presents to the ED complaining, "It's my Crohn's disease acting up again. I overdid it this weekend." She admits to some abdominal pain and diarrhea. "Just give me some prednisone and I will be fine," she states. The priority nursing diagnosis for this patient is which of the following?
    A. Altered nutrition related to less than body requirements.
    B. Altered nutrition related to more than body requirements.
    C. KNOWLEDGE DEFICIT RELATED TO DIET AND MEDICATIONS.
    D. Altered health maintenance.

Rationale:

C. Crohn's disease is a chronic lifelong illness characterized by exacerbations and periods of remission. Because no specific therapy exists, treatment is directed toward symptom relief and controlling the disease process. Patients should eat a well-balanced diet and avoid foods and beverages that exacerbate the symptoms. A long-term risk includes the development of cancer. Prednisone is not without long-term risk and side effects. Knowledge deficit related to diet and medications is the priority diagnosis.

A. Altered nutrition related to less than body requirements is unrelated to eating the incorrect foods and does not address this patient's lack of understanding about medications.

B. Altered nutrition related to more than body requirements is unrelated to eating the incorrect foods and does not address this patient's lack of understanding about medications.

D. Altered health maintenance may apply in this case, but it is not the priority diagnosis.

Content Category: Gastrointestinal

References: Tierney et al., 1999; p. 617; Taptich et al., 1994; p. 775.

132. A patient presents to the ED with a chief complaint of sudden onset of colicky abdominal pain and nausea after eating a meal of fried chicken and French fries. Vital signs are BP 140/80 mm Hg, HR 116/min, respirations 18/min, and temperature 100.4° F (38.0° C). The ED nurse suspects:
    A. diverticulitis.
    B. appendicitis.
    C. CHOLECYSTITIS.
    D. esophagitis.

Rationale:

C. Cholecystitis is an inflammation of the gallbladder. Symptoms include sudden onset of colicky abdominal pain, usually after the ingestion of fried or fatty foods. The patient presents with a low-grade fever, tachycardia, nausea, vomiting, and flatulence.

A. Diverticulitis is an inflammation of the diverticula of the colon. It is caused by weak muscles in the colon leading to blind pouches in the lining and wall of the colon, where bacteria and other irritants are trapped. The patient complains of left lower quadrant pain and constipation and may have blood in the stool. There is no relationship with fried foods and diverticulitis; however, patients should not eat nuts or popcorn, which can become trapped in the diverticula.

B. Appendicitis is an inflammation or obstruction of the appendix. These patients complain of nausea and vomiting followed by pain, which is steady and severe, and finally fever. They tend to have loss of appetite. There is no relationship to eating fried foods.

D. Esophagitis is an inflammatory response by the esophagus. Patients with esophagitis present with slight epigastric tenderness and normal vital signs. The pain is characterized as a burning sensation in the esophagus.

Content Category: Gastrointestinal

References: Kidd et al., 2000; p. 107; Newberry, 1998; pp. 549–550; ENA, Core Curriculum, 2000; pp. 44–45.

133. A 39-year-old female patient presents to the ED with abdominal distention, severe epigastric pain, and hypoactive bowel sounds following a heavy meal. She has a history of alcohol abuse. The ED nurse should be concerned with what potential complications besides fluid volume deficit?
    A. Intestinal obstruction
    B. Ruptured appendix
    C. Sepsis
    D. ACUTE RESPIRATORY DISTRESS SYNDROME

Rationale:

D. Acute respiratory distress syndrome (ARDS), atelectasis, and other pulmonary complications can occur in the patient presenting with acute pancreatitis.

A. Intestinal obstruction is more likely to occur in the patient with adhesions following abdominal surgery, tumors, or peptic ulcer disease.

B. Ruptured appendix is a serious complication of the patient with appendicitis.

C. Sepsis can occur in the patient with diverticulitis, ruptured appendix, and ascending cholangitis.

Content Category: Gastrointestinal

References: Wyatt et al., 1999; pp. 516–533; Newberry, 1998; pp. 550–552.

134. The patient presents with periumbilical pain and fever. Appendicitis is suspected. The diagnosis of appendicitis will largely be derived from:
    A. ultrasonography of the abdomen.
    B. PHYSICAL EXAMINATION.
    C. white blood cell count (WBC).
    D. computed tomography (CT) of the abdomen.

Rationale:

B. Physical examination is usually the basis for the diagnosis of appendicitis. The definitive diagnosis can be made only in the operating room. Therefore, a high index of suspicion, even with negative test results, and a thorough physical examination are most commonly the basis for diagnosis.

A. Ultrasonography of the abdomen has approximately 90% accuracy for diagnosis. However, clinical findings are the most common basis for diagnosis. Appendicitis has been missed on ultrasound.

C. White blood cell count (WBC) is usually not elevated in children or the elderly and can cause a missed diagnosis. This test must be used in combination with clinical findings and other diagnostic measures. Serial white blood cell counts are more helpful in confirming suspected appendicitis.

D. Computed tomography (CT) scan of the abdomen has a 93% accuracy of identifying an inflamed appendix, but can be confusing, as fluid collections can be indicative of other disease processes.

Content Category: Gastrointestinal

References: Kidd et al., 2000; pp. 93–116, 438–445; Porth, 1998; pp. 769–771; Wyatt et al., 1999; pp. 516–533.

135.   Nursing care for the patient who has suspected appendicitis will most likely include:
A. REPEATED PHYSICAL EXAMINATIONS.
B. medicating the patient with a narcotic.
C. discharge instructions to follow up with a surgeon.
D. insertion of a nasogastric tube.

Rationale:

A. Repeated physical examinations provide the most useful care for the patient with suspected appendicitis. Clinical findings are the common basis for diagnosis and are helpful until a surgical evaluation can be done. Appendicitis usually continues to deteriorate and exhibit signs over time.
B. Medicating the patient with a narcotic is usually not done until the diagnosis has been made.
C. Most patients in whom appendicitis is suspected would not be discharged until a surgical evaluation had been performed. Strict observation of the patient's condition is warranted.
D. Insertion of a nasogastric tube would be indicated once surgical evaluation was performed and surgical intervention was the most likely event. Excessive vomiting would indicate the need for nasogastric tube. However, most patients in whom appendicitis is suspected are simply given nothing by mouth (NPO) while awaiting diagnosis.

Content Category: Gastrointestinal

References: ENA, Core Curriculum, 1994; pp. 29–45; Kidd et al., 2000; pp. 93–116, 438–445; Wyatt et al., 1999; pp. 516–533.

136.   A snake handler is bitten on the left arm by a rattlesnake. He presents to the ED for treatment, but tells you that he is OK. He states this has happened many times and all he needs is a shot, after which he will be ready to go back to work. Which of the following symptoms would lead you to believe that he has had a systemic reaction to the venom and will require more extensive treatment than he describes?
A. Two puncture wounds located on the left forearm, approximately 8 mm apart
B. A burning sensation at the site of the puncture wounds
C. HE ASKS FOR A GLASS OF WATER TO CLEANSE THE METALLIC TASTE IN HIS MOUTH.
D. He is very dry mouthed and has unequal pupils.

Rationale:

C. Systemic reactions to snakebite include nausea, vomiting, diaphoresis, syncope, and a metallic or rubber taste. The patient may develop paralysis, excessive salivation, difficulty speaking, visual disturbances, muscle twitching, and ptosis.
A. The fact that two puncture wounds may be present is not indicative of a systemic reaction. Some snakebites occur without envenomation; some cause only a local reaction.
B. The burning sensation at the site of the bite is common with snakebite and is a sign of a local reaction to the venom.
D. Systemic reactions denote excessive salivation. Pupil changes are not associated with snakebites.

Content Category: Substance Abuse & Toxicological & Environmental

Reference: Newberry, 1998.

137.   A patient is being discharged from the ED following a cat bite and scratch by a neighbor's cat the patient was emptying the garbage. Instructions should include which of the following?
   A.   "RETURN IF YOU NOTE SWELLING OF YOUR ARM, EVEN SEVERAL WEEKS LATER."
   B.   "Cat bites and scratches are fairly clean, but local antibiotics will be helpful."
   C.   "Rates of infection are fairly low, but observe for a fever for the next 3 days."
   D.   "Although the scratch is near your elbow, any bacteria would be limited to the skin."

Rationale:

   A.   The incidence of wound infections from cat bites and scratches is higher than that from dog bites. Cats are hunters and often come in contact with bacteria-infested rodents, which contaminate their mouths and claws with *Pasteurella multocida*. Because of the presence of bacteria and the fact that cats use their claws to groom, rapid onset of infection may be observed. Cat-scratch disease may cause lymphadenitis of the extremity days to weeks after the scratch occurs.
   B.   Cat bites and scratches are not clean injuries and have a tendency to become infected.
   C.   Rates of infection are not fairly low. The risk is greater than with a dog bite.
   D.   Osteomyelitis, septic arthritis, and tenosynovitis have been associated with cat bites because the bite or scratch may cause a deep wound due to the sharpness of the claws and teeth.

Content Category: Substance Abuse & Toxicological & Environmental

Reference: Newberry, 1998.

138.   You are a camp nurse providing emergency care to a group on an outing. Which of the following campers would you suspect to have the highest likelihood of experiencing frostbite?
   A.   An 18-year-old female who jogs frequently
   B.   A 25-YEAR-OLD BLACK MALE WHO SMOKES LESS THAN 1 PACK PER DAY
   C.   A 45-year-old female with a history of recent cataract surgery
   D.   A 60-year-old male with asthma and a cold

Rationale:

   B.   Factors affecting the severity of frostbite include skin color. Dark-skinned people are more prone to frostbite, as are people with a previous history of frostbite injury, poor peripheral vascular status, anxiety, and exhaustion.
   A.   This patient does not have any of the proven factors to increase the risk of frostbite.
   C.   Recent cataract surgery would not make this individual more prone to frostbite.
   D.   Asthma and a cold would not increase this individual's risk for frostbite.

Content Category: Substance Abuse & Toxicological & Environmental

Reference: Newberry, 1998.

139.   Which of the following bites has the highest rate of infection?
   A.   Cat
   B.   Dog
   C.   Snake
   D.   HUMAN

Rationale:

   D.   Human bites have the highest rate of infection and tissue damage of all bite injuries. The human mouth has great crushing ability and harbors more than 40 potential pathogens. Treatment of human bites always includes prophylactic antibiotics.
   A.   Cat bites are more prone to infection than are dog bites.
   B.   Human bites have the highest rate of infection.
   C.   Snake bites may display systemic signs as well, but human bites have the highest rate of infection.

Content Category: Substance Abuse & Toxicological & Environmental

Reference: Newberry, 1998.

140. Immediate treatment for a skier presenting to the ED with suspected frostbite to the foot would include:
     A. Removing the boot and rubbing the foot and ankle
     B. Opening the blisters and applying antibiotic cream to the entire area
     C. APPLICATION OF WARM SOAKS TO THE EXTREMITY
     D. Placing the foot in immobilization lower than the heart

Rationale:

C. Frostbite-injured tissue is friable. Recovery depends on gentle handling. The affected area should not be rubbed. Warm soaks at 104°–110° F (40°–43° C) should be applied toward slow rewarming. The patient's room should be warm. Heavy blankets should be avoided because friction and weight on the affected area could increase the tendency toward sloughing.

A. The wet clothing should be removed gently, but the extremity should not be rubbed.

B. The blisters should remain intact and the extremity should be rewarmed with warm soaks.

D. The foot should be immobilized but elevated.

Content Category: Substance Abuse & Toxicological & Environmental

Reference: Newberry, 1998.

141. In evaluating the chart of a patient brought to the ED with hypothermia, you note a treatment that is not appropriate for this patient. The following chart entry was part of your evaluation: "Patient admitted to the ED after being found under bridge early this A.M. Vital signs are BP 140/90 mm Hg, HR 120/min, respirations 24/min, and temperature 90° F (32.2° C). The wet cloths were removed and warm blankets were applied. The patient was given a cola to drink and warmed IV lactated Ringer's was started at 125 ml/hour. Warmed humidified oxygen was started via mask at 6 L. An NG tube was inserted with warm lavage, completed after about 30 minutes. Lab analysis and an ECG were completed. After 30 minutes, repeated vital signs were BP 140/80 mm Hg, HR 100/min, respirations 20/min, and temperature 91° F (32.8° C)." You would have a concern about which entry?
     A. WARMED GASTRIC LAVAGE
     B. Administration of oral cola
     C. Warmed IV lactated Ringer's
     D. Performance of an electrocardiogram

Rationale:

A. The goal in mild hypothermia (84°–94° F or 29°–24° C) is to prevent further heat loss and rewarm the patient. Passive rewarming techniques such as warm blankets, warm fluids, and warm oxygen should be used. Active rewarming efforts such as warmed gastric lavage are generally indicated in moderate to severe hypothermia.

B. Oral cola or other sugar-containing solution is used because shivering consumes glucose stores, exacerbating hypothermia. Heat is provided via calories.

C. Warmed IV fluids would be appropriate for a patient with mild hypothermia.

D. An electrocardiogram would be an appropriate diagnostic test, as a cold heart is often prone to irritability and dysrhythmias. The characteristic Osborne or J wave may be seen on the cardiogram of a patient with hypothermia.

Content Category: Substance Abuse & Toxicological & Environmental

Reference: Newberry, 1998.

142. What proportion of people die when infected with West Nile virus?
      A. CASE FATALITY RATES RANGE FROM 3–15% AND ARE HIGHEST IN THE ELDERLY.
      B. The case fatality rate is 100%.
      C. Case fatality rates range from 25% to 50% and are highest in children under 5 years of age.
      D. The case fatality rate is 80% and is highest in the adult population.

Rationale:

      A. Based on epidemiologic data obtained from the Centers for Disease Control and Prevention, the case fatality rate for the West Nile virus is 3–15% and is highest in the elderly population.
      B. The fatality rate is not 100%.
      C. The percentages are too high. The elderly have the highest fatality range.
      D. The fatality rate is not 80%.

Content Category: Substance Abuse & Toxicological & Environmental

Reference: CDC, 2001.

143. Which of the following statements concerning snakebites is TRUE?
      A. Of the approximately 50,000 snakebites recorded annually, approximately 30% patients die.
      B. MOST POISONOUS SNAKEBITES IN THE UNITED STATES ARE MADE BY PIT VIPERS, USUALLY RATTLESNAKES.
      C. Pit viper venom is neurotoxic and is delivered from the fangs of the snake.
      D. The U.S. has only one family of poisonous snakes: the *Crotalidae*.

Rationale:

      B. Of more than 50,000 snakebites in the U.S. annually, envenomation occurs in only about 8,000 cases. The most common poisonous snake in the U.S. is the pit viper (copperhead, rattlesnake, and cottonmouth), with the most common bite occurring from the rattlesnake, although snake-bite types are regional.
      A. Of the approximately 50,000 snakebites annually, only about 8,000 involve envenomation. Fewer than 15 deaths occur per year.
      C. Pit viper venom is hemotoxic and is delivered from the fangs.
      D. The U.S. harbors two primary families of poisonous snake: *Crotalidae*, the pit vipers (copperheads, rattlesnakes, and cottonmouth), and *Elapidae* (coral snakes).

Content Category: Substance Abuse & Toxicological & Environmental

Reference: Newberry, 1998.

144. A teenager who is visiting a roadside animal show places a hand in the Gila monster (Heloderma) cage. The teen is bitten on the arm and the lizard has to be physically removed from the arm. On the patient's arrival in the ED, you would anticipate:
      A. mild irritation, since lizard bites are benign
      B. an order for immediate administration of antivenin.
      C. NAUSEA, VOMITING, HYPOTENSION, SYNCOPE, AND SHOCK.
      D. only local symptoms, with irritation, swelling, bruising, and petechiae.

Rationale:

      C. There are two venomous varieties of lizards, the Gila monster (Heloderma) and the Mexican bearded lizard. Gila toxin is released in saliva. Symptoms may begin with pain and swelling and progress to systemic symptoms of nausea, vomiting, weakness, hypotension, syncope, and shock.
      A. Although most lizard bites are benign, the two poisonous ones, Gila monster and Mexican bearded lizard, cause serious systemic reactions.

B. There is no known antivenin for a Gila monster bite.

D. Local symptoms may be present, but systemic reactions are noted as well. Petechiae are not common with Gila monster bites.

Content Category: Substance Abuse & Toxicological & Environmental

Reference: Newberry, 1998.

145.   An unconscious patient is being treated for the ingestion of an unknown quantity of hydrocodone tablets. The patient is given naloxone (Narcan). The ED nurse would suspect which of the following actions from the naloxone?

A. Increase the duration of the amphetamine

B. Decrease the intracranial pressure

C. Alter the peripheral vascular resistance

D. REVERSE THE NARCOTIC EFFECT

Rationale:

D. Naloxone (Narcan) is an opioid antagonist. It is used to reverse the effects of an opioid product such a hydrocodone.

A. Naloxone is not used in amphetamine toxicity.

B. Naloxone does not act on intracranial pressure.

C. Naloxone does not alter peripheral vascular resistance.

Content Category: Substance Abuse & Toxicological & Environmental

Reference: Skidmore-Roth, 2001.

146.   As ED Nurse Educator, you are invited to speak at an industry concerning various first aid procedures. During your presentation, an employee asks you to discuss emergency treatment for chemicals on the skin, especially hydrofluoric acid. Which of the following statements would demonstrate an understanding of the immediate treatment for hydrofluoric acid contact?

A. THE SKIN SHOULD BE COATED WITH A CALCIUM GLUCONATE GEL.

B. Copious water irrigation should be performed.

C. Neutralization should begin with baking soda and water.

D. Evaluation by a physician should occur within 2–4 hours.

Rationale:

A. Hydrofluoric acid is one of the few chemicals for which water is not the antidote, but may in fact cause further skin irritation and pain. The appropriate antidote is to coat the skin with a calcium gluconate gel, which stops the effects of the acid. If companies use hydrofluoric acid, the first responder team should be trained in exposure management.

B. Water irrigation should not be performed.

C. Neutralization would not be the solution for this problem.

D. The wound should be evaluated by a physician as soon as possible, as hydrofluoric acid burns can have serious effects.

Content Category: Substance Abuse & Toxicological & Environmental

Reference: Sheehy & Lenehan, 1999.

147. Following admission for a new onset of atrial fibrillation, a patient's discharge medications included warfarin (Coumadin). Upon arriving home, the patient became confused and took the entire bottle. Once the patient's adult daughter learned what had happened, she immediately returned the patient to the ED. You would prepare which of the following for the patient?
    A. Protamine sulfate
    B. PHYTONADIONE (AQUA-MEPHYTON) (VITAMIN K)
    C. Thiamine (vitamin B_1)
    D. Nicotinic acid (Nicobid) (vitamin B_3)

Rationale:

B. A potentially toxic level of warfarin is treated with rapid administration of phytonadione. Vitamin K reverses the inhibitory action of warfarin on blood clotting factors II, VII, IX, and I in the liver.
A. Protamine is the reversal for heparin overdose.
C. Thiamine (vitamin B_1) is given for vitamin B_1 deficiency.
D. Nicotinic acid (vitamin B_3) is given for pellagra, hyperlipidemia, and peripheral vascular disease.

Content Category: Substance Abuse & Toxicological & Environmental

Reference: Skidmore-Roth, 2001.

148. Mild radiation exposure occurs with radiation levels of less than 125 units of absorbed radiation (rads). Symptoms of mild radiation exposure include:
    A. gastrointestinal bleeding.
    B. NAUSEA AND VOMITING.
    C. tremors and muscle weakness.
    D. tachycardia and hypertension.

Rationale:

B. Nausea and vomiting are the most frequent initial manifestations of radiation exposure. Nausea and vomiting within 3 hours of exposure indicate a significant dose.
A. Exposure to more than 600 rads causes significant hematologic and gastrointestinal effects. Bone marrow is completely suppressed. This results in thrombocytopenia, decreased platelet levels, and hemorrhage.
C. Tremors and seizure activity follow massive doses of radiation—usually doses larger than 1000 rads.
D. Cardiovascular symptoms are not seen in mild radiation exposure.

Content Category: Substance Abuse & Toxicological & Environmental

Reference: Sheehy & Lenehan, 1999.

149.   A 25-year-old male is returning home after a weekend scuba expedition. He suddenly develops throbbing pain over the shoulders and upper torso. He is brought to the ED with those complaints in addition to that of a burning sensation with intense itching. As the ED nurse, you would suspect:
       A. barotrauma.
       B. DECOMPRESSION SICKNESS.
       C. nitrogen narcosis.
       D. air embolism.

Rationale:

   B. Decompression sickness occurs during rapid ascent, which causes nitrogen to form bubbles in blood and tissue. The condition is characterized by pain in the large joints, prickling or burning sensation of the skin, and rashes. It may also cause cough, shortness of breath, and substernal discomfort. Symptoms usually occur within 6 hours after ascent.
   A. Barotrauma occurs as a result of gas expansion during ascent. Symptoms include pain and possible rupture of the tympanic membrane.
   C. Nitrogen narcosis develops as a result of breathing gases at pressures that are higher than normal atmospheric pressure. Increased nitrogen levels cause an anesthetic effect similar to that of alcohol. Effects are usually evident at depths of 70–100 feet.
   D. During ascent, air trapped in the lungs begins to expand. The air is forced into the pulmonary circulation and creates an air embolism. Symptoms include blindness, confusion, chest pain, dysrhythmias, sudden loss of consciousness, stroke, and seizure.

Content Category: Substance Abuse & Toxicological & Environmental

Reference: Sheehy & Lenehan, 1999.

150.   A patient has been treated in the ED for decompression sickness. Upon discharge, which of the following statements would indicate the need for additional discharge teaching?
       A. "Next time, I will shorten the length of my dive."
       B. "From now on, I will carry a scuba identification card."
       C. "I NEED TO WATCH HOW FAST I REACH THE BOTTOM."
       D. "I will never try a long scuba dive alone."

Rationale:

   C. This patient needs to control the speed of ascent rather than that of descent. How fast the patient reaches the bottom does not affect the development of decompression sickness, which occurs only with an overly swift ascent.
   A. The severity of decompression sickness depends on the relationship of time to depth for each dive. The shorter the dive, the less the risk of decompression sickness.
   B. All divers should carry a scuba identification card to assist medical personnel with evaluation of presenting symptoms.
   D. Scuba divers should always dive with a companion who can identify any adverse effects from the dive and provide early access to medical management.

Content Category: Substance Abuse & Toxicological & Environmental

Reference: Sheehy & Lenehan, 1999.

Examination 5:
Self-Diagnostic Profile

Instructions

Step 1: Check your answers against the correct answers provided in Part 2 of this chapter. Then calculate your total score.

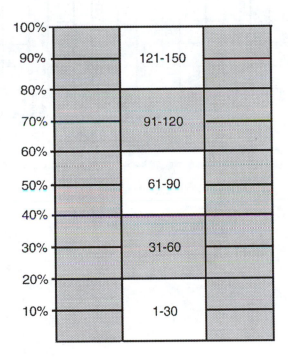

Figure 1: Total Score

Step 2: For each category of the practice examination, determine the number of items that you answered correctly and plot that number in Figure 2. The result will assist you in diagnosing your areas of knowledge strength and in determing which areas benefit from review.

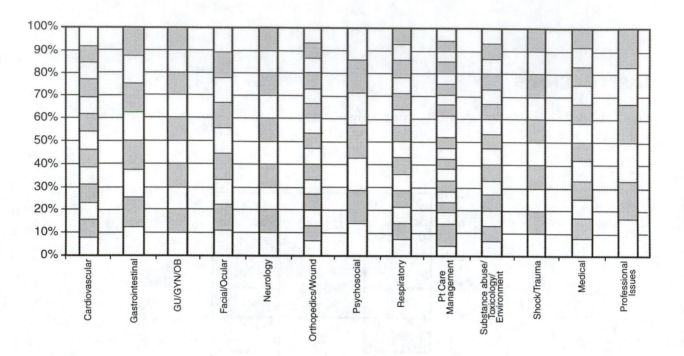

Figure 2: Practice Examination Content Areas

CHAPTER 11

Practice Examination Discussion

• •

Two companion computer-based CEN examinations accompany this review manual. Besides serving as excellent study aids, these examinations can earn Continuing Education Contact Hours (CECH) for each user.

Using Computer-Based Practice CEN Examinations

Each of the two CEN practice tests consists of 175 items, the same number that appear on the actual examinations. Of these, 150 are representative of the content areas specified on the CEN blueprint. The additional 25 items on the examination are interspersed throughout the examination. Those items will not count in the final score of the examination, but represent practice items. To assist users in pacing themselves, the computer-based CEN practice examinations incorporate a 3-hour timing device that indicates the amount of time remaining as the participant progresses with the computer version of the examination. Three hours is the time frame allotted to CEN examinees.

Obtaining Continuing Education Contact Hours

Manual users can obtain CECH from the Emergency Nurses Association by sending the results of their computer-based CEN examinations to the ENA at the address below. To be eligible for contact hours, you must have achieved a score of at least 70%.

Each examination has been approved to provide 3.6 CECH: 2.9 hours in the category Clinical and 0.7 hours in the category Other. One or both of the 175-item practice examinations in this manual (numbers 6 and 7) may be submitted for CECH. Each examination must be accompanied with a $15 processing fee. A certificate awarding CECH will be mailed within 2 weeks of receipt.

To take advantage of this offer, mail one or both of your filled-in examination result printouts with $15 *per examination,* paid by personal check, bank check, or money order, to:

> Emergency Nurses Association
> Education Department
> 915 Lee St.
> Des Plaines, IL 60016

If you have any questions, please contact the Education Department at the Emergency Nurses Association: 1-800-900-9659.

ANSWER SHEETS FOR PRACTICE EXAMINATIONS

Practice Examination #1: Answer Sheet

1. ○ A ○ B ○ C ○ D	31. ○ A ○ B ○ C ○ D	61. ○ A ○ B ○ C ○ D	91. ○ A ○ B ○ C ○ D	121. ○ A ○ B ○ C ○ D
2. ○ A ○ B ○ C ○ D	32. ○ A ○ B ○ C ○ D	62. ○ A ○ B ○ C ○ D	92. ○ A ○ B ○ C ○ D	122. ○ A ○ B ○ C ○ D
3. ○ A ○ B ○ C ○ D	33. ○ A ○ B ○ C ○ D	63. ○ A ○ B ○ C ○ D	93. ○ A ○ B ○ C ○ D	123. ○ A ○ B ○ C ○ D
4. ○ A ○ B ○ C ○ D	34. ○ A ○ B ○ C ○ D	64. ○ A ○ B ○ C ○ D	94. ○ A ○ B ○ C ○ D	124. ○ A ○ B ○ C ○ D
5. ○ A ○ B ○ C ○ D	35. ○ A ○ B ○ C ○ D	65. ○ A ○ B ○ C ○ D	95. ○ A ○ B ○ C ○ D	125. ○ A ○ B ○ C ○ D
6. ○ A ○ B ○ C ○ D	36. ○ A ○ B ○ C ○ D	66. ○ A ○ B ○ C ○ D	96. ○ A ○ B ○ C ○ D	126. ○ A ○ B ○ C ○ D
7. ○ A ○ B ○ C ○ D	37. ○ A ○ B ○ C ○ D	67. ○ A ○ B ○ C ○ D	97. ○ A ○ B ○ C ○ D	127. ○ A ○ B ○ C ○ D
8. ○ A ○ B ○ C ○ D	38. ○ A ○ B ○ C ○ D	68. ○ A ○ B ○ C ○ D	98. ○ A ○ B ○ C ○ D	128. ○ A ○ B ○ C ○ D
9. ○ A ○ B ○ C ○ D	39. ○ A ○ B ○ C ○ D	69. ○ A ○ B ○ C ○ D	99. ○ A ○ B ○ C ○ D	129. ○ A ○ B ○ C ○ D
10. ○ A ○ B ○ C ○ D	40. ○ A ○ B ○ C ○ D	70. ○ A ○ B ○ C ○ D	100. ○ A ○ B ○ C ○ D	130. ○ A ○ B ○ C ○ D
11. ○ A ○ B ○ C ○ D	41. ○ A ○ B ○ C ○ D	71. ○ A ○ B ○ C ○ D	101. ○ A ○ B ○ C ○ D	131. ○ A ○ B ○ C ○ D
12. ○ A ○ B ○ C ○ D	42. ○ A ○ B ○ C ○ D	72. ○ A ○ B ○ C ○ D	102. ○ A ○ B ○ C ○ D	132. ○ A ○ B ○ C ○ D
13. ○ A ○ B ○ C ○ D	43. ○ A ○ B ○ C ○ D	73. ○ A ○ B ○ C ○ D	103. ○ A ○ B ○ C ○ D	133. ○ A ○ B ○ C ○ D
14. ○ A ○ B ○ C ○ D	44. ○ A ○ B ○ C ○ D	74. ○ A ○ B ○ C ○ D	104. ○ A ○ B ○ C ○ D	134. ○ A ○ B ○ C ○ D
15. ○ A ○ B ○ C ○ D	45. ○ A ○ B ○ C ○ D	75. ○ A ○ B ○ C ○ D	105. ○ A ○ B ○ C ○ D	135. ○ A ○ B ○ C ○ D
16. ○ A ○ B ○ C ○ D	46. ○ A ○ B ○ C ○ D	76. ○ A ○ B ○ C ○ D	106. ○ A ○ B ○ C ○ D	136. ○ A ○ B ○ C ○ D
17. ○ A ○ B ○ C ○ D	47. ○ A ○ B ○ C ○ D	77. ○ A ○ B ○ C ○ D	107. ○ A ○ B ○ C ○ D	137. ○ A ○ B ○ C ○ D
18. ○ A ○ B ○ C ○ D	48. ○ A ○ B ○ C ○ D	78. ○ A ○ B ○ C ○ D	108. ○ A ○ B ○ C ○ D	138. ○ A ○ B ○ C ○ D
19. ○ A ○ B ○ C ○ D	49. ○ A ○ B ○ C ○ D	79. ○ A ○ B ○ C ○ D	109. ○ A ○ B ○ C ○ D	139. ○ A ○ B ○ C ○ D
20. ○ A ○ B ○ C ○ D	50. ○ A ○ B ○ C ○ D	80. ○ A ○ B ○ C ○ D	110. ○ A ○ B ○ C ○ D	140. ○ A ○ B ○ C ○ D
21. ○ A ○ B ○ C ○ D	51. ○ A ○ B ○ C ○ D	81. ○ A ○ B ○ C ○ D	111. ○ A ○ B ○ C ○ D	141. ○ A ○ B ○ C ○ D
22. ○ A ○ B ○ C ○ D	52. ○ A ○ B ○ C ○ D	82. ○ A ○ B ○ C ○ D	112. ○ A ○ B ○ C ○ D	142. ○ A ○ B ○ C ○ D
23. ○ A ○ B ○ C ○ D	53. ○ A ○ B ○ C ○ D	83. ○ A ○ B ○ C ○ D	113. ○ A ○ B ○ C ○ D	143. ○ A ○ B ○ C ○ D
24. ○ A ○ B ○ C ○ D	54. ○ A ○ B ○ C ○ D	84. ○ A ○ B ○ C ○ D	114. ○ A ○ B ○ C ○ D	144. ○ A ○ B ○ C ○ D
25. ○ A ○ B ○ C ○ D	55. ○ A ○ B ○ C ○ D	85. ○ A ○ B ○ C ○ D	115. ○ A ○ B ○ C ○ D	145. ○ A ○ B ○ C ○ D
26. ○ A ○ B ○ C ○ D	56. ○ A ○ B ○ C ○ D	86. ○ A ○ B ○ C ○ D	116. ○ A ○ B ○ C ○ D	146. ○ A ○ B ○ C ○ D
27. ○ A ○ B ○ C ○ D	57. ○ A ○ B ○ C ○ D	87. ○ A ○ B ○ C ○ D	117. ○ A ○ B ○ C ○ D	147. ○ A ○ B ○ C ○ D
28. ○ A ○ B ○ C ○ D	58. ○ A ○ B ○ C ○ D	88. ○ A ○ B ○ C ○ D	118. ○ A ○ B ○ C ○ D	148. ○ A ○ B ○ C ○ D
29. ○ A ○ B ○ C ○ D	59. ○ A ○ B ○ C ○ D	89. ○ A ○ B ○ C ○ D	119. ○ A ○ B ○ C ○ D	149. ○ A ○ B ○ C ○ D
30. ○ A ○ B ○ C ○ D	60. ○ A ○ B ○ C ○ D	90. ○ A ○ B ○ C ○ D	120. ○ A ○ B ○ C ○ D	150. ○ A ○ B ○ C ○ D

CEN Practice Examination #2 Answer Sheet

1. ○ A ○ B ○ C ○ D	31. ○ A ○ B ○ C ○ D	61. ○ A ○ B ○ C ○ D	91. ○ A ○ B ○ C ○ D	121. ○ A ○ B ○ C ○ D
2. ○ A ○ B ○ C ○ D	32. ○ A ○ B ○ C ○ D	62. ○ A ○ B ○ C ○ D	92. ○ A ○ B ○ C ○ D	122. ○ A ○ B ○ C ○ D
3. ○ A ○ B ○ C ○ D	33. ○ A ○ B ○ C ○ D	63. ○ A ○ B ○ C ○ D	93. ○ A ○ B ○ C ○ D	123. ○ A ○ B ○ C ○ D
4. ○ A ○ B ○ C ○ D	34. ○ A ○ B ○ C ○ D	64. ○ A ○ B ○ C ○ D	94. ○ A ○ B ○ C ○ D	124. ○ A ○ B ○ C ○ D
5. ○ A ○ B ○ C ○ D	35. ○ A ○ B ○ C ○ D	65. ○ A ○ B ○ C ○ D	95. ○ A ○ B ○ C ○ D	125. ○ A ○ B ○ C ○ D
6. ○ A ○ B ○ C ○ D	36. ○ A ○ B ○ C ○ D	66. ○ A ○ B ○ C ○ D	96. ○ A ○ B ○ C ○ D	126. ○ A ○ B ○ C ○ D
7. ○ A ○ B ○ C ○ D	37. ○ A ○ B ○ C ○ D	67. ○ A ○ B ○ C ○ D	97. ○ A ○ B ○ C ○ D	127. ○ A ○ B ○ C ○ D
8. ○ A ○ B ○ C ○ D	38. ○ A ○ B ○ C ○ D	68. ○ A ○ B ○ C ○ D	98. ○ A ○ B ○ C ○ D	128. ○ A ○ B ○ C ○ D
9. ○ A ○ B ○ C ○ D	39. ○ A ○ B ○ C ○ D	69. ○ A ○ B ○ C ○ D	99. ○ A ○ B ○ C ○ D	129. ○ A ○ B ○ C ○ D
10. ○ A ○ B ○ C ○ D	40. ○ A ○ B ○ C ○ D	70. ○ A ○ B ○ C ○ D	100. ○ A ○ B ○ C ○ D	130. ○ A ○ B ○ C ○ D
11. ○ A ○ B ○ C ○ D	41. ○ A ○ B ○ C ○ D	71. ○ A ○ B ○ C ○ D	101. ○ A ○ B ○ C ○ D	131. ○ A ○ B ○ C ○ D
12. ○ A ○ B ○ C ○ D	42. ○ A ○ B ○ C ○ D	72. ○ A ○ B ○ C ○ D	102. ○ A ○ B ○ C ○ D	132. ○ A ○ B ○ C ○ D
13. ○ A ○ B ○ C ○ D	43. ○ A ○ B ○ C ○ D	73. ○ A ○ B ○ C ○ D	103. ○ A ○ B ○ C ○ D	133. ○ A ○ B ○ C ○ D
14. ○ A ○ B ○ C ○ D	44. ○ A ○ B ○ C ○ D	74. ○ A ○ B ○ C ○ D	104. ○ A ○ B ○ C ○ D	134. ○ A ○ B ○ C ○ D
15. ○ A ○ B ○ C ○ D	45. ○ A ○ B ○ C ○ D	75. ○ A ○ B ○ C ○ D	105. ○ A ○ B ○ C ○ D	135. ○ A ○ B ○ C ○ D
16. ○ A ○ B ○ C ○ D	46. ○ A ○ B ○ C ○ D	76. ○ A ○ B ○ C ○ D	106. ○ A ○ B ○ C ○ D	136. ○ A ○ B ○ C ○ D
17. ○ A ○ B ○ C ○ D	47. ○ A ○ B ○ C ○ D	77. ○ A ○ B ○ C ○ D	107. ○ A ○ B ○ C ○ D	137. ○ A ○ B ○ C ○ D
18. ○ A ○ B ○ C ○ D	48. ○ A ○ B ○ C ○ D	78. ○ A ○ B ○ C ○ D	108. ○ A ○ B ○ C ○ D	138. ○ A ○ B ○ C ○ D
19. ○ A ○ B ○ C ○ D	49. ○ A ○ B ○ C ○ D	79. ○ A ○ B ○ C ○ D	109. ○ A ○ B ○ C ○ D	139. ○ A ○ B ○ C ○ D
20. ○ A ○ B ○ C ○ D	50. ○ A ○ B ○ C ○ D	80. ○ A ○ B ○ C ○ D	110. ○ A ○ B ○ C ○ D	140. ○ A ○ B ○ C ○ D
21. ○ A ○ B ○ C ○ D	51. ○ A ○ B ○ C ○ D	81. ○ A ○ B ○ C ○ D	111. ○ A ○ B ○ C ○ D	141. ○ A ○ B ○ C ○ D
22. ○ A ○ B ○ C ○ D	52. ○ A ○ B ○ C ○ D	82. ○ A ○ B ○ C ○ D	112. ○ A ○ B ○ C ○ D	142. ○ A ○ B ○ C ○ D
23. ○ A ○ B ○ C ○ D	53. ○ A ○ B ○ C ○ D	83. ○ A ○ B ○ C ○ D	113. ○ A ○ B ○ C ○ D	143. ○ A ○ B ○ C ○ D
24. ○ A ○ B ○ C ○ D	54. ○ A ○ B ○ C ○ D	84. ○ A ○ B ○ C ○ D	114. ○ A ○ B ○ C ○ D	144. ○ A ○ B ○ C ○ D
25. ○ A ○ B ○ C ○ D	55. ○ A ○ B ○ C ○ D	85. ○ A ○ B ○ C ○ D	115. ○ A ○ B ○ C ○ D	145. ○ A ○ B ○ C ○ D
26. ○ A ○ B ○ C ○ D	56. ○ A ○ B ○ C ○ D	86. ○ A ○ B ○ C ○ D	116. ○ A ○ B ○ C ○ D	146. ○ A ○ B ○ C ○ D
27. ○ A ○ B ○ C ○ D	57. ○ A ○ B ○ C ○ D	87. ○ A ○ B ○ C ○ D	117. ○ A ○ B ○ C ○ D	147. ○ A ○ B ○ C ○ D
28. ○ A ○ B ○ C ○ D	58. ○ A ○ B ○ C ○ D	88. ○ A ○ B ○ C ○ D	118. ○ A ○ B ○ C ○ D	148. ○ A ○ B ○ C ○ D
29. ○ A ○ B ○ C ○ D	59. ○ A ○ B ○ C ○ D	89. ○ A ○ B ○ C ○ D	119. ○ A ○ B ○ C ○ D	149. ○ A ○ B ○ C ○ D
30. ○ A ○ B ○ C ○ D	60. ○ A ○ B ○ C ○ D	90. ○ A ○ B ○ C ○ D	120. ○ A ○ B ○ C ○ D	150. ○ A ○ B ○ C ○ D

CEN Practice Examination #3 Answer Sheet

1. ○ A ○ B ○ C ○ D	31. ○ A ○ B ○ C ○ D	61. ○ A ○ B ○ C ○ D	91. ○ A ○ B ○ C ○ D	121. ○ A ○ B ○ C ○ D
2. ○ A ○ B ○ C ○ D	32. ○ A ○ B ○ C ○ D	62. ○ A ○ B ○ C ○ D	92. ○ A ○ B ○ C ○ D	122. ○ A ○ B ○ C ○ D
3. ○ A ○ B ○ C ○ D	33. ○ A ○ B ○ C ○ D	63. ○ A ○ B ○ C ○ D	93. ○ A ○ B ○ C ○ D	123. ○ A ○ B ○ C ○ D
4. ○ A ○ B ○ C ○ D	34. ○ A ○ B ○ C ○ D	64. ○ A ○ B ○ C ○ D	94. ○ A ○ B ○ C ○ D	124. ○ A ○ B ○ C ○ D
5. ○ A ○ B ○ C ○ D	35. ○ A ○ B ○ C ○ D	65. ○ A ○ B ○ C ○ D	95. ○ A ○ B ○ C ○ D	125. ○ A ○ B ○ C ○ D
6. ○ A ○ B ○ C ○ D	36. ○ A ○ B ○ C ○ D	66. ○ A ○ B ○ C ○ D	96. ○ A ○ B ○ C ○ D	126. ○ A ○ B ○ C ○ D
7. ○ A ○ B ○ C ○ D	37. ○ A ○ B ○ C ○ D	67. ○ A ○ B ○ C ○ D	97. ○ A ○ B ○ C ○ D	127. ○ A ○ B ○ C ○ D
8. ○ A ○ B ○ C ○ D	38. ○ A ○ B ○ C ○ D	68. ○ A ○ B ○ C ○ D	98. ○ A ○ B ○ C ○ D	128. ○ A ○ B ○ C ○ D
9. ○ A ○ B ○ C ○ D	39. ○ A ○ B ○ C ○ D	69. ○ A ○ B ○ C ○ D	99. ○ A ○ B ○ C ○ D	129. ○ A ○ B ○ C ○ D
10. ○ A ○ B ○ C ○ D	40. ○ A ○ B ○ C ○ D	70. ○ A ○ B ○ C ○ D	100. ○ A ○ B ○ C ○ D	130. ○ A ○ B ○ C ○ D
11. ○ A ○ B ○ C ○ D	41. ○ A ○ B ○ C ○ D	71. ○ A ○ B ○ C ○ D	101. ○ A ○ B ○ C ○ D	131. ○ A ○ B ○ C ○ D
12. ○ A ○ B ○ C ○ D	42. ○ A ○ B ○ C ○ D	72. ○ A ○ B ○ C ○ D	102. ○ A ○ B ○ C ○ D	132. ○ A ○ B ○ C ○ D
13. ○ A ○ B ○ C ○ D	43. ○ A ○ B ○ C ○ D	73. ○ A ○ B ○ C ○ D	103. ○ A ○ B ○ C ○ D	133. ○ A ○ B ○ C ○ D
14. ○ A ○ B ○ C ○ D	44. ○ A ○ B ○ C ○ D	74. ○ A ○ B ○ C ○ D	104. ○ A ○ B ○ C ○ D	134. ○ A ○ B ○ C ○ D
15. ○ A ○ B ○ C ○ D	45. ○ A ○ B ○ C ○ D	75. ○ A ○ B ○ C ○ D	105. ○ A ○ B ○ C ○ D	135. ○ A ○ B ○ C ○ D
16. ○ A ○ B ○ C ○ D	46. ○ A ○ B ○ C ○ D	76. ○ A ○ B ○ C ○ D	106. ○ A ○ B ○ C ○ D	136. ○ A ○ B ○ C ○ D
17. ○ A ○ B ○ C ○ D	47. ○ A ○ B ○ C ○ D	77. ○ A ○ B ○ C ○ D	107. ○ A ○ B ○ C ○ D	137. ○ A ○ B ○ C ○ D
18. ○ A ○ B ○ C ○ D	48. ○ A ○ B ○ C ○ D	78. ○ A ○ B ○ C ○ D	108. ○ A ○ B ○ C ○ D	138. ○ A ○ B ○ C ○ D
19. ○ A ○ B ○ C ○ D	49. ○ A ○ B ○ C ○ D	79. ○ A ○ B ○ C ○ D	109. ○ A ○ B ○ C ○ D	139. ○ A ○ B ○ C ○ D
20. ○ A ○ B ○ C ○ D	50. ○ A ○ B ○ C ○ D	80. ○ A ○ B ○ C ○ D	110. ○ A ○ B ○ C ○ D	140. ○ A ○ B ○ C ○ D
21. ○ A ○ B ○ C ○ D	51. ○ A ○ B ○ C ○ D	81. ○ A ○ B ○ C ○ D	111. ○ A ○ B ○ C ○ D	141. ○ A ○ B ○ C ○ D
22. ○ A ○ B ○ C ○ D	52. ○ A ○ B ○ C ○ D	82. ○ A ○ B ○ C ○ D	112. ○ A ○ B ○ C ○ D	142. ○ A ○ B ○ C ○ D
23. ○ A ○ B ○ C ○ D	53. ○ A ○ B ○ C ○ D	83. ○ A ○ B ○ C ○ D	113. ○ A ○ B ○ C ○ D	143. ○ A ○ B ○ C ○ D
24. ○ A ○ B ○ C ○ D	54. ○ A ○ B ○ C ○ D	84. ○ A ○ B ○ C ○ D	114. ○ A ○ B ○ C ○ D	144. ○ A ○ B ○ C ○ D
25. ○ A ○ B ○ C ○ D	55. ○ A ○ B ○ C ○ D	85. ○ A ○ B ○ C ○ D	115. ○ A ○ B ○ C ○ D	145. ○ A ○ B ○ C ○ D
26. ○ A ○ B ○ C ○ D	56. ○ A ○ B ○ C ○ D	86. ○ A ○ B ○ C ○ D	116. ○ A ○ B ○ C ○ D	146. ○ A ○ B ○ C ○ D
27. ○ A ○ B ○ C ○ D	57. ○ A ○ B ○ C ○ D	87. ○ A ○ B ○ C ○ D	117. ○ A ○ B ○ C ○ D	147. ○ A ○ B ○ C ○ D
28. ○ A ○ B ○ C ○ D	58. ○ A ○ B ○ C ○ D	88. ○ A ○ B ○ C ○ D	118. ○ A ○ B ○ C ○ D	148. ○ A ○ B ○ C ○ D
29. ○ A ○ B ○ C ○ D	59. ○ A ○ B ○ C ○ D	89. ○ A ○ B ○ C ○ D	119. ○ A ○ B ○ C ○ D	149. ○ A ○ B ○ C ○ D
30. ○ A ○ B ○ C ○ D	60. ○ A ○ B ○ C ○ D	90. ○ A ○ B ○ C ○ D	120. ○ A ○ B ○ C ○ D	150. ○ A ○ B ○ C ○ D

CEN Practice Examination #4 Answer Sheet

1. ○ A ○ B ○ C ○ D	31. ○ A ○ B ○ C ○ D	61. ○ A ○ B ○ C ○ D	91. ○ A ○ B ○ C ○ D	121. ○ A ○ B ○ C ○ D
2. ○ A ○ B ○ C ○ D	32. ○ A ○ B ○ C ○ D	62. ○ A ○ B ○ C ○ D	92. ○ A ○ B ○ C ○ D	122. ○ A ○ B ○ C ○ D
3. ○ A ○ B ○ C ○ D	33. ○ A ○ B ○ C ○ D	63. ○ A ○ B ○ C ○ D	93. ○ A ○ B ○ C ○ D	123. ○ A ○ B ○ C ○ D
4. ○ A ○ B ○ C ○ D	34. ○ A ○ B ○ C ○ D	64. ○ A ○ B ○ C ○ D	94. ○ A ○ B ○ C ○ D	124. ○ A ○ B ○ C ○ D
5. ○ A ○ B ○ C ○ D	35. ○ A ○ B ○ C ○ D	65. ○ A ○ B ○ C ○ D	95. ○ A ○ B ○ C ○ D	125. ○ A ○ B ○ C ○ D
6. ○ A ○ B ○ C ○ D	36. ○ A ○ B ○ C ○ D	66. ○ A ○ B ○ C ○ D	96. ○ A ○ B ○ C ○ D	126. ○ A ○ B ○ C ○ D
7. ○ A ○ B ○ C ○ D	37. ○ A ○ B ○ C ○ D	67. ○ A ○ B ○ C ○ D	97. ○ A ○ B ○ C ○ D	127. ○ A ○ B ○ C ○ D
8. ○ A ○ B ○ C ○ D	38. ○ A ○ B ○ C ○ D	68. ○ A ○ B ○ C ○ D	98. ○ A ○ B ○ C ○ D	128. ○ A ○ B ○ C ○ D
9. ○ A ○ B ○ C ○ D	39. ○ A ○ B ○ C ○ D	69. ○ A ○ B ○ C ○ D	99. ○ A ○ B ○ C ○ D	129. ○ A ○ B ○ C ○ D
10. ○ A ○ B ○ C ○ D	40. ○ A ○ B ○ C ○ D	70. ○ A ○ B ○ C ○ D	100. ○ A ○ B ○ C ○ D	130. ○ A ○ B ○ C ○ D
11. ○ A ○ B ○ C ○ D	41. ○ A ○ B ○ C ○ D	71. ○ A ○ B ○ C ○ D	101. ○ A ○ B ○ C ○ D	131. ○ A ○ B ○ C ○ D
12. ○ A ○ B ○ C ○ D	42. ○ A ○ B ○ C ○ D	72. ○ A ○ B ○ C ○ D	102. ○ A ○ B ○ C ○ D	132. ○ A ○ B ○ C ○ D
13. ○ A ○ B ○ C ○ D	43. ○ A ○ B ○ C ○ D	73. ○ A ○ B ○ C ○ D	103. ○ A ○ B ○ C ○ D	133. ○ A ○ B ○ C ○ D
14. ○ A ○ B ○ C ○ D	44. ○ A ○ B ○ C ○ D	74. ○ A ○ B ○ C ○ D	104. ○ A ○ B ○ C ○ D	134. ○ A ○ B ○ C ○ D
15. ○ A ○ B ○ C ○ D	45. ○ A ○ B ○ C ○ D	75. ○ A ○ B ○ C ○ D	105. ○ A ○ B ○ C ○ D	135. ○ A ○ B ○ C ○ D
16. ○ A ○ B ○ C ○ D	46. ○ A ○ B ○ C ○ D	76. ○ A ○ B ○ C ○ D	106. ○ A ○ B ○ C ○ D	136. ○ A ○ B ○ C ○ D
17. ○ A ○ B ○ C ○ D	47. ○ A ○ B ○ C ○ D	77. ○ A ○ B ○ C ○ D	107. ○ A ○ B ○ C ○ D	137. ○ A ○ B ○ C ○ D
18. ○ A ○ B ○ C ○ D	48. ○ A ○ B ○ C ○ D	78. ○ A ○ B ○ C ○ D	108. ○ A ○ B ○ C ○ D	138. ○ A ○ B ○ C ○ D
19. ○ A ○ B ○ C ○ D	49. ○ A ○ B ○ C ○ D	79. ○ A ○ B ○ C ○ D	109. ○ A ○ B ○ C ○ D	139. ○ A ○ B ○ C ○ D
20. ○ A ○ B ○ C ○ D	50. ○ A ○ B ○ C ○ D	80. ○ A ○ B ○ C ○ D	110. ○ A ○ B ○ C ○ D	140. ○ A ○ B ○ C ○ D
21. ○ A ○ B ○ C ○ D	51. ○ A ○ B ○ C ○ D	81. ○ A ○ B ○ C ○ D	111. ○ A ○ B ○ C ○ D	141. ○ A ○ B ○ C ○ D
22. ○ A ○ B ○ C ○ D	52. ○ A ○ B ○ C ○ D	82. ○ A ○ B ○ C ○ D	112. ○ A ○ B ○ C ○ D	142. ○ A ○ B ○ C ○ D
23. ○ A ○ B ○ C ○ D	53. ○ A ○ B ○ C ○ D	83. ○ A ○ B ○ C ○ D	113. ○ A ○ B ○ C ○ D	143. ○ A ○ B ○ C ○ D
24. ○ A ○ B ○ C ○ D	54. ○ A ○ B ○ C ○ D	84. ○ A ○ B ○ C ○ D	114. ○ A ○ B ○ C ○ D	144. ○ A ○ B ○ C ○ D
25. ○ A ○ B ○ C ○ D	55. ○ A ○ B ○ C ○ D	85. ○ A ○ B ○ C ○ D	115. ○ A ○ B ○ C ○ D	145. ○ A ○ B ○ C ○ D
26. ○ A ○ B ○ C ○ D	56. ○ A ○ B ○ C ○ D	86. ○ A ○ B ○ C ○ D	116. ○ A ○ B ○ C ○ D	146. ○ A ○ B ○ C ○ D
27. ○ A ○ B ○ C ○ D	57. ○ A ○ B ○ C ○ D	87. ○ A ○ B ○ C ○ D	117. ○ A ○ B ○ C ○ D	147. ○ A ○ B ○ C ○ D
28. ○ A ○ B ○ C ○ D	58. ○ A ○ B ○ C ○ D	88. ○ A ○ B ○ C ○ D	118. ○ A ○ B ○ C ○ D	148. ○ A ○ B ○ C ○ D
29. ○ A ○ B ○ C ○ D	59. ○ A ○ B ○ C ○ D	89. ○ A ○ B ○ C ○ D	119. ○ A ○ B ○ C ○ D	149. ○ A ○ B ○ C ○ D
30. ○ A ○ B ○ C ○ D	60. ○ A ○ B ○ C ○ D	90. ○ A ○ B ○ C ○ D	120. ○ A ○ B ○ C ○ D	150. ○ A ○ B ○ C ○ D

CEN Practice Examination #5: Answer Sheet

1. ○ A ○ B ○ C ○ D	31. ○ A ○ B ○ C ○ D	61. ○ A ○ B ○ C ○ D	91. ○ A ○ B ○ C ○ D	121. ○ A ○ B ○ C ○ D
2. ○ A ○ B ○ C ○ D	32. ○ A ○ B ○ C ○ D	62. ○ A ○ B ○ C ○ D	92. ○ A ○ B ○ C ○ D	122. ○ A ○ B ○ C ○ D
3. ○ A ○ B ○ C ○ D	33. ○ A ○ B ○ C ○ D	63. ○ A ○ B ○ C ○ D	93. ○ A ○ B ○ C ○ D	123. ○ A ○ B ○ C ○ D
4. ○ A ○ B ○ C ○ D	34. ○ A ○ B ○ C ○ D	64. ○ A ○ B ○ C ○ D	94. ○ A ○ B ○ C ○ D	124. ○ A ○ B ○ C ○ D
5. ○ A ○ B ○ C ○ D	35. ○ A ○ B ○ C ○ D	65. ○ A ○ B ○ C ○ D	95. ○ A ○ B ○ C ○ D	125. ○ A ○ B ○ C ○ D
6. ○ A ○ B ○ C ○ D	36. ○ A ○ B ○ C ○ D	66. ○ A ○ B ○ C ○ D	96. ○ A ○ B ○ C ○ D	126. ○ A ○ B ○ C ○ D
7. ○ A ○ B ○ C ○ D	37. ○ A ○ B ○ C ○ D	67. ○ A ○ B ○ C ○ D	97. ○ A ○ B ○ C ○ D	127. ○ A ○ B ○ C ○ D
8. ○ A ○ B ○ C ○ D	38. ○ A ○ B ○ C ○ D	68. ○ A ○ B ○ C ○ D	98. ○ A ○ B ○ C ○ D	128. ○ A ○ B ○ C ○ D
9. ○ A ○ B ○ C ○ D	39. ○ A ○ B ○ C ○ D	69. ○ A ○ B ○ C ○ D	99. ○ A ○ B ○ C ○ D	129. ○ A ○ B ○ C ○ D
10. ○ A ○ B ○ C ○ D	40. ○ A ○ B ○ C ○ D	70. ○ A ○ B ○ C ○ D	100. ○ A ○ B ○ C ○ D	130. ○ A ○ B ○ C ○ D
11. ○ A ○ B ○ C ○ D	41. ○ A ○ B ○ C ○ D	71. ○ A ○ B ○ C ○ D	101. ○ A ○ B ○ C ○ D	131. ○ A ○ B ○ C ○ D
12. ○ A ○ B ○ C ○ D	42. ○ A ○ B ○ C ○ D	72. ○ A ○ B ○ C ○ D	102. ○ A ○ B ○ C ○ D	132. ○ A ○ B ○ C ○ D
13. ○ A ○ B ○ C ○ D	43. ○ A ○ B ○ C ○ D	73. ○ A ○ B ○ C ○ D	103. ○ A ○ B ○ C ○ D	133. ○ A ○ B ○ C ○ D
14. ○ A ○ B ○ C ○ D	44. ○ A ○ B ○ C ○ D	74. ○ A ○ B ○ C ○ D	104. ○ A ○ B ○ C ○ D	134. ○ A ○ B ○ C ○ D
15. ○ A ○ B ○ C ○ D	45. ○ A ○ B ○ C ○ D	75. ○ A ○ B ○ C ○ D	105. ○ A ○ B ○ C ○ D	135. ○ A ○ B ○ C ○ D
16. ○ A ○ B ○ C ○ D	46. ○ A ○ B ○ C ○ D	76. ○ A ○ B ○ C ○ D	106. ○ A ○ B ○ C ○ D	136. ○ A ○ B ○ C ○ D
17. ○ A ○ B ○ C ○ D	47. ○ A ○ B ○ C ○ D	77. ○ A ○ B ○ C ○ D	107. ○ A ○ B ○ C ○ D	137. ○ A ○ B ○ C ○ D
18. ○ A ○ B ○ C ○ D	48. ○ A ○ B ○ C ○ D	78. ○ A ○ B ○ C ○ D	108. ○ A ○ B ○ C ○ D	138. ○ A ○ B ○ C ○ D
19. ○ A ○ B ○ C ○ D	49. ○ A ○ B ○ C ○ D	79. ○ A ○ B ○ C ○ D	109. ○ A ○ B ○ C ○ D	139. ○ A ○ B ○ C ○ D
20. ○ A ○ B ○ C ○ D	50. ○ A ○ B ○ C ○ D	80. ○ A ○ B ○ C ○ D	110. ○ A ○ B ○ C ○ D	140. ○ A ○ B ○ C ○ D
21. ○ A ○ B ○ C ○ D	51. ○ A ○ B ○ C ○ D	81. ○ A ○ B ○ C ○ D	111. ○ A ○ B ○ C ○ D	141. ○ A ○ B ○ C ○ D
22. ○ A ○ B ○ C ○ D	52. ○ A ○ B ○ C ○ D	82. ○ A ○ B ○ C ○ D	112. ○ A ○ B ○ C ○ D	142. ○ A ○ B ○ C ○ D
23. ○ A ○ B ○ C ○ D	53. ○ A ○ B ○ C ○ D	83. ○ A ○ B ○ C ○ D	113. ○ A ○ B ○ C ○ D	143. ○ A ○ B ○ C ○ D
24. ○ A ○ B ○ C ○ D	54. ○ A ○ B ○ C ○ D	84. ○ A ○ B ○ C ○ D	114. ○ A ○ B ○ C ○ D	144. ○ A ○ B ○ C ○ D
25. ○ A ○ B ○ C ○ D	55. ○ A ○ B ○ C ○ D	85. ○ A ○ B ○ C ○ D	115. ○ A ○ B ○ C ○ D	145. ○ A ○ B ○ C ○ D
26. ○ A ○ B ○ C ○ D	56. ○ A ○ B ○ C ○ D	86. ○ A ○ B ○ C ○ D	116. ○ A ○ B ○ C ○ D	146. ○ A ○ B ○ C ○ D
27. ○ A ○ B ○ C ○ D	57. ○ A ○ B ○ C ○ D	87. ○ A ○ B ○ C ○ D	117. ○ A ○ B ○ C ○ D	147. ○ A ○ B ○ C ○ D
28. ○ A ○ B ○ C ○ D	58. ○ A ○ B ○ C ○ D	88. ○ A ○ B ○ C ○ D	118. ○ A ○ B ○ C ○ D	148. ○ A ○ B ○ C ○ D
29. ○ A ○ B ○ C ○ D	59. ○ A ○ B ○ C ○ D	89. ○ A ○ B ○ C ○ D	119. ○ A ○ B ○ C ○ D	149. ○ A ○ B ○ C ○ D
30. ○ A ○ B ○ C ○ D	60. ○ A ○ B ○ C ○ D	90. ○ A ○ B ○ C ○ D	120. ○ A ○ B ○ C ○ D	150. ○ A ○ B ○ C ○ D

REFERENCES

Abramson, J. S., & Givner, L. B. (1999). Rocky Mountain spotted fever. *Pediatric Infectious Disease Journal, 18* (6), 539–540.

Aghababian, R., et al. (Eds.). (1998). *Emergency medicine: The core curriculum.* New York: Lippincott Raven.

American Association of Critical-Care Nurses (AACN). (1998). *Core curriculum for critical care nursing* (5th ed.). Philadelphia: Saunders.

American College of Surgeons. (1997). *Advanced trauma life support for doctors.* Chicago: Author.

American Heart Association. (2000). Guidelines 2000 for cardiopulmonary resuscitation and emergency cardiovascular care. *Circulation, 102* (8) (Supplement I). I-1 to I-384.

American Heart Association. (1994). *Textbook of Pediatric Advanced Life Support.* Dallas: Author.

Archibald, L. K., & Sexton, D. J. (1995). Long-term sequelae of Rocky Mountain spotted fever. *Clinical Infectious Diseases, 20,* 1122–1125.

Bahr, R. (1998). The concept and the development of chest pain emergency departments as a strategy in the war against heart attack. *Critical Care Nursing Clinics of North America, 10* (41).

Ballard, R., et al. (1999). An algorithm to reduce the incidence of false-negative FAST examinations in patients at high risk for occult injury. Focused assessment for the sonographic examination of the trauma patient. *Journal of the American College of Surgeons, 189* (2), 145–151.

Barkin, R. M., Hayden, S. R., Schaider, J. J., & Wolfe, R. (1999). *The 5 minute emergency medicine consult.* Philadelphia: Lippincott Williams & Wilkins.

Barkin, M., & Rosen, P. (Eds.). (1998). *Emergency medicine: Concepts and clinical practice* (4th ed.). St. Louis: Mosby—Year Book.

Barton, S. (Ed.). (2000). *Clinical Evidence 4.* London: BMJ Publishing Group.

Bayley, E., & Turcke, S. A. (Eds.). (1998). *A comprehensive curriculum for trauma nursing.* Park Ridge, IL: Roadrunner Press.

Beers, M. H., & Berkow, R. (Eds.). (1999). *The Merck manual,* 17th ed. Whitehouse Station, NJ: Merck Research Laboratories.

Black, J., & Matassarin-Jacobs, E. (Eds.). (1997). *Medical–surgical nursing: Clinical management for continuity of care* (5th ed.). Philadelphia: Saunders.

Blansfield, J., Danis, D., & Gervasini, A. (1999). *Manual of clinical trauma care: The first hour* (3rd ed.). St. Louis: Mosby.

Bracken, M. B., et al. (1997). Administration of methylprednisolone for 24 or 48 hours or tirilazad mesylate for 48 hours in the treatment of acute spinal cord injury. *JAMA, 277,* 1597–1604.

Brown, C., Henderson, S., & Moore, S. (1998). Surgical treatment of patients with open tibial fractures. *AORN Journal, 63* (5), 875–895.

Buttaravoli, P., & Stair T. (2000). *Minor emergencies: Splinters to fractures.* St. Louis: Mosby.

Centers for Disease Control and Prevention. (2001). *Monthly statistical overview, infectious diseases.* Atlanta: Author.

Centers for Disease Control and Prevention. (1998). Bioterrorism alleging use of anthrax and interim guidelines for management—United States. *MMWR Morbidity Mortality Weekly Report, 48,* 4.

Carpenito, L. J. (1999). *Handbook of nursing diagnosis* (8th ed.). Philadelphia: Lippincott.

Cinat, M., et al. (1999). Improved survival following massive transfusion in patients who have undergone trauma. *Archives of Surgery, 134* (9), 964–970.

Colliers, L., Balows, A., Sussman, M., & Hausles, W. J. (Eds.). (1998). *Topley and Wilson's microbiology and microbiological infections* (Vol. 3). London: Edward Arnold Press.

Copel, L. C. (1999). *Nurse's clinical guide: Psychiatric and mental health care* (2nd ed.). Springhouse, PA: Springhouse.

Cornwell III, E. (1998). Trauma and critical care. *Journal of the American College of Surgeons, 186,* 115–121.

Dains, J. E., Baumann, L. C. & Scheibel, P. (Eds.). (1998). *Advanced health assessment and clinical diagnosis in primary care.* St. Louis: Mosby.

Dart, R. C., Hulburt, K. M., Kaffner, E. K., & Yip, L. (Eds). (2000). *The 5 minute toxicology consult.* Philadelphia: Lippincott Williams & Wilkins, pp. 330–331.

Dennison, R. (2000). *Pass CCRN.* St. Louis: Mosby.

Department of Transportation. (2000). *Breath Alcohol Technician Training Manual.* Washington, DC: Author.

D'Heere, M. S., Houghton, D., & Ginzburg, E. (1999). Fat embolism syndrome. *Journal of Trauma Nursing, 6* (3), 73–76.

Dieckmann, R. (Ed.) (2000). *Pediatric education for hospital professionals.* Sudbury, MA: Jones & Bartlett.

Dolan, B., & Holt, L. (2000). *Accident and emergency theory into practice.* Edinburgh: Bailliere Tindall and the Royal College of Nursing.

Ehrle, R., Shafer, T., & Nelson, K. (1999). Referral, request and consent for organ donation: Best practice—a blueprint for success. *Critical Care Nurse, 19* (2), 21–33.

Emergency Nurses Association. (2000). *Emergency nursing core curriculum* (5th ed.). Philadelphia: Saunders.

Emergency Nurses Association. (2000) *Trauma nursing core course: Provider manual* (5th ed.). Des Plains, IL: Author.

Emergency Nurses Association. (2000). *Triage: Meeting the challenge* (2nd ed.). Chicago: Author.

Emergency Nurses Association. (1999). *Emergency nursing pediatric course* (2nd ed.). Chicago: Author.

Emergency Nurses Association. (1999). *National emergency department benchmark and staffing database guide.* Des Plaines, IL: Author.

Fahey, V. (Ed.). *Vascular nursing* (3rd ed.). Philadelphia: Saunders.

Frank, G. (2001). EMTALA: An expert tells us what it's all about. *Journal of Emergency Nursing, 27,* 65.

Garcia, R. (1999). Preventing human rabies before and after exposure. *Nurse Practitioner, 24* (4), 91–107.

Gilbert, D. N., Moellering, R. C., & Sande, M. A. (2001). *The Sanford guide to antimicrobial therapy.* Hyde Park, VT: Antimicrobial Therapy.

Goldy, D. (1998). Diaphragmatic rupture: How to recognize this insidious, potentially fatal complication of chest trauma. *American Journal of Nursing, 98,* 33.

Guyton, A. C., & Hall, J. E. (1996). *Textbook of medical physiology* (9th ed.). Philadelphia: Saunders.

Hacker, N., & Moore, J. (1998). *Essentials of obstetrics and gynecology* (3rd ed.). Philadelphia: Saunders.

Hammond, W. A., Kay, R. M., & Skaggs, D. L. (1998). Supracondylar humerus fractures in children. *AORN,* 68 (2), 186–199.

Handysides, G. (1996). *Triage in emergency practice.* St. Louis: Mosby, 162–166.

Hanlon, D., & Duriseti, R. (May–June, 2001). Current concepts in the management of the pregnant trauma patient. *Trauma Reports, 2* (3), 1–10.

Hayes, K. S. (2000). Challenges in emergency care: The geriatric patient. *Journal of Emergency Nursing, 26* (5), 430–435.

Health Care Financing Administration. (1998). *HCFA revised interpretive guidelines: State operations manual provider certification* (HCFA Transmittal No. 2). Washington, DC.

Herington, T., & Morse, L. (1995). *Occupational injuries evaluation management and prevention.* St. Louis: Mosby.

Hickey, J. V. (Ed.). (1997). *The clinical practice of neurological and neurosurgical nursing.* Philadelphia: Saunders.

Hodgson, B., & Kizor, R. (Eds.). (2000). *Saunders nursing drug handbook 2000.* Philadelphia: Saunders.

Holleran, R. S. (Ed.). (1996). *Flight nursing: Principles and practice* (2nd ed.). St. Louis: Mosby-Year Book.

Holleran, R. S. (1994). *Prehospital nursing: A collaborative approach.* St. Louis: Mosby-Year Book.

Holmquist, M., Chabalweski, F., Blout, T., Edwards, C., McBride, V., & Pietroski, R. (1999). A critical pathway: Guiding care for organ donors. *Critical Care Nurse, 19* (2), 84–98.

Howell, J., Altieri, M., Jagoda, A., Prescott, J., Scott, J., and Stair, T. (1998). *Emergency medicine.* Philadelphia: Saunders.

Humes, H. D. (ed.). (2000). *Kelly's textbook of internal medicine* (4th ed.). Philadelphia: Lippincott Williams & Wilkins, pp. 1370–1375, 1350, 1889–1890, 1963.

Jaimovich, D. G., & Vidyasagar, D. (Eds.). (1996). *Handbook of pediatric and neonatal transport medicine.* Philadelphia: Hanley & Belfus.

Jairath, N. (2001). Implications of gender differences on coronary artery disease risk reduction women. *AACN Clinical Issues, 12* (1), 17–28.

Jarvis, C. (1996). *Physical examination and health assessment* (2nd ed.). Philadelphia: Saunders.

Joint Commission on Accreditation of Healthcare Organizations. (2000). *2000 Hospital accreditation standards.* Oakbrook Terrace, IL: Author.

Kalish, R. A., Leong, J. M., & Steere, A. C. (1993). Association of treatment-resistant chronic Lyme arthritis with HLA-DR4 and antibody reactivity to OspA and OspB of *Borrelia burgdorferi. Infection and Immunity, 61,* 2774–2779.

Kasper D. L., et al. (Eds.). (1998). *Harrison's principles of internal medicine* (14th ed.). New York: McGraw–Hill.

Kee, J., & Hayes, E. (2000). *Pharmacology: A nursing process approach.* Philadelphia: Saunders.

Kidd, P., Sturt, P., & Fultz, J. (2000). *Emergency nursing reference* (2nd ed.). St. Louis: Mosby, pp. 668–669.

Kidd, P., & Wagner, K. (Eds.). (1997). *High acuity nursing* (2nd ed.). Stamford, CT: Appleton & Lange.

Kinney, M., Dunbar, S., Brooks-Brunn, J., Molter, N., & Vitello-Cicciu, J. (Eds.) (1998). *AACN clinical reference for critical care nursing* (4th ed.). St. Louis: Mosby.

Kirchoff, L. V. (1996). American trypanosomiasis (Chagas' disease). *Gastroenterology Clinics of North America, 25,* 517–532.

Kirkpatrick, A. W., Chun, R., Brown, R., & Simon, R. (1999). Hypothermia and the trauma patient. *Canadian Journal of Surgery, 42,* 333–343.

Kitt, S., Selfridge-Thomas, J., Proehl, J., & Kaiser, J. (1995). *Emergency nursing: A physiologic and clinical perspective* (2nd ed.). Philadelphia: Saunders.

Knoop, K. J., Stack, L. B., & Storrow, A. B. (Eds.). (1997). *Atlas of emergency medicine.* New York: McGraw-Hill.

Kuhn, M.A. (1998). *Pharmacotherapeutics a nursing process approach* (4th ed.). Philadelphia: F. A. Davis.

Logan, P. (Ed) *Principles of practice for the acute care nurse practitioner.* Stamford, CT: Appleton & Lange.

Lombardi, J., Sheehy, S. (1995). *Manual of emergency care* (4th ed.). St. Louis: Mosby.

Mattox, K. L., Feliciano, D. V., & Moore, E. E. (Eds.). (2000). *Trauma* (4th ed.). New York: McGraw-Hill.

McCance, K. & Huether, S. (Eds.). (1998). *Pathophysiology the biologic basis for disease in adults and children.* St. Louis: Mosby.

McCloskey, K. A. L., & Orr, R. A. (1995). *Pediatric Transport Medicine.* St. Louis: Mosby–Year Book.

Melander, S., & Bucher, L. (1999). *Pocket companion for critical care nursing.* Philadelphia: Saunders.

Montgomery, M. T. (2000). Extraoral facial pain. *Emergency Medicine Clinics of North America, 18,* 577–600.

Moreau, D. (Ed) (2001). *Disease* (3rd ed.). Springhouse, PA: Springhouse.

Moy, M. M. (2000). *The EMTALA Answer Book.* Gaithersburg, MD: Aspen.

Murray, P. R., Baron, E. J., Pfaller, M. A., Tenover, F. C., & Yolken, R. H. (Eds.). (1995). *Manual of Clinical Microbiology* (6th ed.). Washington, DC: American Society for Microbiology Press.

Newberry, L. (Ed.). (1998). *Sheehy's emergency nursing principles and practice* (4th ed.). St. Louis: Mosby—Year Book.

O'Hanlon-Nichols, T. (1995). Adult respiratory distress syndrome: What you need to know to provide support and prevent complications. *American Journal of Nursing, 95* (8), 42.

Oman, K., Kozoll-McLain, J., Scheetz, L. (Eds.). (2001). *Emergency nursing secrets.* Philadelphia: Hanley & Belfus.

Pagana, K. D., & Pagana, J. T. (1998). *Mosby's manual of diagnostic and laboratory tests* (4th ed.). St. Louis: Mosby.

Palay, D. A., & Krachmer, J. H. (Eds.). (1997). *Ophthalmology for the primary care physician.* St. Louis: Mosby.

Porth, C. M. (1998). *Pathophysiology: Concepts of altered health states* (5th ed.). Philadelphia.: Saunders.

Proehl, J. A. (Ed.). (1999). *Emergency Nursing Procedures.* Philadelphia: Saunders.

Reilly, B. (1991). *Practical strategies in outpatient medicine* (2nd ed.). Philadelphia: Saunders.

Reynolds, J., & Apple, S. (2001). A systematic approach to pacemaker assessment. *AACN Clinical Issues, 12* (1), 121.

Rhee, D. J., & Pyfer, M. F. (Eds.). (1999). *The Wills eye manual.* Philadelphia: Lippincott Williams & Wilkins.

Roettig, M., & Tanabe, P. (2000). Emergency management of acute coronary syndromes. *Journal of Emergency Nursing, 28* (6), 8.

Rosen, P., et al. (Eds). (1998). *Emergency medicine: concepts and clinical practice* (4th ed). St. Louis: Mosby.

Royner, M. (1998). The person with dementia: ED assessment tips for this at-risk patient. *Journal of Emergency Nursing, 24* (4), 331–332.

Salluzzo, R., et al. (1997). *Emergency Department management principles and applications.* St. Louis: Mosby.

Seidel, H. M., Ball, J. W., Dains, J. E., & Benedict, G. W. (1999). *Mosby's guide to physical examination* (4th ed.). St. Louis: Mosby.

Shapiro, R. L., Hatheway, C., Becher, J., & Swerdlow, D. L. (1997). Botulism surveillance and emergency response: a public health strategy for a global challenge. *JAMA 278,* 433–435.

Shapiro, R. L., Hatheway, C., & Swerdlow, D. L. (1998). Botulism in the United States: A clinical and epidemiologic review. *Annals of Internal Medicine, 129,* 221–228.

Sheehy, S., Danis, D., Blansfield, J., & Gervasini, A. (1999). *Manual of clinical trauma care* (3rd ed.). St. Louis: Mosby.

Sheehy, S. B., & Lenehan, G. P. (1999). *Manual of emergency care* (5th ed.). St. Louis: Mosby-Harcourt.

Skidmore-Roth, L. (2001). *Mosby's Nursing Drug Reference.* St. Louis: Mosby.

Smego, R., Gebrian, B., & Desmangels, G. (1998).Cutaneous manifestations of anthrax in rural Haiti. *Clinical Infectious Diseases, 26,* 97–102.

Smith, J. S. (1996). New aspects of rabies with emphasis on epidemiology, diagnosis, and prevention of the disease in the United States. *Clinical Microbiology Reviews, 9,* 166–176.

Snider, R. (Ed.). (1997). *Essentials of musculoskeletal care.* Rosemont, IL: American Academy of Orthopedic Surgeons.

Snyder, L. (1993). *Emergency nursing across the lifespan.* Park Ridge, IL: Emergency Nurses Association.

Sondhi, D. S., Hussain, S. A., Munir, A., Dhingra, H., Ayinla, R., & Rosner, F. (2001). Heroin lung: Case report and brief review. *Resident & Staff Physician, 47* (3), 30–32.

Soud, T., & Rogers, J. (1998). *Manual of pediatric emergency nursing.* St. Louis: Mosby.

Stine, R. J., Chudnofsky, C. R., & Aaron, C. K. (1994). *A practical approach to emergency medicine* (2nd ed.). Boston: Little, Brown.

Stuart, G. W., & Laraia, M. T. (1998). *Principles and practice of psychiatric nursing* (7th ed.). St. Louis: Mosby, p. 474.

Suffin, S., Carnes, W., Kaufmann, A. (1998). Inhalation anthrax in a home craftsman. *Clinical Infectious Diseases, 26,* 97–102.

Talan, D. A., Moran, G. J., & Pinner, R. W. (1999). Update on emerging infections from the Centers for Disease Control and Prevention. *Annals of emergency medicine, 33* (5), 590–596.

Taptich, B., Iyer, P., & Bicnocch-Losey, D. (1994). *Nursing diagnosis and care planning.* Philadelphia: Saunders.

Tarascon pocket pharmacopoeia. (2001). Loma Linda, CA: Tarascon.

Tierney, L., McPhee, S., & Papadakis, M. (Eds). (1999). *Current medical diagnosis and treatment* (38th ed). Stamford, CT: Appleton & Lange.

Tintinalli, J. E., Kelen, G. D., & Stapczynski, J. S. (Eds.). (2000). *Emergency medicine: A comprehensive study guide* (6th ed.). New York: McGraw–Hill.

Townsend, M. C. (1999). *Essentials of psychiatric/mental health nursing.* Philadelphia: F. A. Davis, pp. 423–428.

Trott, A. T. (1997). *Wounds and lacerations: Emergency care and closure.* St. Louis: Mosby.

Tumbarella, C. (2000). Acute extremity compartment syndrome. *Journal of Trauma Nursing, 7* (2), 30–35.

Turkoski, B. B., Lance, B. R., & Bonfiglio, M. F. (2000). *Drug information handbook for advanced practice nursing.* Cleveland: Lexi-Comp.

Urquhart, B. S., & Kearney, K. (2001). Anterior shoulder dislocation. *American Journal of Nursing, 101* (2), 33–35.